Breastfeeding
the Newborn

Clinical Strategies for Nurses

Breastfeeding *the* Newborn

Clinical Strategies for Nurses

Second Edition

Marie Biancuzzo, RN, MS, IBCLC
President, Baby-Friendly USA
Perinatal Clinical Nurse Specialist
Herndon, Virginia

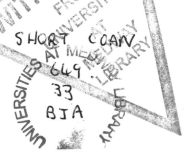
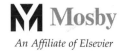 Mosby

An Affiliate of Elsevier

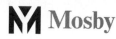

Mosby

An Affiliate of Elsevier

11830 Westline Industrial Drive
St. Louis, Missouri 63146

Breastfeeding the Newborn: Clinical Strategies for Nurses
Copyright © 2003, Mosby Inc. All rights reserved.

NOTICE

Pharmacology is an ever-changing field. Standard safety precautions must be followed, but as new research and clinical experience broaden our knowledge, changes in treatment and drug therapy may become necessary or appropriate. Readers are advised to check the most current product information provided by the manufacturer of each drug to be administered to verify the recommended dose, the method and duration of administration, and contraindications. It is the responsibility of the licensed prescriber, relying on experience and knowledge of the patient, to determine dosages and the best treatment for each individual patient. Neither the publisher nor the editor assumes any liability for any injury and/or damage to persons or property arising from this publication.

Previous edition copyrighted 1999.

Library of Congress Cataloging-in-Publication Data
Biancuzzo, Marie.
  Breastfeeding the newborn : clinical strategies for nurses / Marie Biancuzzo.—2nd ed.
    p. ; cm.
  Includes bibliographical references and index.
    ISBN-13: 978-0-323-01745-9   ISBN-10: 0-323-01745-2
    1. Breast feeding. 2. Infants (Newborn)—Nutrition. 3. Infants (Newborn)—Care. 4. Lactation. I. Title.
    [DNLM: 1. Breast Feeding. 2. Maternal-Child Nursing. 3. Health Education–methods. 4. Infant Nutrition. 5. Nursing Process. WY 157.3 B578b 2003]
RJ516 .B536 2003
649'.33—dc21   2002029386

Vice President, Publishing Director: Sally Schrefer
Executive Editor: Michael S. Ledbetter
Senior Developmental Editor: Laurie K. Muench
Publishing Services Manager: Catherine Jackson
Project Manager: Clay S. Broeker
Designer: Amy Buxton

KI / MVY
ISBN-13: 978-0-323-01745-9
ISBN-10: 0-323-01745-2

Printed in the United States of America.

Last digit is the print number: 9 8 7 6

To my parents, who provided education and support for all of my endeavors
To my husband, David, who gives me unconditional love
And for the greater glory of God

Reviewers

Terry S. Busch, RNC, BS, BSN, MS, LCCE, IBCLC, CBE
Parent and Family Education Coordinator
Shawnee Mission Medical Center
Overland Park, Kansas

Kathleen F. Clasen, RN, BSN, IBCLC
Staff Nurse
Wake Medical Center
Raleigh, North Carolina

Susan J. Garpiel, RNC, BSN, MN, IBCLC
Perinatal Clinical Nurse Specialist
Covenant Health Care System
Saginaw, Michigan

Theresa Baccoli Harte, MS, RD
Clinical Nutrition Specialist
University of Rochester Medical Center
Rochester, New York

Jill Janke, RN, MS, DNSc
Professor
University of Alaska—Anchorage
Anchorage, Alaska

Rebecca Matthews, RN, BSN, MNSc, NP, LCCE, IBCLC
Executive Director, Parenting and Childbirth Education Services
Lactation Consultant in private practice
Jonesboro, Arkansas

Lynne M. Sylvia, PharmD
Associate Professor of Pharmacy Practice
Massachusetts College of Pharmacy and Health Services
Boston, Massachusetts

Susan E. Taylor, RN, BSN, MA, CLE, IBCLC
Breastfeeding Coordinator
Gadsden County WIC; Gadsden County Health Department
Quincy, Florida

Patricia A. Thomas, RN, BFA, BA, IBCLC
Public Health Nurse
Winona County Community Health Department
Winona, Minnesota

Cynthia Turner-Maffei, BS, MA, IBCLC
National Coordinator, Baby-Friendly USA
Sandwich, Massachusetts

Reviewers are for the second edition.

Preface

The idea for this book was conceived in a corridor of the Georgetown University Levey Conference Center. At the time, I was a clinical nurse specialist at the University of Rochester Medical Center and had flown to Washington, DC, to give a lecture. After the lecture, Karen Rechnitzer, RN, IBCLC (who later became my colleague at Georgetown University Hospital), said to me: "I've been doing this for years, and I learned a lot from your presentation. All of that good information should be in one handy place. You should write a book!" I was amused by the idea but had no intention of writing a book. On the return flight, however, I found myself creating one more handout for a class, developing one more policy for the department, and later scurrying to the library for one more article that might help solve our latest clinical crisis. It took a few years before I realized that I had several drawers full of articles, handouts, and related materials that could be assembled into a book.

This book was born out of necessity. From my earliest days as a staff nurse, I needed a book that told me how to provide nursing care for the lactating woman, similar to the dozens of books that told me how to provide nursing care for the laboring woman. My early years in clinical practice were fraught with many frustrations; hospital policies and protocols that restricted breastfeeding made little sense to me. I soon began reading articles in medical journals but found them difficult to comprehend. I wanted a book on my shelf that would help me with my everyday role and responsibilities as a staff nurse. My role changed over the years, and my need for knowledge increased. As the breastfeeding coordinator at the University of Rochester Medical Center, I found myself providing direct patient care; developing policies, procedures, and protocols; and coordinating interdisciplinary efforts on a topic that I needed to know more about—breastfeeding. I wanted a book for nurses that would give evidence-based clinical strategies.

This book reflects my own philosophy about the nurse's role and responsibilities. I believe the nurse must use all of her knowledge, skills, and resources to meet the patient's physical, emotional, and spiritual needs as completely as possible. Nurses cannot pick and choose which needs to meet based on their current knowledge or personal biases. I hope that this book will become a starting point for advanced practice nurses who function in the expanded role. When advanced practice nurses assume care for women and infants who are breastfeeding under difficult circumstances, they need to gain the same level of specialization and expertise as they would when working with groups of patients who have other complex needs, for example, those with diabetes or those undergoing renal dialysis. It is my hope that the advanced practice nurse gains sufficient knowledge about breastfeeding to become a clinical expert for individual patients, as well as a change agent within the health care setting and an advocate for national policy.

This book will be enlightening to some and unsettling to others. Although I have tried to provide clear directives in some cases, I have also tried to avoid giving the impression that there is only one right answer or strategy. Readers are encouraged to use clinical judgment. Furthermore, I presume that readers are like me, continually generating questions and seeking further clarity. Therefore I encourage readers to send their questions and comments to me at bookcomments @wmc-worldwide.com.

My struggle to become both scholar and clinical expert becomes evident in these pages. Yet, after many years as a staff nurse, clinical nurse specialist, and university instructor, I wrote this book not to help the nurse *know* more but to help her *do* something that will effect better patient outcomes. I like to imagine myself standing next to the reader, showing techniques, suggesting strategies, and asking provocative questions about cases that require a decision but have no easy answers. At the same time, I want to inspire the reader to yearn for the library and spend hours there reading about breastfeeding, but relatively few of us need to *generate* new research, but all of us need to *apply* the existing research to clinical practice to achieve better clinical outcomes.

I labored through the first edition of this book during 2 of the most exciting and difficult years of my life. The first four chapters were written amid the paint fumes and nail pounding that occurred during the extensive repair of our storm-damaged home. Just after I completed Chapter 8, my father died and it became very difficult for me to write. Knowing that my father didn't have much respect for people who waste time, however, I pressed on. The text was written on planes and trains while I was criss-crossing the country from Virginia to California. I wrote in hotel rooms in Alaska and next to swimming pools in Florida. Mothers, nurses, and colleagues continually inspired me to write a book that went straight to the heart of clinical matters. I thought the revision of this book, which occurred during a comparatively calmer time in my life, would be fast and easy, with a few updates here and a few corrections there. Of course, it was not that simple. I added four new chapters, and completely overhauled Chapters 5, 10, and 13.

This book was nurtured by numerous people. Two of my former students at Georgetown University School of Nursing, Megan McGratty, RN, and Cathy Zilinskas, RN, assisted me with the first edition. The appendix was masterfully organized by my sister-in-law, Barbara Savins. She verified the titles, cost, and availability of the patient education materials and contact information listed in the appendices for both editions—an awesome task. Without Barbara, the information in the appendix would still be just a collection of 20 years' worth of disorganized files in my bottom drawer. My friend, Mary Beauchamp, PharmD, with her superb organizational skills, attention to detail, and ability to stay calm in my chaotic and cluttered office, also helped me enormously.

I am completely indebted to Debi Bocar, RNC, PhD, IBCLC, who has reviewed more than half of the chapters in the book and has made numerous constructive suggestions. Moreover, Debi's creativity appears throughout these pages; her photographs and other materials have greatly enhanced the quality of this book. Debi is an admired colleague and a cherished friend; without her inspiration, encouragement, and active assistance in the preparation of both editions, the book might never have existed.

I am deeply grateful to Ann Davis, RPh, for her thoughtful review and willingness to respond to multiple panicked phone calls regarding Chapter 13. Karin Cadwell, RN, PhD, has been a great source of inspiration and encouragement to me over the years, and I continued to tap her expertise for this book. I'd also like to thank Sarah Coulter Danner, whose expertise and publications about breastfeeding the infant with cleft or neurologic defects have greatly influenced my clinical approach.

Numerous colleagues at the University of Rochester Medical Center have helped me, including Kathy Della Porta, who has reviewed various portions of this book and responded to multiple phone calls and requests for help. My friend and former colleague, Ruth Lawrence, MD, was a tremendous influence on me during my years at University of Rochester Medical Center and continues to mentor me. She has graciously loaned articles and responded to multiple e-mail, fax, and phone queries since I started writing this book. I am enormously indebted to her not only for her expertise but also for her ongoing support of my endeavors to provide direct care for patients and continuing education for nurses.

My editor at Mosby, Michael Ledbetter, transformed my dream into a reality. He believed in my vision for the book, and he believed in me. My developmental editor for the first edition, Nancy O'Brien, encouraged me with her consistently positive attitude and ability to put up with my numerous quirks. Her incredible gift for recognizing the fine line between pushing me and challenging me was a true blessing. My developmental editor for this edition, Laurie Muench, sustained me through days when I could not see or even look for the light at the end of the tunnel. Moreover, no matter how many times I asked Laurie to solve the biggest problems or handle the most trivial requests, she would always respond, with a lilt in her voice, "Of course!"

My parents have been a tremendous source of inspiration. My mother went against the grain, breastfeeding her children in the 1940s and 1950s when bottle-feeding was the social norm. She was often horrified by my tales of how we restrict breastfeeding in the hospital and wholeheartedly supported my efforts to reduce barriers to breast-feeding within the hospital and on the national front. Without her insistence that every woman can breastfeed, I would have undoubtedly believed that it was reserved for the chosen few. My father always insisted that education was cheaper than ignorance. If this book educates just one nurse, I will never count the cost of the time, energy, and money that went into creating it.

My husband, David W. Vaklyes, has been a pillar of strength for me. Beyond his daily reminder of "you can do this, dear," he took many evenings, weekends, and vacation days to give hands-on sup-port for the project. I shudder to think how many small errors might have gone unnoticed if he had not carefully reviewed the calculations and graphs within these pages. Many times he made the 380-mile trip with me to the Miner Library at the University of Rochester Medical Center. He has dutifully found, copied, and even read articles for me at the National Library of Medicine here in the Washington, DC, metro area. He has also spent hours on the Internet identifying pertinent web sites, finding e-mail addresses for authors of arti-cles, and downloading citations from MedLine. He also plowed through newspapers, finding every-thing from articles about breastfeeding legislation to cartoons about authors, editors, and breastfeed-ing mothers. (The cartoons helped me keep my sense of humor.) Without his help and encourage-ment, I would still be complaining about the need for this book, rather than writing it.

Contents

Breastfeeding as a Public Health Priority

BREASTFEEDING SHOULD BE A PUBLIC HEALTH PRIORITY

In the United States, most public health priorities focus on two things: the goal of good health and the benefits of embracing or avoiding certain health practices. Breastfeeding should be a high public health priority; it is one way to achieve optimal health because it confers many benefits.

Good Health: A Precious Resource in a Land of Wealth

Good health is the most important resource we have. Although we can buy more and better health care products and services and enjoy the benefits of health care insurance, we cannot buy good health. This becomes evident from our casual observations; we see plenty of wealthy but ailing men and women here in the United States. It becomes more apparent—even frightening—when formal epidemiologic statistics show that the United States ranks twenty-fifth in infant mortality. The mortality rates in this land of wealth are only a beginning to understanding how this is not a land of health. For example, although healthy infants are born at reputable hospitals, morbidity is soon a problem. One large study carried out in nine metropolitan hospitals showed that more than 12% of the infants born there were readmitted during the first 2 weeks; the three most frequent reasons for hospital readmission were infection, hyperbilirubinemia, and feeding/gastrointestinal problems.[1] When mortality and morbidity rates are so striking, it becomes apparent that a wealthy and affluent nation is experiencing a great poverty. A question might be, Is there anything that would help reduce the morbidity and mortality of newborns, older infants, and adults?

In a capitalist society like the United States, there is an underlying value that money is to be saved and wisely spent, and presumably that would include health care dollars as well. Oddly, that is not the case. Health care expenditures have increased from 5% of the U.S. gross domestic product in 1960 to more than 13% in 1999.[2] Even more interesting is the government's spending of taxpayer dollars to purchase artificial milk. Approximately 40% of the formula sold in the United States is purchased by the government.[3] The cost of this—most of which is for the Special Supplemental Nutrition Program for Women, Infants, and Children (WIC)—runs in the millions. For example, in 1997 the WIC program spent $567 million (after company rebates) on formula.[3] In the private sector, too, the costs of not breastfeeding are astounding. Ball and Wright report astonishing figures: "In the first year of life, after adjusting for confounders, there were 2033 excess office visits, 212 excess days of hospitalization, and 609 excess prescriptions for these three illnesses [lower respiratory illness, otitis media, and gastrointestinal illness] per 1000 never-breastfed infants compared with 1000 infants exclusively breastfed for at least 3 months. These additional health care services cost the managed care health system between $331 and $475 per never-breastfed infant during the first year of life."[4] A question might be, Is there any way that we could save billions of dollars on health care and millions of taxpayer dollars?

Health care professionals who have recently espoused the idea of evidence-based practice have begun to look at the literature before implementing treatment regimens for patients. Evidence-based practice is clearly the way modern health care will advance. Oddly, however, some practices have become so culturally acceptable that they are presumed to have been proven effective for achieving or maintaining good health. For example, artificial milk is assumed to be harmless, maybe even good. This assumption is inaccurate, however, and "the explosive expansion of artificial feeding of infants is an extraordinary example of a large in vivo experiment performed without any research protocol, including a control series."[5]

Indeed, the time has come to tackle the tough questions and issues. A recent government report estimates that $3.6 billion could be saved if breastfeeding were the norm in this country.[3] Unquestionably, government and private sectors and individual health care providers and consumers recognize that health is a precious resource; health care dollars are limited, and evidence-based practice must be implemented for all practices, not just a select few. Similarly, these same people need to recognize the means by which we might achieve and maintain optimal health, save health care dollars, and implement evidence-based practices that focus not only on cures but also on prevention. Herein lies a strong reason for why breastfeeding must be a public health priority. Those who advocate strategies to prevent acute and chronic illness must recognize that breastfeeding accomplishes this, and more. Those who want to reduce costs of hospital readmission, outpatient visits, insurance rates, and employee absenteeism would further their objective by supporting breastfeeding as a simple but highly effective cost-saving measure. Those who fly the flag in support of evidence based practice need to recognize that the benefits of breastfeeding will ultimately improve the nation's health and wealth. Indeed, the time has come for breastfeeding to be a public health priority.

Research has shown the uniqueness of human milk as a valuable resource throughout the

 # RESEARCH HIGHLIGHT

Artificially Fed Infants: A Financial Drain for Parents and Health Care Plans

Citation: Ball TM, Wright AL. Health care costs of formula-feeding in the first year of life. *Pediatrics* 1999;103:870-876.

Ball and Wright[4] aimed to estimate the total costs of care for artificially fed infants compared with breastfed infants who had lower respiratory infection (LRI), otitis media (OM), and gastrointestinal illnesses. Using two already existing studies, they analyzed data from physician visits in the first year of life. Infants were then classified into three categories, based on the duration of exclusive breastfeeding: never-breastfed, partially breastfed, and exclusively breastfed for at least 3 months.

During the first year, 1022 children were followed. A total of 33.2% had LRI; of those, 251 had only one episode but 73 had two episodes, and 15 had more than two. In the first data set, acute OM was diagnosed 1679 times. In the second data set they observed that "Compared with 1000 infants who were breastfed exclusively for ≥3 months, the never-breastfed group experienced 60 more episodes of LRI and 580 more episodes of OM after adjusting for maternal education and smoking. These children also experienced 1053 more episodes of gastrointestinal illness. For 1000 never-breastfed infants, there were >609 excess prescriptions and 80 excess hospitalizations, relative to 1000 infants breastfed exclusively for 3 months." These "extra" visits to the physician were costly. Among the never-breastfed groups, investigators estimated expenses to be $331,051 greater than for those who were exclusively breastfed for at least 3 months. They considered this estimate to be conservative and said that services that were feeding related could cost from $331 to $475 per infant never breastfed. They emphasized that the costs presented in the study reflected only direct medical costs and not the indirect costs of lost work for the parent, transportation, and other expenses that would be incurred as a result of increased illness.

ℋistorical Highlight

Artifically Fed Children Inferior Physically and Mentally

In 1929 Hoefer and Hardy[30] conducted a study of 383 children; 38 were artificially fed and 345 were exclusively breastfed. The aim of the study was to compare the results of tests and measurements among artificially fed children with those who were exclusively breastfed. Outcome measures were attainment of growth and developmental milestones, results of anthropometric measurements, and performance on educational and psychologic examinations. At the time of the study, the children ranged in age from 7 to 13 years and were classified into four groups: (1) artificially fed, (2) exclusively breastfed 3 or fewer months, (3) exclusively breastfed 4 to 10 months, or (4) exclusively breastfed 10 to 20 months. Investigators gathered data from a questionnaire, medical records, parents' "baby books," and a personal interview with the parents.

No tall children were in the artificially fed group, and all of them walked and talked later than any in the breastfed groups. Although there was no significant difference in the intelligence of the parents, the intelligence of the children differed dramatically. The smallest percentage of children with intelligence quotients (IQs) ≥120 were in the artificially fed group. Compared with the breastfed groups, only half as many of the artificially fed children had IQs above 120. None of the children in the artificially fed group had IQs above 130. (The researchers noted that children who were exclusively breastfed for 4 to 9 months ranked best of all of the groups on all of the outcome measures.)

From Hoefer C, Hardy MC. *J Am Med Assoc* 1929;92:615-620.

world. Literally hundreds of studies have shown the benefits conferred to the infant, the mother, and society. Some benefits have not been fully described, and some existing studies have yielded conflicting results. However, when a clear health benefit has not been shown, it is often because studies are lacking a clear definition of breastfeeding. Studies that lack a definition of breastfeeding usually describe the effects of the "never-ever" breastfeeding experience (i.e., those who were never breastfed compared with those who received at least some human milk for an unspecified length of time); therefore it may be difficult to identify the benefits of breastfeeding. However, the benefits of breastfeeding may be apparent if the infant has received only human milk, whereas such benefits may remain unidentified if the infant has been supplemented with artificial milk or breastfed for only a very short time. Fortunately, definitions for breastfeeding—partial, full, or token—have been developed, and more recent research has therefore yielded more meaningful results. The most commonly used definition of breastfeeding is shown in Fig. 1-1.[6]

A recent study has clearly shown that a dose-response relationship exists; the more human milk an infant consumes, the more bountiful the benefits conferred.[7] Even in studies with unclear definitions, breastfeeding has been shown to confer multiple benefits to the infant and mother.

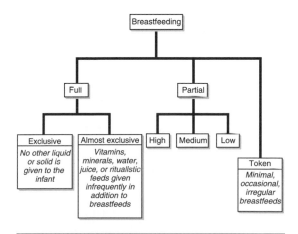

FIGURE 1-1 Schema for breastfeeding definition. *(From Labbok M, Krasovec K.* Stud Fam Plann *1990;21:226-230.)*

Benefits of Breastfeeding

Breastfeeding offers significant health and socio-economic benefits. Often, the health benefits conferred to the infant are highly publicized, but the benefits of breastfeeding abound for adults as well. Women who breastfeed gain multiple personal health benefits for themselves, and adults who were breastfed as infants have significantly reduced risk for developing certain diseases, as described later. Many nurses and other health care providers are unaware of the many advantages of breastfeeding. A quiz in Box 1-1 may be useful as a self-inventory of knowledge.

The Surgeon General's *Blueprint for Action on Breastfeeding*[8] has summarized the advantages of breastfeeding as shown in Box 1-2. With much recognition of the benefits of breastfeeding and human milk, the government and private sector have begun to promote, protect, and support breastfeeding.

EFFORTS TO MAKE BREASTFEEDING A PUBLIC HEALTH PRIORITY

During the last few decades, research has shown the health and socioeconomic advantages of breastfeeding as just described. Few, therefore, would question whether breastfeeding *should* be a public health priority. The more pressing question is, Has breastfeeding become a public health priority in the United States?

Box 1-1   Do You Know the Benefits of Breastfeeding?

The following self-test is designed to help you discover whether you know the advantages of breastfeeding. (Modified from the Curriculum in Support of the Ten Steps to Successful Breastfeeding.[31])

1. In the United States, how many yearly deaths from diarrhea are attributed to artificial feeding?
   a. 50-100
   b. 100-250
   c. 250-300
   d. 400-500
2. Which of the following gastrointestinal diseases is *not* associated with artificial feeding?
   a. Crohn's disease
   b. Inflammatory bowel disease
   c. Celiac disease
   d. Duodenal ulcers
3. What is the increased risk of fatal or nonfatal respiratory infection in nonbreastfed infants?
   a. None
   b. Twofold to fivefold
   c. Threefold to eightfold
   d. Greater than tenfold
4. Which of the following statements regarding otitis media is *false*?
   a. Artificially fed babies have double the rate of ear infections compared with breastfed babies.
   b. Artificially fed babies have more recurrent ear infections than breastfed babies.
   c. Feeding method does not affect the rate of ear infections.
   d. Costs to treat ear infections are higher for artificially fed children.
5. Compared with breastfed babies, artificially fed babies have how much increased risk of bacteremia and meningitis?
   a. 2 times higher
   b. 3 times higher
   c. 4 times higher
   d. 5 times higher
6. Not breastfeeding, or exposure to formula, is attributed to how much increased risk of juvenile (insulin-dependent) diabetes?
   a. 10%
   b. 15%
   c. 20%
   d. 25%
7. Artificially fed children have how much increased risk of childhood (up to 15 years) malignant lymphomas?
   a. 2% to 4%
   b. 4% to 6%
   c. 6% to 8%
   d. 8% to 10%

Box 1-1   Do You Know the Benefits of Breastfeeding?—cont'd

8. Women older than 40 who were breastfed as children have how much *less* risk for breast cancer according to one comprehensive study?
   a. 10%
   b. 15%
   c. 20%
   d. 25%

9. Which statement about allergies related to feeding methods is *false*?
   a. Forty-two percent of gastroesophageal reflux is related to allergy to cow's milk.
   b. Breastfed children have delayed onset of allergic disease.
   c. Breastfeeding prevents allergies.
   d. Breastfed children have less wheezing.

10. All of the following conditions are positively associated with artificial feeding *except:*
   a. Muscular dystrophy
   b. Chronic respiratory disease
   c. Coronary artery disease
   d. Higher cholesterol in young adulthood

11. All of the following nutrients in human milk are responsible for improved cognitive and neurologic development *except:*
   a. Lactose
   b. Long-chain polyunsaturated fatty acids
   c. Proteins
   d. Lactoferrin

12. Higher cognitive and neuromotor test scores of children in middle-income families are related to all of the following *except:*
   a. Length of exclusive breastfeeding
   b. Age when solids were introduced
   c. Ever having breastfed
   d. Duration of breastfeeding

13. When tested at age 7 to 8 years, premature babies who received their mother's milk by feeding tube had which of the following (compared with artificially fed premature babies)?
   a. Same IQ
   b. 5 points higher IQ
   c. 10 points higher IQ
   d. 15 points higher IQ

14. Human milk accomplishes all of the following neuromotor functions *except:*
   a. Improves hearing
   b. Mitigates deficits in congenital cretinism
   c. Improves visual acuity
   d. Higher neuromotor skills in impaired children

15. Which of the following would a breastfeeding woman expect in the postpartum period?
   a. Increased postpartum bleeding
   b. Slow uterine involution
   c. Difficulty returning to prepregnant weight
   d. Delayed return of menstruation and fertility

16. Maternal benefits of breastfeeding extend past the childbearing age. Which of the following are *not* related to breast feeding?
   a. Reduction in hip fractures
   b. Reduction in ovarian cancer
   c. Reduction in risk of premenopausal breast cancer
   d. Earlier menopause

17. Economic benefits of breastfeeding include all of the following *except:*
   a. Increased costs for special breastfeeding garments
   b. Reduced health care costs
   c. Reduced employee absenteeism to care for sick infants
   d. Reduced expenses for infant formula in the WIC program

18. Human milk composition does *not* contribute to which of the following?
   a. Growth and proliferation of tissues
   b. Maturation of tissue function
   c. Protection from infectious disease
   d. Dehydration

19. Which of the following statements about breastfeeding patterns is true?
   a. Exclusive breastfeeding is required to see any benefits.
   b. Benefits are conferred to the infant in a dose-response relationship.
   c. Complete protection of the infant is conferred by token breastfeeding.
   d. The breastfeeding pattern makes no difference in research studies that address benefits.

Answers (Answers are based on the Curriculum in Support of the Ten Steps to Successful Breastfeeding,[31] other sources,[32] and newer literature.)

1. **C.** About 250 to 300 infant deaths have been attributed to artificial feeding here in the United States.[33,34] In developing countries and in situations or locations with poor sanitary conditions, the rates associated with artificial feeding are even higher.

Continued

Box 1-1   Do You Know the Benefits of Breastfeeding?—cont'd

2. **D.** The incidence of duodenal ulcers has not been associated with artificial feeding. Crohn's disease, inflammatory bowel disease, and celiac disease are avoided, minimized, or delayed among adults who were breastfed.[35-41]

3. **B.** Cunningham, Jelliffe, and Jelliffe's careful review showed that the risk of fatal or nonfatal respiratory infections is twofold to fivefold higher among nonbreastfed infants.[42] Respiratory illness is a major public health problem in the United States. Approximately 500 to 600 infants die here each year from acute respiratory problems that have been associated with not being breastfed.[42]

4. **C.** Artificially fed infants have far more ear infections than breastfed infants, especially when compared with infants who have been breastfed for longer periods of time.[43]

5. **C.** Compared with breastfed infants, artificially fed infants have a fourfold increased incidence of bacteremia and meningitis.[44]

6. **D.** Approximately 25% of cases of juvenile-onset diabetes can be attributed to not being breastfed or by being exposed to artificial milk.[45]

7. **C.** Artificially fed children face a 6% to 8% increase in risk of childhood lymphoma.[46,47] (Lymphoma, a tumor of the cells of the lymphoid tissue, is usually benign but can be malignant. The two categories of malignant lymphomas are Hodgkin and non-Hodgkin lymphoma. The etiology of both is not well understood.)

8. **D.** The risk of breast cancer in women older than 40 is reduced by 25% if they were breastfed as children.[48]

9. **C.** Breastfeeding has not been shown to *prevent* allergies. However, it does appear that infants whose parents both have allergic disease experience a delay in the onset of allergic symptoms, and wheezing is less severe.[49]

10. **A.** Existing studies have not shown a relationship between breastfeeding and muscular dystrophy. Chronic respiratory disease in adults is often preceded by lower respiratory infections and wheezing in infants and children and has been associated with nonbreastfeeding.[50] Coronary disease is often preceded by other conditions such as ischemic heart disease,[51] which appears greater among exclusively bottle-fed infants. Furthermore, lower cholesterol in young adulthood seems to be a benefit of breastfeeding.[52]

11. **D.** Lactoferrin has not been associated with improved cognition or neurologic development.

12. **B.** Introduction of solids was not associated with improved test scores. However, test scores of cognitive and motor development increase in proportion to the duration of breastfeeding during infancy.[53]

13. **C.** Lucas and his colleagues in England gained international attention from the popular media when they showed that preterm children who were not given human milk for their early feeds had IQs that were 10 points lower than their breastfed cohorts.[54] In this well-controlled study, 300 children were followed until they were 7½ to 8 years old. Differences between IQ scores persisted even after investigators adjusted for differences between groups in mother's education and social class ($p < .0001$).

14. **A.** Existing data do not relate improved hearing function to breastfeeding, but other sensory benefits have been associated with breastfeeding. Children who have not been breastfed or those who have been breastfed for only a very short time have less visual acuity than those who have been breastfed.[55] The effects of congenital cretinism are mitigated through breastfeeding.[56] Even in children who are neurologically impaired, neuromotor skills are measurably less when they have received no human milk or when they have received human milk for only a short time.[57]

15. **D.** Compared with nonlactaters, lactating mothers have a delayed return of menses and fertility.[58] Some women use this lactational amenorrhea (LAM) to achieve child-spacing. This particular method of child-spacing is especially effective if the woman is exclusively breastfeeding.

Box 1-1   Do You Know the Benefits of Breastfeeding?—cont'd

16. **D.** Earlier menopause has not been associated with breastfeeding. However, women who have breastfed are at lower risk for fractures as a result of osteoporosis, presumably because of improved bone remineralization.[59,60] In some studies breastfeeding has been associated with reduced risk of ovarian cancer[61] and premenopausal breast cancer.[62]

17. **A.** Breastfeeding mothers do not need to buy special clothing, although some women do.

18. **D.** Human milk does *not* contribute to dehydration. To the contrary, human milk is about 87% water, and healthy infants, except under extreme circumstances, get enough water by breastfeeding.

19. **B.** The benefits of breastfeeding have been shown to be in a dose-response relationship.[7]

Box 1-2   Benefits of Breastfeeding

Extensive research on the biology of human milk and on the health outcomes associated with breastfeeding has established that breastfeeding is more beneficial than formula-feeding. Breastfed infants experience fewer cases of infectious and noninfectious diseases, as well as less severe cases of diarrhea, respiratory infections, and ear infections.[4,46,63-74] Mothers who breastfeed experience less postpartum bleeding, earlier return to prepregnancy weight, and a reduced risk of ovarian cancer and premenopausal breast cancer.[62,75-83] Furthermore, breastfeeding is cost beneficial to families.[4] Based on this evidence, the American Academy of Pediatrics has stated that "The breastfed infant is the reference or normative model against which all alternative feeding methods must be measured with regard to growth, health, development, and all other short- and long-term outcomes."[18] Thus human milk is uniquely suited for human infants.

RESISTANCE TO INFECTIOUS DISEASES

Human milk contains an abundance of factors that are active against infection. Because the infant's immune system is not fully mature until about 2 years of age, the transfer of these factors from human milk provides a distinct advantage that infants fed formula do not experience. Specifically, human milk contains immunologic agents and other compounds, such as secretory antibodies, leukocytes, and carbohydrates; these agents act against viruses, bacteria, and parasites.[84,85] Overall, research shows that breastfeeding may decrease the incidence of several acute bacterial and viral infections in infants (Box 1-3).

ENHANCED IMMUNE SYSTEM

Breastfed infants, compared with formula-fed infants, produce enhanced immune responses to polio, tetanus, diphtheria, and *Haemophilus influenzae* immunizations and to respiratory syncytial virus infection, a common infant respiratory infection.[81,86,87] Human milk contains antiinflammatory factors and other factors that regulate the response of the immune system against infection.[84] There is also evidence that breastfeeding results in earlier development of the infant immune system.[88]

Protection against infection is strongest during the first several months of life for infants who are breastfed exclusively.[7,64,66,72,89-91] Several studies suggest that the benefits continue even after breastfeeding ceases[64,66,92] and a few studies have found that breastfeeding into the second 6 months of life protects against infection.[72,73,93] Longer durations of breastfeeding may provide an even stronger protective effect.[64,66,92,94,95] Finally, children who were breastfed exclusively have fewer illnesses than those who were never breastfed.[64,89,90]

NUTRITIONAL AND GROWTH BENEFITS

Human milk contains a balance of nutrients that more closely matches human infant

Continued

Box **1-2**   Benefits of Breastfeeding—cont'd

requirements for growth and development than does the milk of any other species.[96] For example, compared with cow's milk, human milk is low in total protein and low in casein, making it more readily digestible and less stressful on immature infant kidneys. The lipids and enzymes in human milk promote efficient digestion and utilization of nutrients.[96,97]

Scientific evidence suggests that the normal pattern for breastfed infants is to gain less weight and to be leaner at 1 year of age than formula-fed infants, while maintaining normal activity level and development.[98] This early growth pattern may influence later growth patterns, resulting in less overweight and obesity among children who were breastfed.[98-104] Despite the finding that many African-American infants are premature or small at birth, premature babies fare better when breastfed compared with premature babies who are fed formula.[105]

REDUCED RISK FOR CHRONIC DISEASES

Many studies in infant feeding have found lower rates of several chronic childhood diseases among children who were breastfed. Recent findings suggest that breastfeeding may reduce the risk of type 1 and 2 diabetes[106-110] celiac disease,[35-38] inflammatory bowel disease,[39,111,112] childhood cancer,[71,113,114] and allergic disease/asthma.[74] Mixed results from some studies suggest that further research is needed to establish some of these benefits.[40,49,115-121]

DEVELOPMENTAL BENEFITS

Considerable interest has been raised about the potential effect of breastfeeding on cognitive development.[54,122-128,149] Long-chain polyunsaturated fatty acids, available in breast milk, are important for brain growth and development.[54,125-128] Observations in some studies on neurologic and cognitive outcomes in breastfed children have led to a hypothesis that the early visual acuity and cognitive function of these children is greater than in nonbreastfed children.[54,122,126] However, this hypothesis has not been conclusively proven.[123,127]

IMPROVED MATERNAL HEALTH

Breastfeeding has several positive hormonal, physical, and psychosocial effects on the mother. Breastfeeding increases levels of oxytocin, a hormone that stimulates uterine contractions, helping to expel the placenta, to minimize postpartum maternal blood loss, and to induce a more rapid uterine involution.[22,129] Breastfeeding, particularly exclusive breastfeeding, delays the resumption of normal ovarian cycles and the return of fertility in most women.[130] Mothers who breastfeed their infants may also experience psychologic benefits, such as increased self-confidence and facilitated bonding with their infants.[131-133]

Studies have shown that breastfeeding for longer time periods (up to 2 years) and among younger mothers (early twenties) may reduce the risk of premenopausal and possibly postmenopausal breast cancer.[62,77-81] In addition, the risk of ovarian cancer may be lower among women who have breastfed their children.[82,83,134]

SOCIOECONOMIC BENEFITS

Breastfeeding provides economic and social benefits to the family, the health care system, the employer, and the nation.[135] Families can save several hundred dollars over the cost of feeding breast-milk substitutes, even after accounting for the costs of breast pump equipment and additional food required by the nursing mother.[136] Breastfed infants typically require fewer sick care visits, prescriptions, and hospitalizations, especially if breastfed exclusively or almost exclusively.[4] Consequently, total medical care expenditures were approximately 20% lower for fully breastfed infants than for never-breastfed infants.[137] Because of the high occurrence of poverty among African-Americans, these families would benefit substantially from breastfeeding their infants.[138]

Employers also benefit when their employees breastfeed. Breastfed infants are sick less often; therefore maternal absenteeism from work is significantly lower in companies with established lactation programs.[139] In addition, employer medical costs are lower and employee productivity is higher.

Reprinted from HHS Blueprint for Action on Breastfeeding. Washington, DC: Department of Health and Human Services, Office on Women's Health; 2000.

Box **1-3** Infections That Are Lower in Incidence or Severity in Breastfed Infants Than in Formula-Fed Infants

Diarrhea[63,66,72,73,89]
Respiratory tract infection[7,63,66,89,90,140]
Otitis media[64,72,94,141]
Pneumonia[93,142]
Urinary infection[143,144]
Necrotizing enterocolitis[145,146]
Invasive bacterial infection[84,91,92,147]

Reprinted from HHS Blueprint for Action on Breastfeeding. Washington, DC: Department of Health and Human Services, Office on Women's Health; 2000.

Public Policy Statements and Initiatives

During the last three decades, several events and initiatives have taken place with the goal of making breastfeeding a public health priority. Most of these have been expressed either as public health policy statements or initiatives or as legislative efforts.

International and National Levels

Initiatives were undertaken on both the national and international levels, and in some cases, developments occurred concurrently on both levels. These initiatives are discussed first on the international level and then on the national level.

International Level. In 1974 the Twenty-seventh World Health Assembly noted the general decline in breastfeeding in many parts of the world. This decline was related to sociocultural factors and other factors, including the promotion of manufactured breast-milk substitutes. The Assembly urged "Member countries to review sales promotion activities on baby food and to introduce appropriate remedial measure, including advertisement codes and legislation where necessary" (resolution WHA27.43).

Following, in 1977, the World Health Organization (WHO) recognized that the lofty goal for the "highest attainable standard of health" as set out in its 1946 constitution was more theoretic than real. In an attempt to achieve this goal, the "Health for All" concept was launched in 1978 at a conference in Alma-Ata. This conference acted as a catalyst for countries, including the United States, to return to and apply "Health for All" principles at home.

In the same year that "Health for All" was initiated, the Thirty-first World Health Assembly identified prevention of infant malnutrition as a public health priority and breastfeeding as an important way to achieve this priority (resolution WHA31.47).

A year later, in 1979, WHO and the United Nations Children's Fund (UNICEF) convened a meeting on infant and young child feeding. This meeting brought together some 150 representatives of governments, the United Nations system and other intergovernmental bodies, nongovernmental organizations, the infant-food industry, and experts in related disciplines. Of the five interrelated themes discussed, the marketing and distribution of breast-milk substitutes attracted the most media attention. Among the recommendations emerging from this joint WHO/UNICEF meeting was the statement that "there should be an international code of marketing of infant formula and other products used as breast-milk substitutes."

In 1980 the Thirty-third World Health Assembly endorsed the statement and recommendations of the joint WHO/UNICEF meeting. The Assembly requested the director-general of WHO to prepare, "in close consultation with Member States and with all other parties concerned" (resolution WHA33.32), a code regarding the marketing and distribution of breast-milk substitutes. Several distinct drafts were sent out for comment. In 1981 WHO's executive board endorsed the fourth draft and recommended to the Thirty-fourth World Health Assembly its adoption in the form of a recommendation rather than as a regulation.

In May 1981 the World Health Assembly adopted the International Code of Marketing of Breast-milk Substitutes, by 118 votes in favor to 1 against, with 3 abstentions (the single vote against the Code came from the United States). The aim of the Code is "to contribute to the provision of safe and adequate nutrition for infants, by the protection and promotion of breast-feeding, and by ensuring the proper use of breast-milk substitutes, when those are necessary, on the basis of adequate information and through appropriate marketing and distribution."[9] The Code's main points are summarized in Appendix D.

In 1989 WHO/UNICEF put forth their statement *Protecting, Promoting, and Supporting Breast-Feeding: The Special Role of Maternity Services.*[10] This statement, which outlined universally relevant principles and action steps, was intended as a summary of what needed to be done to improve perinatal breastfeeding efforts throughout the world. (The definition of "protecting, promoting, and supporting" was not specified at that time.) The "Ten Steps to Successful Breastfeeding" contained in that document was intended as an executive summary and later became the cornerstone for the Baby-Friendly™ Hospital Initiative (BFHI) in 1991 (see Chapter 8). This important document also contained the Checklist for Evaluating the Adequacy of Support for Breastfeeding, which served as the backbone and impetus for breastfeeding promotion in the 1990s.

In the early 1990s, breastfeeding gained much momentum as a public health priority. Sponsored by the U.S. Agency for International Development and the Swedish International Development Authority, the meeting "Breastfeeding in the 1990s: A Global Initiative" was held from July 30 to August 1, 1990. From this critical meeting of

WHO/UNICEF policy makers came the WHO/UNICEF joint statement the "Innocenti Declaration."[11] The statement addressed the protection, promotion, and support of breastfeeding, although those terms were not specifically defined at the time. (Definitions developed later,[12] shown in Box 1-4, may be helpful.) It described the current state of breastfeeding promotion worldwide and outlined goals to be reached by 1995. Specifically, it required all governments to have accomplished the tasks noted in Box 1-5 by the year 1995.

In 1991 UNICEF and WHO launched the BFHI, which sought to overcome some of the general barriers that hospitals imposed on women throughout the world. At the heart of the BFHI were the 10 steps listed in the WHO/UNICEF statement. Subsequently, more than 15,000 hospitals throughout the world attained Baby-Friendly status. In the United States the movement was spearheaded by the U.S. Committee for UNICEF (which provided the funding for the project) and Wellstart International (which provided the technical expertise). Although the United States signed the Innocenti Declaration, efforts to implement the Ten Steps were delayed (see following discussion).

National Level. In 1978, the year when the "Health for All" concept was launched by WHO, the U.S. government began to recognize the cen-

Box **1-4**   DEFINITIONS OF PROMOTION, PROTECTION, AND SUPPORT

Although the Innocenti emphasized the need for promotion, protection, and support of breastfeeding, those terms were not defined. Later, Cadwell[12] defined those terms so that others might better operationalize them.

Breastfeeding promotion efforts focus on the advantages of breastfeeding to the individual baby and mother. Also included as promotion efforts are the dissemination of the advantages of breastfeeding in regard to the global ecology: decreased waste from bottles and manufacturing process and the diminished environmental cost of the care and feeding of dairy cattle.

Breastfeeding protection involves the legislated rights of women and children that enable breastfeeding. Included are adequate maternity leaves and appropriate child care facilities. Protection of breastfeeding also involves prohibiting certain marketing practices of companies manufacturing breast-milk substitutes.

Support of breastfeeding is accomplished through evidence-based hospital policies, health worker practices, and community programs that increase breastfeeding initiation and duration.

From Cadwell K. *Clin Perinatol* 1999;26:527-537.

Box 1-5   Main Points of the Innocenti Declaration

By the year 1995, all governments should have the following:

- Appointed a national breastfeeding coordinator of appropriate authority and established a multisectoral national breastfeeding committee composed of representatives from government departments, nongovernmental organizations, and health professional associations
- Ensured that every facility providing maternity services fully practices all 10 of the "Ten Steps to Successful Breastfeeding" set out in the joint WHO/UNICEF statement, "Protecting Promoting and Supporting Breastfeeding: The Special Role of Maternity Services"
- Took action to give effect to the principles and aims of all Articles of the International Code of Marketing of Breast-milk Substitutes and subsequent relevant World Health Assembly resolutions in their entirety
- Enacted imaginative legislation protecting the breastfeeding rights of working women and established means for its enforcement

From World Health Organization and United Nations Children's Fund. *Innocenti Declaration: 30 July to 1 August, 1990, Florence, Italy.* Geneva, Switzerland: World Health Organization; 1990.

trality of breastfeeding to the health and nutrition of our nation. The Carter administration appointed a committee to develop the first "Goals for the Nation"; one of these goals was increasing breastfeeding incidence and duration. The committee set a goal that, by 1990, breastfeeding would be initiated for 75% of infants and that 35% would still be breastfeeding at age 6 months.[13] Although a small administrative group developed this first set of goals, subsequent goals, revised every 10 years, have come from every level of government and, before they are released, are posted for public comment. The goals for breastfeeding, which have been revised twice, are intended to promote breastfeeding as a way to achieve optimal health and nutrition (Box 1 6).

During the 1980s, while much was happening on the international scene, several significant national events that aimed to increase breastfeeding incidence and continuation in the United States were taking place. In 1982 the American Academy of Pediatrics (AAP) issued a policy statement titled "The Promotion of Breast-feeding," which strongly favored breastfeeding.[14] It followed

Box 1-6   Goals for the Nation

In 1978 goals were set that stated that by the year 1990:

- 75% of women would initiate breastfeeding
- 35% of women would continue breastfeeding for at least 6 months

In 1988 goals were set that stated that by the year 2000:

- 75% of women would initiate breastfeeding
- 50% of women would continue breastfeeding for at least 6 months

The current goals state that by the year 2010:

- 75% of women will initiate breastfeeding
- 50% of women will continue breastfeeding for at least 6 months
- 25% of women will continue breastfeeding for at least 12 months

From US Department of Health Education and Welfare. *Healthy people: The Surgeon General's report on health promotion and disease prevention.* Washington, DC: Department of Health Education and Welfare, Government Printing Office HHS #79-55071; 1979; US Department of Health and Human Services. *Healthy people 2000: National health promotion and disease prevention objectives.* Washington, DC: Government Printing Office, 1991; and US Department of Health and Human Services. *Healthy people 2010: National health promotion and disease prevention objectives.* Washington, DC: Government Printing Office; 2000. Also available at http://www.health.gov/healthypeople/Document/.

an earlier statement,[15] titled "Encouraging Breast-Feeding," which was somewhat less directive; the earlier statement drew general conclusions, whereas the 1982 statement made four clear recommendations. Later, the AAP reaffirmed its statement in conjunction with the American College of Obstetricians.[16,17] In 1997 the AAP strengthened its original statement. The title, "Breastfeeding and the Use of Human Milk,"[18] emphasizes the use of human milk even when breastfeeding is not possible, and the statement itself delivers a strong assertion that artificial milk is clearly inferior in all cases.

In 1984 the U.S. government undertook a major effort to improve breastfeeding. The Maternal and Child Health Bureau (MCHB) of the U.S. Department of Health and Human Services (USDHHS) convened the Surgeon General's Workshop. This workshop was the first formal attempt to facilitate breastfeeding at the national level through a multidisciplinary group. Its purpose was to assess the current status of breastfeeding in the United States and to develop strategies to facilitate reaching the 1990 breastfeeding goal for the nation. At the workshop, then U.S. Surgeon General, C. Everett Koop, said, "We must identify and reduce the barriers which keep women from beginning or continuing to breastfeed their infants."[19] To that end, work groups were formed to identify and prioritize issues related to breastfeeding and lactation and to develop recommendations that would remove the barriers to breastfeeding and better enable the United States to meet breastfeeding goals. A report[19] summarizing the themes and recommendations was generated at the conclusion of the meeting, and two follow-up reports were written in subsequent years.[20,21]

In 1987 the Institute of Medicine Subcommittee on Nutrition During Lactation convened and generated several recommendations[22] and an official statement that endorsed breastfeeding under ordinary circumstances. Around the same time, various national organizations began writing official position statements about breastfeeding as a response to the directive given at the Surgeon General's 1984 meeting. Many position statements by various nursing, medical, and other professional organizations

have since been written; they are listed in Appendix D. In addition, new U.S.-based organizations that focused solely on breastfeeding were founded, including the International Lactation Consultant Association (founded in 1985), Human Milk Banking Association of North America (HMBANA) (founded in 1985), and the International Society for Research in Human Milk and Lactation (founded in 1988). Other national and international organizations focusing solely on breastfeeding were established after the end of that decade.

In 1988, in a follow-up to the 1978 effort initiated by the Carter administration, the first Bush administration appointed a committee to develop goals for the nation for the year 2000. A goal was established to increase to 75% the number of mothers who breastfeed their newborns on discharge from the hospital (same as in 1978) and to 50% those who continue breastfeeding for the first 6 months of life (increased 15% from 1978).[23]

In 1990, as a follow-up to the 1984 Surgeon General's workshop, the National Center for Education in Maternal and Child Health, in consultation with MCHB staff, conducted a pilot study to gather descriptive data on breastfeeding promotion.[21] Although the study identified some promotion activities, many barriers were also revealed in the following categories: (1) professional education, (2) public education, (3) support in the health care system, (4) support services in the community, (5) support in the workplace, and (6) research. Although some of these barriers have been reduced or removed, many still exist more than a decade later.

In 1990 the USDHHS, through MCHB, held a national workshop titled "Call to Action: Better Nutrition for Mothers, Children, and Families."[24] One of the recommendations of the workshop was "to promote breastfeeding among all women to achieve the year 2000 National Health Promotion and Disease Prevention objectives for breastfeeding, and establish breastfeeding as the societal norm for infant feeding."[24] To meet this recommendation, specific strategies were developed at the workshop and include the points listed in Box 1-7. Other recommendations also addressed issues such as the marketing of artificial milk, the

Box 1-7   Strategies for Achieving the Year 2000 Objectives for Breastfeeding

- Promote breastfeeding as the preferred method of infant feeding to the memberships of all health professional organizations
- Continue efforts to develop more effective strategies to promote breastfeeding through hospitals, maternal-child health programs, WIC and other food assistance programs, industry, and other work sites (including federal agencies)
- Explore ways to promote breastfeeding through community programs, such as the Expanded Food and Nutrition Education Program, food stamps, and other community-based interventions
- Encourage federal agencies to serve as models for providing support of breastfeeding women in the federal work site

- Ensure that health care professionals who interact with pregnant women, including hospital personnel, communicate breastfeeding as the norm
- Continue to develop and implement ways to support and provide incentives for breastfeeding in the WIC program
- Include specific methods of supporting breastfeeding in the standards of practice for health professionals
- Provide lactation management training to all health care professionals who interact with pregnant and breastfeeding women to enhance their ability to support breastfeeding, and involve hospitals in networking for the promotion of breastfeeding

From Sharbaugh CS. *Call to action: Better nutrition for mothers, children, and families.* Washington, DC: National Center for Education in Maternal and Child Health; 1990.

need for reliable and standardized data on infant feeding practices, and research priorities as related to infant feeding.

In 1997 Baby-Friendly USA was founded as the official organization to implement the 1991 UNICEF and WHO BFHI in the United States (see Appendix D). Hospitals that changed protocols to reflect the BFHI have had excellent results; initiation of breastfeeding, artificial milk supplementation, and support from hospital staff improve markedly when these principles are implemented.[25,26]

In 1998 the U.S. Breastfeeding Committee (USBC) was formed with representatives from many organizations. Charter members of the USBC included two nursing organizations: the Association of Women's Health, Obstetric and Neonatal Nurses (AWHONN) and the American College of Nurse-Midwives (ACNM). The mission of the USBC is to improve the nation's health by working collaboratively to protect, promote, and support breastfeeding. To accomplish that mission, the USBC has developed a strategic plan for breastfeeding in the United States and this plan was

appended to the Surgeon General's USDHHS "Call to Action for Breastfeeding."[8]

The United States has progressed slowly in meeting national goals and international directives. The most notable downfalls have been in relation to meeting the goals for the nation and implementing the Innocenti Declaration. The goals for the nation for 1990 and for the year 2000 still have not been met. Through protection, promotion, and support efforts described earlier, however, the incidence and duration of breastfeeding in the United States have improved over the past two decades, as shown by statistics in Chapter 2.

Sadly, the United States continues to be slow to implement the directive set forth by the Innocenti Declaration. A national breastfeeding coordinator has never been appointed, and such an appointment is unlikely to occur in the future. Presumably, the Secretary of Health and Human Services, or his or her designee, might logically fill that role. However, even if the Secretary did undertake that responsibility, the role would not be enacted like it has been in other countries. Fortunately, a related point of the Innocenti Declaration was finally fulfilled when the U.S. Breastfeeding Committee was formed. (Visit http://www.usbreastfeeding.org.)

Another goal of the Innocenti Declaration was for governments to ensure "that every facility providing maternity services fully practices all 10 of the Ten Steps to Successful Breastfeeding set out in the joint WHO/UNICEF statement *Protecting, Promoting, and Supporting Breast-Feeding: The Special Role of Maternity Services.*" Only 33 U.S. hospitals have been designated as Baby-Friendly at press time, with others actively working toward achieving the award, but this is only a small fraction of "all facilities" in the United States.

The first edition of this book, multiple other printed sources, and literally hundreds of breastfeeding advocates have stated that the United States "endorsed" the WHO Code in May of 1994, but this interpretation is questionable. The language of "endorsing" is inaccurate because the Code, or any recommendation from WHO, is not a document that member states can ratify. (Unlike a treaty that is signed, a WHO recommendation is more akin to an automobile manufacturer's recommendation to change a car's oil every 3000 miles; because it is not a regulation, it is not legally binding, nor does it carry a penalty for member states that do not comply with or implement it.) Moreover, how delegates from member states "reaffirmed" this recommendation in 1994 was vastly different from how it was originally adopted. In 1981 the Code was adopted after a roll-call vote, whereas in 1994 the U.S. government and other member states rescinded their proposed amendments and the Code was "reaffirmed" by consensus, not by vote. Because no vote was taken, the best that can be said is that the United States and other member states did not object to reaffirming the Code without modifications. This passive agreement rather than active "endorsement" may help explain why the U.S. government has not "taken action to give effect to the principles and aim"[9] of the Code. Multiple companies continue to violate the Code, but they have received no reprimand from the U.S. government, and it is unlikely that any reprimand will be forthcoming.

The fourth point of the Innocenti, having to do with legislation to protect, promote, and support breastfeeding, has been implemented here in the United States. Federal and state legislation is described in the following section and in Appendix D.

State and Local Level

Historically, state health departments have been involved in many matters related to health, but they have been minimally involved in breastfeeding promotion. Now, many years after the directives from the Surgeon General's conference, many states, although not all, have done little to remove the barriers to breastfeeding at the state level.

Some of the most serious barriers to breastfeeding in the hospital have been overcome in New York, however; their success is attributable to the specific breastfeeding directives incorporated into the state health code (see Appendix D). Because hospitals are required to comply with all aspects of the state health code, hospital personnel took these directives seriously and many improvements in breastfeeding management followed. The New York state health code mandates that a breastfeeding coordinator be identified in every hospital and every WIC agency. Furthermore, the New York State Department of Health has sponsored training programs for health care professionals and has included information about breastfeeding in grade school curricula. These state-mandated directives have done much to bring about social change. Other states have also implemented some of these mandates.

Several states have enacted legislation to protect breastfeeding. Appendix D outlines state legislation related to a woman's right to breastfeed in public, jury duty exemption, employment situations, and family law. Some states have established a task force on breastfeeding, providing an opportunity for health care providers to interact with policy makers to identify barriers to breastfeeding and ways to overcome those barriers.

Federal Legislation

Federal legislation has focused on two areas: protecting the rights of breastfeeding mothers and supporting breastfeeding through federally funded grants and programs.

Legislation to Protect Breastfeeding Mothers

Because breastfeeding is no longer the social norm, women who have breastfed in public during the last few decades have encountered multiple problems. Others, including officers and others who are responsible for enforcing the law, have prohibited women from "illegally" breastfeeding. Women who have breastfed in public places have frequently been asked to leave, harassed, or even arrested for indecent exposure. Certainly, it is not illegal to breastfeed anywhere in the United States, and state legislation has been enacted to protect a woman's right to breastfeed, as described in Appendix D.

Federal legislation to explicitly protect the rights of breastfeeding women occurred at the close of the twentieth century. In 1999 the Right to Breastfeed Act was enacted into law. This act ensures a woman's right to breastfeed anywhere on federal property where she and her child are authorized to be.

Further legislation is currently pending. Bills have been introduced into the federal legislature that address issues such as employment termination of a woman who breastfeeds, the right to express milk in the workplace, tax credits for employers who provide the optimal circumstances for mothers who breastfeed, and minimum quality standards for breast pumps. (Updates on legislation can be found at http://thomas.loc.gov.)

Women, Infants, and Children Program

The WIC program was legislated by Congress as a pilot program in 1972 and authorized as a permanent program in 1975. WIC was initiated for pregnant, lactating, or postpartum women and their infants and children up to 5 years of age. The goal of this federally funded program is to improve birth outcomes and early childhood development by providing nutrient-dense supplemental foods, nutrition education, and health care referrals. Women and their children are eligible for WIC benefits when their gross family income is at or below 185% of the poverty level and a nutritionally related medical condition and/or nutritional risk

exists. The program has benefited from numerous legislative and regulatory acts over the years. An excellent history of WIC and discussion of its effects on women and their children are found elsewhere.[27]

The WIC program provides supplemental foods that are high in protein, iron, vitamins A and C, and calcium for women, infants, and children. Because WIC serves more than 40% of all infants born in the United States, it is a major purchaser of artificial milk. In the early years, WIC paid the full retail price for artificial milk; it later bid for contracts and then received rebates. This change strengthened the program's ability to serve additional participants; in fact, today this cost-saving measure supports about one fourth of WIC's 7.3 million participants. In addition, WIC's nutrition education and counseling efforts, particularly related to breastfeeding promotion and support, have shown significant improvement. Breastfeeding rates are growing faster among WIC participants than among the general population.[28]

Unlike other organizations and circumstances that perpetuated the barriers, WIC has actively facilitated breastfeeding. In 1989 the U.S. Department of Agriculture (USDA) set aside $8 million each year, which WIC state agencies were required to spend on breastfeeding promotion and support. Furthermore, each state WIC agency is required to designate a breastfeeding coordinator. Breastfeeding women have a higher priority for enrollment in the WIC program, their benefits are more varied (more supplemental food benefits), and they have a longer participation period (1 year as opposed to 6 months) than those who choose artificial feeding. Furthermore, mothers receive an expanded food package if they exclusively breastfeed and do not receive any artificial milk from WIC.

In the late 1990s WIC stepped up efforts to provide education and support for breastfeeding. In 1994 Public Law 103-448, the Healthy Meals for Healthy Americans Act, revised the method for determining the amount of funds to be spent for WIC breastfeeding promotion and support. The act replaced the $8 million target level with a national maximum for breastfeeding promotion and supported expenditures of $25.21 per year for each pregnant and breastfeeding woman. This amount is adjusted annually based on inflation.

Staff training is required by WIC state agencies to ensure staff members' ability to assist mothers through all phases of breastfeeding, from prenatal decision making to weaning. Furthermore, WIC has endeavored to be seen as a referral center and resource within the community. In August 1997 the USDA launched the WIC National Breastfeeding Promotion Campaign together with Best Start (a social marketing organization). This campaign includes television and radio spots, billboards, and pamphlets that advertise breastfeeding. The campaign's motto, "Loving support makes breastfeeding work," is designed to send a positive message not only to breastfeeding mothers but also to families and friends who support them.

SUMMARY

Good health is the most important resource we have. The health and socioeconomic benefits of breastfeeding are a vital part of good health not only for infants but also for their mothers and society. These benefits, most apparent during the perinatal period, have long-lasting effects that promote optimal health throughout the life span of the breastfed infant and his mother. However, identifying the benefits of breastfeeding is only the first step. As Ball and Bennett point out, "To reap the health and economic benefits associated with breastfeeding, society must support breastfeeding promotion, which most likely will necessitate a coordinated U.S. breastfeeding program"[29] (p. 260).

International, national, state, and local efforts to promote breastfeeding have included the creation of many policy statements and goals. The United States has been slow to implement directions that have been issued by WHO, and these delays have likely been related to the slow progress we have experienced. Although the incidence and duration of breastfeeding has improved somewhat here in the United States, the Goals of the Nation for 1990 and 2000 were not achieved. Whether the goals for the year 2010 are achieved may depend on how breastfeeding is protected, promoted, and supported in the United States over the next several years.

REFERENCES

1. Brown AK, Damus K, Kim MH et al. Factors relating to readmission of term and near-term neonates in the first two weeks of life. Early Discharge Survey Group of the Health Professional Advisory Board of the Greater New York Chapter of the March of Dimes. *J Perinat Med* 1999;27:263-275.
2. Health Care Financing Administration. *National health expenditures aggregate and per capita amounts, percent distribution and average annual percent growth, by source of funds: selected calendar years 1960-98.* Washington, DC: Health Care Financing Administration; 1999.
3. Weimer J. *The economic benefits of breastfeeding: a review and analysis.* Washington, DC: Economic Research Service, US Department of Agriculture, Report #13; 2001.
4. Ball TM, Wright AL. Health care costs of formula-feeding in the first year of life. *Pediatrics* 1999;103:870-876.
5. Hambraeus L. Proprietary milk versus human breast milk in infant feeding. A critical appraisal from the nutritional point of view. *Pediatr Clin North Am* 1977;24:17-36.
6. Labbok M, Krasovec K. Toward consistency in breastfeeding definitions. *Stud Fam Plann* 1990;21:226-230.
7. Raisler J, Alexander C, O'Campo P. Breast-feeding and infant illness: a dose-response relationship? *Am J Public Health* 1999;89:25-30.
8. US Department of Health and Human Services. *HHS blueprint for action on breastfeeding.* Washington, DC: Office on Women's Health, US Department of Health and Human Services; 2000.
9. World Health Organization. *International code of marketing of breast-milk substitutes.* Geneva: World Health Organization; 1981.
10. World Health Organization and United Nations Children's Fund. *Protecting, promoting, and supporting breast-feeding: the special role of maternity services.* Geneva, Switzerland: World Health Organization; 1989.
11. World Health Organization and United Nations Children's Fund. *Innocenti Declaration: 30 July to 1 August, 1990, Florence Italy.* Geneva, Switzerland: World Health Organization; 1990.
12. Cadwell K. Reaching the goals of "*Healthy People 2000*" regarding breastfeeding. *Clin Perinatol* 1999;26:527-537.
13. US Department of Health Education and Welfare. *Healthy people: the Surgeon General's report on health promotion and disease prevention.* Washington, DC: Department of Health Education and Welfare, Government Printing Office, DHHS #79-55071; 1979.
14. American Academy of Pediatrics. The promotion of breastfeeding. Policy statement based on task force report. *Pediatrics* 1982;69:654-661.

15. American Academy of Pediatrics Committee on Nutrition. Encouraging breast-feeding. *Pediatrics* 1980;65:657-658.

16. American Academy of Pediatrics and The American College of Obstetricians and Gynecologists. *Guidelines for perinatal care.* 3rd ed. Elk Grove Village, IL: American Academy of Pediatrics; 1992.

17. American Academy of Pediatrics and the American College of Obstetricians and Gynecologists. *Guidelines for perinatal care.* 4th ed. Elk Grove Village, IL: American Academy of Pediatrics; 1997.

18. American Academy of Pediatrics Work Group on Breastfeeding. Breastfeeding and the use of human milk. *Pediatrics* 1997;100:1035-1039.

19. US Department of Health and Human Services. *Report of the Surgeon General's workshop on breastfeeding and human lactation.* Rockville, MD: Health Resources and Services Administration; 1984.

20. US Department of Health Education and Welfare. *Followup report: the Surgeon General's workshop on breastfeeding and human lactation.* Rockville, MD: Health Resources and Services Administration, DHHS Publication #HRS-D-85-2; 1985.

21. Spisak S, Gross SS. *Second followup report: the Surgeon General's workshop on breastfeeding and human lactation.* Washington, DC. National Center for Education in Maternal and Child Health; 1991.

22. Institute of Medicine. *Nutrition during lactation.* Washington, DC: National Academy Press; 1991.

23. US Department of Health and Human Services. *Healthy people 2000: national health promotion and disease prevention objectives.* Washington, DC: Government Printing Office; 1991.

24. Sharbaugh CS. *Call to action: better nutrition for mothers, children, and families.* Washington, DC: National Center for Education in Maternal and Child Health; 1990.

25. Philipp BL, Merewood A, Miller LW et al. Baby-Friendly Hospital Initiative improves breastfeeding initiation rates in a U.S. hospital setting. *Pediatrics* 2001;108:677-681.

26. Kramer MS, Chalmers B, Hodnett ED et al. Promotion of breastfeeding intervention trial (PROBIT): a randomized trial in the Republic of Belarus. *JAMA* 2001;285: 413-420.

27. Owen AL, Owen GM. Twenty years of WIC: a review of some effects of the program. *J Am Diet Assoc* 1997; 97: 777-782.

28. Ryan A. The resurgence of breastfeeding in the United States. *Pediatrics* 1997;99:e1-5.

29. Ball TM, Bennett DM. The economic impact of breastfeeding. *Pediatr Clin North Am* 2001;48:253-262.

30. Hoefer C, Hardy MC. Later development of breast fed and artificially fed infants. *J Am Med Assoc* 1929;92: 615-620.

31. Cadwell K, Arnold LDW, Turner-Maffei C et al, editors. *The curriculum in support of the ten steps to successful breastfeeding: interdisciplinary breastfeeding management course for the United States.* Rockville, MD: US Department of Health and Human Services, Health Resources & Services Administration, Maternal & Child Health Bureau (Available from Baby-Friendly USA); 1999; Order #98-0264 (P).

32. Stuart-Macadam P, Dettwyler KA, editor. *Breastfeeding: biocultural perspectives.* Hawthorne, NY: Aldine de Gruyter; 1995.

33. Newburg DS, Peterson JA, Ruiz-Palacios GM et al. Role of human-milk lactadherin in protection against symptomatic rotavirus infection. *Lancet* 1998;351:1160-1164.

34. Ho MS, Glass RI, Pinsky PF et al. Diarrheal deaths in American children. Are they preventable? *JAMA* 1988; 260:3281-3285.

35. Greco L, Auricchio S, Mayer M et al. Case control study on nutritional risk factors in celiac disease. *J Pediatr Gastroenterol Nutr* 1988;7:395-399.

36. Auricchio S, Follo D, de Ritis G et al. Does breast feeding protect against the development of clinical symptoms of celiac disease in children? *J Pediatr Gastroenterol Nutr* 1983;2:428-433.

37. Falth-Magnusson K, Franzen L, Jansson G et al. Infant feeding history shows distinct differences between Swedish celiac and reference children. *Pediatr Allergy Immunol* 1996;7:1-5.

38. Ivarsson A, Persson LA, Nystrom L et al. Epidemic of coeliac disease in Swedish children. *Acta Paediatr* 2000;89: 165-171.

39. Koletzko S, Sherman P, Corey M et al. Role of infant feeding practices in development of Crohn's disease in childhood. *BMJ* 1989;298:1617-1618.

40. Rigas A, Rigas B, Glassman M et al. Breast-feeding and maternal smoking in the etiology of Crohn's disease and ulcerative colitis in childhood. *Ann Epidemiol* 1993; 3:387-392.

41. Davis MK. Breastfeeding and chronic disease in childhood and adolescence. *Pediatr Clin North Am* 2001; 48:125-141.

42. Cunningham AS, Jelliffe DB, Jelliffe EF. Breast-feeding and health in the 1980s: a global epidemiologic review. *J Pediatr* 1991;118:659-666.

43. Duffy LC, Faden H, Wasielewski R et al. Exclusive breastfeeding protects against bacterial colonization and day care exposure to otitis media. *Pediatrics* 1997;100:E7.

44. Fallot ME, Boyd JL III, Oski FA. Breast-feeding reduces incidence of hospital admissions for infection in infants. *Pediatrics* 1980;65:1121-1124.

45. Mayer EJ, Hamman RF, Gay EC et al. Reduced risk of IDDM among breast-fed children. The Colorado IDDM Registry. *Diabetes* 1988;37:1625-1632.

46. Davis MK, Savitz DA, Graubard BI. Infant feeding and childhood cancer. *Lancet* 1988;2:365-368.

47. Shu XO, Clemens J, Zheng W et al. Infant breastfeeding and the risk of childhood lymphoma and leukaemia. *Int J Epidemiol* 1995;24:27-32.

48. Freudenheim JL, Marshall JR, Graham S et al. Exposure to breastmilk in infancy and the risk of breast cancer. *Epidemiology* 1994;5:324-331.

49. Saarinen UM, Kajosaari M. Breastfeeding as prophylaxis against atopic disease: prospective follow-up study until 17 years old. *Lancet* 1995;346:1065-1069.

50. McConnochie KM, Roghmann KJ. Breast feeding and maternal smoking as predictors of wheezing in children age 6 to 10 years. *Pediatr Pulmonol* 1986;2:260-268.

51. Fall CH, Barker DJ, Osmond C et al. Relation of infant feeding to adult serum cholesterol concentration and death from ischaemic heart disease. *BMJ* 1992;304:801-805.

52. Marmot MG, Page CM, Atkins E et al. Effect of breast-feeding on plasma cholesterol and weight in young adults. *J Epidemiol Community Health* 1980;34:164-167.

53. Rogan WJ, Gladen BC. Breast-feeding and cognitive development. *Early Hum Dev* 1993;31:181-193.

54. Lucas A, Morley R, Cole TJ et al. Breast milk and subsequent intelligence quotient in children born preterm. *Lancet* 1992;339:261-264.

55. Birch E, Birch D, Hoffman D et al. Breast-feeding and optimal visual development. *J Pediatr Ophthalmol Strabismus* 1993;30:33-38.

56. Bode HH, Vanjonack WJ, Crawford JD. Mitigation of cretinism by breast-feeding. *Pediatrics* 1978;62:13-16.

57. Lanting CI, Fidler V, Huisman M et al. Neurological differences between 9-year-old children fed breast-milk or formula-milk as babies. *Lancet* 1994;344:1319-1322.

58. Labbok MH. Effects of breastfeeding on the mother. *Pediatr Clin North Am* 2001;48:143-158.

59. Krebs NF, Reidinger CJ, Robertson AD et al. Bone mineral density changes during lactation: maternal, dietary, and biochemical correlates. *Am J Clin Nutr* 1997;65:1738-1746.

60. Kalkwarf HJ, Specker BL. Bone mineral loss during lactation and recovery after weaning. *Obstet Gynecol* 1995;86:26-32.

61. Whittemore AS. Characteristics relating to ovarian cancer risk: implications for prevention and detection. *Gynecol Oncol* 1994;55:S15-S19.

62. Newcomb PA, Storer BE, Longnecker MP et al. Lactation and a reduced risk of premenopausal breast cancer. *N Engl J Med* 1994;330:81-87.

63. Beaudry M, Dufour R, Marcoux S. Relation between infant feeding and infections during the first six months of life. *J Pediatr* 1995;126:191-197.

64. Duncan B, Ey J, Holberg CJ et al. Exclusive breast-feeding for at least 4 months protects against otitis media. *Pediatrics* 1993;91:867-872.

65. Frank AL, Taber LH, Glezen WP et al. Breast-feeding and respiratory virus infection. *Pediatrics* 1982;70:239-245.

66. Howie PW, Forsyth JS, Ogston SA et al. Protective effect of breast feeding against infection. *BMJ* 1990;300:11-16.

67. Kovar MG, Serdula MK, Marks JS et al. Review of the epidemiologic evidence for an association between infant feeding and infant health. *Pediatrics* 1984;74:615-638.

68. Popkin BM, Adair L, Akin JS et al. Breast-feeding and diarrheal morbidity. *Pediatrics* 1990;86:874-882.

69. Saarinen UM. Prolonged breast feeding as prophylaxis for recurrent otitis media. *Acta Paediatr Scand* 1982;71:567-571.

70. Moreland J, Coombs J. Promoting and supporting breast-feeding. *Am Fam Physician* 2000;61:2093-2100, 2103-2104.

71. Davis MK. Review of the evidence for an association between infant feeding and childhood cancer. *Int J Cancer Suppl* 1998;11:29-33.

72. Dewey KG, Heinig MJ, Nommsen-Rivers LA. Differences in morbidity between breast-fed and formula-fed infants. *J Pediatr* 1995;126:696-702.

73. Duffy LC, Byers TE, Riepenhoff-Talty M et al. The effects of infant feeding on rotavirus-induced gastroenteritis: a prospective study. *Am J Public Health* 1986;76:259-263.

74. Wright AL, Holberg CJ, Taussig LM et al. Relationship of infant feeding to recurrent wheezing at age 6 years. *Arch Pediatr Adolesc Med* 1995;149:758-763.

75. Chua S, Arulkumaran S, Lim I et al. Influence of breast-feeding and nipple stimulation on postpartum uterine activity. *Br J Obstet Gynaecol* 1994;101:804-805.

76. Dewey KG, Heinig MJ, Nommsen LA. Maternal weight-loss patterns during prolonged lactation. *Am J Clin Nutr* 1993;58:162-166.

77. Enger SM, Ross RK, Paganini-Hill A et al. Breastfeeding experience and breast cancer risk among postmenopausal women. *Cancer Epidemiol Biomarkers Prev* 1998;7:365-369.

78. Marcus PM, Baird DD, Millikan RC et al. Adolescent reproductive events and subsequent breast cancer risk. *Am J Public Health* 1999;89:1244-1247.

79. Weiss HA, Potischman NA, Brinton LA et al. Prenatal and perinatal risk factors for breast cancer in young women. *Epidemiology* 1997;8:181-187.

80. Brinton LA, Potischman NA, Swanson CA et al. Breastfeeding and breast cancer risk. *Cancer Causes Control* 1995;6:199-208.

81. Newcomb PA, Egan KM, Titus-Ernstoff L et al. Lactation in relation to postmenopausal breast cancer. *Am J Epidemiol* 1999;150:174-182.

82. Gwinn ML, Lee NC, Rhodes PH et al. Pregnancy, breast feeding, and oral contraceptives and the risk of epithelial ovarian cancer. *J Clin Epidemiol* 1990;43:559-568.

83. Rosenblatt KA, Thomas DB. Lactation and the risk of epithelial ovarian cancer. The WHO collaborative study of neoplasia and steroid contraceptives. *Int J Epidemiol* 1993;22:192-197.

84. Goldman AS. The immune system of human milk: antimicrobial, antiinflammatory and immunomodulating properties. *Pediatr Infect Dis J* 1993;12:664-671.

85. Goldman AS, Goldblum RM, Hanson LA. Anti-inflammatory systems in human milk. *Adv Exp Med Biol* 1990;262:69-76.

86. Hahn-Zoric M, Fulconis F, Minoli I et al. Antibody responses to parenteral and oral vaccines are impaired by conventional and low protein formulas as compared to breastfeeding. *Acta Paediatr Scand* 1990;79:1137-1142.

87. Pabst HF. Immunomodulation by breast-feeding. *Pediatr Infect Dis J* 1997;16:991-995.
88. Garofalo RP, Goldman AS. Expression of functional immunomodulatory and anti-inflammatory factors in human milk. *Clin Perinatol* 1999;26:361-377.
89. Scariati PD, Grummer-Strawn LM, Fein SB. A longitudinal analysis of infant morbidity and the extent of breast-feeding in the United States. *Pediatrics* 1997;99:E5.
90. Cushing AH, Samet JM, Lambert WE et al. Breastfeeding reduces risk of respiratory illness in infants. *Am J Epidemiol* 1998;147:863-870.
91. Istre GR, Conner JS, Broome CV et al. Risk factors for primary invasive *Haemophilus influenzae* disease: increased risk from day care attendance and school-aged household members. *J Pediatr* 1985;106:190-195.
92. Takala AK, Eskola J, Palmgren J et al. Risk factors of invasive *Haemophilus influenzae* type b disease among children in Finland. *J Pediatr* 1989;115:694-701.
93. Levine OS, Farley M, Harrison LH et al. Risk factors for invasive pneumococcal disease in children: a population-based case-control study in North America. *Pediatrics* 1999;103:E28.
94. Owen MJ, Baldwin CD, Swank PR et al. Relation of infant feeding practices, cigarette smoke exposure, and group child care to the onset and duration of otitis media with effusion in the first two years of life. *J Pediatr* 1993;123:702-711.
95. Nafstad P, Jaakkola JJ, Hagen JA et al. Breastfeeding, maternal smoking and lower respiratory tract infections. *Eur Respir J* 1996;9:2623-2629.
96. Picciano MF. Human milk: nutritional aspects of a dynamic food. *Biol Neonate* 1998;74:84-93.
97. Hernell O, Blackberg L. Human milk bile salt-stimulated lipase: functional and molecular aspects. *J Pediatr* 1994;125:S56-S61.
98. Dewey KG. Growth characteristics of breast-fed compared to formula-fed infants. *Biol Neonate* 1998;74:94-105.
99. von Kries R, Koletzko B, Sauerwald T et al. Breast feeding and obesity: cross-sectional study. *BMJ* 1999;319:147-150.
100. Ravelli AC, van der Meulen JH, Osmond C et al. Infant feeding and adult glucose tolerance, lipid profile, blood pressure, and obesity. *Arch Dis Child* 2000;82:248-252.
101. Kramer MS. Do breast-feeding and delayed introduction of solid foods protect against subsequent obesity? *J Pediatr* 1981;98:883-887.
102. Strbak V, Skultetyova M, Hromadova M et al. Late effects of breast-feeding and early weaning: seven-year prospective study in children. *Endocr Regul* 1991;25:53-57.
103. Hamosh M. Does infant nutrition affect adiposity and cholesterol levels in the adult? *J Pediatr Gastroenterol Nutr* 1988;7:10-16.
104. Elliott KG, Kjolhede CL, Gournis E et al. Duration of breastfeeding associated with obesity during adolescence. *Obes Res* 1997;5:538-541.
105. Centers for Disease Control and Prevention. *Pediatric nutrition surveillance, 1997 full report.* Atlanta: US Department of Health and Human Services, Centers for Disease Control and Prevention; 1998.
106. Perez-Bravo F, Carrasco E, Gutierrez-Lopez MD et al. Genetic predisposition and environmental factors leading to the development of insulin-dependent diabetes mellitus in Chilean children. *J Mol Med* 1996;74:105-109.
107. Gerstein HC. Cow's milk exposure and type I diabetes mellitus. A critical overview of the clinical literature. *Diabetes Care* 1994;17:13-19.
108. Hammond-McKibben D, Dosch HM. Cow's milk, bovine serum albumin, and IDDM: can we settle the controversies? *Diabetes Care* 1997;20:897-901.
109. Norris JM, Scott FW. A meta-analysis of infant diet and insulin-dependent diabetes mellitus: do biases play a role? *Epidemiology* 1996;7:87-92.
110. Pettitt DJ, Forman MR, Hanson RL et al. Breastfeeding and incidence of non-insulin-dependent diabetes mellitus in Pima Indians. *Lancet* 1997;350:166-168.
111. Acheson ED, Truelove SC. Early weaning in the aetiology of ulcerative colitis: a study of feeding in infancy in cases and controls. *BMJ* 1961;2:929-933.
112. Whorwell PJ, Holdstock G, Whorwell GM et al. Bottle feeding, early gastroenteritis, and inflammatory bowel disease. *BMJ* 1979;1:382.
113. Shu XO, Linet MS, Steinbuch M et al. Breast-feeding and risk of childhood acute leukemia. *J Natl Cancer Inst* 1999;91:1765-1772.
114. Smulevich VB, Solionova LG, Belyakova SV. Parental occupation and other factors and cancer risk in children: I. Study methodology and non-occupational factors. *Int J Cancer* 1999;83:712-717.
115. Ascher H, Krantz I, Rydberg L et al. Influence of infant feeding and gluten intake on coeliac disease. *Arch Dis Child* 1997;76:113-117.
116. Gilat T, Hacohen D, Lilos P et al. Childhood factors in ulcerative colitis and Crohn's disease. An international cooperative study. *Scand J Gastroenterol* 1987;22:1009-1024.
117. Gruber M, Marshall JR, Zielezny M et al. A case-control study to examine the influence of maternal perinatal behaviors on the incidence of Crohn's disease. *Gastroenterol Nurs* 1996;19:53-59.
118. Kramer MS. Does breast feeding help protect against atopic disease? Biology, methodology, and a golden jubilee of controversy. *J Pediatr* 1988;112:181-190.
119. Oddy WH, Holt PG, Sly PD et al. Association between breast feeding and asthma in 6 year old children: findings of a prospective birth cohort study. *BMJ* 1999;319:815-819.
120. Bjorksten B, Kjellman NI. Perinatal environmental factors influencing the development of allergy. *Clin Exp Allergy* 1990;20(Suppl 3):3-8.
121. Burr ML, Limb ES, Maguire MJ et al. Infant feeding, wheezing, and allergy: a prospective study. *Arch Dis Child* 1993;68:724-728.

122. Anderson JW, Johnstone BM, Remley DT. Breast-feeding and cognitive development: a meta-analysis. *Am J Clin Nutr* 1999;70:525-535.

123. Jacobson SW, Chiodo LM, Jacobson JL. Breastfeeding effects on intelligence quotient in 4- and 11-year-old children. *Pediatrics* 1999;103:e71.

124. Jensen CL, Prager TC, Zou Y et al. Effects of maternal docosahexaenoic acid supplementation on visual function and growth of breast-fed term infants. *Lipids* 1999;34(Suppl):S225.

125. Jensen RG. Lipids in human milk. *Lipids* 1999;34: 1243-1271.

126. Jorgensen MH, Hernell O, Lund P et al. Visual acuity and erythrocyte docosahexaenoic acid status in breast-fed and formula-fed term infants during the first four months of life. *Lipids* 1996;31:99-105.

127. Richards M, Wadsworth M, Rahimi-Foroushani A et al. Infant nutrition and cognitive development in the first offspring of a national UK birth cohort. *Dev Med Child Neurol* 1998;40:163-167.

128. Hamosh M, Salem N Jr. Long-chain polyunsaturated fatty acids. *Biol Neonate* 1998;74:106-120.

129. Heinig MJ. Health effects of breast feeding for mothers: a critical review. *Nutrition Research Reviews* 1997;10:35-56.

130. McNeilly AS. Lactational amenorrhea. *Endocrinol Metab Clin North Am* 1993;22:59-73.

131. Kuzela AL, Stifter CA, Worobey J. Breastfeeding and mother-infant interactions. *J Reprod Infant Psychol* 1990;8:185-194.

132. Widstrom AM, Wahlberg V, Matthiesen AS et al. Short-term effects of early suckling and touch of the nipple on maternal behavior. *Early Hum Dev* 1990;21:153-163.

133. Virden SF. The relationship between infant feeding method and maternal role adjustment. *J Nurse Midwifery* 1988;33:31-35.

134. Whittemore AS, Harris R, Itnyre J. Characteristics relating to ovarian cancer risk: collaborative analysis of 12 US case-control studies. II. Invasive epithelial ovarian cancers in white women. Collaborative Ovarian Cancer Group. *Am J Epidemiol* 1992;136:1184-1203.

135. Riordan JM. The cost of not breastfeeding: a commentary. *J Hum Lact* 1997;13:93-97.

136. Montgomery DL, Splett PL. Economic benefit of breast-feeding infants enrolled in WIC. *J Am Diet Assoc* 1997;97:379-385.

137. Hoey C, Ware JL. Economic advantages of breast-feeding in an HMO: setting a pilot study. *Am J Manag Care* 1997;3:861-865.

138. US Department of Commerce. *Poverty 1998.* Washington, DC: US Department of Commerce, Census Bureau; 1999.

139. Cohen R, Mrtek MB, Mrtek RG. Comparison of maternal absenteeism and infant illness rates among breast-feeding and formula-feeding women in two corporations. *Am J Health Promot* 1995;10:148-153.

140. Wright AL, Holberg CJ, Martinez FD et al. Breast feeding and lower respiratory tract illness in the first year of life. Group Health Medical Associates. *BMJ* 1989;299:946-949.

141. Aniansson G, Alm B, Andersson B et al. A prospective cohort study on breast-feeding and otitis media in Swedish infants. *Pediatr Infect Dis J* 1994;13:183-188.

142. Gessner BD, Ussery XT, Parkinson AJ et al. Risk factors for invasive disease caused by *Streptococcus pneumoniae* among Alaska native children younger than two years of age. *Pediatr Infect Dis J* 1995;14:123-128.

143. Pisacane A, Graziano L, Mazzarella G et al. Breast-feeding and urinary tract infection. *J Pediatr* 1992;120:87-89.

144. Marild S, Jodal U, Hanson LA. Breastfeeding and urinary-tract infection [letter; comment]. *Lancet* 1990;336:942.

145. Lucas A, Cole TJ. Breast milk and neonatal necrotising enterocolitis. *Lancet* 1990;336:1519-1523.

146. Kurscheid T, Holschneider AM. Necrotizing enterocolitis (NEC)—mortality and long-term results. *Eur J Pediatr Surg* 1993;3:139-143.

147. Cochi SL, Fleming DW, Hightower AW et al. Primary invasive *Haemophilus influenzae* type b disease: a population-based assessment of risk factors. *J Pediatr* 1986;108:887-896.

148. US Department of Health and Human Services. *Healthy people 2010: national health promotion and disease prevention objectives.* Washington, DC: US Department of Health and Human Services; 2000. Available at http://www.health.gov/healthypeople/Document/

149. Mortensen EL et al. The association between duration of breastfeeding and adult intelligence. *JAMA* 2002;287:2365-2371.

CHAPTER

2

Social and Cultural Trends Influencing Breastfeeding

HISTORICAL AND SOCIAL TRENDS

Infants and children have been breastfed since the dawn of humankind. Drawings show that primitive peoples breastfed their infants,[1] and ancient written accounts, most notably those in the Bible, clearly describe the suckling of one's own and other's children. Breastfeeding one's own child, particularly the firstborn, was not only accepted but also required: A Spartan woman, even if she were the wife of a king, was required to breastfeed her eldest son, while plebeians were required to breastfeed all of their offspring.[2] Although feeding devices were used in the Greek culture and burial rites of infants, wet-nursing—suckling another woman's infant (often as a work-for-hire)—was the more common alternative to suckling one's own infant. Hammurabi's code, from about 1800 BC, contained regulations on the practice of wet-nursing, and the Bible gives a clear account that Pharaoh's daughter, who found Moses, immediately sought a wet nurse to suckle him.

Wet-nursing continued to figure prominently in the history of breastfeeding, but it began to fall into disfavor in the seventeenth century, when the Dowager Countess of Lincoln wrote about the duty to breastfeed one's own children.[3] Although she had borne 18 children, all had been suckled by a wet nurse and only one survived. When her son's wife suckled her own child, the Countess then regretted that her children had been fed by wet nurses. Writing in 1662 about the "duty of nursing, due by mothers to their children," she emphasized that the Bible describes Eve as having breastfed her children. She went on to use the biblical quote from Job 29:16, "to withhold a full breast is to be more savage than dragons and more cruel than ostriches to their little ones." Nonetheless, wet-nursing continued as the primary alternative for women who did not suckle their own infants.

During the eighteenth century, wet-nursing continued but was more highly scrutinized. Quoting Cogan's 1748 "Essay upon the Nursing and Management of Children," Wickes[4] points out, "there is great reason to fear these Nurses, who . . . often do much harm where they intended to do good, by fancying Nature has left a great deal to their Skill and Contrivance." Wickes observes that the same might be said of physicians and the makers of artificial milk later on.

In that same century, the uniqueness of human milk began to be recognized. English physician Hugh Smith was important because he described the constituent properties of human milk, noting that it lacked a tough curd and cream as found in other mammalian milk. William Moss, a Liverpool surgeon, wrote "Essay on the Management Nursing and Disease of Children," published in 1794, in which he regards human milk as a perfect.

By the mid-nineteenth century, physicians began to formulate a substitute for human milk as a replacement for wet nurses,[3] and later, chemists began to do the same. In Switzerland, Henri Nestlé began to develop a bovine-milk formula that was advertised to be "scientifically correct so as to leave nothing to be desired."[5]

During the late nineteenth century, breastfeeding rates began to decline in the United States as other options became readily available. Nestlé had manufactured and distributed its Milk Food for Infants in the 1870s throughout the United States and Europe and in other areas. Shortly after the turn of the century, American medical researchers were also involved in creating artificial milk for infants.[6] Thereafter, infants could be either breast-fed or bottle-fed in American society. However, artificial milk could not be prepared at home because "formula preparation was so complex that it was commonly performed in commercial laboratories dedicated to this purpose"[7] (p. 410-s). Eventually, because of this complex preparation, pediatrics emerged as a specialty in the late nineteenth century, based primarily on its expertise in infant feeding.[6]

Around this same time, the infant mortality rate gained national attention as both a health and a political issue, and massive public health efforts were undertaken in the United States to reduce it.[8] Although public health officials and statisticians found it difficult to identify all of the reasons for the high infant mortality rate, "everyone agreed that breastfeeding was important, because artificially-fed infants died at a much higher rate from gastrointestinal diseases than did breastfed infants"[8] (p. 480).

At the turn of the twentieth century, breastfeeding was almost universal.[9] Not only was breast-feeding initiated, but it also continued throughout most of the first year of life, even though some infants received some artificial milk as well.[7] Between 1911 and 1915, approximately 70% of women initiated breastfeeding, but between 1926 and 1930, approximately 50% of women initiated breastfeeding.[10] These declines may be explained by some of the social, cultural, and technological changes that began and continued to occur in American society.[9]

Statistics[10] on feeding methods used from 1930 to 1950 are incomplete, but there is "no question that the [breastfeeding] trend was downward"[7] (p. 411-s). More and more women began giving birth in hospitals with central nurseries, and the ease of sterilization processes made bottle-feeding possible there and at home. Furthermore, physicians and commercial companies throughout the world were making more and more precise "formulas" for infants. Formula, meaning artificial milk or human milk substitute, soon became widely avail-

able. Even the word *formula* connoted a scientific method, and these milk substitutes gained favor as the scientific way of feeding. Eventually, the mother was able to make the "formula" at home because the directions for mixing were simply printed on the container. Physicians, worried their influence on infant feeding would be usurped by "commercial men," began to have talks with artificial milk companies about advertising. Between 1929 and 1932 the American Medical Association exerted pressure on the formula industry to advertise only to physicians.[12] This understanding between the professional and corporate worlds continued for nearly 50 years.

In the 1940s the dairy industry exploded, resulting in an abundance of leftover whey. Rather than let it go to waste, the industry used the whey to create a huge industry for artificial milk. Increasing numbers of women delivered in hospitals, a change which brought with it the use of anesthesia and the fact that mothers were therefore separated from their newborns until they recovered. Similarly, separate nurseries added to the separation of mothers and newborns. At least one attempt was made to reverse this trend: The Yale New Haven Rooming-In Project was initiated. This project was enthusiastically received by mothers and subsequently improved breastfeeding efforts.[13] Few hospitals adopted this model, however, and central nurseries and bottle-feeding predominated. The downward trend continued into the 1950s.

Statistics for breastfeeding rates before the early 1950s are sketchy, but with home-prepared formulas so readily accepted by the public, the makers of these artificial milks soon recognized the need to gain information for marketing purposes. Breastfeeding rates began to be monitored and recorded in the 1950s by Abbott Laboratories, the parent company of Ross Laboratories and makers of artificial milk. The survey was begun in 1951 and continues each year, as shown in Fig. 2-1. (Very recent data are yet unpublished.)

In 1955 the Ross Laboratories Mother Survey (RLMS) showed that only 29.2% of infants were breastfed at 1 week. Clearly, women who breastfed were in the minority. That same year, a group of breastfeeding mothers attending a church picnic

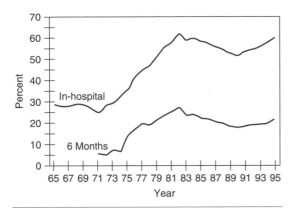

FIGURE 2-1 U.S. breastfeeding rates: 1965 through 1995. *(From Ryan AS.* Pediatrics *1997;99:2.)*

recognized the need to support one another. They also recognized that with few breastfeeding role models and sources of support, a mother-to-mother support network was needed throughout the country. These women began the organization La Leche League (*leche* is Spanish for "milk"). The support group soon grew, and La Leche League International now has local chapters throughout the world. (To find a local chapter, see Appendix A.)

Artificial feeding, which predominated throughout the 1950s, 1960s, and 1970s, was often viewed as superior, or at least equal, to breastfeeding. One physician, a breastfeeding advocate, noted that the decline in breastfeeding was caused by perception: "Formula feeding has become so simple, safe and uniformly successful that breastfeeding no longer seems worth the bother."[14] As a result of effective marketing strategies, artificial milk and bottles became a status symbol for those who could afford them. Americans hailed the scientific advances of artificial milk, considering it equal to or better than human milk. With virtually no studies on human milk and an emphasis on "science-based" artificial milk, breastfeeding management was soon based more on myth than on science; hence, inaccurate information from health care providers and changing social norms later led to a decline in breastfeeding.

Breastfeeding rates reached a low level in 1971. That year, breastfeeding initiation was at 24.7%,

breastfeeding at 1 week was 22.8%, and breastfeeding at 6 months was 5.4%.[15,16] Thereafter, breastfeeding rates began to climb, and by 1982, rates had more than doubled: 61.9% initiated breastfeeding, while 60.5% were breastfeeding at 1 week, and 27.1% were breastfeeding at 6 months.[17,18] Exactly what explains this dramatic rise in breastfeeding, which has not occurred before or since, is difficult to determine. Changes in birth practices and the advent of prenatal classes were likely most influential.[19]

In the late 1970s, attitudes and practices related to childbearing began to undergo dramatic changes. The movement toward home birth and birthing centers in the San Francisco Bay area fueled the fires to promote natural methods as desirable and superior to the overmedicalized styles of perinatal management. Psychoprophylaxis, rather than medication, became popular for pain management during labor. To learn psychoprophylaxis, such as the Lamaze or Bradley method, pregnant women attended antenatal childbirth classes, and breastfeeding was often included in the curriculum as part of the "natural" childbirth experience. Furthermore, providers of perinatal health care began to change. Certified nurse-midwives were more frequently involved in perinatal care, nurse practitioners were beginning to perform well-baby assessments, and the number of female obstetricians and pediatricians was increasing. These changes in the general philosophy and the gender of health care providers bolstered efforts to focus on the woman's capabilities and needs rather than the medical management of natural processes.

During the 1980s, breastfeeding gained more attention as a public health issue, as described in Chapter 1. During the decade, multiple statements and position papers were put forth. From 1982 to 1991, breastfeeding rates once again sank.[20] In-hospital initiation rates in 1991 were at 51.3%, and breastfeeding at 6 months was 18.2%. Thereafter, breastfeeding rates once again began to climb, although this time much more slowly than from the late 1970s to early 1980s.

In 1995 the breastfeeding initiation rate was 59.7%, and it was 21.6% at 6 months.[21] Although the increase in incidence and continuation from 1991 to 1995 was unremarkable, breastfeeding initiation rates increased more than 14%, and continuation until 6 months rose sharply from 18.1% to 21.6% from 1989 to 1995.[21] Presumably, some of the improvements in breastfeeding rates are attributable to the promotional activities that have occurred during the last decade. However, notable in this last published data set is the increase in incidence among the Women, Infants, and Children (WIC) population. From 1989 to 1995, a 36% *increase* in breastfeeding initiation rates and a 51% *increase* in continuation at 6 months occurred among the WIC participants.[21]

When one looks at nearly a half-century of data from the RLMS, a few trends are especially noteworthy. First, the incidence of in-hospital breastfeeding is not appreciably different than at 1 week. Second, the number of women who discontinue breastfeeding at age 2 months is substantial and has been corroborated by noncommercial statistics.[22] Third, and perhaps most important, is a trend that has yet not been noted in published literature: The "retention" rate for longer-term breastfeeding has not changed significantly over the decades. That is, of the mothers who initiate breastfeeding, the percentage who continue to breastfeed until the infant is 6 months old has not changed appreciably over nearly 50 years. This trend suggests that although initiation rates have varied significantly with societal changes, those changes have had little, if any, effect on the percentage of breastfeeding mothers who are retained in the breastfeeding group. From this trend, it is tempting to conclude that personal, rather than societal, factors are most influential in the mother's ability to continue breastfeeding.

The RLMS continues to be a reliable source for breastfeeding data here in the United States. The survey has been conducted annually for nearly 50 years; collection methods are clear and consistent, and surveys are mailed to 10,000 subjects from all 50 states. (The National Survey for Family Growth collects breastfeeding data also, but not on an annual basis; trends are similar.[23]) However, looking only at the aggregate described in this chapter has limited usefulness for clinical application in one particular hospital or clinic. The survey

reports differences in several subgroups. For example, mothers who are well educated, affluent, and older are more likely to initiate breastfeeding[21] and breastfeed exclusively.[24] Conversely, mothers who are less educated, economically disadvantaged, younger, and members of minority ethnic groups are less likely to breastfeed. Women on the West Coast, particularly California, are most likely to breastfeed, whereas women in the deep South are least likely. Understanding the demographics of who does or does not breastfeed is useful. For the most part, however, the health care system cannot change the demographics. Rather, a focus on the cultural assessment of individuals and their families is more likely to improve the incidence and duration of breastfeeding.

CULTURAL ASSESSMENT OF INDIVIDUALS AND FAMILIES

Perhaps no two topics are more rooted in culture than food and sex. In the United States, breasts are thought of primarily as sexual objects, rather than objects designed to nourish society's young. Admittedly, everyone agrees that breastfeeding provides food. However, the lactating woman is involved in something much more than simply producing food; breastfeeding has a significant emotional impact for mother and child. Feeding is the first and perhaps most enduring function of the mothering role.

Breastfeeding occurs within a cultural context. The woman lives within the context of her family's values, beliefs, norms, and practices that are likely to be similar or identical to her own. She also receives health care from nurses and others who have their own set of values, beliefs, norms, and practices, which may differ dramatically from her own or that of her family. Caregivers need to first grasp a definition of culture and recognize their own cultural biases. They then need to develop a systematized way to assess the cultural framework within which the woman breastfeeds.

Giger and Davidhizar[25] define *culture* as "a patterned behavioral response that develops over time as a result of imprinting the mind through social and religious structures and intellectual and artistic manifestations. Culture is also the result of acquired mechanisms that may have innate influences but are primarily affected by internal and external environmental stimuli. Culture is shaped by values, beliefs, norms and practices that are shared by members of the same cultural group. Culture guides our thinking, doing and being and becomes patterned expressions of who we are. These patterned expressions are passed down from one generation to the next. Culture provides implicit and explicit codes of behavior."

In the United States, members of the dominant culture tend to be white, educated, and of the middle socioeconomic class; this is clearly the group in which breastfeeding has been most popular in recent decades. By contrast, ethnic groups are distinct from the dominant culture. More than 100 ethnic groups are found in the United States, and breastfeeding typically is less popular among these groups than among the dominant culture. It is not possible here to address the needs of cultural groups throughout the world, nor is it possible to describe every nuance of various cultures. To examine the concept of culture as it relates to mothers who are breastfeeding in America, it is helpful to recognize the overlap of culture, ethnicity, and religion and to use Giger and Davidhizar's model[25] for cultural assessment of the client. The components of their model include (1) a culturally unique individual, (2) communication, (3) space, (4) social organization, (5) time, (6) environmental control, and (7) biologic variations. These components identify several important concepts to be addressed for the breastfeeding mother.

Culturally Unique Individual

Certain cultural norms drive practices related to feeding in general and to breastfeeding in particular. From a clinical standpoint, it is useful to identify norms but not to rely on stereotypes. Knowing that a certain ethnic group embraces a particular norm is helpful when anticipating someone's possible needs and preferences. This knowledge, however, must be tempered with the recognition that not all members of the ethnic group embrace that norm or practice.

Those who have been acculturated into the American way of life may not exhibit the norm from the "old country" at all. In one study, initiation of breastfeeding was highest among women least acculturated (52.9%) and lowest in those most acculturated (36.1%).[26] In another study, acculturation was seen as a complex process in which clear trends are not easily categorized.[27] Thus norm recognition is important but should not replace respect for individual variation and choice. Some cultural beliefs, values, and practices related to childbirth and breastfeeding are described in Table 2-1. New immigrants may perceive bottle-feeding as the cultural norm and may be eager to assimilate practices of their new culture in the United States. Immigrants may perceive that formula is superior to human milk because they see it used so frequently. Similarly, they may equate the cost of the product with its superiority. (If it costs a lot of money, it must be desirable.) Furthermore, they may draw conclusions about American products that have no basis in reality. A colleague described one Asian woman who said she wanted to use artificial milk "so the baby will grow tall like Americans."

Communication

Communication includes verbal exchange, nonverbal communication, and the use of silence. Certainly, initiation and continuation of breastfeeding can be affected if language barriers exist, as shown recently with Vietnamese-speaking mothers.[28] In a much broader sense, however, it is an outward manifestation of inner values and beliefs. For example, in some cultures it is inappropriate to outwardly disagree with a nurse or other health care professional, so the client may respond affirmatively or be silent, implying agreement. Words that have one meaning for one culture may have a different meaning for another. For example, African-Americans may describe the newborn's eating behavior as "greedy"; because the word *greedy* may have a negative connotation for the white nurse, she may misinterpret the mother's meaning. Actually, the mother's description of the baby's "greedy" behavior at the breast should be understood as "eager" or "vigorous."

Table 2-1 CULTURAL BEHAVIORS RELATED TO ASSESSMENT OF CHILDBIRTH AND BREASTFEEDING

Nations of Origin	Important Cultural Considerations	Clinical Strategy
Native American (170 Native American tribes, Aleuts, Eskimos)	Extremely family-oriented and likely to value traditional healing methods	Capitalize on the family as a support for breastfeeding
Asian (China, Hawaii, Philippines, Korea, Japan), Southeast Asia (Laos, Cambodia, Vietnam)	Earlier generations more likely to breastfeed, but second-generation Asian-Americans may not; may delay breastfeeding or do "breast and bottle"; belief in yin and yang	Determine whether delay in breastfeeding is practiced because it is part of a strong belief system or if the woman would be receptive to knowing of early the benefits breastfeeding
African	African-American women in today's America are products of mothers who gave birth at a time when bottle-feeding was viewed or as a status symbol; often, friends grandmothers provided primary support; breastfeeding is popular among African-Americans in the southern United States, but not in the northern states	Involve close friend or family member in discussions about breastfeeding; be aware of media that frequently do not depict African-American women who breastfeed
Hispanic (Spain, Cuba, Mexico, Central and South America)	Primary belief that breastfeeding is good; woman's mother or mother-in-law is often the primary support person if modern-day mother must return to work; belief in the hot and cold theory	Involve mother or mother-in-law or female relatives in discussions about breastfeeding; show respect for belief in hot and cold theory and facilitate woman's consumption of appropriate foods during pregnancy and lactation

Eye contact is part of communication in general, and some specific norms about eye contact pertain to infant care. For example, in some cultures it is inappropriate for a nurse or other health care professional to make eye contact with an infant without touching him. Some Hispanics, for instance, believe that such a practice results in a curse known as *mal de ojo*. Those who hold this belief also think that the curse can be cured by having the person touch the infant.

Another aspect of communication is touch and, along with it, modesty. In American culture, for example, it is considered immodest to breastfeed in public, even though little or no breast tissue may be visible. In other cultures, women may wear long sleeves to cover their arms and veils to cover their faces, yet at the same time partially expose their breasts while suckling an infant.

Space

The amount of personal space considered appropriate varies among cultures. The most general example pertains to the distance maintained during a conversation. For the breastfeeding mother, some specific examples come into play. For example, the mother whose infant is in the neonatal intensive care unit may have difficulty breastfeeding her infant if she knows that other people are just on the other side of a flimsy curtain. This may be more than a matter of modesty; the sights and sounds of the environment may inhibit her as well.

Social Organization and Orientation

A basic structure of social organization is the family, and the social support of family becomes especially important during the childbearing period.

RESEARCH HIGHLIGHT

Formula-Fed Black Infants Are Five Times More Likely to Die Than if Breastfed

Citation: Forste R et al. The decision to breastfeed in the United States: does race matter? *Pediatrics* 2001;108:291-296.

Forste and colleagues aimed "to estimate the effects of maternal and birth characteristics on the decision to breastfeed, and to relate breastfeeding practices to racial differences in infant mortality." The National Survey of Family Growth (NSFG) Cycle V, 1995, was used to obtain data on 1088 subjects for this study.

A descriptive data analysis showed that percentages of mothers who breastfed were lower for black (30%) than for white (65%) mothers. All maternal sociodemographic characteristics were correlated to the decision to breastfeed, as were birth characteristics.

Later, in the multivariate analysis when investigators controlled for background variables known to be associated with black mothers, they found that regardless of education, income, and other maternal sociodemographic factors, black mothers were 2.5 times less likely to breastfeed than white mothers. The most common reason for their decision was the preferred to bottle-feed." After controlling for feeding method, investigators found that breastfeeding "accounts for as much of the race difference in infant mortality rates as does low birth weight." The take-home message is simple: Black infants do not die more frequently because they are black; they die more frequently because they are less likely to be breastfed and more likely to be low birth weight.

A weakness of the study, namely that all infants who were ever breastfed were counted as "breastfed," actually made the results more impressive. Presumably, results would have been more dramatic if breastfeeding had been confined to exclusive or prolonged breastfeeding.

This is the first study to show that breastfeeding explains part of the racial differences in infant mortality; low birth weight has been a known factor for some time. The compelling results show that "by increasing breastfeeding among black women the racial gap in infant mortality should narrow—a gap that is currently (1997) about 1.3 times higher for blacks than for whites.

A shift from an extended to a nuclear family gradually occurred as the United States became more urban. The effect of this trend on breastfeeding can only be inferred, but fewer women have breastfed since this change has occurred. Today, it is entirely possible that a woman has never seen a sister or a cousin or any other woman breastfeeding. Furthermore, how a woman was fed may influence her decision for how to feed her own child[29-34] and whether she is successful.[35]

Apologizing for a personal anecdote, I feel compelled to mention my own mother, who is a good example of how the extended family influences breastfeeding success and how she, in turn, has influenced my values, beliefs, and practices related to breastfeeding. My mother was born in Italy in 1918. She came to the United States around 1928. Unlike most women living in the United States in the 1940s and 1950s, she breastfed her children because bottle-feeding "didn't make sense" to her.

She grew up in an extended family, seeing her older sister and other family members and friends suckle their children. She is frequently taken aback at the notion of "teaching" women to breastfeed; to her breastfeeding seems like something "all women just know how to do." She appears to have been completely unencumbered by the rules and dicta given to American mothers, and it simply never occurred to her that she might not succeed. She considers a baby at the breast, a pot of sauce simmering on the stove, a loaf of bread in the oven, and a kiss on the cheek essential gifts a mother provides for her family.

One's family or friends can provide social support. Baranowski's study[36] differentiates between social support and social influence. Quoting Caplan and colleagues, he asserts, "Social support is defined as any input directly provided by another person (or group) which moves the receiving person towards goals which the receiver desires."[36]

He implies that social support is primarily a process, whereas social influence is the result—to choose or not choose breastfeeding. Although *social influence* may result in the decision to breast-feed, *social support* of family and friends is as likely to sustain the breastfeeding mother's efforts later.[37] It is helpful to identify the primary support person for the breastfeeding mother. This person tends to differ from culture to culture. African-American mothers generally identify a close friend as the primary support person for breastfeeding, whereas Mexican-Americans are more likely to turn to their mothers for breastfeeding support. Anglo-Americans are most likely to seek support from their male partners.[36]

Time

Time is influential in every culture, and the importance of the clock in American culture is discussed in the section on values. However, two central ideas that vary tremendously among cultures are the time of initiation of breastfeeding and the time of weaning.

Time of Initiation

In some cultures breastfeeding is not initiated until the milk "comes in." For example, Mexican-American women, who may believe that colostrum is dirty or bad, do not begin breastfeeding at the time of birth. If this cultural norm is not understood, there can be miscommunication between the newly delivered mother and the nurse. One should not presume that the woman has chosen to bottle-feed if she folds her arms over her chest and announces, *"No leche."* She is not saying, "I don't want to breastfeed." She is giving a message that she is not going to breastfeed at this point, but she may and usually does go home and begin to breast-feed after her milk comes in. Similarly, Asian women often delay the initiation of breastfeeding.

Time of Weaning

In other parts of the world, children typically are weaned when they are 3 to 4 years old, but in the United States, infants typically are weaned before 6 months of age. Hervada and Newman[38] provide an extensive review of weaning practices. Weaning is

one of the most culturally charged issues related to breastfeeding in America today. Nearly half of mothers reported "no negative aspect" is associated with breastfeeding at 6 months, but only about one fourth say there is no negative aspect to breastfeeding a 1-year-old. Approximately 25% cite "social stigma" (i.e., negative attitudes of others) as a negative aspect of breastfeeding at 6 months, and approximately 40% cite it as a negative aspect of breastfeeding past 1 year.[39]

Environmental Control

Environmental control includes beliefs and values about health and illness and how to overcome adverse situations related to the health or illness that one is experiencing.

Beliefs

Perhaps the most basic belief is about life and health. Those who believe they can influence their own health by good health care practices—such as breastfeeding—are likely to embrace such practices. Some cultures have specific beliefs about human milk and breastfeeding. For example, many of the dominant culture groups in America still believe that artificial milk is truly equivalent to human milk. Often in ethnic groups, the younger members of the cultures—those of childbearing age—are not as likely to be as entrenched in a belief as their elders. If a cultural belief that breastfeeding is intrinsically good is strong, however, the woman is likely to initiate and continue breastfeeding. However, more specific beliefs influence the choices a woman makes about breastfeeding.

Beliefs about Colostrum and Mature Milk. Some ethnic groups believe that colostrum is "bad" but that mature milk is "good." Some, including the dominant culture here in the United States, may also mistakenly believe that the ability to lactate is related to the appearance of the breasts; these myths and others are explored in Chapter 5. Other beliefs may never be voiced but may underlie a parent's feeding decision. For example, the bottle-feeding mind-set may lead the parent to believe that when the bottle is empty, the feeding is over. The uninformed may believe the same is true for breastfeeding, which it is not. In addition, it is important to realize that infants (or older children) often come to the breast for comfort as much as nutrition, and breastfeeding mothers experience a pleasure that is not attainable through bottle-feeding.

Beliefs about the Effect of Maternal Food Consumption. It is difficult to separate the idea of food preferences from the beliefs one holds about certain foods' effect on health in general or on lactation specifically. Some cultures have specific beliefs about foods that are helpful or harmful to the mother's milk. The most notable example is the hot and cold theory that influences dietary choices during the childbearing cycle, as discussed in the following sections. Other examples are common in the dominant American culture. Health care professionals and women themselves have developed long lists of foods that are presumably bothersome to infants, but few foods have as much effect on the milk as they are presumed to have (see Chapter 5). For example, in American culture chocolate is thought to be "bad" for the mother's milk, but in other cultures it is thought to enhance the milk supply.

Some ethnic groups have specific beliefs about the consumption of hot and cold foods to improve health conditions. The theory of hot and cold is based on the four bodily humors (blood, phlegm, black bile, and yellow bile), which manifest themselves in dry, wet, hot, and cold. The basic premise is that the elements must be balanced, and the food that is ingested helps balance the condition. Over the years, the wet and dry components of the theory have become insignificant, but the hot and cold components remain important in some cultures that believe that a "cold" condition requires a person to eat only "hot" foods and vice versa. The "hot" or "cold" designation has nothing to do with the actual temperature or spiciness of the food; it is an arbitrary designation. Asians and Hispanics often espouse the hot and cold theory. Hispanics refer to conditions or foods as *frío* or *fresco* (cold) and *caliente* (hot); examples are shown in Box 2-1. Similarly, Asians refer to the *yin* (cold) and *yang* (hot); examples are shown in Box 2-2.

Belief in the hot and cold theory influences dietary practices during the childbearing cycle.

Pregnancy is viewed as a "hot" condition requiring "cold" foods. Once delivered, both mother and newborn are considered to be in a cold state for about 100 days and should consume hot foods for at least 30 days.[40] Human milk is thought to be neutral because ideally the woman is in a state of balance. However, an important consideration cannot be overlooked: Some women are actually

Box 2-1   Hot and Cold Food Classifications among Puerto Ricans

Frío (Cold)	Caliente (Hot)
Milk	Alcoholic beverages
Avocado	Chili peppers
Coconut	Chocolate
Lima beans	Coffee
Sugarcane	Cornmeal
White beans	Evaporated milk
Barley water	Kidney beans
Chicken	Onions
Fruits	Peas
Honey	Tobacco
Raisins	
Salt cod	
Watercress	

Box 2-2   Hot and Cold Food Classifications among Chinese

Yin (Cold)	Yang (Hot)
Watercress	Soups
Water chestnuts	Herbs
Bamboo shoots	Broccoli
Mustard greens	Liver
Bok choy	Mushrooms
Chrysanthemum tea	Peanuts
Fruits	Peppers
Vegetables	Ginger
Seaweed	Chicken
Soybean	Meat
Sprouts	Pig's feet
Cola drinks	Broth
Rice milk	Nuts
Juices	Fried food
Milk	Coffee
Beer	Spices
	Infant formula

CLINICAL SCENARIO

Responding to Culturally Diverse Breastfeeding Women

SITUATION A

You are the nurse on the postpartum unit. Your patient, Ms. S., is a breastfeeding mother of Asian descent. She appears to have eaten little. On her lunch tray you see an apple, a ham sandwich, a crisp garden salad, and a carton of low-fat milk. The nurse on the shift ahead of you said that she tried to tell Ms. S. how important it is for lactating mothers to eat and drink, but to no avail. What would you do?

SITUATION B

You are the clinical instructor in the newborn nursery. One of your undergraduate students is caring for Mrs. C., a 39-year-old white, middle-class multipara. The student tells you that she cannot possibly teach Mrs. C. anything about breastfeeding because the woman "nursed her other baby." You caution the student that sometimes women nurse for only a couple of weeks but report that they have "nursed before," so you recommend that the student find out a little more about Mrs. C.'s past breastfeeding experience. The student comes back and reports that she is convinced that Mrs. C. nursed "for a fair chunk of time." You ask when Mrs. C. weaned her first baby, and the student responds, "I couldn't get that out of her." What do you think is going on. What would you recommend that the student do next?

ANSWERS

These scenarios describe real-life situations. There is seldom only one "right" answer to a clinical situation. The following answers are provided to give the reader guidance, with the full recognition that other answers may be appropriate.

Situation A

The fruit, vegetables, and milk are "cold" foods that are typically avoided by traditional Chinese postpartum women because the postpartum period is considered a "cold" condition. One strategy is to simply observe what has happened and talk with the woman about it. An example might be, "Ms. S., I notice you haven't eaten much on your lunch tray. I would be happy to order a different lunch for you. What kind of food would you prefer?" If she declines, encourage her to have family members bring in soup or other food from home. If she does not elaborate on her preferences, call the dietary department and ask for a meal that contains many of the "hot" foods.

Situation B

The woman was reluctant to answer because she was still breastfeeding a toddler at home. She felt that the student nurse might think this was "weird" and did not wish to reveal the real situation. There are several options for how to handle this. Students, who are always allowed to be in the learning role, have a wonderful opportunity to put the woman at ease by simply saying, "Mrs. C., you never really told me when you had weaned your last child. I'm wondering if you are still nursing her. If so, maybe you can tell me a little about how you've been able to be so successful." This is a good lead-in because it shows approval for the behavior and helps the woman share her experience.

relieved to be in the United States, far away from elders who may hold these beliefs about the bodily humors. They may not wish to abstain from certain foods, so it is important to recognize that the hot and cold theory may or may not be part of their belief system.

Another important belief is related to galactogogues, that is, food and drink thought to increase milk supply. Box 2-3 lists several common galactogogues for various ethnic groups. Somewhat surprisingly, foods that are presumed to be "bad" in some cultures may be considered galactogogues in others. One new mother reported that her mother-in-law, who lived in northern Mexico, gave her a hot drink made with chocolate, *masa* (cornmeal), cinnamon, sugar, and condensed milk to help her milk supply. This is in contrast to the frequent recommendation in American culture to avoid chocolate.

Box 2-3   Traditional Galactogogues

- Broth made from blue cornmeal (Navajo Indians)
- Brewer's yeast or beer (whites)
- Anise and sesame seed (Hispanics)
- Chocolate (Guatemalans)
- Rice, gruel, fish soup, lotus, roots (Japanese, Chinese)
- Fish soup (Vietnamese, Cambodians, Laotians)

Values

The general values within a society are reflected in specific values about health and health care, and hence about breastfeeding. Leininger41 identifies seven cultural values that influence American health care (presumably for either consumers or providers). Taking her work one step further, we can see how breastfeeding may be influenced by values.

1. Americans value optimal health as a human right and a civil right. We have often tried to convince women that "breast is best," based on the idea that breastfeeding promotes optimal health. Curiously, however, bottle-feeding mothers tend to choose bottle-feeding for reasons other than achieving optimal health.[39] Similarly, Americans have made breastfeeding a civil right, with a good deal of publicity and legislation surrounding the idea of whether women may breastfeed in public (see Appendix D).

   More Americans have recently come to value natural foods, good nutrition, and safer environments, so it logical that the decision to breastfeed should follow. For example, women who bake their own whole-grain bread and recycle their newspapers have already demonstrated that they value high-quality nutrition and saving resources. It would be wonderful if society could see how breastfeeding epitomizes "health food" and preserves the environment.

2. The value of democracy implies majority-driven decisions and equality-driven treatment. This majority-wins mentality may influence women to make feeding decisions based on what they see most women doing. (Although a slim majority *do* breastfeed, few are *seen* breastfeeding.) This equality-driven value comes across in communication by health care providers who sometimes ask, "Are you going to breastfeed or bottle-feed?" with the implication that those two "treatments" are equal.

3. American culture values individualism; that is, the individual is more highly respected and valued than the group. In the case of breastfeeding, this seems to play out as an emphasis on a woman's breasts as sexual objects. In our culture it is acceptable for the individual to expose her breasts—as long as the nipples and areolas are covered—when advertising a commercial product, sunbathing at the beach, or trying to attract male attention at a party. It is not acceptable, however, to breastfeed in public, even though the nipples and areola are indeed covered by the baby and probably less breast tissue is exposed than on the beach. When the breasts are used for individual or commercial gain, the culture approves, but using them to nourish another person is not favored in American culture these days.

   Historically and in other cultures, this sex-object value has not necessarily been relevant. For example, women in Mali are bemused or horrified that men would be aroused by women's breasts or that women would find breast-to-mouth contact pleasurable.[42] It is difficult to imagine anyone today admiring a celebrity and exclaiming, as in Luke 11:27, "Happy the womb that bore you and the breasts that nursed you!" When a contemporary researcher asked a Scottish woman how she felt about breastfeeding, the reply was "Euch, those are for your husband."[43] (*Euch* is a Scottish word that expresses disgust beyond that conveyed by the American word *yuk*.)

   Women are more likely to breastfeed in cultures where the group is valued and where groups of women publicly breastfeed. This notion of the influence of the group on the individual's breastfeeding decision is one aspect of social support. For example, La Leche League International has provided one mechanism for helping women see the value that a group attaches to breastfeeding.

4. Americans value achieving and doing. Women often say they are going to "try" breastfeeding, with the implication that they consider failure entirely possible, or even likely. Often, terminology used by professionals throughout the childbearing cycle has had negative connotations. Phrases such as *incompetent cervix, trial of labor, failed induction, failure to progress,* and *lactation failure* have reinforced this pass-fail mentality. The literature is replete with the term *lactation failure* in reference to the lactating woman when it would often be more accurate to refer to the health care professional's failure to provide adequate education and support for the woman. (In this text, the phrase *lactation failure* is reserved for those rare situations in which the woman's physiologic functions interfere with milk production, much as *renal failure* refers to physiologic dysfunctions of urine production.)

5. Our value of "cleanliness" being next to godliness may have had detrimental effects on breastfeeding. Americans have been indoctrinated into believing that artificial nipples should be sterilized, that artificial milk will spoil if it is unrefrigerated, and that anything disposable (e.g., disposable bottles or milk bags) is therefore cleaner than reusable. This value makes some erroneous advice seem plausible. For example, women have been instructed or have inferred that they should wash their nipples with sterile water, that they should discontinue breastfeeding if they are sick or have cracked nipples, and that certain foods taint human milk. Perhaps a better focus for this "cleanliness" value would be the environmental waste created by the use of artificial milk, bottles, and related paraphernalia.

6. American culture values time and time schedules, whereas some other cultures place little importance on time; in fact, some cultures have no clocks or calendars whatsoever. "Scheduled" feedings, limited-time feedings, delayed feedings—however detrimental these may be to breastfeeding—have until recently been easily accepted in this culture. A review of the literature clearly shows that pediatric textbooks used the clock as the primary frame of reference for clinical management for over 100 years.[44] However, health care providers seldom mention that breastfeeding requires no time to prepare or reheat milk or to store leftovers. Similarly, with breastfeeding there are no bottles to buy, wash, and dry, and no cans to recycle. Our culture has valued convenience foods but has often overlooked breast milk, the original "fast food."

7. Americans value technology and automation. This is perhaps the most important value that has contributed to our preferences for bottle-feeding. Artificial milk is a product of improved technology and automation. It is mass-produced and shipped to consumers. Bottles, too, are the result of technology, and it is easy to be persuaded that this technology must be intrinsically good.

Biologic Variations

It is sometimes difficult to delineate sociocultural factors from psychologic and biologic factors because they are highly interrelated. For example, native American Indian populations are at especially high risk for developing diabetes; one study showed that subjects who had been breastfed were less likely to develop non–insulin-dependent diabetes later in life.[45] Rickets are more common in Alaskan natives than among the general population.[46] Some ethnic groups, most notably those of African descent, are at risk for anemia. Infants of African descent who are exclusively breastfed are likely to have iron prescribed for them because of this deficiency. Asians, Africans, and Hispanics are often lactose intolerant. All of these infants can be breastfed, but some special considerations may need to be made in clinical management for them or their mothers.

SUMMARY

Breastfeeding was the cultural norm from antiquity until the latter nineteenth century. Multiple influences during the late nineteenth century and early twentieth century led to the decline of breastfeeding in the United States. Breastfeeding is more than just a biologic matter of fact: Individual, family, and social values and beliefs also influence practice. Culturally sensitive care, regardless of origin, is imperative. The first step is recognizing that clients' attitudes, beliefs, values, and social norms may be different from those embraced by the provider. Assessing the beliefs, values, and social norms of the breastfeeding mother and her family and responding in ways that are respectful and support the mother's choices are helpful for improving breastfeeding incidence and continuation.

REFERENCES

1. Wickes IG. A history of infant feeding. Part I. Primitive peoples, ancient works, Renaissance writers. *Arch Dis Child* 1953;28:151-158.
2. Taylor J. The duty of nursing children. *Child Fam* 1949; 8:19.
3. Wickes IG. A history of infant feeding. Part II. Seventeenth and eighteenth centuries. *Arch Dis Child* 1953;28:232-240.
4. Wickes IG. A history of infant feeding. Part III. Eighteenth and nineteenth century writers. *Arch Dis Child* 1953;28:332-340.
5. Wickes IG. A history of infant feeding. Part IV. Nineteenth century continued. *Arch Dis Child* 1953;38:416-422.
6. Apple RD. *Mothers and medicine: a social history of infant feeding.* Madison WI: University of Wisconsin Press, 1987.
7. Fomon S. Infant feeding in the 20th century: formula and beikost. *J Nutr* 2001;131:409S-420S.
8. Brosco JP. The early history of the infant mortality rate in America: A reflection upon the past and a prophecy of the future. *Pediatrics* 1999;103:478-485.
9. Wright A, Schanler R. The resurgence of breastfeeding at the end of the second millennium. *J Nutr* 2001;131:421S-425S.
10. Hirschman C, Butler M. Trends and differentials in breast feeding: an update. *Demography* 1981;18:39-54.
11. Hirschman C, Hendershot GE. Trends in breast feeding among American mothers. *Vital Health Stat* 1979;23:1-39.
12. Greer FR, Apple RD. Physicians, formula companies, and advertising. A historical perspective. *Am J Dis Child* 1991;145:282-286.
13. Jackson EB, Olmsted RW, Foord A et al. A hospital rooming-in unit for four newborn infants and their mothers: Descriptive account of background, development and procedures with a few preliminary observations. *Pediatrics* 1948;1:28-43.
14. Hill LF. A salute to La Leche League International. *J Pediatr* 1968;73:161-162.
15. Martinez GA, Nalezienski JP. 1980 update: The recent trend in breast-feeding. *Pediatrics* 1981;67:260-263.
16. Martinez GA, Nalezienski JP. The recent trend in breast-feeding. *Pediatrics* 1979;64:686-692.
17. Martinez GA, Dodd DA. 1981 milk-feeding patterns in the United States during first 12 months of life. *Pediatrics* 1983;71:166-170.
18. Martinez GA, Krieger FW. 1984 milk-feeding patterns in the United States. *Pediatrics* 1985;76:1004-1008.
19. Wright AL. The rise of breastfeeding in the United States. *Pediatr Clin North Am* 2001;48:1-12.
20. Ryan AS, Rush D, Krieger FW et al. Recent declines in breast-feeding in the United States, 1984 through 1989. *Pediatrics* 1991;88:719-727.
21. Ryan AS. The resurgence of breastfeeding in the United States. *Pediatrics* 1997;99:E12.
22. Ertem I. The timing and predictors of the early termination of breastfeeding. *Pediatrics* 2001;107:543-548.
23. Ryan AS, Pratt WF, Wysong JL et al. A comparison of breast-feeding data from the National Surveys of Family Growth and the Ross Laboratories Mothers Surveys. *Am J Public Health* 1991;81:1049-1052.
24. Ryan AS, Wysong JL, Martinez GA et al. Duration of breast-feeding patterns established in the hospital. Influencing factors. Results from a national survey. *Clin Pediatr (Phila)* 1990;29:99-107.
25. Giger JN, Davidhizar RE. *Transcultural nursing.* 3rd ed. St. Louis: Mosby; 1999.
26. Rassin DK, Markides KS, Baranowski T et al. Acculturation and the initiation of breastfeeding. *J Clin Epidemiol* 1994;47:739-746.
27. Byrd TL, Balcazar H, Hummer RA. Acculturation and breast-feeding intention and practice in Hispanic women on the US Mexico border. *Ethn Dis* 2001;11:72-79.
28. Rossiter JC, Yam BM. Breastfeeding: how could it be enhanced? The perceptions of Vietnamese women in Sydney, Australia. *J Midwifery Womens Health* 2000;45: 271-276.
29. Bentley ME, Caulfield LE, Gross SM et al. Sources of influence on intention to breastfeed among African-American women at entry to WIC. *J Hum Lact* 1999;15:27-34.
30. Gabriel A, Gabriel KR, Lawrence RA. Cultural values and biomedical knowledge: choices in infant feeding. Analysis of a survey. *Soc Sci Med* 1986;23:501-509.
31. James DC, Jackson RT, Probart CK. Factors associated with breast-feeding prevalence and duration among international students. *J Am Diet Assoc* 1994;94:194-196.
32. Libbus MK, Kolostov LS. Perceptions of breastfeeding and infant feeding choice in a group of low-income mid-Missouri women. *J Hum Lact* 1994;10:17-23.
33. Perez-Escamilla R, Himmelgreen D, Segura-Millan S et al. Prenatal and perinatal factors associated with breast-feeding initiation among inner-city Puerto Rican women. *J Am Diet Assoc* 1998;98:657-663.
34. Sayers G, Thornton L, Corcoran R et al. Influences on breast feeding initiation and duration. *Ir J Med Sci* 1995;164:281-284.
35. Sloper K, McKean L, Baum JD. Factors influencing breast feeding. *Arch Dis Child* 1975;50:165-170.
36. Baranowski T, Bee DE, Rassin DK et al. Social support, social influence, ethnicity and the breastfeeding decision. *Soc Sci Med* 1983;17:1599-1611.
37. Bryant CA. The impact of kin, friend and neighbor networks on infant feeding practices. Cuban, Puerto Rican and Anglo families in Florida. *Soc Sci Med* 1982;16: 1757-1765.

38. Hervada AR, Newman DR. Weaning: Historical perspectives, practical recommendations, and current controversies. *Curr Probl Pediatr* 1992;22:223-240.

39. Reamer SB, Sugarman M. Breast feeding beyond six months: mothers' perceptions of the positive and negative consequences. *J Trop Pediatr* 1987;33:93-97.

40. Fishman C, Evans R, Jenks E. Warm bodies, cool milk: Conflicts in postpartum food choice for Indochinese women in California. *Soc Sci Med* 1988;26:1125-1132.

41. Leininger M. The significance of cultural concepts in nursing. *J Transcultural Nurs* 1990;2:52-59.

42. Dettwyler KA: Beauty and the breast: The cultural context of breastfeeding in the United States. In Stuart-Macadam P, Dettwyler KA, editors. *Breastfeeding: Biocultural perspectives*. New York: Aldine De Gruyter; 1995.

43. Morse JM. "Euch, those are for your husband:" examination of cultural values and assumptions associated with breast-feeding. *Health Care for Women International* 1989;11:223-232.

44. Millard AV. The place of the clock in pediatric advice: rationales, cultural themes, and impediments to breastfeeding. *Soc Sci Med* 1990;31:211-221.

45. Pettitt DJ, Forman MR, Hanson RL et al. Breastfeeding and incidence of non-insulin-dependent diabetes mellitus in Pima Indians. *Lancet* 1997;350:166-168.

46. Gessner BD, deSchweinitz E, Petersen KM et al. Nutritional rickets among breast-fed black and Alaska Native children. *Alaska Med* 1997;39:72-74, 87.

Psychologic Factors

Too often, nurses and other health care providers select strategies for breastfeeding management as though breastfeeding were only a matter of milk production and synthesis for infant consumption. The breastfeeding experience, however, is reflective of the attitudes, beliefs, and values of the woman or her family and the broader parenting experience. This chapter examines the psychologic aspects of the woman's feeding decisions and her experience of breastfeeding and the context of parenting within which breastfeeding occurs.

PSYCHOLOGIC ASPECTS OF LACTATION

In her classic article, psychologist Niles Newton and her husband, physician Michael Newton,[1] identified three psychologic aspects of lactation: group-derived emotions and attitudes, individual emotions and attitudes, and psychophysiologic mediating mechanisms. The Newtons' writings and observations were based on studies available when they wrote the article in 1967 and on their vast clinical experience. Their paper addressed how the psychologic aspects of lactation influence milk *production,* but the framework continues to be useful now that studies have shown how emotions and attitudes affect the woman's feeding choice and, subsequently, the breastfeeding experience.

Group-Derived Emotions and Attitudes

Emotions and attitudes that women experience because of others are called *group-derived* emotions and attitudes. Newton[1] identified feelings related to female status; feelings related to region, education, social class, and work; and feelings of others.

Feelings Related to Female Status

Niles Newton observed that the break-up of the extended family unit as the main economic unit of society has had profound effects on the role of woman and the value of her unique biologic contributions.[1] She further postulates that the status of women as bearers of children has fallen because having large families is no longer economically advantageous; to the contrary, large families pull down the family's economic standing. Therefore "women's joy and acceptance of the female biologic role in life may be an important factor in their psychosexual behavior, which includes lactation"[1] (p. 1183). She points out that historically, women of royal or aristocratic backgrounds chose to have their infants wet-nursed and that, for the most part, royal women were objects of men's amusement rather than real contributors to the work of the society.

Were Dr. Newton here today, she likely would expound on this idea and point out the broader issue of women's feelings about themselves and their breasts. In the United States women are encouraged to limit family size through artificial contraception and have truly lost their standing as childbearers. Paraphrasing Penny Van Esterik, Dettwyler observes that breastfeeding promotion means "a change in a culture's valuation of child rearing as an activity, and a change in the valuation of the important contributions that only women can make to the social reproduction of a society"[2] (p. 204). Indeed, breasts and breastfeeding are related to women's roles in society.

In the current U.S. culture, women and women's breasts are often seen as objects for entertainment,

Historical Highlight

Breast or Bottle: Not Psychologically Equivalent

Citation: Newton N, Newton M. Psychologic aspects of lactation. *N Engl J Med* 1967; 277:1179-1188.

Few would dispute the psychologic benefit of breastfeeding over bottle-feeding. However, few have articulated these benefits as clearly as the late Niles Newton, a professor of psychiatry and behavioral sciences. Newton states, "It is a common assumption in our society today that the bottle-fed baby held in his mother's arms is receiving an experience equivalent to that of breastfeeding" (p. 993). She further clarifies that common restrictions placed on breastfeeding—limiting the number of feedings, duration of feedings, interval between feedings, and maternal contact—limit the psychologic benefits of breastfeeding and mimic the bottle-feeding experience. These practices still exist, and Newton's paper, a review of the existent literature nearly three decades ago, still holds implications for caregivers in today's society. Newton enumerates several points that differ psychologically for both mother and infant. She describes pschologic benefits for the mother in terms of the initial experience, psychophysiologic

reactions, maternal interests and behavior, sexual behavior and attitude toward men, personality and adjustment, and social variations. She describes psychologic benefits for the infant in terms of initial experience, assuagement of hunger, mother-baby interaction, oral gratification and anal sensation, activity and learning, and personality adjustment. She expounds upon each of these benefits. Perhaps the most compelling benefit she describes is the mother-baby interaction. She emphasizes how the mother interprets and meets her infant's need and that the infant's toes curl and feet move in rhythm during a satisfying breastfeeding interaction. She says, "Comfort sucking and feeding are regularly presented along with the mother as one united total experience" (p. 998), and goes on to say that "in restricted breastfeeding, nourishment and comfort sucking are split." Clearly, breast and bottle are not equivalent, and the mother who restricts breastfeeding provides food but not comfort or pleasure. Have you ever seen a newborn curl his toes or move his feet in rhythm while bottle-feeding?

---

as evidenced by the huge pornographic industry. Cleavage is used in advertisements for everything from cigarettes to motorcycles. Dettwyler points out that this fixation on women's breasts is not common in non-U.S. cultures, where breasts are thought of as nourishing organs rather than sexual playthings.[2]

Feelings Related to Region, Education, Social Class, and Work

Newton made the observation that region, education, social class, and work were components of the psychologic impact of breastfeeding. Interestingly, formal data collected since then have shown that these factors are associated with not only the incidence but also the duration of breastfeeding.[3,4] Unfortunately, no government effort has been

made to monitor these statistics, so efforts have been fragmented or left to the artificial milk companies to collect. For the most part, however, the health care provider cannot modify the woman's geographic location, educational level, social class, or employment status. Other personal characteristics, such as attitude, can be influenced tremendously, and attitudes, not demographics, are a better predictor of the woman's choice to initiate or continue breastfeeding.[5]

Effect of Feelings of Others

A woman's family often influences her attitudes, beliefs, and behaviors. For the white woman, the most influential person is her husband or male partner; for Mexican women, their mothers or mothers-in-law are most influential, and for African-American women, their sister or close friend has the most influence.[6]

Partner's Beliefs and Attitudes. Exploring the father's attitudes, either positive or negative, is useful. Fathers who show a positive attitude about breastfeeding may focus on the physiologic and psychologic advantages for the mother and infant (Box 3-1).[7,8] A recent review of the literature shows that fathers with positive attitudes influence the choice and the duration of breastfeeding.[9] Exclusive breastfeeding during the first month, as well as continuation of breastfeeding at 3 months, was greater when fathers had more knowledge of breastfeeding.[10]

Negative attitudes among fathers may be based simply on misconceptions; for example, some men may think that breastfeeding will make the woman's breasts ugly.[7] Often, these misconceptions can be cleared up fairly easily in a class or a one-to-one interaction with the mother or father. Other negative attitudes are more difficult to deal with. Some men have made candid remarks that included issues related to jealousy, competition, and "ownership" of the mother's breasts.[11] (A classic study on this topic helps put such comments in perspective.[12]) Fathers do not seem to mind if their partner breastfeeds in front of relatives, but they do not like them to feed in front of nonfamily members or in a public place.[13] It is often difficult to address these concerns, but one central responsibility emerges: Helping the father overcome his negative attitudes improves chances for the mother to initiate and continue breastfeeding.

Paternal attitudes may significantly influence the maternal feeding decision. As previously noted, among white women, the most influential person in the feeding decision is her male partner.[14,15] In one study the *only* significant factor related to maternal breastfeeding intention pertained to the father's level of education and his approval of breastfeeding.[16] Another study showed that the best predictor of formula-feeding was that the male partner reported wanting to be involved in the feeding.[17] It is likely that the partner's request to be involved in the feeding really expresses a desire to establish a relationship with the baby and overlooks alternative ways to do so. William Sears, a noted pediatrician, asserts that the role of the father is twofold: (1) to develop comforting skills to calm the infant and (2) to support the new mother, relieving her of many household tasks that drain her energy.[18] Sears gives some practical strategies to help fathers more fully function in that role and in a way that benefits the mother and infant as well. Furthermore, it appears that women who have supportive husbands continue breastfeeding longer.[19]

Box **3-1**   FACTORS AFFECTING A FATHER'S DECISION TO SUPPORT BREASTFEEDING

KNOWLEDGE[7,8]

Disease protection
Improved bonding
Natural method

POSITIVE ATTITUDES[7,8]

Better for the baby
Respect for women who breastfeed
Healthier for the baby

NEGATIVE ATTITUDES[7,8,11,67]

Less attractive
Bad for breasts
A reason that breasts are ugly
No opportunity to develop relationship with child
Feeling of inadequacy
Separation from the mate
Feelings of being left out
Fears that it will interfere with sex
Envious of special bonding with mother
Dislike for breastfeeding in public
Perception that artificial feeding is easier
Better growth with artificial feeding

Modified from Sharma M, Petosa R. *J Am Dietetic Assoc* 1997;97:1311-1313.

Attitudes and Behaviors of Mothers and Mothers-in-Law. Women who have been breastfed themselves are likely to choose breastfeeding for their own infants.[20-25] Presumably, the woman who was breastfed has a mother who is in favor of breastfeeding; she is therefore more likely to choose breastfeeding.[8] Conversely, if the woman's mother has negative attitudes or beliefs about breastfeeding, the woman is more likely to choose artificial feeding. However, primiparae seem to be more vulnerable because if their mothers express negative opinions toward breastfeeding, they are less likely to choose breastfeeding. This is not true, however, among multiparae.[26] The influence of mothers-in-law has not been well studied, but it may be that their influence is on their sons, the infants' father.

Beliefs and Attitudes of Health Care Providers. Nurses, physicians, or other health care providers come to their practices with either positive or negative attitudes, and personal breastfeeding experience or lack thereof. The attitude of the health care provider has a potential effect on the mother's decision to initiate or continue breastfeeding.

Those who have positive beliefs and attitudes or positive past personal experience tend to actively promote breastfeeding. Female pediatric house staff are more likely to agree that pediatricians should encourage breastfeeding; male pediatric house staff are more likely to see breastfeeding as "instinctive."[27] Those who have had personal experience breastfeeding or who have a spouse who has breastfed consistently promote the initiation and continuation of breastfeeding.[28-31] Physicians are more likely to encourage women to initiate breastfeeding if they believe in the immune properties of human milk and if they were confident in their own ability to counsel the breastfeeding mother.[32] Health care providers who have positive attitudes and encourage women to breastfeed may be advantageous, but this alone is not sufficient to persuade women to breastfeed; family, primarily fathers, are more influential than health care providers in the woman's ultimate decision.[33] Among women who breastfeed, however, provider support has been associated with exclusive breastfeeding.[34]

Conversely, a negative attitude or past experience or ignorance may negatively influence the mother's decision to initiate and continue breastfeeding. Some nurses perceive breastfeeding support as too time-consuming, given the restraints of early postpartum discharges.[31] Attitude, however, is only part of the picture. Often, physicians are not knowledgeable about the superiority of human milk, contraindications to breastfeeding, and other issues related to breastfeeding management, so they do not promote breastfeeding. A further discussion of knowledge and education and how they influence clinical recommendations is found in Chapter 5.

Media. Media may be one of the most powerful and least studied influences on the decision to initiate or continue breastfeeding. Media was first identified in the early 1980s as a major factor in decision making,[35,36] but few studies since have evaluated the content of popular media or analyzed its possible impact.

Not surprisingly, midwives in Australia found that an overwhelming majority of popular magazines available to women there contained information about birth and breastfeeding issues.[37] However, the content of such media was not always helpful and, in some cases, gave negative messages. In Hong Kong, bottle-feeding women were more influenced by television messages, whereas breastfeeding women were more influenced by their social network.[38] In Bangladesh, both women who breastfed and those who bottle-fed were more influenced by messages on television than those in the newspaper.[39] Furthermore, the use of television has been associated with rises in breastfeeding initiation.[40] Adolescents, who watch a substantial amount of television, are especially influenced by it. Adolescents in Alabama reported that television was a major source for information on feeding.[41] Similarly, Canadian teenagers were more influenced by advertisements for breastfeeding on television, rather than newspaper advertisements.[42]

Henderson and her colleagues conducted a qualitative study in the United Kingdom[43] and analyzed 235 references to breastfeeding in television and 38 references in newspapers. Significantly fewer references to breastfeeding appeared in the printed media compared with references to bottle-feeding. In the television shows, more references were made to bottle-feeding than to breastfeeding, but more important, the content of verbal and visual references to breastfeeding were presented differently. In the health or parenting programs in which feeding was mentioned, 142 references were to bottle-feeding, whereas only 2 references were to breastfeeding. Bottle-feeding, including preparation of formula, was shown in 170 scenes and was depicted as simple and problem free. Breastfeeding, on the other hand, was depicted as problematic: Mastitis, engorged breasts, painful nipples, weight gain, and sagging breasts were highlighted as potential problems. Furthermore, the sexuality of the breasts, embarrassment, or the idea that the lactating woman did not have control of her own body was used as a means to provide humor for the story line. For example, "a barmaid (whose breasts had been leaking) asked a startled male customer whether he could see that her bra was stuffed with toilet paper."[43]

Interestingly, in 1990 there was a clear call for an international commitment to use the popular media to promote breastfeeding.[44] To date, however, that effort is lacking, even though American women report that they would be more likely to breastfeed if they heard messages about it on television.[45] In the United States not only has the popular mass media been grossly underused but also, with the exception of Ray's 1984 study,[36] none of the published studies describing the content or effects of the popular mass media have been conducted in the United States.

Individual Emotions, Attitudes, and Behaviors

Individual emotions, attitudes, and behaviors affect not only milk production, as Newton and Newton[1] first described, but also the entire breastfeeding experience, including the mother's decision to initiate and continue breastfeeding. The mother's attitude and emotions are especially important when generating strategies to support and encourage breastfeeding. Finally, the woman's life experiences and personality, as well as her infant's emotions and behaviors can affect the breastfeeding experience.

Maternal Attitude

Attitude clearly and consistently predicts subsequent behavior,[5] including the decision to breastfeed. Those who have positive attitudes about breastfeeding are more likely to select that as the feeding method for their infants, and conversely, those with negative attitudes are more likely to choose artificial feeding.

Reasons Named: Bottle-Feeding Mothers. As first identified by Newton, and borne out by subsequent studies described later, women who choose to bottle-feed name reasons for their decision that are largely self-centered, rather than infant-centered. Furthermore, when asked why they chose the method they chose, bottle-feeding mothers do not list the benefits of artificial feeding so much as they list the barriers to breastfeeding. The most common barriers to breastfeeding are perceived pain or discomfort, the notion that breastfeeding "ties me down," or the father's preferences.

Perceived Pain or Discomfort. Women who choose artificial feeding have identified pain or discomfort as a reason why they do not want to breastfeed.[46] (Women who breastfeed also believe this.[13]) Although sore nipples should not be an expected consequence of breastfeeding, sore nipples are commonly experienced, and women who have heard this from friends or family can be easily "turned off" by these reports.

Embarrassment. Bottle-feeding mothers often name embarrassment about breastfeeding as a factor when making their feeding decision.[13,41,47-59] It is likely that fears about embarrassment are based on the presumption that the woman will need to breastfeed in public and the erroneous belief that breastfeeding requires her to expose her breasts. In addition, breastfeeding in public places is less than ideal.[60]

"Ties Me Down." Women who decide against breastfeeding often say that breastfeeding "ties me down."[46,52,58,61,62] This idea is expressed in different ways; they may speak of being "tied down" as an inconvenience or point out that with artificial feeding, someone else can assume responsibility for feeding.

Father's Needs/Preferences. Unlike women who choose breastfeeding, mothers who choose bottle-feeding often name the father's attitude or preference as a reason for their choice. They may express their decision as "the baby's father wants me to bottle-feed" or "my boyfriend doesn't want me breastfeeding" or "my husband wants to feed the baby, too." Although all fathers influence all mothers, it appears that negative paternal attitudes are more influential in the mother's feeding decision than are positive paternal attitudes.

Reasons Named: Breastfeeding Mothers. Mothers who breastfeed name reasons that collectively might be called *infant-reasons* for their choice. The first reason is usually that breastfeeding is best for the infant.[35,63] These women can often recite a litany of benefits for the infant; some can name benefits for themselves as well.

Although breastfeeding mothers may name the advantages of breastfeeding as their primary reason for doing so, the mere ability to recite these advantages does not result in the decision to breastfeed. Women who choose artificial feeding often acknowledge that breastfeeding is better for the infant.[64-66]

Mother's Behaviors and Life Experiences

The mother's life experiences are likely to weigh heavily on whether she chooses breastfeeding. Important factors include first exposures to breastfeeding, previous breastfeeding experience, the birth experience, and postpartum depression.

Early Experiences with Breastfeeding. Early experiences with breastfeeding appear to influence the feeding choice. Similarly, the first time that a woman observes another woman breastfeeding is likely to have a profound impact on her feeding decision, even if she makes that decision many years later.[68] Women who have had positive first impressions are more likely to choose breastfeeding than women who have had negative first impressions of other women breastfeeding.

Previous Attempts to Breastfeed. Mothers who have breastfed a previous child are likely to breastfeed the child they are expecting.[24,26,69] However, if they did breastfeed other children, it is important to review past experiences—positive and negative— to better prepare both parents and providers for future breastfeeding outcomes. For example, a woman whose previous experience had been to breastfeed until her child weaned himself is more likely to foster a subsequent positive breastfeeding experience, whereas the mother who gave up in defeat at 2 weeks will have some apprehensions about breastfeeding that require extensive support and follow-up. The duration of breastfeeding of a second child has been positively correlated with the duration of breastfeeding for the first child.[70]

The Birth Experience. Bentovim[71] identifies several variables that affect breastfeeding, including ones related to factors surrounding delivery. These factors include length of delivery, need for anesthesia, sleepiness of the mother and infant, joyfulness of response to the infant, prolongation of state of excitation, management of first mother-infant contact, emotional contact and regressive experiences, prematurity, separation, and malformation. Clinical experience shows that, indeed, those mothers who antepartally decided to breastfeed can sometimes change their minds if adverse circumstances happen during the intrapartum experience. Labor in a clinical environment may undermine a woman's confidence to give birth and to breastfeed,[72] and a meta-analysis suggested that women giving birth by cesarean delivery were less likely to breastfeed.[73]

Postpartum Depression. Postpartum depression occurs in at least 1 in every 10 women, and its exact cause is unknown. It is likely, however, that major depression is related to lower serum levels of prolylendopeptidase (PEP).[74] It is sometimes assumed that breastfeeding, as part of the reproductive cycle, puts a woman at risk for postpartum depression because "[v]irtually no life event rivals the neuroendocrine and psychosocial changes associated with pregnancy and childbirth."[75] However, no cause-and-effect relationship has been established between lactation and the incidence of postpartum depression and lactation. To the contrary, most women diagnosed with depression have reported that the depression began when they stopped breastfeeding; relatively few women stated that their depression was present before weaning.[76] Similarly, there is some association between early weaning and subsequent depression.

RESEARCH HIGHLIGHT

Positive Experience and Self-Confidence Predict Commitment to Breastfeeding

Citation: Hoddinott P, Pill R. Qualitative study of decisions about breastfeeding among women in east end of London. *BMJ* 2000;318:30-34.

Hoddinott and Pill conducted a qualitative study in London to determine how knowledge and previous exposure to infant feeding affects the first-time mother's decision-making process. Twenty-one pregnant women were interviewed soon after their pregnancies were confirmed; they were told that the study was about choices women make for their firstborn children. They were visited in their homes after giving birth.

Two themes emerged from the interviews: a woman's confidence in her ability to breastfeed and her commitment to a particular method. The investigators classified self-confidence and commitment into five categories: (1) committed breastfeeders, (2) probable breastfeeders, (3) possible breastfeeders, (4) probable formula feeders, and (5) committed formula-feeders.

A woman's past experience of watching or interacting with other women who breastfed was strongly associated with her antenatal commitment and self-confidence to do so herself and to actually initiate breastfeeding after giving birth. Whether past observations or interactions influenced her to breastfeed, depended on whether she perceived these experiences as positive or negative. Embarrassment was often mentioned as a deterrent to breastfeeding. All women in the study were aware of the benefits of breastfeeding, yet some chose to use formula. The investigators noted that women demonstrated "ownership" of the goodness of breastfeeding by using the personal pronoun "I," for example, "*I* feel it would be better for the baby." On the other hand, women who were not committed to breastfeeding used the second or third person pronoun, for example, "But *you* don't know how much they are getting" or "*They* say it's best for a baby."

A clear strength of this study is the detailed analysis of the interview transcripts so that the five categories could be delineated. A limitation is that the study looked only at women living in the lower east end of London; most were white and socioeconomically disadvantaged. Therefore it may not be fair to generalize these results to other populations.

Results of this study guide two areas of practice. First, education that focuses on the theoretical benefits of breastfeeding may not be nearly as important as helping women to see positive role models. Second, the clinician should be alerted to language mothers use that shows "ownership" and commitment to breastfeeding.

From Biancuzzo M. *Helping mothers choose and initiate breastfeeding.* Herndon, VA: WMC Worldwide; 2001.

Conversely, "longer continuation of breastfeeding has been associated with lower levels of anxiety and depression, as well as increased self-esteem and coping capacity and stronger social health."[77]

Nurses should be alert for signs of clinical depression when the mother stops breastfeeding. Women who exhibit signs of postpartum depression should be referred for professional help and/or to support groups. Postpartum Support International, headquartered in California, can be reached at 805-967-7636 (927 N. Kellogg Avenue, Santa Barbara, CA 93111). Depression After Delivery, a nonprofit organization headquartered in Morrisville, Pennsylvania, can be reached at 800-944-4773.

Domestic Violence and Abuse. Recently, nurses and other health care professionals have become more concerned about the effects of physical and sexual abuse on all women, and particularly on the obstetric patient. Typically, battering begins or escalates when a woman is pregnant. Existing research does not describe the effect of battering on a woman's prenatal feeding decision or her postpartum ability to produce or eject milk. One study correlated a decrease in the incidence of domestic violence among breastfeeding families.[78] Anecdotally, it has been noted that abused women might willingly suckle a female infant but not a male infant; one could assume that the sexual partner's jealousy of an infant having access to the woman's breasts might be a deterrent for deciding to breastfeed.

Mother's Personality

The concepts of commitment, confidence, and self-esteem are closely related, and all have received relatively little attention with respect to breastfeeding in the professional literature. At present, few studies address how these affect the initiation and continuation of breastfeeding.

Confidence. Many years ago, Derrick Jelliffe observed that breastfeeding is "a confidence game."[79] The woman's confidence level is a factor in both the prenatal decision making and the postpartum breastfeeding experience.

Low confidence is a major factor among women who decide not to breastfeed.[80,81] Some of this may be explained by the fact that women consider breastfeeding "difficult to learn"[59] and because health care providers have often made it seem complicated.

Lack of self-confidence and self-esteem contributes to breastfeeding problems, including a perceived lack of milk.[82] Low confidence has also been associated with early termination of breastfeeding[53,83,84]; conversely, mothers who have higher levels of self-confidence wean later.[77] Some evidence indicates that mothers who have conceived by in vitro fertilization have lower self-esteem,[85] so they may be at greater risk for discontinuation of breastfeeding. Although often maligned, early discharge does not appear to hamper the woman's confidence to feed her baby.[86] Dennis[87] has addressed the theoretic underpinnings of confidence and has developed a tool to measure maternal confidence to breastfeed and identify women who are at risk for discontinuation.[88]

Confidence is a peculiar thing; it is not something that we can give to the woman, the way we would give a treatment or an injection. However, confidence is something that we can take away or undermine. Communication that affirms the woman's ability to successfully breastfeed is likely to be helpful, whereas comments or inferences that she is doing something "wrong" are likely to be counterproductive.

Commitment. Commitment, although closely linked to stated intention, is different from intention only. Women who intend to do something have a plan in mind; women who are committed have more completely embraced the endeavor they are about to embark upon, and they are more invested. There is little research on this topic. In an effort to identify those who are not completely committed, however, it is important to listen carefully to the language that the woman uses when she discusses breastfeeding. Pregnant women who are more committed talk about breastfeeding in the first person, that is, "*I* believe . . . " rather than the second person (e.g., "you can have a baby with fewer earaches . . .) or third person (e.g., "They say that . . . "). These verbal clues, although sometimes subtle, may be the best for early identification of weak commitment to breastfeeding. Mothers who are more committed to breastfeeding are more likely to continue when problems or concerns arise.[89]

Infant's Behavior and Emotions

Often, when thinking of the psychologic impact of breastfeeding, we look at it from an adult perspective and presume that the infant is devoid of psychologic feelings and mechanisms from birth. This viewpoint is incorrect; we need to look at the effect breastfeeding has on the infant's behaviors and emotions, namely, on the psychologic experience of imprinting, pheromones, crying, and how the mother responds to his needs.

Imprinting, Nipple Confusion, Pacifiers. *Imprinting* (or *stamping* as it was called in the 1930s) suggests that the young animal finds an object of a particular shape. In mammals the mouth is the most well-developed body part— both from a motor and a sensory standpoint—and the object that is first recognized is the maternal nipple. Hence, infants who are first introduced to the artificial nipple rather than the mother's nipple may be more apt to "recognize" it early and favor it. This could give rise to the idea of a nipple preference, or nipple confusion.

Nipple confusion is a term that is neither completely understood nor accepted by the medical community. So-called nipple confusion supposedly happens when the newborn is introduced to artificial nipples (and bottles) and then "forgets" how to suckle the breast correctly or, rather, uses the piston-like tongue motion and negative pressure to attempt transfer of milk. Some self-help books imply that as little as one bottle will result in this so-called confusion, but a well-controlled prospective study showed that mothers who are highly motivated to nurse can give one bottle per day with no significant effect on the duration of breastfeeding.[90] Perhaps both are right, and the difference lies in the skill of the infant or the motivation of the mother.

Well-respected experts have suggested that the term *nipple confusion* should be limited to describing only newborns who have not learned to suckle well (not older infants). They specify that the term be used only for situations in which an infant may or may not have breastfed successfully but was offered an artificial nipple and subsequently had difficulty achieving good latch-on at the breast; the term should not be used for the infant who displays a primary inability to suckle the breast effectively without prior exposure to an artificial teat.[91] These researchers have formulated the only hypotheses to date to explain the phenomenon of nipple confusion, and they are summarized in Box 3-2. Readers are strongly encouraged to read the original source because it is the only work to date that deals with this phenomenon from a scientific standpoint, completely unadulterated by personal experience and myth.

An understanding of imprinting and nipple confusion usually evokes the question of whether to use artificial nipples or pacifiers. Before deciding to use artificial nipples or pacifiers, however, both parents and clinicians should understand that nipple confusion is but one of many factors that should be considered. Pacifiers and artificial nipples have multiple adverse effects, as discussed in Chapters 8 and 16.

Pheromones. Newton[92] defines *pheromones* as "substances that are secreted by an animal to the

---

Box 3-2 HYPOTHESES TO EXPLAIN NIPPLE CONFUSION

1. A neonate may have limited ability to adapt to various oral configurations. When a newborn infant who has been breastfed is given an artificial teat to suck, such as a pacifier, bottle nipple, or adult finger, this stimulus may intercept the physiologic action of normal breastfeeding, and the infant may readjust to a sucking pattern that compresses and controls the teat. In addition, if a higher volume and faster flow of fluid is obtained by bottle-feeding than by breastfeeding, the infant may adapt his oral configuration to control the increased fluid flow.
2. A form of "imprinting" may occur in the immediate postpartum period. If the first feeding after birth is given by bottle, the artificial nipple may be imprinted in the infant and make subsequent attempts at breastfeeding more difficult.
3. Newborn infants may be vulnerable to nipple confusion because of the relatively low volume of colostrum available with breastfeeding in the first few days of life. Before full lactogenesis, the amount of colostrum available is small, and even after the true milk comes in, infants must nurse correctly to obtain generous quantities during breastfeeding. Measurements of milk intake by breastfed newborn infants have documented intakes of about 1 oz (30 ml) in the first 24 hours after birth. Thus, if a neonate is given the opportunity to feed from a 3- or 4-oz (90- to 120-ml) bottle on the first day of life, at a time when only a minimum quantity of milk would be available during a single breastfeeding session, the infant might act fretful during attempts at breastfeeding.
4. Infants who have difficulty with their initial attempts at breastfeeding may be more prone to manifest nipple confusion. Not only is the poorly feeding infant more likely to receive supplemental bottle-feedings, but an infant who has not learned to grasp and suckle the maternal nipple correctly is likely to perceive bottle-feeding as easier and more rewarding than the breast.

From Neifert M, Lawrence R, Seacat J. *J Pediatr* 1995;126:S126-S127.

outside and that cause a specific reaction in a receiving individual of the same species." Giving the example of how female dogs in heat give off an odor that attracts male dogs and citing Russell's work,[93] Newton postulates that it is likely that the lactating mother gives off an odor that attracts the baby to the breast. Newton was perhaps ahead of her time because later research has shown this to be correct.

Numerous other studies describe how the newborn's sense of smell is an integral part of the breastfeeding experience.[93-106] It is likely that human milk is simply an attractant for the infant who has just been born. A recent study has shown that even if other maternal stimuli are absent, the odor of the mother's breast is sufficient to attract the infant.[98] A 3- to 4-day-old newborn instinctively turns toward a pad that has been worn on the breast, rather than a "clean" pad. More amazingly, this is true not only for breastfed newborns but also for bottle-feeding infants.[97]

Crying. Some mothers and health care providers believe that artificially fed infants cry less because they have longer sleep episodes. This has yet to be proven. One study showed that mode of feeding was not related to the overall duration of crying. Mode of feeding did relate to the point in time when crying duration peaked: The duration of crying peaked around 2 weeks for artificially fed infants, whereas it was around 6 weeks for breastfed infants.[107] During the first 2 weeks, newborns are more visually attentive and have more opportunities for intimate contact when breastfed rather than bottle-fed.[108] Breastfed babies actually do cry less; contact with the mother is a key element in the overall amount of crying.[109]

Infants who are separated from their mothers cry 10 times more than those who are skin-to-skin during the first 1 to 2 hours after birth.[110] Furthermore, it appears that infants cry more when they are separated from their mothers, and this cry mimics the separation distress call that animals exhibit when they are away from their mothers.[111]

Maternal Responsiveness. The mother's response is likely a critical part of the newborn's reaction, whether pleasurable or unpleasurable. Uvnas-Moberg points out there this is evidence

that "non-noxious stimuli induces a psychophysiologic response pattern involving sedation, relaxation, decreased sympathoadrenal activity, and increased vagal nerve tone and thereby an endocrine and metabolic pattern favoring the storage of nutrients and growth."[112] Furthermore, it appears that maternal oxytocin is a major factor in relaxation for the mother.[113]

Although research has not provided definitive answers for how the mother's responsiveness influences the infant's pleasurable experience, we can make inferences from related data. For example, crying behavior, mentioned earlier, seems to indicate that an infant is unhappy when he or she is separated from the mother; breastfeeding is a way to be completely in the presence of his mother. Similarly, the theory of symbolic interaction, presented in the following sections, helps explain the feeding experience from the infant's perspective. In addition, clinical observations are important here: When mammals are having a particularly good and pleasurable feeding, they exhibit behaviors showing their pleasure. Little kittens meow, little piglets wiggle their tails, and human newborns curl their toes!

Psychologic Mediating Mechanisms

Newton and Newton[1] emphasized that psychologic mediating mechanisms, those that govern milk production and ejection, can be affected by psychologic factors. These effects are described in Chapter 4. However, the reverse situation—the effects of breastfeeding on feelings of stress or well-being—also needs to be considered.

Stress and Anxiety

Some women report feeling tense and overwhelmed by breastfeeding.[114] Mothers have many stressful internal and external pressures, however, that are more related to the transition to parenthood, the multitasking that women tend to take on, or just the stress of urban living. Internal pressures might include anything from maintaining high standards to being "in charge" of a completely dependent infant. External stress might be related to paying the bills, experiencing marital or relationship discord, or sandblasting the house next door. It is important to help women cope with these stressors and to not "blame" breastfeeding because they are having difficulty coping. Women can and do have stressful situations that make breastfeeding especially challenging, however,

Good interviewing skills, as discussed in Chapter 5, and astute observation provide clues to stressful situations. Mothers often minimize stressful situations when asked, as a few anecdotes demonstrate. One legally blind mother who told me of her perceived low milk supply denied there was any stress in her life. This woman, however, boarded a city bus every day to visit her 27-week gestation infant at a hospital on the other side of town. Another mother reported that she was unable to get any milk into the collection container attached to a hospital-grade pump. Her breasts were obviously full, so it was apparent that something was interfering with her milk-ejection reflex. She was in a private room adjacent to the intensive care nursery, so privacy was not a problem, but in talking with her it soon became evident that she was anxious about the uncertainty surrounding her infant's well-being. Warm compresses and hand massage helped a little, but she was still unable to release her milk. Finally, with a locked door and her husband massaging her breasts, she had an enormous milk-ejection reflex and enough milk to feed several newborns!

Breastfeeding does seem to result in positive psychologic experiences. Most women report feelings of well-being or tranquility as a result of breastfeeding. This feeling can be explained by the higher prolactin levels that occur during lactation. Breastfeeding, an activity designed for survival of the species, is usually as pleasurable for the mother as it is for the infant.

MOTHERHOOD AND SYMBIOSIS

In recent years much attention has been given to the goodness of breastfeeding and the superiority of human milk over artificial milk. However, breastfeeding provides more than food; breastfeeding is intricately woven into the experience of motherhood, maternal role attainment, symbolic interaction of the families, and the transition to parenthood.

In her classic article, psychiatrist Dr. Therese Benedek says, "Mothering, the suckling, feeding, succoring of the young, is a complex behavior pattern; its motivation is 'innate' and regulated by hormones. The pattern of maternal behavior is rigidly set and characteristic of the species throughout the animal kingdom."[115] She maintains that growth, neurophysiologic maturation, and psychosexual development are interwoven and that cultural patterns repress the natural motives that ensure survival of the species. Furthermore, she says, "The psychodynamic tendencies which motivate maternal behavior—the wish to feed, to succor the infant—originate in the alimentary (symbiotic) relationship which the mother-individual has experienced with her own mother. . . . The term symbiosis signifies a *continual reciprocal interaction* between mother and child."[115] Indeed the breastfeeding relationship is reciprocal, with both mother and infant enjoying its psychophysiologic benefits, as described in the previous Historical Highlight box. Some women, however, do not experience this reciprocal joy.[116]

Benedek has articulated a biologic basis for the psychologic maturation of the mother as an individual and the maturation of the mother-infant relationship. This biologic basis (rooted in hormones associated with pregnancy and lactation) and the continual reciprocal interaction between mother and child are critical. Benedek wrote her article more than four decades ago, when most women were artificially feeding their infants, which makes her message even more compelling. She defines *mothering* as "the suckling, feeding, succoring of the young." Like breastfeeding experts who look to the animal kingdom for information about components of milk, imprinting, and other data about lactating mammals, Benedek looks beyond the *Homo sapiens* species to the entire animal kingdom to explain how this suckling behavior *is* mothering.

Her words "continual reciprocal interaction between mother and child" are more perfectly fulfilled in breastfeeding than in any other context. In essence, Benedek explains that hormones are the basis for taking on the mothering role and that such hormones predispose the woman to assume the caregiver role.

FAMILIES AND SYMBOLIC INTERACTION

Although Benedek would not have considered herself an interactionist, she emphasizes that suckling, the act, is intrinsically bound to mothering, the role. An understanding of role is inherent in the theory of symbolic interactionism and its relationship to the breastfeeding experience.

The theory of symbolic interaction assumes that all interactions are purposeful and meaningful and that each person's action or relationship is dependent on the other. For example, if you are learning something from the words (symbols) on this page, you consider me to be a teacher; hence I become a teacher by virtue of the fact that you are a learner. If you are not learning, I am not teaching. Symbols may include words, actions, voice inflection, and touch. Burr and colleagues, who illuminated the concept of symbolic interaction as it relates to the family, assert that "humans decide what to do and not to do primarily on the basis of the symbols they have learned in interaction with others and their beliefs about the importance of these meanings."[117] The symbols that we receive drive actions and reactions. If we were in a classroom, for example, I would interpret the scowl on your face as a symbol of confusion or the nodding of your head as a symbol of understanding; from that information I would decide what to do next. A scowl would cue me to clarify my explanation; I might even feel badly that I was unsuccessful in explaining the material. Conversely, if I saw you nodding, I would be likely to continue with my next point and would feel successful in my role as teacher. This mutual giving and receiving of symbols and subsequent actions and reactions are what the relationship is all about.

Perhaps no relationship is more dependent on symbolism than the breastfeeding relationship, for behaviors (and later, words) are especially symbolic in this intimate, reciprocal relationship. The mother who correctly interprets her infant's hunger cues offers the breast. Similarly, her behaviors hold meaning for the infant. When she readily offers the breast, the infant assigns meaning to it; he or she learns that here is warmth, comfort, and nourishment. Early on, the mother assigns meaning to the behaviors of the infant; for example, she learns to recognize cues of satiety. (Later on, when the child can talk, he or she will have a word, such as *ma* or *tah-tah,* which represents breastfeeding, and both mother and child will know what this means.) Most of us have seen mothers who show signs that they feel contented, gratified, and successful when the infant peacefully falls asleep at the end of feeding. Conversely, a mother may appear uneasy and full of self-doubt when the infant awakens and exhibits hunger cues again in 2 hours. It is important to recognize that her reaction is not related to breastfeeding per se but rather her interpretation that she has "failed" to adequately meet the infant's needs. The mother who understands how breastfeeding works is likely to interpret this behavior as a matter-of-fact message: The baby is hungry. A mother who has seen older infants or artificially fed newborns sleep for a longer duration has already assigned a different meaning to this wakefulness. She is likely to interpret this as a reflection of her inability to adequately meet the infant's needs.

Imogene King[118] discusses not only interaction but also interaction as it relates to goal attainment. Her main premise is that all interaction is meaningful and that the nurse's responsibility is to help the client achieve the client's goal. For example, in the case of the lactating mother, the nurse's role is to provide information and support to set and achieve a goal by helping the mother understand the cues and communication from her infant in relation to the breastfeeding experience.

TRANSITION TO PARENTHOOD

Alice Rossi's classic article takes Benedek's premise a bit further. She asserts that the real transition in life is not from being single to being married but from being childless to being a parent.[119] This is an important point as one interacts with a breastfeeding primipara. Much of what may sometimes be labeled as a "breastfeeding problem" is often more a reflection of the transition to parenthood. Rossi states, "The birth of a child is not followed by any gradual taking on of responsibility, as in the case of a professional work role. It is as if the woman shifted from graduate student to full professor with little intervening apprenticeship experience of slowly increasing responsibility. The new mother starts out immediately on 24-hour duty, with responsibility for a fragile and mysterious infant totally dependent on her care."[119]

Rossi acknowledges Benedek's idea that the infant's need for dependence is absolute, whereas the woman's need to mother is relative. However, Rossi goes on to say that lack of mothering can be compensated for by the extended family, but in our culture women typically are isolated from extended families at the time the infant is most dependent on mothering. This observation assumes that the newborn is completely dependent on someone to meet his needs, including feeding, diapering, and cuddling. If a woman is breastfeeding, all of these needs, except feeding, can be met by the extended family or other caregivers. In American culture a strange paradox appears: Feeding is viewed as the central caregiving activity, and everyone wants to participate. A woman who chooses artificial feeding, however, gives up her exclusive rights to this central caregiving activity.

Understanding this idea of transition to parenthood is critical when assisting the breastfeeding mother because it enables one to accurately identify nonbreastfeeding problems. As a clinical nurse specialist, I have often been asked to solve a "breastfeeding problem," only to find that the real problem was a new mother struggling with the transition to parenthood. The mother may voice her feelings couched in breastfeeding language, but the real problem is likely to relate to the transition to parenthood and attaining the maternal role.

Maternal Role Attainment

Reva Rubin, author of several classic articles, describes maternal role attainment. For decades, Rubin's works have been revered as insightful and practical by nurses who wish to gain a better understanding of the maternity experience. Her work has suffered some criticism.[120] This is unfortunate because Rubin has clearly delineated phases relative to maternity, and these phases can be observed easily in today's breastfeeding mother.

Rubin[121] used the terms *taking-in* and *taking-hold* to describe the mother during the first few days after birth. These terms have some similarity to the bonding and attachment definitions, but with a clearer description of how this significant time in the woman's life affects not only how she relates to the infant but also how she relates to others.

Rubin asserts that "taking-in" lasts for 2 to 3 days; during this period the woman is focused on food—her own hunger and her infant's intake. She often relives and retells the details of her labor. Rubin says that during this taking-in period, the mother exhibits passive and dependent behavior. (Benedek would say that this is biologically induced through hormones.) "She is a receiver at this point. She accepts what she is given, tries to do what she is told, awaits the actions of others and initiates very little herself."[121] Taking-in is a time when the mother herself needs to be "mothered." This is significant for the breastfeeding mother because she is often still in this taking-in period when she is cut off from the nurturing behaviors of the hospital nurse and is instead expected to "take hold," that is, assume full responsibility for the infant.

The taking-in phase is in contrast to the taking-hold phase, during which the mother becomes the initiator, the producer. The taking-hold phase, which is marked by rapid and frequent mood swings, lasts about 10 days. Rubin says that during this period a woman needs to get on with things, to give up passivity for an active role. During the taking-hold phase, she is especially concerned with having control of her own body. It is at this time that she is able to take hold of the tasks of mothering. Rubin's observations about the woman's behaviors parallel Benedek's assertion that the mother needs to be a caregiver. Interestingly, the time line that she suggests for the taking-in phase is roughly equivalent to the time when the mother has colostrum, and the taking-hold phase begins at approximately when transitional milk appears.

Parenthood and the Family

Communication between individuals is often referred to as *engrossment, bonding,* and *attachment.*

Engrossment refers to the relationship between the father and his newborn.[122] In the past *bonding* has been used to refer to the maternal aspect of the relationship.[123] The early literature used *attachment* to refer to the infant aspect of the relationship between mother and newborn, with the opposite of attachment being loss. Bowlby[124] and Ainsworth[125] are most commonly recognized for their early contributions to the concept of attachment, but this literature was derived in part from studies of maternally deprived infants; hence, attachment was viewed as the opposite of loss. (Interestingly, Ainsworth never mentions breastfed babies.) More recent literature has used the word *attachment* when referring to *either* the infant or the maternal aspect of the relationship. All sources seem to agree, however, that bonding is unique in that there is a sensitive period immediately after birth when this relationship is influenced. (Note that this is a sensitive period, not a critical period; a critical period implies that irreparable harm may occur if the interaction is not achieved during that time.) Attachment, on the other hand, is thought of as being more linear; it starts prenatally and continues throughout life. Attachment behaviors include establishing eye-to-eye contact (enface position); providing physical contact of holding, touching, cuddling, or stroking; talking to the infant; and initiating care for the baby. Except for talking to the baby, all of these behaviors are inherent in the breastfeeding process.

BREASTFEEDING ATTRITION

The published literature uses various words to describe quitting breastfeeding early. Few of these words or phrases have adequately captured the essence of quitting breastfeeding because of the psychologic and cultural barriers that inhibit continuation. In the very early literature, the term *lactation failure* was used to describe women who gave up breastfeeding after only a short time. That term, in addition to being negative and implying blame or inability to lactate, is inaccurate. (In this text, *lactation failure* refers to a primary physiologic inability to successfully lactate, in much the same way as the term cardiac failure or renal failure would be used.) Later, words such as *early termination* or *early cessation of breastfeeding, premature*

weaning, discontinuation of breastfeeding, and *unsuccessful breastfeeding* have all shown up in the literature.

The definition of *success* can be rather subjectively defined. "Success" in breastfeeding is often discussed as though everyone agrees on the operational definition, which they do not. For example, success is sometimes defined as a subjective "report of success,"[126] or more objectively as breastfeeding at 4 to 6 weeks.[127] Perhaps a more pragmatic definition is "breastfeeding with less than 4 ounces of formula (supplementation) at 4 to 6 weeks postpartum."[128] This definition is useful in light of the fact that lactation is fairly well established by this time and the use of artificial milk is the exception rather than the norm.

Perhaps the most accurate term is *breastfeeding attrition,* used by Janke and based on the Theory of Planned Behavior. Janke's tool to predict breastfeeding attrition[129] focuses more on the barriers to continuation of breastfeeding (e.g., the woman's belief that breastfeeding is difficult or lack of social support) and acknowledges that a successful breastfeeding experience is defined by the mother's intentions, not an arbitrary number of weeks or months. Janke's emphasis on the woman's meeting her own goals and barriers that interfere with meeting those goals helps the nurse generate strategies to overcome potential barriers.

System-level barriers include lack of social support and lack of evidence-based hospital policies (see Chapter 8). Beyond these system-level factors, however, breastfeeding attrition has been linked to individual factors, such as weak commitment,[130-134] whereas continuation of breastfeeding has been associated with high motivation.[135,136] Some of these individual-level barriers can be changed through positive interactions, as described in Chapter 5.

CONCLUSION

Attitudes, both those derived from others and individual attitudes, have a significant psychologic impact on the woman's decision to breastfeed and the breastfeeding experience. The psychologic impact of breastfeeding is not limited to the mother, or the father, but very much includes the newborn's early experience. Breastfeeding is a continual, reciprocal relationship. The mother learns to interpret cues and meet the needs of her infant, and the infant learns that the mother's breasts provide warmth and nourishment. The process of attachment is perfectly fulfilled in the act of breastfeeding. Multiple factors can positively or negatively influence the breastfeeding relationship. The nurse's interactions with the mother should support the positive influences and counteract the negative influences.

REFERENCES

1. Newton N, Newton M. Psychologic aspects of lactation. *N Engl J Med* 1967;277:1179-1188.
2. Dettwyler KA. Beauty and the breast: The cultural context of breastfeeding in the United States. In Stuart-Macadam P, Dettwyler KA, editors. *Breastfeeding: Biocultural perspectives.* New York: Aldine De Gruyter; 1995.
3. Ryan AS. The resurgence of breastfeeding in the United States. *Pediatrics* 1997;99:E12.
4. Piper S, Parks PL. Predicting the duration of lactation: evidence from a national survey. *Birth* 1996;23:7-12.
5. Losch M, Dungy CI, Russell D et al. Impact of attitudes on maternal decisions regarding infant feeding. *J Pediatr* 1995;126:507-514.
6. Baranowski T, Bee DE, Rassin DK et al. Social support, social influence, ethnicity and the breastfeeding decision. *Soc Sci Med* 1983;17:1599-1611.
7. Freed GL, Fraley JK, Schanler RJ. Attitudes of expectant fathers regarding breast-feeding. *Pediatrics* 1992;90:224-227.
8. Kessler LA, Gielen AC, Diener-West M et al. The effect of a woman's significant other on her breastfeeding decision. *J Hum Lact* 1995;11:103-109.
9. Bar-Yam NB, Darby L. Fathers and breastfeeding: A review of the literature. *J Hum Lact* 1997;13:45-50.
10. Susin LR, Giugliani ER, Kummer SC et al. Does parental breastfeeding knowledge increase breastfeeding rates? *Birth* 1999;26:149-156.
11. Jordan PL, Wall VR. Breastfeeding and fathers: Illuminating the darker side. *Birth* 1990;17:210-213.
12. Waletzky LR. Husbands' problems with breast-feeding. *Am J Orthopsychiatry* 1979;49:349-352.
13. Shepherd CK, Power KG, Carter H. Examining the correspondence of breastfeeding and bottle-feeding couples' infant feeding attitudes. *J Adv Nurs* 2000;31:651-660.
14. McClurg Hitt D, Olsen J. Infant feeding decisions in the Missouri WIC Program. *J Hum Lact* 1994;10:253-256.
15. Scott JA, Binns CW, Aroni RA. The influence of reported paternal attitudes on the decision to breast-feed. *J Paediatr Child Health* 1997;33:305-307.
16. Littman H, Medendorp SV, Goldfarb J. The decision to breastfeed. The importance of father's approval. *Clin Pediatr Phila* 1994;33:214-219.
17. Dungy CI, Losch M, Russell D. Maternal attitudes as predictors of infant feeding decisions. *J Assoc Acad Minor Phys* 1994;5:159-164.
18. Sears W. The father's role in breastfeeding. *NAACOGS Clin Issu Perinat Womens Health Nurs* 1992;3:713-716.
19. Isabella PH, Isabella RA. Correlates of successful breastfeeding: A study of social and personal factors. *J Hum Lact* 1994;10:257-264.
20. Bentley ME, Caulfield LE, Gross SM et al. Sources of influence on intention to breastfeed among African-American women at entry to WIC. *J Hum Lact* 1999;15:27-34.
21. Gabriel A, Gabriel KR, Lawrence RA. Cultural values and biomedical knowledge: choices in infant feeding. Analysis of a survey. *Soc Sci Med* 1986;23:501-509.
22. James DC, Jackson RT, Probart CK. Factors associated with breast-feeding prevalence and duration among international students. *J Am Diet Assoc* 1994;94:194-196.
23. Libbus MK, Kolostov LS. Perceptions of breastfeeding and infant feeding choice in a group of low-income mid-Missouri women. *J Hum Lact* 1994;10:17-23.
24. Perez-Escamilla R, Himmelgreen D, Segura-Millan S et al. Prenatal and perinatal factors associated with breast-feeding initiation among inner-city Puerto Rican women. *J Am Diet Assoc* 1998;98:657-663.
25. Sayers G, Thornton L, Corcoran R et al. Influences on breast feeding initiation and duration. *Ir J Med Sci* 1995;164:281-284.
26. Kieffer EC, Novotny R, Welch KB et al. Health practitioners should consider parity when counseling mothers on decisions about infant feeding methods. *J Am Diet Assoc* 1997;97:1313-1316.
27. Williams EL, Hammer LD. Breastfeeding attitudes and knowledge of pediatricians-in-training. *Am J Prev Med* 1995;11:26-33.
28. Freed GL, Clark SJ, Sorenson J et al. National assessment of physicians' breast-feeding knowledge, attitudes, training, and experience. *JAMA* 1995;273:472-476.
29. Freed GL, Clark SJ, Lohr JA et al. Pediatrician involvement in breast-feeding promotion: a national study of residents and practitioners. *Pediatrics* 1995;96:490-494.
30. Freed GL, Clark SJ, Cefalo RC et al. Breast-feeding education of obstetrics-gynecology residents and practitioners. *Am J Obstet Gynecol* 1995;173:1607-1613.
31. Patton CB, Beaman M, Csar N et al. Nurses' attitudes and behaviors that promote breastfeeding. *J Hum Lact* 1996;12:111-115.
32. Burglehaus MJ, Smith LA, Sheps SB et al. Physicians and breastfeeding: beliefs, knowledge, self-efficacy and counseling practices. *Can J Public Health* 1997;88:383-387.
33. Giugliani ER, Caiaffa WT, Vogelhut J et al. Effect of breastfeeding support from different sources on mothers' decisions to breastfeed. *J Hum Lact* 1994;10:157-161.

34. Lu MC, Lange L, Slusser W et al. Provider encouragement of breast-feeding: evidence from a national survey. *Obstet Gynecol* 2001;97:290-295.

35. Ekwo EE, Dusdieker LB, Booth BM. Factors influencing initiation of breast-feeding. *Am J Dis Child* 1983;137:375-377.

36. Ray DV, Estok PJ. Infant feeding choice and the adolescent mother. *J Obstet Gynceol Neonatal Nurs* 1984;13:115-118.

37. Handfield B, Bell R. What are popular magazines telling young women about pregnancy, birth, breastfeeding and parenting? *J Aust Coll Midwives* 1996;9:10-14.

38. Hung BK, Ling L, Ong SG. Sources of influence on infant feeding practices in Hong Kong. *Soc Sci Med* 1985;20:1143-1150.

39. Kabir M, Islam MA. The impact of mass media family planning programmes on current use of contraception in urban Bangladesh. *J Biosoc Sci* 2000;32:411-419.

40. McDivitt JA, Zimicki S, Hornik R et al. The impact of the Healthcom mass media campaign on timely initiation of breastfeeding in Jordan. *Stud Fam Plann* 1993;24:295-309.

41. Forrester IT, Wheelock G, Warren AP. Assessment of students' attitudes toward breastfeeding. *J Hum Lact* 1997;13:33-37.

42. Friel JK, Hudson NI, Banoub S et al. The effect of a promotion campaign on attitudes of adolescent females towards breastfeeding. *Can J Public Health* 1989;80:195-199.

43. Henderson L, Kitzinger J, Green J. Representing infant feeding: content analysis of British media portrayals of bottle feeding and breast feeding. *BMJ* 2000;321:1196-1198.

44. Parlato MB. The use of mass media to promote breastfeeding. *Int J Gynaecol Obstet* 1990;31(Suppl 1):105-10; discussion 111-113.

45. Arora S, McJunkin C, Wehrer J et al. Major factors influencing breastfeeding rates: Mother's perception of father's attitude and milk supply. *Pediatrics* 2000;106:E67.

46. Bevan ML, Mosley D, Solimano GR. Factors influencing breast feeding in an urban WIC program. *J Am Diet Assoc* 1984;84:563-567.

47. Marchand L, Morrow MH. Infant feeding practices: understanding the decision-making process. *Fam Med* 1994;26:319-324.

48. Jones DA. Attitudes of breast-feeding mothers: a survey of 649 mothers. *Soc Sci Med* 1986;23:1151-1156.

49. Gregg JE. Attitudes of teenagers in Liverpool to breast feeding. *BMJ* 1989;299:147-148.

50. Jones DA. The choice to breast feed or bottle feed and influences upon that choice: a survey of 1525 mothers. *Child Care Health Dev* 1987;13:75-85.

51. Bacon CJ, Wylie JM. Mothers' attitudes in infant feeding at Newcastle General Hospital in summer 1975. *BMJ* 1976;1:308-309.

52. Matthews K, Webber K, McKim E et al. Maternal infant-feeding decisions: reasons and influences. *Can J Nurs Res* 1998;30:177-198.

53. Holmes W, Thorpe L, Phillips J. Influences on infant-feeding beliefs and practices in an urban aboriginal community. *Aust NZ J Public Health* 1997;21:504-510.

54. Sullivan P. Breast-feeding still faces many roadblocks, national survey finds. *Can Med Assoc J* 1996;154:1569-1570.

55. Connolly C, Kelleher CC, Becker G et al. Attitudes of young men and women to breastfeeding. *Ir Med J* 1998;91:88-89.

56. Fein SB, Roe B. The effect of work status on initiation and duration of breast-feeding. *Am J Public Health* 1998;88:1042-1046.

57. McIntyre E, Hiller JE, Turnbull D. Determinants of infant feeding practices in a low socio-economic area: identifying environmental barriers to breastfeeding. *Aust NZ J Public Health* 1999;23:207-209.

58. Guttman N, Zimmerman DR. Low-income mothers' views on breastfeeding. *Soc Sci Med* 2000;50:1457-1473.

59. Hannon PR, Willis SK, Bishop-Townsend V et al. African-American and Latina adolescent mothers' infant feeding decisions and breastfeeding practices: a qualitative study. *J Adolesc Health* 2000;26:399-407.

60. Sheeska J, Potter B. Womens experiences breastfeeding in public places. *J Hum Lact* 2001;17:31-38.

61. Mackey S, Fried PA. Infant breast and bottle feeding practices: some related factors and attitudes. *Can J Public Health* 1981;72:312-318.

62. Yoos L. Developmental issues and the choice of feeding method of adolescent mothers. *J Obstet Gynecol Neonatal Nurs* 1985;14:68-72.

63. Novotny R, Kieffer EC, Mor J et al. Health of infant is the main reason for breast-feeding in a WIC population in Hawaii. *J Am Diet Assoc* 1994;94:293-297.

64. Dix DN. Why women decide not to breastfeed. *Birth* 1991;18:222-225.

65. Graffy JP. Mothers' attitudes to and experience of breast feeding: a primary care study. *Br J Gen Pract* 1992;42:61-64.

66. Leeper JD, Milo T, Collins TR. Infant feeding and maternal attitudes among mothers of low-income. *Psychol Rep* 1983;53:259-265.

67. Voss S, Finnis L, Manners J. Fathers and breast feeding: a pilot observational study. *J R Soc Health* 1993;113:176-180.

68. Hoddinott P, Pill R. Qualitative study of decisions about infant feeding among women in east end of London. *BMJ* 1999;318:30-34.

69. Carmichael SL, Prince CB, Burr R et al. Breast-feeding practices among WIC participants in Hawaii. *J Am Diet Assoc* 2001;101:57-62.

70. Nagy E, Orvos H, Pal A et al. Breastfeeding duration and previous breastfeeding experience. *Acta Paediatr* 2001;90:51-56.

71. Bentovim A. Shame and other anxieties associated with breast-feeding: a systems theory and psychodynamic approach. *Ciba Found Symp* 1976;45:159-178.

72. Hofmeyr GJ, Nikodem VC, Wolman WL et al. Companionship to modify the clinical birth environment: effects on progress and perceptions of labour, and breast-feeding. *Br J Obstet Gynaecol* 1991;98:756-764.

73. DiMatteo MR, Morton SC, Lepper HS et al. Cesarean childbirth and psychosocial outcomes: a meta-analysis. *Health Psychol* 1996;15:303-314.

74. Maes M, Libbrecht I, Lin A et al. Effects of pregnancy and delivery on serum prolyl endopeptidase (PEP) activity: Alterations in serum PEP are related to increased anxiety in the early puerperium and to postpartum depression. *J Affect Disord* 2000;57:125-137.

75. Llewellyn AM, Stowe ZN, Nemeroff CB. Depression during pregnancy and the puerperium. *J Clin Psychiatry* 1997; 58(Suppl 15):26-32.

76. Misri S, Sinclair DA, Kuan AJ. Breast-feeding and postpartum depression: is there a relationship? *Can J Psychiatry* 1997;42:1061-1065.

77. Papinczak TA, Turner CT. An analysis of personal and social factors influencing initiation and duration of breastfeeding in a large Queensland maternity hospital. *Breastfeed Rev* 2000;8:25-33.

78. Acheson L. Family violence and breast-feeding. *Arch Fam Med* 1995;4:650-652.

79. Jelliffe DB, Jelliffe EFP. Breast feeding is best for infants everywhere. *Nutrition Today* 1978:12-16.

80. Buxton KE, Gielen AC, Faden RR et al. Women intending to breastfeed: predictors of early infant feeding experiences. *Am J Prev Med* 1991;7:101-106.

81. O'Campo P, Faden RR, Gielen AC et al. Prenatal factors associated with breastfeeding duration: recommendations for prenatal interventions. *Birth* 1992;19:195-201.

82. Hill PD, Aldag J. Potential indicators of insufficient milk supply syndrome. *Res Nurs Health* 1991;14:11-19.

83. Coreil J, Murphy J. Maternal commitment, lactation practices, and breastfeeding duration. *J Obstet Gynecol Neonat Nurs* 1988;17:273-278.

84. Loughlin HH, Clapp-Channing NE, Gehlbach SH et al. Early termination of breast-feeding: identifying those at risk. *Pediatrics* 1985;75:508-513.

85. McMahon CA, Ungerer JA, Tennant C et al. Psychosocial adjustment and the quality of the mother-child relationship at four months postpartum after conception by in vitro fertilization. *Fertil Steril* 1997;68:492-500.

86. Brown S, Lumley J, Small R. Early obstetric discharge: does it make a difference to health outcomes? *Paediatr Perinat Epidemiol* 1998;12:49-71.

87. Dennis CL. Theoretical underpinnings of breastfeeding confidence: a self-efficacy framework. *J Hum Lact* 1999;15:195-201.

88. Dennis CL, Faux S. Development and psychometric testing of the breastfeeding self-efficacy scale. *Res Nurs Health* 1999;22:399-409.

89. Hewat RJ, Ellis DJ. Breastfeeding as a maternal-child team effort: women's perceptions. *Health Care Women Int* 1984;5:437-452.

90. Cronenwett L, Stukel T, Kearney M et al. Single daily bottle use in the early weeks postpartum and breast-feeding outcomes. *Pediatrics* 1992;90:760-766.

91. Neifert M, Lawrence R, Seacat J. Nipple confusion: toward a formal definition. *J Pediatr* 1995;126:S125-129.

92. Newton N. Key psychological issues in human lactation. In Symposium on Human Lactation, Department of Health,

Education & Welfare, Publication No (HSA) 79-5107; 1979:25-37.

93. Russell MJ. Human olfactory communication. *Nature* 1976;260:520-522.

94. Porter RH, Makin JW, Davis LB et al. An assessment of the salient olfactory environment of formula-fed infants. *Physiol-Behav* 1991;50:907-911.

95. Varendi H, Porter RH, Winberg J. Does the newborn baby find the nipple by smell? *Lancet* 1994;344:989-990.

96. Righard L. How do newborns find their mother's breast? *Birth* 1995;22:174-175.

97. Makin JW, Porter RH. Attractiveness of lactating females' breast odors to neonates. *Child Dev* 1989;60:803-810.

98. Varendi H, Porter RH. Breast odour as the only maternal stimulus elicits crawling towards the odour source. *Acta Paediatr* 2001;90:372-375.

99. Varendi H et al. Soothing effect of amniotic fluid smell in newborn infants. *Early Hum Dev* 1998;51:47-55.

100. Eidelman AI, Kaitz M. Olfactory recognition: a genetic or learned capacity? *J Dev Behav Pediatr* 1992;13:126-127.

101. Cernoch JM, Porter RH. Recognition of maternal axillary odors by infants. *Child Dev* 1985;56:1593-1598.

102. Varendi H, Porter RH, Winberg J. Attractiveness of amniotic fluid odor: evidence of prenatal olfactory learning? *Acta Paediatr* 1996;85:1223-1227.

103. Varendi H, Porter RH, Winberg J. Natural odour preferences of newborn infants change over time. *Acta Paediatr* 1997;86:985-990.

104. Marlier L, Schaal B, Soussignan R. Neonatal responsiveness to the odor of amniotic and lacteal fluids: A test of perinatal chemosensory continuity. *Child Dev* 1998;69:611-623.

105. Marlier L, Schaal B, Soussignan R. Orientation responses to biological odours in the human newborn. Initial pattern and postnatal plasticity. *C R Acad Sci III* 1997;320:999-1005.

106. Winberg J, Porter RH. Olfaction and human neonatal behaviour: Clinical implications. *Acta Paediatr* 1998;87:6-10.

107. Lucas A, St. James-Roberts I. Crying, fussing and colic behaviour in breast- and bottle-fed infants. *Early Hum Dev* 1998;53:9-18.

108. Paul K, Dittrichova J, Papousek H. Infant feeding behavior: development in patterns and motivation. *Dev Psychobiol* 1996;29:563-576.

109. Lee K. Crying and behavior pattern in breast- and formula-fed infants. *Early Hum Dev* 2000;58:133-140.

110. Michelsson K, Christensson K, Rothganger H et al. Crying in separated and non-separated newborns: sound spectrographic analysis. *Acta Paediatr* 1996;85:471-475.

111. Christensson K, Cabrera T, Christensson E et al. Separation distress call in the human neonate in the absence of maternal body contact. *Acta Paediatr* 1995;84:468-473.

112. Uvnas-Moberg K. Physiological and endocrine effects of social contact. *Ann N Y Acad Sci* 1997:807:146-163.

113. Uvnas-Moberg K. Oxytocin linked antistress effects—the relaxation and growth response. *Acta Physiol Scand Suppl* 1997;640:38-42.

114. Graef P, McGhee K, Rozycki J et al. Postpartum concerns of breastfeeding mothers. *J Nurse Midwifery* 1988;33: 62-66.

115. Benedek T. Psychobiological aspects of mothering. *Am J Orthopsychiatry* 1956;26:272-278.

116. Schmied V, Barclay L. Connection and pleasure, disruption and distress: women's experience of breastfeeding. *J Hum Lact* 1999;15:325-334.

117. Burr WR, Leigh GK, Day RD et al. Symbolic interaction and the family. In Burr WR, Hill R, Nye FI et al., editors. *Contemporary theories about the family*. Vol III. New York: The Free Press; 1979.

118. King I. *A theory for nursing: Systems, concepts & process*. New York: Wiley; 1981.

119. Rossi A. Transition to parenthood. *Journal of Marriage and the Family* 1968;30:26-40.

120. Gay JT, Edgil AE, Douglass AB. Reva Rubin revisited. *J Obstet Gynceol Neonatal Nurs* 1988;17:394-399.

121. Rubin R. Puerperal change. *Nursing Outlook* 1961;9: 753-755.

122. Greenberg M, Morris N. Engrossment: The newborn's impact upon the father. *Am J Orthopsychiatry* 1974;44: 520-531.

123. Klaus MH, Kennell JH. *Parent-Infant bonding*. 2nd ed. St. Louis: Mosby; 1982.

124. Bowlby J. *Attachment*. Vol 1. New York: Basic Books; 1969.

125. Ainsworth MDS. Object relations, dependency and attachment: A theoretical review of the infant-mother relationship. *Child Development* 1969;40:969-1026.

126. Wiles LS. The effect of prenatal breastfeeding education on breastfeeding success and maternal perception of the infant. *J Obstet Gynceol Neonatal Nurs* 1984;13:253-257.

127. Hall JM. Influencing breastfeeding success. *J Obstet Gynceol Neonatal Nurs* 1978;7:28-32.

128. Hellings P. A discriminant model to predict breast-feeding success. *West J Nurs Res* 1985;7:471-478.

129. Janke JR. Development of the breast-feeding attrition prediction tool. *Nurs Res* 1994;43:100-104.

130. Rousseau EH, Lescop JN, Fontaine S et al. Influence of cultural and environmental factors on breast-feeding. *Can Med Assoc J* 1982;127:701-704.

131. Arafat I, Allen DE, Fox JE. Maternal practice and attitudes toward breastfeeding. *J Obstet Gynceol Neonatal Nurs* 1981;10:91-95.

132. Janke JR. Breastfeeding duration following cesarean and vaginal births. *J Nurse Midwifery* 1988;33:159-164.

133. Ryan AS, Martinez GA. Breast-feeding and the working mother: a profile. *Pediatrics* 1989;83:524-531.

134. Wright HJ, Walker PC. Prediction of duration of breast feeding in primiparas. *J Epidemiol Community Health* 1983;37:89-94.

135. Rentschler DD. Correlates of successful breastfeeding. *Image J Nurs Sch* 1991;23:151-154.

136. Locklin MP, Naber SJ. Does breastfeeding empower women? Insights from a select group of educated, low-income, minority women. *Birth* 1993;20:30-35.

Anatomy and Physiology Related to Lactation

The study of the anatomy and physiology of breastfeeding and lactation could conceivably involve a discussion of the anatomy and physiology of every cell in the body at the cellular, organ, and system level. This is because breastfeeding and lactation involve both biologic factors, such as maternal neuroendocrine mechanisms and infant digestive function, and psychologic mediating mechanisms. The scope of this chapter is more confined, and its aim is to describe the most basic anatomy and physiology of lactation that underlie the clinical management strategies found in subsequent chapters. Readers who wish to have a thorough understanding of anatomy and physiology are urged to read detailed texts.[1-5]

This chapter addresses both breastfeeding (the act of an infant suckling at the mother's breast) and lactation (the process of making milk). A brief overview is presented to describe the overall regulation of lactation, the main hormones involved, and a brief definition of terms related to lactation.

REGULATION OF LACTATION

Lactation is regulated by both endocrine and autocrine factors. That is, hormones operate systemically to regulate the development of sufficient glandular tissue to synthesize and secrete milk, and local factors appear to stimulate or inhibit milk synthesis.

Studies about milk "volume" can be confusing or misleading without a thorough understanding of the terminology used and the physiology of milk production and transfer. Daly and Hartmann make the distinction between *milk synthesis,* which refers to "the accumulation of milk within the breast,"

and *milk production,* which refers to "the volume of milk removed from the breast."[4] Milk *synthesis,* however, is not necessarily related to milk *transfer* (i.e., infant intake). Milk may indeed be accumulating within the breast (i.e., the breast is synthesizing milk), but because the infant self-regulates intake, the milk may simply be stored. Larger breasts may indeed have more storage capacity. Even when storage capacity is low, high production is still possible.[5] An analogy may help clarify this: A certain amount of water accumulates in a well. The volume of water taken out of the well ("production") may be different from the amount of water that is in the well; the water is therefore stored or "accumulating" in the well. This distinction may help explain why the volume of milk during the neonatal period is driven primarily by the frequency of milk removal and the infant's ability to self-regulate intake. The distinctions among milk synthesis (amount of milk created and accumulating), milk production (amount removed from the breast by the infant or by expression), and the amount of milk transferred (the amount of milk the infant actually ingests) are somewhat academic, however. Unless some pathologic or extenuating circumstance exists (e.g., mastitis in which milk accumulates in the breast), any of these terms for volume of milk are fairly interchangeable and this text makes no clear distinction, unless noted.

During early lactation, volume (supply) of milk is indeed related to demand (i.e., removal of milk); frequency of feedings correlates with increased maternal milk volume.[6] The same is not true in later lactation. After breastfeeding has been well established, increasing frequency does not result in increased volume.[7]

HORMONES THAT REGULATE LACTATION

Just as hormones regulate birth, pubertal growth, conception, pregnancy, and delivery, they also regulate lactation, which completes the reproductive cycle. Hormones associated with pregnancy and lactation are summarized in Table 4-1. The two hormones most closely associated with lactation are oxytocin and prolactin. For a comparison of oxytocin and prolactin, see Table 4-2.

Oxytocin

Oxytocin is the primary hormone responsible for the milk-ejection reflex, or "let-down." *Let-down*, a term borrowed from the dairy industry, is more precisely referred to as the *milk-ejection reflex*, but well-respected experts continue to use *let-down*.[1,2]

Oxytocin causes myoepithelial cells to contract—in the uterus during labor, in the genitals during orgasm, and in the ductule system of the lactating breast. In the breasts the contraction occurs about 4 to 10 times during a 10-minute period, and each contraction lasts about 1 minute.[8] Thus mothers can and do have more than one "let-down" during a feeding. The contraction results in a sensation that mothers usually describe as a "tingling" or "sensual" feeling, which apparently varies in intensity from woman to woman and from day to day, just like labor contractions and orgasms.

Similar to what happens elsewhere in the body, an outside *stimulus* occurs to a *receptor*, initiating a reflex—a predictable response to the stimulus. In this case a *stimulus* (usually suckling) occurs to the sensory nerve endings in the nipple and areola

Table **4-1** STAGES OF MAMMARY DEVELOPMENT

Developmental Stage	Hormonal Regulation	Local Factors	Description
Embryogenesis	???	Fat pad necessary for ductal extension	Epithelial bud develops in 18- to 19-week fetus, extending a short distance into mammary fat pad with blind ducts that become canalized; some milk secretion may be present at birth
Pubertal development	—	—	—
Prior to onset of menses	Estrogen, GH	IGF–1, HGF, TGF-β, ???	Ductal extension into the mammary fat pad; branching morphogenesis
After outset of menses	Estrogen, progesterone, PRL?		Lobular development with formation of TDLU
Development in pregnancy	Progesterone, PRL, placental lactogen	HER, ???	Alveolus formation; partial cellular differentiation
Transition: lactogenesis	Progesterone withdrawal, PRL, glucocorticoid	Unknown	Onset of milk secretion Stage I, midpregnancy Stage II, parturition
Lactation	PRL, oxytocin	FIL, stretch	Ongoing milk secretion, milk ejection
Involution	Withdrawal of prolactin	Milk stasis (FIL???)	Alveolar epithelium undergoes apoptosis and remodeling and gland reverts to prepregnant state

From Neville MC. *Pediatr Clin North Am* 2001;48:13-34.

???, Additional factors unknown; *FIL*, feedback inhibitor of lactation; *GH*, growth hormone; *HCF*, hyperglycemic-glycogenolytic factor; *HER*, herregulin; *hPL*, human placental lactogen; *IGF*, insulin-like growth factor; *PRL*, prolactin; *TDLU*, terminal duct lobular unit; *TGF*, transforming growth factor.

Table 4-2   COMPARISON OF OXYTOCIN AND PROLACTIN

	Oxytocin	Prolactin
Function	Essential for milk *ejection*	Essential for milk *production*
Secreted by	Posterior pituitary	Anterior pituitary
Release stimulated by	Hypothalamus	Hypothalamus
Release triggered by	(1) Can be stimulated by visual or auditory stimuli, but strongest release is triggered by suckling; after lactation is established, initial release is within minute of suckling; release continues in a spurtlike fashion (2) Visual or auditory stimuli also trigger release, but not as strongly as suckling	(1) Delivery of placenta, which removes prolactin-inhibiting hormone (PIH), triggers low estrogen and high prolactin level (2) Only tactile stimuli (suckling of the breast) triggers release; suckling provides a continuous stimulation for prolactin release
Relationship to milk volume	Levels of oxytocin not related to milk volume at given feeding	Baseline level probably not related to milk volume Stimulating both breasts simultaneously increases prolactin level approximately 30%, thereby producing greater volume
Clinical implications	Peak and plateau is about every 6-10 min during a feeding Average pituitary contains 1000 mU of oxytocin; only about 0.5 mU are required for the milk-ejection reflex	Baseline levels rise during maternal sleep; this correlates to the fact that infant suckling is greatest in the morning

Modified from Biancuzzo M. *Breastfeeding the healthy newborn: a nursing perspective.* White Plains, NY: March of Dimes Foundation; 1994.

(receptors). Afferent neurons—those that carry messages to the brain and spinal cord—travel along a pathway that is primarily regulated by *neural* control; nerve impulses travel to the spinal cord then to the mesencephalon and hypothalamus in the mother's brain. Messages arriving in the brain then stimulate the release of oxytocin from the posterior pituitary gland. Efferent neurons—those that carry messages away from the brain—travel along a pathway that is primarily regulated by *hormonal* control. At the completion of the reflex arc, some effect happens to the *effector* (a muscle or a gland) (Fig. 4-1). The oxytocin stimulates the myoepithelial (muscle) cells surrounding the alveoli (milk-producing cells). When the myoepithelial cells contract, milk is ejected into the ductal system, propelled into the lactiferous sinuses (milk reservoirs), and ejected through the nipples.

Oxytocin levels rise significantly during the first 45 minutes after delivery, compared with levels 15 minutes before delivery.[9] In the lactating mother, oxytocin release is both pulsatile and variable and can occur before suckling.[10] Sensory stimuli, for example, seeing the infant or hearing him cry, can trigger let-down. However, the *strongest* stimulus for milk let-down is suckling. In addition, recent unpublished research in Sweden suggests that the actual stretching and elongation of the nipple during suckling triggers the reflex, implying that proper latch-on is therefore critical.

Physiologic, psychologic, and substance stimuli and pharmacologic suppressors can all affect release of oxytocin. For example, although suckling significantly elevates levels of oxytocin in mothers who have had no medication or naloxone, mothers who have been given morphine before

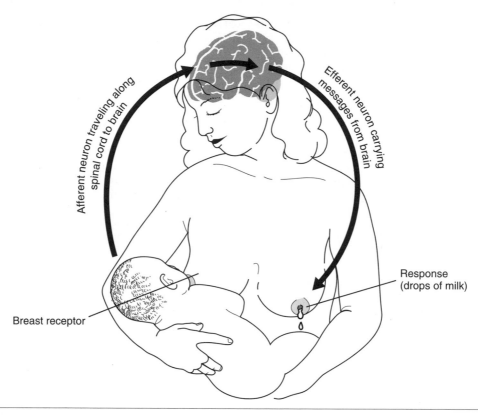

Afferent neuron traveling along spinal cord to brain

Efferent neuron carrying messages from brain

Response
(drops of milk)

Breast receptor

FIGURE **4-1** Reflex arc in the breastfeeding mother.

breastfeeding experience no significant rise in oxytocin levels.[11] The most common physiologic stimulus that inhibits lactation is ice. Ice, commonly recommended to help nipples become erect for easy latch-on, inhibits milk ejection. Cold temperatures reduce the size of the involved blood vessels, thereby reducing the amount of blood flow. Reduced blood flow causes less oxytocin to be at the site, so milk is not ejected. (Ice may be applied to the breasts *after* the feeding as a comfort measure but never to the nipples *before* the feeding.) Some psychologic stimuli, originally identified by Newton in 1948,[12] such as stress or pain, decrease milk output. Thus they were able to see the result but were not able to explain the physiologic basis. Much more recently, Ueda and colleagues explained the phenomena observed by Newton and Newton. They showed that the frequency of pulsatile release of oxytocin was significantly lower in subjects who were exposed to irritating stimuli compared with those who were not.[13] Conversely, relaxation can help the mother experience let-down.

The problem of fatigue is commonly reported as an inhibitor of lactation, but no scientific evidence substantiates that possibility. Why fatigue is or might be an inhibitor of let-down is not entirely understood. However, the hypothalamus is the major relay station between the emotions and changed bodily functions; that is, the hypothalamus governs psychosomatic phenomena. Furthermore, the hypothalamus plays an essential role in maintaining the waking state. Given these facts, it is not surprising that release of oxytocin from the brain is somehow inhibited when the woman is fatigued.

Prolactin

Perhaps prolactin could be described as the "great sensation" hormone. Prolactin (*pro* meaning "for" and *lactin* meaning "milk") can help a woman feel relaxed or even euphoric. Prolactin levels rise during pregnancy and drop for a brief time before birth; they then rise again a few hours after birth or as soon as the neonate is suckled.

Serum prolactin levels are influenced by suckling and by the length of lactation. Regardless of the infant's age, baseline prolactin levels double when suckling occurs.[14] However, baseline serum prolactin levels during lactation gradually decrease over 6 months and presumably beyond until the infant is ultimately weaned.[14] For the first 10 days, baseline prolactin levels are around 200 ng/ml, rising to 400 ng/ml during suckling. In the first 10 to 90 days, baseline levels are 60 to 110 ng/ml, rising to 70 to 220 ng/ml during suckling; at 90 to 180 days, baseline levels are around 50 ng/ml, rising to 100 ng/ml, and from 180 days to 1 year, baseline levels range from 30 to 40 ng/ml and rise to 45 to 80 ng/ml with suckling.[14]

Suckling, not the mere presence of an infant, causes higher prolactin levels. However, during a breastfeeding episode prolactin levels generally double, as shown in Fig. 4-2. Prolactin release can be blocked by prolactin-inhibiting factor. Physiologic and pharmacologic stimuli and pharmacologic suppressors can all affect release of prolactin, as shown in Box 4-1.[1]

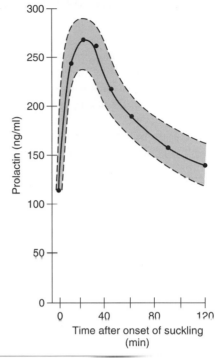

FIGURE 4-2 Effect of suckling (hatched area) on serum prolactin levels. Average values from 20 lactating women suckling for 10 minutes on days 5 and 6 postpartum. (From Neville MC. Regulation of mammary development and lactation. In Neville MC, Neifert MR. Lactation: physiology, nutrition, and breast-feeding. New York, Plenum Press; 1983.)

Box 4-1 FACTORS AFFECTING PROLACTIN RELEASE IN HUMANS

PHYSIOLOGIC STIMULI

Nursing in postpartum women—breast stimulation
Sleep
Stress
Sexual intercourse
Pregnancy

PHARMACOLOGIC STIMULI

Neuroleptic drugs
Thyroid-releasing hormone
Metoclopramide (procainamide derivative)
Estrogens

Hypoglycemia
Phenothiazines, butyrophenones
Norepinephrine
Histamine
Acetylcholine

PHARMACOLOGIC SUPPRESSORS

L-Dopa
Ergot preparations (2-Br-α-ergocryptine)
Clomiphene citrate
Large amounts of pyridoxine
Monoamine oxidase inhibitors
Prostaglandins E and $F_{2\alpha}$

From Lawrence RA, Lawrence RM. *Breastfeeding: a guide for the medical profession.* 5th ed. St. Louis: Mosby; 1999.

STRUCTURE OF THE MAMMARY GLAND (BREAST)

The breasts—paired mammary glands—are actually modified exocrine glands, having a ductule system for secreting outwardly to the surface of the organ.[1] The glands are anchored to the overlying skin and to the pectoral muscles by the suspensory ligaments of Cooper as shown in Fig. 4-3. The three major structures of the breast are the skin, the subcutaneous tissue, and the body of the breast.

Skin

The general skin, nipple, and areola are visible externally. (Chapter 12 describes features that the examiner should note when inspecting the external anatomy of the breast.) The areola, or areola mammae, is a pigmented area that surrounds the nipple. In the areola are Montgomery's glands, which appear as raised projections. These are actually sebaceous glands that provide secretions to protect the areola and nipple.

The nipple (papilla mammae) is a raised projection in the center of the areola. Because the breast is an exocrine gland, the nipple is the external opening through which milk is secreted. The nipple contains smooth muscle fibers and sensory nerve endings that cause it to become erect when stimulated.

Subcutaneous Tissue

The gland as well as fat and connective tissue are contained within the subcutaneous tissue. The size of a woman's breasts reflects the amount of fat and connective tissue, not glandular tissue. Hence, the size of the breast has little or nothing to do with their functionality.

Body of the Breast (Corpus Mammae)

The corpus mammae from the Latin *corpus,* meaning "body," and *mammae* from the Latin *mamma,* meaning "breast," is the glandular organ. Like most organs, the breast is made up of two parts: the glandular tissue (parenchyma) and the supporting tissue (stroma).

Glandular Tissue (Parenchyma)

The parenchyma of the breast consists of the lobular, ductular, and alveolar structures. The breast has 15 to 25 *lobi* (singular, *lobus*). Like lobi in other parts of the body, each lobus is separated from neighboring lobi; in the breast it is separated by connective tissue. The duct from a lobus goes to the nipple. Lobi are subdivided into *lobuli* (about 20 to 40 lobuli in the breast), and each lobulus is again subdivided into 10 to 100 *alveoli.* Fig. 4-4 shows the ductal system within the gland.

The *alveolus* (plural, *alveoli*) is the smallest functioning unit in the mammary gland. Two types of cells are in the alveolus as shown in Fig. 4-5: (1) the *secretory epithelial cells,* which synthesize fat and protein into milk, and (2) the *myoepithelial cells,* which surround the secretory epithelial cells and are responsible for the milk ejection. The myoepithelial cells (*myo,* meaning "muscle") can be either at rest or contracted. When these myoepithelial cells contract, milk is ejected into the ductal system.

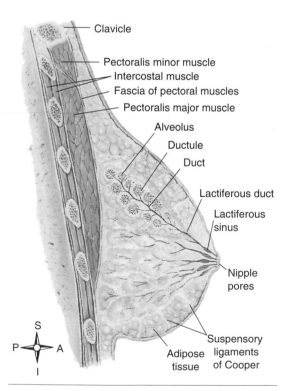

Clavicle
Pectoralis minor muscle
Intercostal muscle
Fascia of pectoral muscles
Pectoralis major muscle
Alveolus
Ductule
Duct
Lactiferous duct
Lactiferous sinus
Nipple pores
Suspensory ligaments of Cooper
Adipose tissue

S
P — A
I

FIGURE **4-3** Sagittal section of a lactating breast. *(From Thibodeau GA, Patton KT. Anatomy and physiology. 4th ed. St. Louis: Mosby; 1999.)*

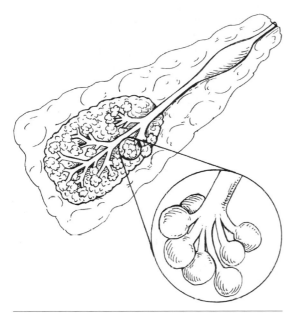

FIGURE 4-4 Lobus (lobe) of the breast, with enlarged view of alveoli.

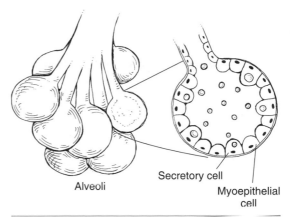

Alveoli

Secretory cell

Myoepithelial cell

FIGURE 4-5 Alveoli showing myoepithelial cells and secretory cells.

Milk flows through a ductular system that is embedded in the connective and fatty tissue. The ductular system is arranged in a treelike fashion, with larger "branches" and smaller "twigs." Ductules empty into ducts, which empty into the lactiferous sinuses, and eventually the milk is secreted through the nipple.

Stroma

The stroma contains the connective tissue, fat tissue, blood vessels, nerves, and lymphatics. The duct system of the breast is located within the connective tissue and fat.

Connective Tissue. Suspensory ligaments (Cooper's ligaments) help support the glandular and connective tissue and anchor them to the pectoral muscles, which are behind the breast.

Blood Vessels. The lactating breast is a highly vascular organ. Not surprisingly, the internal mammary artery and the lateral thoracic artery provide most of the blood supply to the breast. Other arteries and veins are also involved in circulation to the breast.

Nerves. The breast is innervated primarily by branches from the fourth, fifth, and sixth inter-

costal nerves. However, the branch runs from deep to superficial, so the corpus mammae has less innervation than the areola or the nipple. The nipple/areola complex is innervated by the lateral cutaneous branch of the fourth intercostal nerve. The nipple contains smooth muscle fibers, a rich blood supply, and multiple sensory nerve endings. Nerve endings in the nipple are receptive to *pain* and *pressure*. With stimulation, nerve endings send a message via the spinal cord to the brain; the pituitary then triggers the release of the hormones oxytocin and prolactin, and the nipple becomes erect. The nerve endings in the areola are sensitive to *pressure* and *suckling*. From the standpoint of breastfeeding management, this makes sense because the infant should grasp and stimulate primarily the areola; the infant should not nipple suck (see Chapter 7).

Lymphatics. Lymph vessels carry a moving fluid, lymph, which is derived from blood and body fluid. Lymph is drained from the mammary gland and its surrounding tissues by two sets of lymphatic vessels. One set originates in and drains the skin over the breast, with the exception of the areola and nipple. The other set drains the corpus mammae as well as the skin of the areola and nipple. The lymphatic system in the breast is largely unrelated to lactation, although lymphatic fluid accumulates during engorgement, contributing to visible distention.

Box 4-2 Definitions for Stages of Lactation in Humans

Embryogenesis: Growth of mammary bud in the growing embryo

Pubertal development: Growth of the mammary ducts in the adolescent

Lactogenesis: The process by which the mammary gland develops the *capacity* to secrete milk in the pregnant and postpartum mother

Lactation: The process of milk secretion

Involution: Occurs when the regular extraction of milk from the gland ceases or, in humans, when prolactin is withdrawn.

Reference: Neville MC. *Pediatr Clin North Am* 2001; 48:13-34.

Stages of Mammary Function

There are five basic stages of mammary function: (1) embryogenesis, (2) pubertal development, (3) lactogenesis, (4) lactation, and (5) involution (Box 4-2). Embryogenesis and pubertal development are sometimes combined and referred to as *mammogenesis,* which simply means the growth of the mammary gland.

Embryogenesis

A bulb-shaped epithelial mammary bud is present about 18 to 19 weeks in the growing fetus. This bud extends a bit into the mammary fat pad, but the ducts have a "dead end." (Ductal extension occurs at adolescence.) Researchers have not identified the hormones responsible for this structural growth. At the time of birth, the newborn consumes the mother's milk (which contains hormones) and may even secrete a tiny bit of milk from the nipple. After birth, the small branching ducts grow as the child grows.[3]

Pubertal Development

Pubertal development occurs before and after the onset of menses. In early puberty, before the onset of menses, hormonal regulation occurs primarily through estrogen and growth hormone and the bare ducts course through the fat.[3] Later in puberty, with the onset of menses and ovulatory cycles,

progesterone that is present during the luteal phase of each ovulatory cycle appears to create some lobuloalveolar development. Estrogen, progesterone, and possibly prolactin are the primary hormones that influence growth of the mammary ducts. The internal developments that occur within the gland are visible externally as the breast becomes larger. The breast is never fully developed, however, until after it has produced milk.

Lactogenesis

Lactogenesis is "the process by which the mammary gland develops the capacity to secrete milk."[3] Lactogenesis occurs in two stages, referred to as *lactogenesis stage I* and *lactogenesis stage II.*

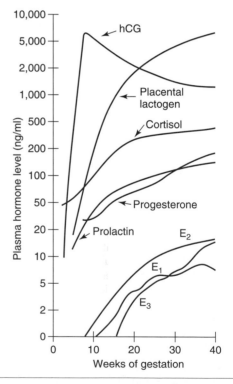

FIGURE 4-6 Plasma hormone levels during pregnancy. *(From Neville MC. Regulation of mammary development and lactation. In Neville MC, Neifert MR. Lactation: physiology, nutrition, and breast-feeding. New York: Plenum Press; 2001.)*

During pregnancy, profound hormonal changes prepare the breast for lactation, as shown in Fig. 4-6. Luteal and placental hormones are responsible for the substantial increase in ductular sprouting, branching, and lobular formation.[1] Placental lactogen, prolactin, and chorionic gonadotrophin also contribute to growth.[1] Final stages of mammary growth and differentiation are accomplished primarily by progesterone, and prolactin or human placental lactogen may be involved. Because of the high serum levels of maternal progesterone, secretion of milk does not occur.

Lactogenesis stage I begins around the middle of pregnancy.[3] Structurally, ductular and lobular proliferation occurs as a result of the influence of hormones. Functionally, the gland merely becomes competent for secretion, but it secretes only a colostrum-like substance. Although the gland is structurally competent to secrete milk, it does not because the hormones associated with pregnancy prevent milk from being synthesized.

At birth and even before birth, mothers secrete colostrum. Thereafter, they secrete transitional milk. These secretions are usually presumed to define the period of lactogenesis stage I. However, Neville and colleagues point out that the terms *colostrum* and *transitional milk* "do not define clear-cut temporal changes in milk composition and are not useful distinctions" (Box 4-3). Rather, the changes in milk composition that occur postpartum should be viewed as part of a continuum wherein rapid changes in composition occur during the first 4 days postpartum, followed by slow changes in various components of milk throughout the course of lactation."[15] Neville specifies a starting time for lactogenesis stage I but does not give a firm temporal definition for when it ends or for when lactogenesis stage II begins or ends.

Lactogenesis stage II is "the onset of copious milk secretion and occurs during the first 4 days postpartum."[3] The onset of copious milk secretion is attributable to the dramatic changes that occur after the placenta is delivered. During the first 4 days or so after birth, *progesterone* levels fall sharply but do not reach the levels seen in nonpregnant women for several days. *Prolactin* levels remain high. Levels of estradiol (the most potent naturally occurring estrogen), progesterone, and prolactin are shown in Fig. 4-7.[18] This is usually referred to as the *coming-in* of milk. The mother

---

Box 4-3 DESCRIPTIONS OF SECRETIONS FROM THE BREAST DURING LACTOGENESIS AND LACTATION

Colostrum, the first "milk," is a thick substance that appears yellow because of its high carotene content. Colostrum is contained in the ducts during the later part of pregnancy and is secreted the first few days postpartum. Colostrum is especially important for the newborn; it is rich in immunoglobulins and has a laxative effect on the gut, aiding with the passage of newborn meconium. Compared with mature milk, colostrum is higher in protein, lower in fat, and lower in carbohydrate. Colostrum is lower in energy than mature milk, containing about 67 kcal/100 ml (about 20 calories per ounce), whereas mature milk has about 75 kcal/100 ml (22.5 calories per ounce).[15]

Transitional milk is produced in the very early postpartum period as the colostrum diminishes and the mature milk develops.

Mature milk is produced after lactogenesis stage II. The energy content is different from colostrum, as are the proportion of many nutrients.

Foremilk—the milk that is produced and stored between feeding and released at the beginning of the next feeding—has an appearance similar to skimmed milk, with a characteristic blue tinge.

Hindmilk—milk that is produced during and released at the end of a feeding—looks much like heavy cream

Reference: Lawrence RA, Lawrence RM. *Breastfeeding: a guide for the medical profession.* 5th ed. St. Louis: Mosby; 1999.

generally recognizes this coming-in of milk because she notices a copious volume of milk. During stage II, changes in milk volume and composition are significant.

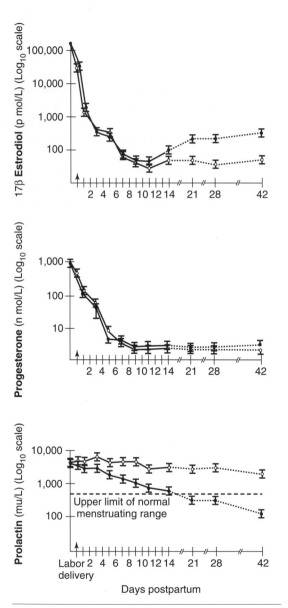

FIGURE 4-7 Maternal hormone levels after birth in breastfeeding and nonbreastfeeding women. Breastfeeding subjects *(open circles)* and non-breastfeeding subjects *(filled circles)*; *p* < .01. *(From Martin RH et al.* Clin Endocrinol *1980;13:223-230.)*

Technically, the measurement of maternal volume of milk (that which is synthesized and therefore available) may be different from infant intake (that which is consumed.) Nonetheless, studies that measure milk volume have done so by test-weighing the infant before and after feeding to determine the volume of milk that has been transferred to the newborn.[19-21] Neville and colleagues showed that the volume of milk transferred to the newborn begins to increase dramatically at approximately 36 hours postpartum and continues to increase for approximately 48 hours.[19] The increase in milk volume, from zero to about 200 ml at 48 hr, is shown in Fig. 4-8.

As noted, composition of milk also changes during lactogenesis. Neville and colleagues describe the sequence of three significant changes in milk composition during lactogenesis.[17] Immediately after delivery, sodium and chloride concentrations decrease, but lactose concentration increases; this change is completed within about 72 hours as shown in Fig. 4-9.[22] About 24 hours after these changes, milk volume becomes copious. Then, concentrations of two important proteins, secretory immunoglobulin A and lactoferrin,

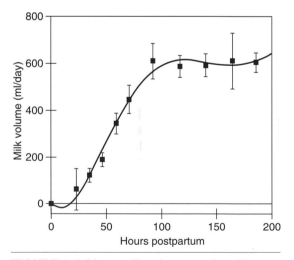

FIGURE 4-8 Mean milk volume produced by American women fully breastfeeding their infants during the first week postpartum. *(From Neville MC. Lactogenesis in women. In Jensen RG. Handbook of milk composition. San Diego: Academic Press; 1995.)*

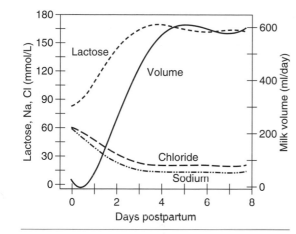

FIGURE 4-9 Time course of changes in the lactose, chloride (Cl), and sodium (Na) concentrations in human milk during the first week postpartum. (From Neville MC. Clin Perinatol 1999;26:251-279.)

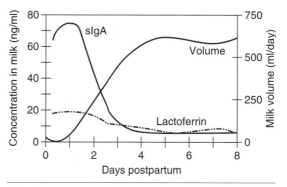

FIGURE 4-10 Changes in the concentration of secretory immunoglobulin A (sIgA) and lactoferrin during the onset of lactation in women. The secretion rate of both substances increases during the first 2 days postpartum. (From Neville MC. Clin Perinatol 1999;26:251-279.)

increase[23] and remain elevated for about the first 48 hours after birth. They then decrease rapidly after the second postpartum day because as the milk volume increases, these proteins become more diluted in the greater volume of milk, as shown in Fig. 4-10. Finally, at about 36 hours after birth, milk volume increases by as much as tenfold, as shown in Figs. 4-9 and 4-10. In terms of volume, this means that the woman has a volume that reaches 50 ml/day by the first 36 hours, which increases to 500 to 600 ml/day during the subsequent 36 hours (see Fig. 4-10). (Neville cautions that the few existing studies of milk volume or composition during this time have all been conducted among middle-class, white women.)

Lactogenesis can sometimes be delayed. Causes of delay include placental retention,[24] cesarean birth,[25] diabetes,[19,20,26] and prolonged second-stage labor.[27] In addition, several demographic factors and formula-feeding are also associated with delayed onset of lactogenesis.[27]

Lactation

Lactation is the "the process of milk secretion and is prolonged as long as milk is removed from the gland on a regular basis."[3] Established lactation is regulated primarily by prolactin and oxytocin, and throughout lactation these two hormones are secreted in response to suckling, as shown in Fig. 4-11.

In addition to the systemic, hormonal regulation of milk, however, volume of milk appears to be regulated locally by the removal of milk; this is sometimes referred to as *autocrine regulation of milk*.[28] A further discussion of how infant suckling and milk removal regulates lactation is provided in Chapter 7.

Volume of milk is remarkably similar among women, although it does vary during the course of lactation. American mothers produce about 500 to 600 ml/day during the first 2 weeks and 700 to 800 ml/day thereafter, up to 6 months.[7,29,30] In the United States, where infants are often given solids after 4 to 6 months, milk volume decreases. Milk volume averages 769 g/day at 6 months, 637 g/day at 9 months, and 445 g/day at 12 months.[31]

Age of the mother appears to have little or no effect on the volume of milk. Despite early concerns of "disuse atrophy" after age 24, studies have shown no correlation between advancing maternal age and milk consumption.[32] At the other end of the spectrum, teenage mothers apparently produce enough milk to satisfy their infants.[33]

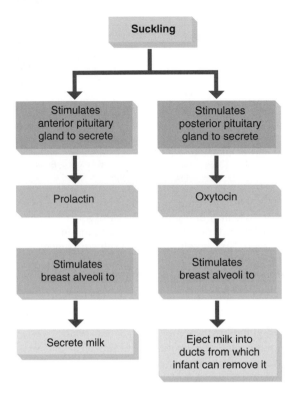

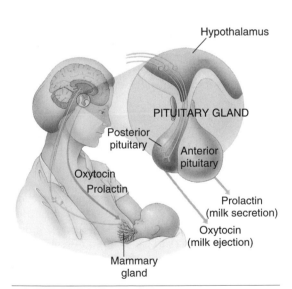

FIGURE **4-11** Lactation. The illustration and accompanying flow chart summarize the mechanisms that control secretion and ejection of milk. *(From Thibodeau GA, Patton KT. Anatomy and physiology. 4th ed. St. Louis: Mosby; 1999.)*

The effect of parity on milk volume, until recently presumed to have no effect, may indeed have an effect. Earlier evidence indicated that multiparous women may produce a greater supply of milk on the fourth postpartum day,[34] and multiparity was the most significant factor at 1 week.[35] After lactation is well established, however, no significant correlation between parity and infant intake has been noted in well-nourished populations.[30,36,37]

Milk volume varies diurnally, with greater volume in the morning; milk volume peaks between 8 AM and 12 noon.[38] Milk volume can be significantly greater in one breast than in the other.[39] Other factors related to maternal health and health habits, especially smoking, can also influence milk production (see Chapter 7).

Most people think of lactation as originating in the breast and being concerned only with milk. Actually, multiple sites are involved in the process of lactation, most notably the pituitary gland, and the effects of lactation permeate the woman's being, including her fertility and behavior.

Newton and Newton point out that "the survival of the human race, long before the concept of 'duty' evolved, depended upon the satisfactions gained from the two voluntary acts of reproduction—coitus and breastfeeding. These had to be sufficiently pleasurable to ensure their frequent occurrence."[40] Multiple physical and psychologic responses that occur during lactation also occur during coitus.[40] Furthermore, multiple physical and psychologic responses experienced during sexual excitement have similarities to those that occur during the act of giving birth.[41] These responses can be explained by the fact that the same hormones—including estrogen, progesterone, oxytocin, and prolactin—are involved in the menstrual cycle, sexual intercourse, pregnancy, birth, and lactation.

Few well-controlled studies address the effect of breastfeeding on sexual desire and behavior. Masters and Johnson, however, found that women who breastfeed are generally more interested in an early return to sexual activity.[42] A more recent study has suggested that while women thought that breastfeeding may have a slightly negative effect on their sexuality, it did not affect their overall sexual relationship.[43] Negative effects can include spraying milk during orgasm or having excessive vaginal dryness. (Some simple strategies, such as using lubricating jelly and feeding the infant before intercourse, minimize these effects.) Dyspareunia is more commonly reported among lactating mothers compared with nonlactating mothers.[44]

Breastfeeding significantly suppresses fertility and contributes to limiting populations.[45] It is well documented that mothers who breastfeed have longer intervals between births.[46] The elevated prolactin levels that occur during lactation suppress ovulation and the reproductive cycle. The time it takes for a woman's menses to return depends in large part on the frequency with which she suckles her infant, meaning this amenorrhea can last for weeks, months, or years. This difference has important teaching implications for child-spacing. The lactational amenorrhea method (LAM) relies on the increased prolactin levels during lactation to avoid the occurrence of a pregnancy. This is further discussed in Chapter 5.

Involution

Involution occurs when "regular extraction of milk from the gland ceases or, in many but not all species, when prolactin is withdrawn"[3] (p. 19). Lactation can therefore continue indefinitely, as long as the breast is suckled. Conversely, when infants fail to suckle well, the mammary glands involute; lactose concentration and therefore milk volume are reduced, while electrolytes are elevated.[47] Regarding lactation worldwide, the average time for complete cessation of breastfeeding may not occur until around 4 years.[48] In some cultures, women long past menopause continue to suckle infants, often more than one infant or child, and continue to lactate; cultural aspects of weaning are discussed in Chapter 2. Ideally, weaning is initiated based on the infant's nutritional needs and developmental milestones, and it then progresses gradually. The focus of this text is on the newborn, however, so the reader is referred to other professional[1] and consumer sources for a more complete discussion of weaning.

Whenever weaning does occur, however, the breast begins a postinvolution much as the uterus involutes after it has performed its intended function. During weaning the mother's milk changes in terms of its volume, nutritional components, and immunologic properties, whether weaning is gradual[49] or abrupt.[47] When the infant suckles less frequently, prolactin levels decrease, and when the breast is not emptied it becomes engorged; blood vessels are compressed, resulting in diminished oxytocin to the myoepithelium. Gradually, the alveoli collapse, although even after the gland has returned to the resting state, the alveoli do not fully involute.

COMPOSITION OF HUMAN MILK

From a broad perspective, the composition of human milk is fairly similar among mothers. That is, milk is similar from one group of mothers (e.g., women who are 8 weeks postpartum) to another, and the same components are present in adequate amounts to meet the infant's needs, regardless of other factors. From a narrower perspective, however, milk varies tremendously in terms of both individual and time-related factors.

Gestation at time of delivery; volume of milk secreted; time of day; age of infant; and the mother's age, parity, and general health status and habits influence the configuration of her milk components. Maternal nutrition has very little to do with the makeup of milk, however. The mother's intake of vitamins and fatty acid content may alter her milk somewhat, but in general nature provides nutrients to the infant at the mother's expense. For this reason, severely undernourished women have been known to provide adequate milk to their infants. Most important, the composition of milk changes as the infant grows older, so that it more perfectly meets his nutritional needs. (Components of milk in relation to the preterm infant's needs is discussed in later chapters.)

Approximately 87% of human milk is water, and all other components are suspended in the water (Fig. 4-12). Other components include fats, proteins, and carbohydrates, along with nonnitrogen compounds and water-soluble and fat-soluble vitamins, cells, minerals, and trace elements as

Box 4-4   Constituents of Human Milk

PROTEINS

α-Lactalbumin
β-Lactoglobulin
Caseins
Enzymes
Growth factors
Hormones
Lactoferrin
Lysozyme
sIgA and other immunoglobulins

NONPROTEIN NITROGEN

α-Amino nitrogen
Creatine
Creatinine
Glucosamine
Nucleic acids
Nucleotides
Polyamines
Urea
Uric acids

CARBOHYDRATES

Lactose
Oligosaccharides
Glycopeptides
Bifidus factors

LIPIDS

Fat-soluble vitamins (A,D, E, and K)
Carotenoids
Fatty acids
Phospholipids
Sterols and hydrocarbons
Triglycerides

WATER-SOLUBLE VITAMINS

Biotin
Choline
Folate

Inositol
Niacin
Pantothenic acid
Riboflavin
Thiamin
Vitamin B_{12}
Vitamin B_6
Vitamin C

MINERAL AND IONIC CONSTITUENTS

Bicarbonate
Calcium
Chloride
Citrate
Magnesium
Phosphate
Potassium
Sodium
Sulfate

TRACE MINERALS

Chromium
Cobalt
Copper
Fluoride
Iodine
Iron
Manganese
Molybdenum
Nickel
Selenium
Zinc

CELLS

Epithelial cells
Leukocytes
Lymphocytes
Macrophages
Neutrophils

From Picciano MF. *Pediatr Clin North Am* 2001;48:56-57.

listed in Box 4-4.[51] Components of milk either are synthesized in the secretory cells of the alveoli, or they are transferred from maternal plasma. The secretory cells synthesize the macronutrients—protein, fat, and carbohydrate (lactose). Maternal plasma transfers the macronutrients plus the macronutrient elements—vitamins and minerals.[50]

Substances can readily cross the alveolar membrane either by diffusion or by active transport because human milk is isotonic with plasma. Calcium, amino acids, glucose, magnesium, and sodium cross the membrane by active transport, whereas water, electrolytes, and water-soluble compounds move by way of diffusion.

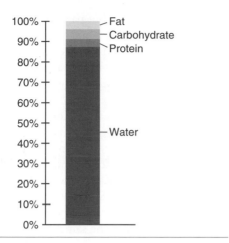

FIGURE 4-12 Water and nutrients in human milk.

The constituents of human milk really have two main functions: to provide nutrition to every cell in the infant's body and to provide a protective and/or developmental effect. Some constituents of human milk accomplish both. Therefore human milk is often discussed in terms of its nutrient value or its bioactive factors. Bernt and colleagues assert that "hormones, growth factors, cytokines and even whole cells are present in breast milk and act to establish biochemical and immunologic communication between mother and child"[52] (p. 27S).

Primary Nutrients in Human Milk

Lipids

Fat is needed in human milk because it is (1) a vehicle for fat-soluble vitamins, (2) necessary for brain development, (3) a precursor of prostaglandin and hormones, and (4) an essential constituent of all cell membranes.[53]

From 40% to 50% of the total calories in human milk are from fat.[54,55] The total fat content of human milk varies from 30 to 50 g/L. Fat is digested by four enzymes: lingual lipase, gastric lipase, bile-salt-stimulated lipase, and pancreatic lipase.

Approximately 98% of human milk fat is composed of triglycerides; cholesterol also is present and clinically important. Although cholesterol is known to have adverse effects on adult cardiovascular function, it has not been shown to have any negative effects on the infant, even though serum levels are higher in breastfed than artificially fed infants. To the contrary, higher levels of cholesterol are desirable because cholesterol is essential for brain growth in infants. Artificial milk has about the same amount of its calories from fat, but it relies solely on vegetable fat, whereas human milk has cholesterol.

Human milk is rich in fatty acids. The essential fatty acids, linoleic acids and α-linolenic acids, and their long-chain derivatives, arachidonic acid (AA) and docosahexaenoic acid (DHA), are the most representative long-chain polyunsaturated fatty acids (LCPUFAs). However, the exact requirements of AA and DHA for growth and development in the exclusively breastfed infant have not yet been established.[56]

LCPUFAs affect infants' growth and neural development,[57] and experts emphasize that those found in human milk are superior to those found in some artificial milks.[58] Present in all lactating women throughout lactation, LCPUFAs are critical for the synthesis and development of retinal[59] and neural tissues.[60,61] Even women who have low intakes of arachidonic acid have about the same amounts in their milk, when compared with that of well nourished women.[62]

Fat is the most variable component of human milk for a variety of reasons. Fat content is higher in mature milk than in colostrum, accounting for approximately 2% of all components of colostrum and approximately 3.6% of mature milk. Fat content is highest in the afternoon and evening (4 to 8 PM) and lowest between 4 to 8 AM.[38,63] Fat content is four to five times higher in hindmilk than in foremilk.[64,65] Fig. 4-13 shows the fat content in foremilk in comparison with the fat content in hindmilk.

Although it does not influence other components of human milk, maternal diet can significantly influence fat in human milk. While the *amount* of fat is about the same and adequately meets the infant's needs, the *constituents* of fat differ when the mother is extremely malnourished or consumes mostly vegetable rather than animal

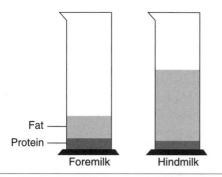

Fat

Protein

Foremilk   Hindmilk

FIGURE **4-13** Variation in composition of human milk. Note the greater amount of fat in hindmilk in comparison with foremilk. *(From the National Center for Education in Maternal and Child Health. The art and science of breastfeeding. Arlington, VA: National Center for Education in Maternal and Child Health; 1986.)*

fat. For example, if the mother consumes lower amounts of polyunsaturated fats, her milk will have a lower fatty acid content. Other factors, including length of gestation and parity, also seem to affect the fat amount.[53]

Proteins

The benefits of human milk and the risks of artificial milk can be best explained by understanding all of the components, but particularly the protein components, of human milk. Protein is synthesized from amino acids in the secretory cells or transferred from the maternal plasma. Amino acids are the "building blocks" of protein. Although the terms *essential amino acids* and *nonessential amino acids* are commonly used, by definition they apply to adult needs, not to newborns' needs. However, human milk contains all amino acids necessary for the nursling, as shown in Box 4-5.[50] Protein levels are most concentrated in colostrum during the first few days after birth.[21] After milk volume increases, however, the "dose" continues to be about the same while the concentration decreases; protein accounts for approximately 2.3% of colostrum but only about 0.9% of mature milk.

Protein intakes are significantly higher for artificially fed infants than for breastfed infants at 3, 6, and 9 months.[66] Human milk has *half* the renal solute load as artificial milk because of lower levels of protein, calcium, sodium, potassium, and other ions. The relatively low levels of these ions require less water for excretion, and hence lower levels of water are lost when the infant consumes human milk. This water conservation results in a more stable body temperature because water is a factor in thermoregulation.

Box **4-5**   AMINO ACIDS PRESENT IN HUMAN MILK

Alanine	Tryptophan
Arginine	Tyrosine
Aspartic acid	Valine
Cystine	
Glutamic acid	When compared with cow's milk, human milk is richer in cystine, which is needed for central nervous system development.
Glycine	
Histidine	
Isoleucine	When compared with cow's milk, human milk is lower in phenylalanine and tyrosine. Higher amounts of phenylalanine and tyrosine may lead to central nervous system damage, especially in preterm infants.
Leucine	
Lysine	
Methionine	
Phenylalanine	
Proline	
Serine	Human milk is rich in taurine; newborns cannot synthesize taurine, and cow's milk does not contain any taurine. Taurine is essential for neurologic development.
Taurine	
Threonine	

Human milk contains two types of proteins: casein (curd) and whey (lactalbumins). Cow's milk contains these two proteins also, but the ratio of casein to whey can be significantly different. Human milk is made up of 60% whey and 40% casein, whereas cow's milk can be 20% whey and 80% casein. Human milk is easily and quickly digested, and its greater proportion of whey produces softer stools. If artificial milk has a greater percentage of casein, it is more difficult to digest and results in a more rubbery curd, and hence more rubbery stools.

Whey Proteins. Whey proteins are synthesized in the mammary gland. The primary whey protein in human milk is a *α-lactalbumin*. Lactalbumin, together with the other key proteins lactoferrin and secretory immunoglobulin A, make up 60% to 80% of human milk protein. Other proteins (serum albumin, β-lactoglobulins, other immunoglobulins, and various glycoproteins) are also present.

Secretory immunoglobulin A (sIgA), a whey protein, is the most abundant immunoglobulin in human milk. Without the secretory component, this immunoglobulin would be digested by proteolysis in the gastrointestinal tract. Furthermore, sIgA is enhanced by protein *complement*—a group of proteins found in human milk. The primary function of sIgA in human milk is to protect the infant against respiratory and enteric bacterial and viral organisms; it also may protect against allergies. Infants are less likely to have allergies to human milk not because of what it contains but because of the absence of food antigens.

Casein Protein. *Casein* is a curd protein. Human milk caseins are predominately the β-type, while bovine casein is approximately 50% α-casein. The high α-casein ratio in bovine milk decreases iron absorption. Because iron is so poorly absorbed, relatively large amounts of it need to be added to artificial milk in order for infants to absorb the amount they need. The high β-casein ratio in human milk allows approximately 80% of iron to be absorbed. This is important because iron is bound to lactoferrin, which inhibits the growth of iron-dependent bacteria in the gastrointestinal tract.

Other Proteins. Other proteins are also present in human milk, including serum albumin and β-lactoglobulins. β-Lactoglobulin makes use of some of the protein and some of the globulins. Cow's milk, in which β-lactoglobulin predominates over α-lactalbumin, can cause insult to the pancreas and predispose the body to diabetes. Immunoglobulins IgG and IgM, which the fetus received through the placenta, are present in small amounts in human milk, along with various glycoproteins and other substances. Complement proteins are a group of proteins found in human milk. The two that are most important in lactation are C3 and C4. Bifidus factor, which is also present in human milk, supports the growth of lactobacillus.

Carbohydrates

The main carbohydrate in human milk is lactose. Lactose (*lact,* meaning "milk," and *ose,* meaning "sugar") is a disaccharide, consisting of two monosaccharides, galactose, and glucose. It is synthesized in the secretory cells from circulating maternal blood glucose and galactose. Approximately 4.8% of human milk is lactose, which represents about 40% of the total calories provided by human milk.[1] Nearly all of the carbohydrate in human milk is lactose, but trace amounts of other carbohydrates—glucose, galactose, glucosamines, and other nitrogen-containing oligosaccharides—are also present. Although there is a greater *amount* of carbohydrate in human milk, most of the total *calories* are from fat because carbohydrate yields approximately 4 kilocalories per gram, and fat yields 9 kilocalories per gram.

Colostrum is lower in lactose (about 5.3 g/100 ml), whereas mature milk is significantly higher (about 6.8 g/100 ml). Unlike fat, the amount of lactose varies little throughout the day. Lactose is unique in that it seems to regulate the volume of milk; that is, when less lactose is synthesized, the mother has a smaller total volume of milk and when more is synthesized, the mother has a larger total volume of milk. Therefore the *concentration* of lactose in human milk is always about the same. Furthermore, lactose dramatically increases from day 4 to day 120,[67] and therefore milk production increases as well.

The percentage of lactose in human milk differs significantly from that in cow's milk. Whereas lactose accounts for about 6.8 g/100 ml of human milk, cow's milk contains only 0.3 g/100 ml. This is important because the higher amount of lactose creates a more acid environment for the gut, thus decreasing the amount of undesirable bacteria there and improving the absorption of calcium, phosphorus, magnesium, and other elements. Lactose assists in the synthesis of the B vitamins and promotes the growth of lactobacilli, which are gram-positive normal flora of the gut that produce lactic acid from carbohydrate.

Vitamins

The vitamin content of human milk is influenced by maternal vitamin status. In general, chronically low maternal vitamin status results in low concentration of that vitamin in her milk. The Institute of Medicine Subcommittee on Nutrition[50] has carefully described the role of vitamins in human milk, so a summary is reviewed briefly here.

Fat-Soluble Vitamins. Fat-soluble vitamins include vitamins A, D, E, and K, all of which are present in human milk. These vitamins vary significantly across the course of lactation. Vitamins A, E, and K all decrease over the course of lactation. (Exogenous vitamin K, higher in colostrum, is still recommended for breastfed infants.[68]) Beta-carotene, a precursor of vitamin A, gives colostrum its characteristic yellow color. Colostrum is approximately twice as high in vitamin K concentration as mature milk.[69] Concentrations of tocopherols, the main component of vitamin E, are highest in colostrum and lower in mature milk.

Vitamin D content of human milk is currently the subject of much controversy, the controversy being whether breastfed infants get enough vitamin D. The amount of vitamin D in human milk varies dramatically and is affected by maternal intake. Mothers who severely restrict their intake of vitamin D, particularly strict vegetarians, are especially at risk for producing milk with a low vitamin D content. Although infants can synthesize vitamin D from sunlight, infants can be deficient in vitamin D,[68] and parents are sometimes hesitant to expose their infants to sunlight.

Breastfed infants can and do get rickets, particularly infants of African descent. A recent report has provoked much discussion among pediatricians and other professionals.[70] Currently, the American Academy of Pediatrics has not issued a statement on supplemental vitamin D for infants, but it is expected that one may be forthcoming.

Water-Soluble Vitamins. Water-soluble vitamins include vitamin C, thiamin, riboflavin, niacin, vitamin B_6, folate, vitamin B_{12}, biotin, and pantothenic acid. The levels of water-soluble vitamins decrease over the course of lactation, with the exception of folacin,[71] but the volume increases, so total intake remains sufficient. Vitamin B_6 has also been given to mothers who follow a reducing diet and exercise in the first 4 to 14 weeks postpartum, and infant growth does not appear to be hampered by the dieting or exercise when mothers take supplemental vitamin B_6.[72]

Minerals and Ionic Constituents

Minerals regulate body function; when minerals have a positive or negative charge, they are called ions. Minerals are often categorized as major minerals or trace minerals.

Major Minerals. The major minerals present in human milk are listed in Box 4-4. Maternal ingestion of calcium, phosphorus, and magnesium has no strong effect on the concentrations found in milk. Most of the calcium, phosphorous, and magnesium is bound to casein. Potassium, sodium, and chloride are largely unaffected by maternal nutritional status.

Trace Minerals. The trace elements are also listed in Box 4-4. Iron, copper, and zinc levels are highest in human milk immediately after birth. Concentrations of copper decline between birth and 5 months and then stabilize, whereas zinc levels continue to decline throughout lactation.[73] Maternal levels of most trace elements,[74] including zinc,[75] appear to have little or no influence on concentrations in milk.

Bioactive Factors in Human Milk

Hamosh explains that the bioactive factors in human milk have not been duplicated in artificial milk. She further explains that the bioactive factors in human milk protect against infection, affect child development, modulate immune function, and have antiinflammatory effects.[76] In a superb review, Hamosh gives a detailed explanation of the bioactive factors in human milk, including proteins, glycoconjugates and oligosaccharides, lipids, immunomodulating agents, antiinflammatory components (including vitamins, enzymes, antienzymes, nucleotides, prostaglandins, growth factors, cytokines, and cytokine receptors), cells, hormones and growth factors (most notably prolactin), and other factors. The most prominent factors are discussed here, and the reader is referred to Hamosh's work[76] for a detailed review.

Proteins

Immunoglobulins. The immunologic benefits of human milk can be best understood in the context of how the immune system works and what immunoglobulins really are. First, the body can have either *nonspecific* immunity or *specific* immunity. *Nonspecific immunity* means that resistance occurs toward threatening pathogens, but the cells exhibit a sort of "shotgun approach" by simply responding to anything that is foreign. *Specific immunity* means that the immune response is focused; it goes about attacking a certain pathogen in a certain way.

The human body has three lines of defense. The first two lines are *nonspecific*. The first line of defense consists of mechanical or chemical barriers (e.g., skin, mucosa, secretions). The second line of defense is an inflammatory response (blocking off the pathogens while a large number of immune cells arrive on the scene of the invader) or phagocytosis (ingesting and destroying the invading cells). The third line of defense involves both specific and nonspecific immunity. Nonspecific immunity includes natural killer (NK) cells. NK cells are a group of nonspecific lymphocytes that take a "shotgun" approach to killing pathogens using direct means to lyse, or break apart, the invading cells. Interferon is a nonspecific protein. Complement is a group of about 20 enzymes that can exhibit specific or nonspecific immune responses. NK cells, interferon, and complement are all present in human milk.

Specific immunity is part of the body's third line of defense. The two major classes of cells that are important are the *B lymphocytes* and *T lymphocytes* (sometimes called *B cells* and *T cells*). B cells do not attack pathogens directly but instead produce *antibodies* to be the direct attackers (antibody-mediated immunity). T cells, however, attack pathogens directly (cell-mediated immunity). Antibodies are plasma proteins of the class called *immunoglobulins*. The major immunoglobulins (abbreviated Ig) include IgA, IgG, IgM, IgD, and IgE. In serum the most abundant immunoglobulin is IgG, but in human milk the predominant immunoglobulin is sIgA. The mother produces sIgA in response to a specific organism and passes it along through her milk. Thus the newborn gradually builds immunities to most pathogens in his immediate environment.

Colostrum is really the first "inoculation." Secretory IgA antibodies are produced locally in the breast, and these antibodies amount to about 0.5 to 1 g/day throughout the course of lactation. They are directed against food proteins and microorganisms often present in the intestine.[77]

Lactoferrin. *Lactoferrin* is also a whey protein that has several infection-protection properties. Present in higher concentrations in colostrum than in mature milk, lactoferrin inhibits the growth of iron-dependent bacteria in the gastrointestinal tract. Therefore organisms that require iron, such as coliforms and yeast, are inhibited by lactoferrin. It also acts synergistically with sIgA to enhance antibacterial activity against *Escherichia coli*, but its effect diminishes when the infant is supplemented with cow's milk–based artificial milk. Lactoferrin also acts on microorganisms by blocking carbohydrate metabolism, attacking the cell wall, and binding calcium and magnesium.[78] Recent evidence suggests that lactoferrin has a fungistatic (rather than fungicidal) effect.[79]

Lysozyme. *Lysozyme* is an enzyme that destroys Enterobacteriaceae and gram-positive bacteria. It also enhances the growth of intestinal flora, namely, lactobacilli, and has antiinflammatory functions. It is higher in human milk than in cow's milk, and concentrations increase as the course of lactation progresses.

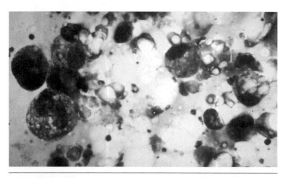

FIGURE **4-14** Stain of human milk under the microscope. *(Courtesy Becky Behre, Moscow, Idaho.)*

Cells

Human milk is dynamic; it is literally a living and life-giving substance that contains thousands of living cells per milliliter (Fig. 4-14). During the early postpartum period, most of the cells are leukocytes in the form of polymorphonuclear cells, macrophages, and lymphocytes[80]; after the first month the predominant cell type is no longer leukocytes but sloughed epithelial cells.[81] In contrast, artificial milk has no cells, as seen under the microscope in Fig. 4-15, because the cells in unpasteurized fresh bovine milk have been destroyed by heat and other processes.

Human milk contains many white blood cells (WBCs). When classified according to structure, granulocytes—having granules in the cytoplasm— include neutrophils, eosinophils, and basophils; agranulocytes include lymphocytes and mono-

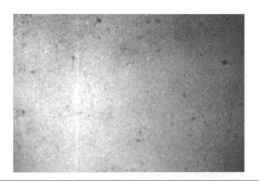

FIGURE **4-15** Stain of artificial milk under the microscope. *(Courtesy Becky Behre, Moscow, Idaho.)*

cytes. Neutrophils, lymphocytes, and monocytic macrophages (a phagocytic type of monocyte) are all present in human milk. Neutrophils are highest in colostrum, and monocytic macrophages are highest later in lactation.

Hormones and Growth Factors

Hormones and growth factors are present in human milk. Hamosh explains that hormones in human milk are structurally different from those in plasma, and therefore some specific effects may not be elicited by the serum hormone, especially for prolactin.[76]

Prolactin is the main hormone present in human milk. Looking at others' work, Hamosh points out that prolactin in milk has neuroendocrine effects that may condition responses in later life.[76] Other hormones in human milk include other pituitary hormones (growth hormone[82] and thyroid-stimulating hormone), as well as hypothalamus, thyroid, parathyroid, and steroid hormones.[76] Researchers are often able to identify the hormones in human milk, but their function in the newborn is sometimes not well-defined. Summarizing the works of others, Hamosh says that many of the hormones and growth factors "affect growth, differentiation, and functional maturation of specific organs, and they may, on ingestion by the infant, affect various aspects of development." She notes that erythropoietin, melatonin, and leptin are also present in human milk, but their function is less certain. Melatonin appears to be important for infant awareness.[76]

CONCLUSION

The mammary gland, formed when the mother herself was only an embryo, undergoes structural changes during pregnancy that enable it to produce and provide milk after giving birth. The components of human milk vary to best accommodate the needs of the infant. Breastfeeding (the act of suckling the infant) and lactation (the process of making milk) provide advantages for infant nutrition, the woman's health, social and economic conservation, and a sense of satisfaction for the mother. It is no wonder, then, that human milk and breastfeeding truly constitute the gold standard by which other methods are measured.

REFERENCES

1. Lawrence RA, Lawrence RM. *Breastfeeding: a guide for the medical profession.* 5th ed. St. Louis: Mosby; 1999.
2. Neville MC. Physiology of lactation. *Clin Perinatol* 1999;26:251-279.
3. Neville MC. Anatomy and physiology of lactation. *Pediatr Clin North Am* 2001;48:13-34.
4. Daly SE, Hartmann PE. Infant demand and milk supply. Part 2: The short-term control of milk synthesis in lactating women. *J Hum Lact* 1995;11:27-37.
5. Newton M, Newton NR. The normal course and management of lactation. *Clin Obstet Gynecol* 1962;5:44-46.
6. DeCarvalho M, Robertson S, Friedman A et al. Effect of frequent breast-feeding on early milk production and infant weight gain. *Pediatrics* 1983;72:307-311.
7. DeCarvalho M, Robertson S, Merkatz R et al. Milk intake and frequency of feeding in breast fed infants. *Early Hum Dev* 1982;7:155-163.
8. Cobo E, De Bernal MM, Gaitan E et al. Neurohypophyseal hormone release in the human. II. Experimental study during lactation. *Am J Obstet Gynecol* 1967;97:519-529.
9. Nissen E, Lilja G, Widstrom AM et al. Elevation of oxytocin levels early postpartum in women. *Acta Obstet Gynecol Scand* 1995;74:530-533.
10. McNeilly AS, Robinson IC, Houston MJ et al. Release of oxytocin and prolactin in response to suckling. *BMJ* 1983;286:257-259.
11. Lindow SW, Hendricks MS, Nugent FA et al. Morphine suppresses the oxytocin response in breast-feeding women. *Gynecol Obstet Invest* 1999;48:33-37.
12. Newton M, Newton NR. The let-down reflex in human lactation. *J Pediatr* 1948;33:698-704.
13. Ueda T, Yokoyama Y, Irahara M et al. Influence of psychological stress on suckling-induced pulsatile oxytocin release. *Obstet Gynecol* 1994;84:259-262.
14. Battin DA, Marrs RP, Fleiss PM et al. Effect of suckling on serum prolactin, luteinizing hormone, follicle-stimulating hormone, and estradiol during prolonged lactation. *Obstet Gynecol* 1985;65:785-788.
15. Neville MC, Neifert MR, editors. *Lactation: physiology, nutrition and breast-feeding.* New York: Plenum Press; 1983.
16. Hartmann PE, Trevethan P, Shelton JN. Progesterone and oestrogen and the initiation of lactation in ewes. *J Endocrinol* 1973;59:249-259.
17. Neville MC, Morton J, Umemura S. Lactogenesis. The transition from pregnancy to lactation. *Pediatr Clin North Am* 2001;48:35-52.
18. Martin RH, Glass MR, Chapman C et al. Human alpha-lactalbumin and hormonal factors in pregnancy and lactation. *Clin Endocrinol Oxf* 1980;13:223-230.
19. Neville MC, Keller R, Seacat J et al. Studies in human lactation: milk volumes in lactating women during the onset of lactation and full lactation. *Am J Clin Nutr* 1988;48:1375-1386.
20. Arthur PG, Smith M, Hartmann PE. Milk lactose, citrate, and glucose as markers of lactogenesis in normal and diabetic women. *J Pediatr Gastroenterol Nutr* 1989;9: 488-496.
21. Saint L, Smith M, Hartmann PE. The yield and nutrient content of colostrum and milk of women from giving birth to 1 month post-partum. *Br J Nutr* 1984;52:87-95.
22. Neville MC, Allen JC, Archer PC et al. Studies in human lactation: milk volume and nutrient composition during weaning and lactogenesis. *Am J Clin Nutr* 1991; 54:81-92.
23. Lewis Jones DI, Lewis Jones MS, Connolly RC et al. Sequential changes in the antimicrobial protein concentrations in human milk during lactation and its relevance to banked human milk. *Pediatr Res* 1985;19:561-565.
24. Neifert MR, McDonough SL, Neville MC. Failure of lactogenesis associated with placental retention. *Am J Obstet Gynecol* 1981;140:477-478.
25. Sozmen M. Effects of early suckling of cesarean-born babies on lactation. *Biol Neonate* 1992;62:67-68.
26. Neubauer SH, Ferris AM, Chase CG et al. Delayed lactogenesis in women with insulin dependent diabetes mellitus. *Am J Clin Nutr* 1993;58:54-60.
27. Chapman DJ, Perez-Escamilla R. Identification of risk factors for delayed onset of lactation. *J Am Diet Assoc* 1999;99:450-454.
28. Wilde CJ, Prentice A, Peaker M. Breast-feeding: matching supply with demand in human lactation. *Proc Nutr Soc* 1995;54:401-406.
29. Lonnerdal B, Forsum E, Hambraeus L. A longitudinal study of the protein, nitrogen, and lactose contents of human milk from Swedish well-nourished mothers. *Am J Clin Nutr* 1976;29:1127-1133.
30. Butte NF, Garza C, Stuff JE et al. Effect of maternal diet and body composition on lactational performance. *Am J Clin Nutr* 1984;39:296-306.
31. Dewey KG, Heinig MJ, Nommsen LA et al. Maternal versus infant factors related to breast milk intake and residual milk volume: the DARLING study. *Pediatrics* 1991;87:829-837.
32. Butte NF, Garza C, Smith EO et al. Human milk intake and growth in exclusively breast-fed infants. *J Pediatr* 1984;104:187-195.
33. Lipsman S, Dewey KG, Lonnerdal B. Breast-feeding among teenage mothers: milk composition, infant growth, and maternal dietary intake. *J Pediatr Gastroenterol Nutr* 1985;4:426-434.
34. Zuppa AA, Tornesello A, Papacci P et al. Relationship between maternal parity, basal prolactin levels and neonatal breast milk intake. *Biol Neonate* 1988;53:144-147.
35. Ingram JC, Woolridge MW, Greenwood RJ et al. Maternal predictors of early breast milk output. *Acta Paediatr* 1999;88:493-499.
36. Dewey KG, Lonnerdal B. Infant self-regulation of breast milk intake. *Acta Paediatr Scand* 1986;75:893-898.

37. Rattigan S, Ghisalberti AV, Hartmann PE. Breast-milk production in Australian women. *Br J Nutr* 1981; 45:243-249.

38. Stafford J, Villalpando S, Urquieta et al. Circadian variation and changes after a meal in volume and lipid production of human milk from rural Mexican women. *Ann Nutr Metab* 1994;38:232-237.

39. Daly SE, Owens RA, Hartmann PE. The short-term synthesis and infant-regulated removal of milk in lactating women. *Exp Physiol* 1993;78:209-220.

40. Newton N, Newton M. Psychologic aspects of lactation. *N Engl J Med* 1967;277:1179-1188.

41. Newton N. Trebly sensuous woman. *Psychol Today* 1971;98(July):68-71.

42. Masters WH, Johnson VE. *Human sexual response.* Boston: Little, Brown; 1966.

43. Avery MD, Duckett L, Frantzich CR. The experience of sexuality during breastfeeding among primiparous women. *J Midwifery Womens Health* 2000;45:227-237.

44. Signorello LB, Harlow BL, Chekos AK et al. Postpartum sexual functioning and its relationship to perineal trauma: a retrospective cohort study of primiparous women. *Am J Obstet Gynecol* 2001;184:881-888.

45. McNeilly AS. Lactational amenorrhea. *Endocrinol Metab Clin North Am* 1993;22:59-73.

46. Perez A, Labbok MH, Queenan JT. Clinical study of the lactational amenorrhoea method for family planning. *Lancet* 1992;339:968-970.

47. Hartmann PE, Kulski JK. Changes in the composition of the mammary secretion of women after abrupt termination of breast feeding. *J Physiol Lond* 1978; 275:1-11.

48. Dettwyler KA. Beauty and the breast: the cultural context of breastfeeding in the United States. In Stuart-Macadam P, Dettwyler KA, editors. *Breastfeeding: biocultural perspectives.* New York: Aldine De Gruyter; 1995.

49. Garza C, Johnson CA, Smith EO et al. Changes in the nutrient composition of human milk during gradual weaning. *Am J Clin Nutr* 1983;37:61-65.

50. Institute of Medicine. *Nutrition during lactation.* Washington, DC: National Academy Press; 1991.

51. Picciano MF. Nutrient composition of human milk. *Pediatr Clin North Am* 2001;48:53-67.

52. Bernt KM, Walker WA. Human milk as a carrier of biochemical messages. *Acta Paediatr Suppl* 1999;88:27-41.

53. Hamosh M, Bitman J. Human milk in disease: lipid composition. *Lipids* 1992;27:848-857.

54. Jensen RG, Jensen GL. Specialty lipids for infant nutrition. I: Milks and formulas. *J Pediatr Gastroenterol Nutr* 1992;15:232-245.

55. Hamosh M. Lipid metabolism in premature infants. *Biol Neonate* 1987;52(Suppl 1):50-64.

56. Xiang M, Alfven G, Blennow M et al. Long-chain polyunsaturated fatty acids in human milk and brain growth during early infancy. *Acta Paediatr* 2000;89:142-147.

57. Carlson SE. Long-chain polyunsaturated fatty acids and development of human infants. *Acta Paediatr Suppl* 1999;88:72-77.

58. Koletzko B, Agostoni C, Carlson SE et al. Long chain polyunsaturated fatty acids (LC-PUFA) and perinatal development. *Acta Paediatr* 2001;90:460-464.

59. Jensen CL, Prager TC, Zou Y et al. Effects of maternal docosahexaenoic acid supplementation on visual function and growth of breast-fed term infants. *Lipids* 1999; 34(Suppl):S225.

60. Uauy R, Mena P, Valenzuela A. Essential fatty acids as determinants of lipid requirements in infants, children and adults. *Eur J Clin Nutr* 1999;53(Suppl 1):S66-S77.

61. Uauy R, Peirano P. Breast is best: human milk is the optimal food for brain development. *Am J Clin Nutr* 1999; 70:433-434 (editorial).

62. Del Prado M, Villalpando S, Elizondo A et al. Contribution of dietary and newly formed arachidonic acid to human milk lipids in women eating a low-fat diet. *Am J Clin Nutr* 2001;74:242-247.

63. Jackson DA, Imong SM, Silprasert A et al. Circadian variation in fat concentration of breast-milk in a rural northern Thai population. *Br J Nutr* 1988;59:349-363.

64. Hall B. Uniformity of human milk. *Am J Clin Nutr* 1979;32:304-312.

65. Dorea JG, Horner MR, Bezerra VL et al. Variation in major constituents of fore- and hindmilk of Brazilian women. *J Trop Pediatr* 1982;28:303-305.

66. Heinig MJ, Nommsen LA, Peerson JM et al. Energy and protein intakes of breast-fed and formula-fed infants during the first year of life and their association with growth velocity: the DARLING study. *Am J Clin Nutr* 1993; 58:152-161.

67. Coppa GV, Gabrielli O, Pierani P et al. Changes in carbohydrate composition in human milk over 4 months of lactation. *Pediatrics* 1993;91:637-641.

68. Greer FR. Do breastfed infants need supplemental vitamins? *Pediatr Clin North Am* 2001;48:415-423.

69. von Kries R, Shearer M, McCarthy PT et al. Vitamin K1 content of maternal milk: influence of the stage of lactation, lipid composition, and vitamin K1 supplements given to the mother. *Pediatr Res* 1987;22:513-517.

70. Kreiter SR, Schwartz RP, Kirkman HN et al. Nutritional rickets in African American breast-fed infants. *J Pediatr* 2000;137:153-157.

71. Cooperman JM, Dweck HS, Newman LJ et al. The folate in human milk. *Am J Clin Nutr* 1982;36:576-580.

72. Lovelady CA, Williams JP, Garner KE et al. Effect of energy restriction and exercise on vitamin B–6 status of women during lactation. *Med Sci Sports Exerc* 2001;33:512-518.

73. Casey CE, Neville MC, Hambidge KM. Studies in human lactation: secretion of zinc, copper, and manganese in human milk. *Am J Clin Nutr* 1989;49:773-785.

74. Lonnerdal B. Regulation of mineral and trace elements in human milk: exogenous and endogenous factors. *Nutr Rev* 2000;58:223-229.

75. Feeley RM, Eitenmiller RR, Jones JB Jr et al. Copper, iron, and zinc contents of human milk at early stages of lactation. *Am J Clin Nutr* 1983;37:443-448.

76. Hamosh M. Bioactive factors in human milk. *Pediatr Clin North Am* 2001;48:69-86.

77. Hanson LA, Ahlstedt S, Andersson B et al. The immune response of the mammary gland and its significance for the neonate. *Ann Allergy* 1984;53(6 Pt 2):576-582.

78. Sanchez L, Calvo M, Brock JH. Biological role of lactoferrin. *Arch Dis Child* 1992;67:657-661.

79. Andersson Y, Lindquist S, Lagerqvist C et al. Lactoferrin is responsible for the fungistatic effect of human milk. *Early Hum Dev* 2000;59:95-105.

80. Ho FC, Wong RL, Lawton JW. Human colostral and breast milk cells. A light and electron microscopic study. *Acta Paediatr Scand* 1979;68:389-396.

81. Brooker BE. The epithelial cells and cell fragments in human milk. *Cell Tissue Res* 1980;210:321-332.

82. Hull KL, Harvey S. Growth hormone: roles in female reproduction. *J Endocrinol* 2001;168:1-23.

CHAPTER 5

Maternal Education Programs

As the Surgeon General's report stated in 1984, a major barrier to breastfeeding initiation and continuation is the lack of good consumer education.[1] Nurses, faced with providing education for parents, often feel bewildered about not only what to include in the curricula but also how and when to present the information. Effective educational programs, developed by a multidisciplinary team, are comprehensive and designed to educate the woman and her family from conception (or before) until weaning. Formal educational programs are best supported when health care professionals possess superb communication skills and integrate breastfeeding education into the larger context of parent education. The purpose of this chapter is to help the nurse refine communication approaches and develop a formal learning program for parents.

COMMUNICATIONS APPROACHES

Effective communication approaches may hinge on how three things are handled: the tone and technique used for sending and receiving messages, teaching of individuals or groups, and the choosing of an appropriate teaching/learning format.

Positive, Participative Approaches

A few general communication principles are critical when teaching about breastfeeding. Short, positive, targeted messages work best.[2,3] Conversely, long or negative messages are ineffective.

Participative learning approaches build on principles of adult education. Monologues are not particularly effective and can be perceived as patronizing. More important, adults retain more information when they are actively involved in the learning process. That is, they retain about 10% to 20% of what they hear; 20% to 30% of what they see; 30% to 50% of what they have heard, written, and repeated; but 70% to 90% of information that they apply. So, for example, mothers who listen to a "talking head" describe how to hold an infant at the breast retain only about 10% to 20% of that information, whereas they retain 70% to 90% of the information if they are actively involved in holding a doll or an infant.

Interviewing Techniques

A skilled interview may still be the best means to gather critical data from new mothers, mothers-to-be, or the families. Establishing rapport, ensuring privacy and confidentiality, explaining the process of the interview, giving the client the lead, and focusing the discussion are essential to conducting a successful interview; other sources have covered these topics in more detail.[4] Two critical components of the interview—posing thoughtful questions and responding with active listening—will help the interviewer understand women's choices and provide guidance in making those choices.

Asking Questions

There are two types of questions: closed-ended questions and open-ended questions. Closed-ended questions require a yes, no, or short-answer response. Closed-ended questions are useful for pertinent negatives (e.g., "Are you on any kind of medication?") or for obtaining specific information (e.g., "How many children do you have?"). If closed-ended questions are not used too soon in the interview, they can facilitate effective communication. For the most part, however, closed-ended questions are ineffective when interviewing the mother about breastfeeding. For example, asking, "Do you plan to breastfeed or bottle-feed?" implies that the choices are equal. Furthermore, the mother is likely to give a one-word answer to this closed-ended question, oftentimes, replying "Bottle." If she does, the interviewer is at a dead end; the one-word response makes it difficult or impossible to explore the woman's reasons for the choice.

Open-ended questions require something other than a one-word or short-answer response. Open-ended questions are useful for gathering a wide range of information (e.g., "Tell me about your last breastfeeding experience"). Open-ended questions give the mother the lead, and the interviewer must be ready to listen to what may be a rambling or tangential response. Nonetheless, the information that the mother shares is often pertinent to further assessment and clinical management. Open-ended questions are helpful because they provide the woman with a chance to give a broad response and the interviewer with an opportunity to listen. Ideally, the question should be incorporated into the context of the physical assessment or general antepartal teaching by asking, *"What do you know about breastfeeding?"* or *"What have you heard about breastfeeding?"* This approach helps the interviewer provide targeted messages that address specific questions or myths that may be barriers to making an informed decision.

Active Listening

Active listening is a way to further the conversation without taking over. One way to accomplish this is by making verbal or nonverbal responses that encourage the woman to keep talking. This might be nodding, maintaining silence, refocusing the interview, or probing. Although probing is usually used too soon, it can be effective in eliciting further information when it is done gently and at the right time. For example, "Tell me more about that" is a probing statement, but it is often successful in eliciting further information.

Reflective listening is a specific type of active listening that verifies content and acknowledges feelings. Before using reflective listening, however, one must determine whether the woman is giving a message primarily about content (a play-by-play account of action) or feelings (deep-rooted feelings about how an action or event influenced her). Reflective listening requires a highly sophisticated interpretation of what has been said, followed by a response that accurately and succinctly captures the content, the feeling, or both. Reflective listening is not parroting. Common mistakes in active listening are listed in Table 5-1.

Teaching Individuals

One-to-one teaching can be especially effective and rewarding for both the parent and the provider. With individual teaching it is easy to assess and respond to the individual's needs. One-to-one teaching is often the most effective approach for achieving individual, affective objectives such as helping a woman overcome a specific barrier in her decision to breastfeed. One-to-one situations are also satisfying for the mother because she has the educator's help in accomplishing some specific psychomotor skill, such as effectively latching her newborn onto her breast. However, one-to-one teaching is time-consuming and expensive when resources are limited.

Teaching Groups: Prenatal and Postnatal Classes

Group classes can be used anytime throughout the perinatal period. Classes should be held in a comfortable environment at times convenient for parents. The group setting has some distinct advantages. It encourages the sharing of ideas and questions. The affective aspects of learning—discussing feelings and fears about breastfeeding—are often best accomplished in this environment, where other mothers may have the same thoughts and feelings, and they frequently offer encouragement and support for difficulties or dilemmas they have successfully resolved.

Classes can help mothers interact with one another and with their partners. This interaction lays the foundation for getting a network of support from others, and it serves as a catalyst for discussion about breastfeeding between a woman and her partner. Furthermore, mothers perceive their partners to be more supportive of breastfeeding if they have attended the class.[5]

Table 5-1   COMMON MISTAKES IN ACTIVE LISTENING FEEDBACK

Example: "I'm sick and tired of getting up to breastfeed this baby twice each night."

Mistake	Description	Example
Exaggerating	Overdoing your feedback of the feelings expressed	*Sounds like you're furious!*
Adding	Adding something or expanding the scope of what was said	*Nothing seems to be going well.*
Anticipating	Leading the speaker by saying what she may express next	*You're about ready to give up breastfeeding.*
Psychoanalyzing	Guessing about unexpressed underlying motives related to problems	*You're worried that your boyfriend will feel neglected in bed.*
Minimizing	Lessening the intensity of the expressed feeling	*You seem a little displeased with night feedings.*
Subtracting	Leaving out or missing the "kernel" of what was said	*You seem pretty unhappy.*
Backtracking	Feeding back something that was said earlier or not keeping up	*You said you hadn't had a good nights rest since the baby was born.*
Echoing	Repeating almost word for word what the speaker said	*You've had it with night feeds.*
Content	Reflecting content when speaker is really talking about feelings	*Your baby consistently wakes you up twice each night to breastfeed.*
Advising	Giving advice when speaker is venting feelings	*He's probably not eating frequently enough during the day. Let's talk about . . .*
Reassuring	Without acknowledging the feeling, telling speaker that this is okay	*Babies do that a lot at first; he'll settle down in a few weeks.*
Refocusing	Getting the focus off the speaker and onto someone or something else	*Oh yes, my baby did the same thing. He drove me crazy the first few weeks and I . . .*
Persuading	Assuming the speaker will take an action that you would rather she didn't	*Yes, but you know, formula-fed babies can do that too.*

Better Responses:
When that happens night after night, you begin to wonder if there's a light at the end of the tunnel.
Waking up night after night can feel like a drag, huh?
My baby did that for the first few weeks. It gets pretty exhausting, doesn't it?

Classes are time-efficient ways to cover material for several persons rather than for just one individual at a time. This works well for addressing commonly asked questions with fairly straightforward answers that vary little or not at all among mothers. For example, nearly all mothers have concerns and questions about achieving or increasing milk supply, and basic answers can be discussed in a group setting. However, specific questions about why a mother with a particular set of circumstances does not have enough milk require one-to-one interaction.

The content for group classes can be determined by asking the group to share their needs, questions, and concerns. For example, it is helpful to open the class by asking participants why they came to the class or what they are hoping to learn. Those who are comfortable in the group setting will offer their reasons; others will remain silent. This approach for identifying teaching priorities can work well and spark discussion if individuals are comfortable with each other and the leader; it can have a distinct downside if individuals feel put "on the spot" or if a sufficient rapport has not been previously established.

Formats for Individual or Group Learning

Several formats that use participative strategies are useful when teaching parents. Group discussions are excellent; they foster camaraderie within the group and help individuals realize that other parents have the same or similar questions or concerns. Games are a great way to get parents involved. (A book of games that can be used for breastfeeding may be helpful for teaching a variety of breastfeeding topics, especially in group situations.[6]) Individual paper-and-pencil exercises can be used to help participants get in touch with their questions, feelings, or answers to questions posed by the instructor. Written responses can remain private or be shared with the woman's partner, the group, or the educator, depending on the nature of the exercise.

RESOURCES

Identifying resources for the breastfeeding mother is a critical part of an effective breastfeeding program. In addition to interactions with health care providers, resources for the mother or her family include consumer educational media and community support.

Consumer Educational Media

Media are useful for reinforcing (not introducing) the main points made during one-to-one or group teaching sessions. A template for evaluating breastfeeding media is found in Appendix B7 and should be reviewed because only the main points are included here:

- Is the media appropriate for *this* audience?
- Does the media address the main need?
- What is the cost for the media?
- Is the media biased?
- Who produces the media? (Artificial milk companies?)
- Is the information accurate and up-to-date?

- Are there strong positive messages about breastfeeding?
- Are the graphics accurate?

Books, pamphlets, and videotapes[7] are all helpful teaching aids. Appendix B lists multiple sources, and Appendix E lists how to contact the publisher or distributor. Appendix B also presents ways to summarize the content of the media and points for consideration when purchasing the materials.

When selecting or using media, some judgment is required. First, be aware that the sheer number of books, pamphlets, and other materials given to parents can be overwhelming, and parents who receive fewer materials are more likely to actually read them. Second, determine whether the parents who are receiving the media can actually read the words as described later in this chapter. Finally, avoid recommending or distributing education material produced by corporations that want to advertise and promote a product. Some of these materials have carefully targeted and often subtle messages that benefit the company, but not necessarily the mother or the newborn.

Community Support

Community support, broadly defined, could include the woman's family and friends. Because this type of support is discussed in other sections, the focus here is on locating and choosing support groups and products and services.

Community Resources: Products and Services

Multiple community resources, both in terms of personnel and material resources, are now available for breastfeeding mothers. Organizations that provide outpatient services—private physicians' offices, hospital clinics, health department clinics, Women, Infants, and Children (WIC) clinics, and home care services—are available in most communities. Other resources, such as lactation clinics staffed by nurses and/or lactation consultants, along with telephone hotlines or warm lines, are available in some communities. In addition, pharmacies, medical supply houses, and specialized stores or depots have breast pumps and related products for the breastfeeding mother. Many community resources are listed in Appendix A.

Support Programs

Ideally, women should start building a support network early in pregnancy and continue this throughout the period of lactation. The woman may need help identifying family and friends who have enjoyed breastfeeding, health care providers who are knowledgeable about breastfeeding, and availability of mother-to-mother support groups.

Support programs differ considerably. Some use a one-to-one situation with one peer counselor working with one or a few mothers. Other programs use primarily a group format, with a leader and other mothers. The La Leche League model perhaps best embodies this format; it is primarily a mother-to-mother support group. Women who wish to find a La Leche League group in their area should contact 1-800-LA-LECHE to find a local chapter.

Mother-to-mother or peer support groups, when they contain the essential characteristics for a positive impact, can be especially powerful.[8] In one study, 53% of women who had formal support groups initiated and continued breastfeeding for 6 weeks compared with only 33% of those who did not.[9] In another study an intervention group received weekly visits from trained volunteers who had had at least one positive previous breastfeeding experience; informal contact was maintained at other times. In the intervention group, 82% of mothers initiated breastfeeding, whereas only 31% did so in the control group. Continuation of breastfeeding also differed significantly among the groups; women helped by volunteers breastfed for a mean of 5.7 weeks, whereas those in the control group breastfed for a mean of only 2.5 weeks.[10] Because these studies and other studies[9-17] strongly suggest the effectiveness of the mother-to-mother support groups, mothers should be made aware of available support groups in the community, or if such groups are nonexistent, they should be established.

ESTABLISHING GOALS, OBJECTIVES, AND CONTENT

Educational programs to support breastfeeding initiation and continuation must include broad, overarching goals, and specific learning objectives. In general, the program should be developed using goals and objectives that aim to support healthy mothers and newborns. (Considerations for women and newborns with special circumstances are described in the next section.) Box 5-1 lists specific learning objectives.

Antepartum

During the antepartum period, the main goal is to have the mother choose a feeding method.[18] Approximately 50% to 75% of women choose a feeding method during the first trimester of pregnancy[19-24] or even before conception.[24,25] By the time they give birth, most women have decided on a feeding method[26]; occasionally, a mother does not choose a feeding method until after giving birth. In any of these situations, it is important to continue giving short, targeted, positive messages about breastfeeding, but not to force her to verbalize her decision. When women feel forced to verbalize a choice, they might not choose to breastfeed, and after declaring the original plan, it may be harder to later announce a different plan.[27] It is better to create a nonjudgmental environment in which the woman and her family can continue to explore the issues for as long as they need.

Feelings, Expectations, Contacts

Achieving affective objectives—those that focus on feelings, expectations, and contacts who positively influence breastfeeding—is critical during pregnancy. Once the mother can successfully achieve the objectives listed in Box 5-1, she is better able to make an informed decision and respond to the anticipatory guidance.

Feelings. As explained in Chapter 3, women have deep positive and negative emotional feelings about their feeding choices and their breasts. So it is important to help them get in touch with their own feelings and those of their significant others. There are many ways to help the woman achieve this. One way is by using reflective listening techniques, responding to the "feeling" message that she transmits when discussing the idea of feeding or her breasts. Another way is to use paper-and-

Box **5-1**   Learning Objectives for Mothers

ANTEPARTUM

Main Goal

During the antepartum period, the main goal is to have the mother make an informed choice about feeding method.[18] Before giving birth, the pregnant woman will:

Affective

- Explore her own and her significant others' feelings about infant feeding methods
- Verbalize specific attitudes, beliefs, or values that influence her feeding decision
- Gather accurate information to make an informed decision
- Experience enthusiasm and support from health care providers
- Identify women who have enjoyed breastfeeding and who could become part of a supportive network
- Develop a plan to combine breastfeeding and employment outside the home (if applicable)

Cognitive

- Describe benefits of breastfeeding for herself and her infant
- Recognize existing factors that may contraindicate breastfeeding and identify workable alternatives (if applicable)
- Recognize that common questions and concerns about breastfeeding—for both mother and infant—can be overcome with information and support
- List community resources to support breastfeeding

Psychomotor

- Demonstrate (with doll) optimal positioning for *comfortable* milk transfer

IMMEDIATE POSTPARTUM

The main goal in the immediate postpartum period (i.e., during the hospital stay) is for optimal latch-on and effective transfer of milk.[18] Before discharge from the hospital, the breastfeeding mother will be able to:

Affective

- Determine how to feed her infant (if not determined earlier)
- Express confidence in her ability to provide adequate milk for her newborn
- Reevaluate any prior decisions about breastfeeding initiation and continuation
- With partner, explore her feelings related to the transition to parenthood

Cognitive

- Recognize reassuring signs that the infant is getting enough milk
- Recognize signs and symptoms of existing or impending problems (e.g., engorgement) and verbalize when and where to seek help
- Interpret and appropriately respond to behavioral cues that reflect infant states of consciousness, hunger/satiety, and distress
- Develop strategies to maintain her energy level and identify effective stress-management techniques

Psychomotor

- Demonstrate optimal latch-on technique
- Demonstrate effective hand-expression technique

CONTINUING POSTPARTUM

Main Goal

The main goal after hospital discharge is for exclusive breastfeeding and lactation to continue uneventfully for at least 6 months. Before weaning, the breastfeeding mother will be able to:

Affective

- With health care provider, determine optimal time for introduction of solids
- Identify resources that may be helpful for postpartum adjustment

Cognitive

- List signs and symptoms of impending problems (e.g., candidiasis, mastitis)
- Identify health care professionals who could help her make an informed decision and choose an appropriate alternative if situations arise that may require temporary interruption of breastfeeding

Box 5-1   Learning Objectives for Mothers—cont'd

- Select a reliable family-planning method that minimally affects milk production and is congruent with the family's spiritual beliefs and cultural preferences
- Identity strategies to maintain lactation if she is or expects to be separated from her infant

- Describe optimal weaning techniques after she meets her breastfeeding goals

Psychomotor
- Report ability to effectively express milk (by hand and with pump)

pencil activities in group classes where she can write what she is feeling about certain issues.

Expectations. Women often have unrealistic expectations about breastfeeding. Quite possibly, they may never have seen a woman breastfeeding, and they may think that breastfeeding means completely disrobing. Similarly, they often have unrealistic expectations about how often breastfed newborns need to eat, based on their observations of older infants, or infants who are formula-fed. Talking with women about what they think the experience will be like is the key to helping them develop more realistic expectations.

Contacts and Sources of Support. Women need to begin building their support network during pregnancy. Asking the question, "Do you know anyone who has enjoyed breastfeeding?" usually serves as a good start in helping the woman identify such a network. Families and friends can be an important source of support for breastfeeding mothers.[28] Conversely, they can be counterproductive to the mother's efforts or undermine her confidence if they are misinformed or if they have a negative attitude about breastfeeding. Therefore it is helpful for the woman to identify someone in her family or among her friends who had an enjoyable breastfeeding experience because that person is most likely to be a supportive resource.

Making an Informed Choice

Sometimes a woman assumes that her everyday health habits will need to be dramatically altered or that less healthy habits preclude breastfeeding. Erroneous beliefs such as these and others shown in Box 5-2 can be deterrents to either the initiation or the continuation of breastfeeding. Such beliefs should be replaced with science-based information

Box 5-2   Breastfeeding: Making an Informed Decision

ERRONEOUS BELIEFS ABOUT BREASTFEEDING EXPERIENCE

Myth: Breastfeeding hurts.
Science: Sore nipples are not an expected consequence of breastfeeding. Nipples should not be sore when the infant is positioned correctly. Furthermore, breastfeeding is meant to be a pleasurable experience. If it were not, the human species might never have survived!
Myth: Breastfeeding will make my breasts sag.
Science: There is no support for the idea that breastfeeding will make a woman's breasts sag. Wearing a bra during pregnancy or lactation to support the ligaments of the breast, however, may be helpful.

ERRONEOUS BELIEFS ABOUT "SPECIAL" REQUIREMENTS OF BREASTFEEDING

Myth: I can't breastfeed because I didn't prepare my nipples.
Science: No special preparation is necessary.
Myth: I can't breastfeed because I don't like to drink milk.
Science: One does not need to drink milk to make milk.
Myth: I can't breastfeed because I don't want to give up [whatever food].
Science: Diet should be self-selected.

so that the expectant mother can make an informed decision.

Food and Fluid: Myths and Realities

Erroneous beliefs, expectations, and assumptions about breastfeeding are common. The nurse needs to confront misunderstandings about maternal fluid requirements, nutrient and energy needs, effects of food on the infant, and lifestyle and other issues as described in the following sections.

Fluid Requirements. Contrary to popular myth, no arbitrary number of glasses of fluid is required to maintain or enhance lactation. It is best for breastfeeding mothers to drink enough to satisfy thirst. For some, this might indeed be eight glasses of fluid, but for others it may be more or fewer. In the first few days postpartum, thirst may be intense; mothers who have had a long labor, multiple episodes of vomiting during labor, or a cesarean delivery are likely to have some degree of dehydration, and hence a high degree of thirst.

As the postpartum course progresses, the lactating mother will feel thirstier than the nonlactating mother. This can be explained by the simple concept of intake and output; milk is output from her system just as perspiration or blood loss is output. The mother often puts her infant's needs ahead of her own, however, and may neglect to drink when she is thirsty. Therefore having a glass of liquid nearby when the infant suckles is a good idea, not because it is related to the act of breastfeeding but because this is a relaxing time for the mother to sip on a drink.

Women often erroneously believe that increasing fluids will improve their milk supply. Health professionals who give this advice, which is not supported by research, do the woman a great disservice because the root of a supply problem, and hence the corrective strategy, may never be addressed. (See Chapter 7 for strategies to improve milk supply.) When women increase their fluid intake by at least 25%, no change in milk volume occurs and fluid intake and milk volume are not correlated (Fig. 5-1).[29,30] When women increase their fluid intake by 50%, milk supply increases somewhat, but not significantly.[31]

Nutrient Requirements. Nutrient requirements for the lactating woman are nearly the same as for other women. The Institute of Medicine states, "Lactating women who meet the RDA [recommended daily allowance] for energy are likely to meet the RDA for all nutrients except calcium and zinc if the nutrient density of their diets is close to the average for young U.S. women. At energy levels less than 2700 kcal/day, the nutrients for which intake is most likely to be low, relative to need, include calcium, magnesium, zinc, vitamin B_6, and folate."[32] For the most part therefore, lactating women should have a self-selected diet, choosing

Table 5-2   Foods Containing Nutrients Needed during Lactation

Nutrient Needed	Foods Rich in This Nutrient
Calcium	Milk, cheese and yogurt; fish with edible bones; tofu processed with calcium sulfate; bok choy, broccoli and kale; collard, mustard, and turnip greens; breads made with milk
Zinc	Meat, poultry, seafood, eggs, seeds, legumes, yogurt, whole grains (bioavailability from this source is variable)
Magnesium	Nuts, seeds, legumes, whole grains, green vegetables, scallops, oysters (in general, this mineral is widely distributed in food rather than concentrated in a small number of foods)
Vitamin B_6	Bananas, poultry, meat, fish, potatoes, sweet potatoes, spinach, prunes, watermelon, some legumes, fortified cereals, and nuts
Thiamine	Pork, fish, whole grains, organ meats, legumes, corn, peas, seeds, nuts, fortified cereal grain (widely distributed in foods)
Folate	Leafy vegetables, fruit, liver, green beans, fortified cereals, legumes, and whole-grain cereals

Source: Institute of Medicine. *Nutrition during lactation.* Washington, DC: National Academy Press; 1991.

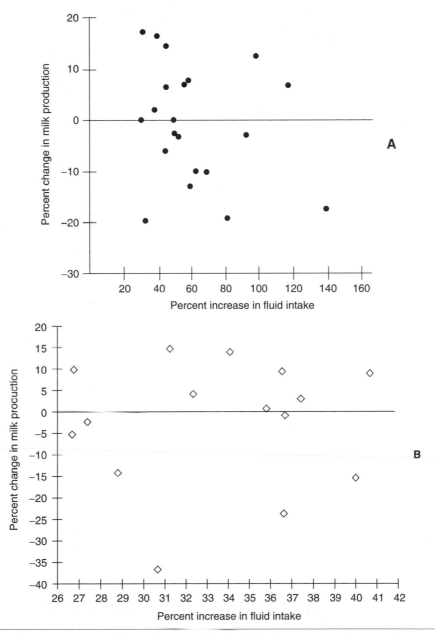

FIGURE **5-1** These scattergrams show there is no significant relationship between percentage of fluid intake and percentage change in milk production over baseline. The studies were nearly identical, except that **A** shows percentages when mothers increased their fluid intake for 3 days, whereas **B** shows percentages when mothers increased their intake over a 7-day period. (**A** *from Dusdieker LB et al.* J Pediatr *1985;106:209.* **B** *from Dusdieker LB et al.* Pediatrics *1990;86:739.)*

foods from the food pyramid shown in Fig. 5-2. Women who are at risk for low intake of calcium, magnesium, zinc, vitamin B_6, and folate should be encouraged to eat the foods listed in Table 5-2. Groups particularly at risk for nutritional deficits, namely those with restricted eating patterns (e.g.,

Table 5-3   SUGGESTED MEASURES FOR IMPROVING NUTRIENT INTAKE OF WOMEN WITH RESTRICTIVE EATING PATTERNS

Type of Restrictive Eating Pattern	Corrective Measures
Excessive restriction of food intake (i.e., ingestion of <1800 kcal of energy per day), which ordinarily leads to unsatisfactory intake of nutrients compared with the amounts needed by lactating women	Encourage increased intake of nutrient-rich foods to achieve an energy intake of at least 1800 kcal/day; if the mother insists on curbing food intake sharply, promote substitution of foods rich in vitamins, minerals, and protein for those lower in nutritive value; in individual cases, it may be advisable to recommend a balanced multivitamin-mineral supplement; discourage use of liquid weight loss diets and appetite suppressants
Complete vegetarianism (i.e., avoidance of all animal foods, including meat, fish, dairy products, and eggs)	Advise intake of a regular source of vitamin B_{12} such as special vitamin B_{12}–containing plant food products or a 2.6 µg vitamin B_{12} supplement daily
Avoidance of milk, cheese, or other calcium-rich dairy products	Encourage increased intake of other culturally appropriate dietary calcium sources, such as collard greens for blacks from the southeastern United States; provide information on the appropriate use of low-lactose dairy products if milk is being avoided because of lactose intolerance; if correction by diet cannot be achieved, it may be advisable to recommend 600 mg of elemental calcium per day taken with meals
Avoidance of vitamin D–fortified foods, such as fortified milk or cereal, combined with limited exposure to ultraviolet light	Recommend 10 µg of supplemental vitamin D per day

From *Nutrition during lactation.* Copyright 1991 by the National Academy of Sciences. Courtesy the National Academy Press, Washington, DC.

vegetarians, women who diet to lose weight, those who avoid dairy products), adolescents, and low-income women,[32] may need special counseling. These women need suggestions on how to improve nutrient intake, and Table 5-3 offers specific ideas. A woman whose counseling needs appear to be extraordinary should be referred to a registered dietitian. Recommendations for calorie intake, weight loss, exercise, and use of caffeine, alcohol, and cigarettes are listed in Box 5-3.

Energy Requirements. The energy requirements of lactating women differ little from the requirements of those who are not lactating. Nonpregnant adults need about 2200 kcal per day to maintain optimal nutrition. The pregnant woman needs about 2500 kcal per day, and the lactating woman

needs about 2700 kcal per day. This need for 2700 kcal per day translates to about 500 kcal per day more than a woman's prepregnant needs. Contrary to myths the woman may have heard, she does not need any special foods to meet this need. She may eat whatever nutritious food she would enjoy to obtain the extra 500 kcal. (For a thorough discussion of nutritional needs during pregnancy, see Worthington-Roberts and Williams[33] and the Institute of Medicine.[32])

Effects of Maternal Foods on Infant Behavior. Mothers often talk among themselves about foods they believe to be bothersome to their infants. One example is garlic. However, although infants are apparently sensitive to the odor of garlic, they actually ingest more milk when the garlic odor is pres-

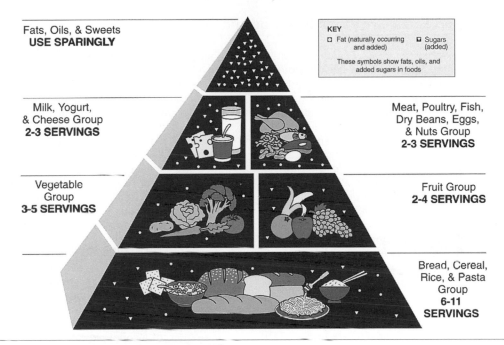

KEY
☐ Fat (naturally occurring
    and added)   ◼ Sugars
                      (added)

These symbols show fats, oils, and
added sugars in foods

Fats, Oils, & Sweets
USE SPARINGLY

Milk, Yogurt,
& Cheese Group
2-3 SERVINGS

Meat, Poultry, Fish,
Dry Beans, Eggs,
& Nuts Group
2-3 SERVINGS

Vegetable
Group
3-5 SERVINGS

Fruit Group
2-4 SERVINGS

Bread, Cereal,
Rice, & Pasta
Group
**6-11
SERVINGS**

FIGURE 5-2 Food guide pyramid. *(From US Department of Agriculture, Washington, DC.)*

ent.[34] One study suggests that cruciferous vegetables, including those listed in Box 5-4 and other "common offenders," may be associated with fussy behavior.[35] This is not meant to be a list of "don'ts" but rather one that may be helpful as a mother keeps a log of foods she has ingested.

Other reportedly "bothersome" foods are peanuts, milk, and milk products. Infants of mothers who frequently consume peanuts during pregnancy or while breastfeeding are at increased risk for developing allergies to peanuts.[36] Often, reducing or eliminating maternal consumption of peanuts is helpful for the infant. Milk and milk products have been associated with fussy behaviors in infants who are especially sensitive to these products. If the infant exhibits fussy behaviors, the mother should understand that the milk products she is ingesting may be the culprit, and the problem often disappears when she eliminates or significantly reduces dairy products from her diet. She should also understand that the infant is reacting to the foods the mother has eaten, not to her breast milk per se.

Questions about bothersome foods are commonly raised by mothers and require some practical recommendations. If a new mother asks how these or other foods may affect her infant, acknowledge that some foods may indeed bother some infants, but they may or may not have an effect on hers. Suggest that she avoid reportedly bothersome foods for the first week or so while she and the newborn are getting used to one another. This approach acknowledges that symptoms may appear but does not restrict the woman in her consumption of nutritious foods she may enjoy. Fussy infant behavior typically appears about 8 to 12 hours after the mother ingests the bothersome food and symptoms subside after 24 hours. Keeping a log is often helpful in identifying specific foods that cause problems.

Body and Body-Image Issues. Body and body-image issues commonly enter into the woman's feeding decision. Embarrassment, as discussed in Chapter 3, is a primary reason given for not breastfeeding. Other issues are many and varied, but the prominent issues appear to be exercise

Box 5-3   RECOMMENDATIONS FOR INTAKE DURING LACTATION

Note: Nutritional status of lactating women in the United States has not been thoroughly or extensively studied; therefore data are lacking on all aspects of this subject.

Normal weight loss: Advise women that the average rate of weight loss postpartum appears to be consistent with maintaining adequate milk volume. On average, lactating women who eat to appetite lose weight at the rate of 0.6 to 0.8 kg (1.3 to 1.6 lb) per month in the first 4 to 6 months of lactation, but there is wide variation in the weight loss experience of lactating women (some women gain weight during lactation). Those who continue breastfeeding beyond 4 to 6 months ordinarily continue to lose weight, but at a slower rate than during the first 4 to 6 months.

Reducing diets: If a lactating woman is overweight, a weight loss of up to 2 kg (~4.5 lb) per month is unlikely to adversely affect milk volume, but such women should be alert for any indications that the infant's appetite is not being satisfied. Rapid weight loss (>2 kg/mo after the first month postpartum) is not advisable for breastfeeding women. Because the impact of curtailing maternal energy intake during the first 2 to 3 weeks postpartum is unknown, dieting during this period is not recommended.

Weight loss and milk volume: Advise women that the average rate of weight loss postpartum (0.5 to 1.0 kg, or 1 to 2 lb, per month after the first month) appears to be consistent with maintaining adequate milk volume.

Nutritional assessments: Identify factors that predict whether women are at risk for adverse outcomes (such as low socioeconomic status) or predict a beneficial effect (such as low weight for height). Obtaining measurements of skinfold thickness or conducting laboratory tests as part of the routine assessment of the nutritional status is not recommended because of difficulties with accuracy and expense for these assessments.

Energy intake and physical activity: Advise women about energy (calorie) intake based on a thorough understanding of their level of physical activity. Intakes below 1500 kcal/day are not recommended at any time during lactation, although brief fasts (lasting less than 1 day) are unlikely to decrease milk volume. Liquid diets and weight loss medications are not recommended.

Alcohol: If alcohol is used, advise the lactating woman to limit her intake to no more than 0.5 g of alcohol per kilogram of maternal body weight per day. Intake over this level may impair the milk-ejection reflex. For a 60-kg (132-lb) woman, 0.5 g of alcohol per kilogram of body weight corresponds to approximately 2 to 2.5 oz of liquor, 8 oz of table wine, or two 12-oz cans of beer.

Cigarette smoking: Actively discourage cigarette smoking among lactating women, not only because it may reduce milk volume but also because of harmful effects on the mother and her infant.

Caffeine: Discourage intake of large quantities of coffee and other caffeine-containing beverages, including decaffeinated coffee, and foods that contain caffeine, such as chocolate.

Condensed and modified from Institute of Medicine. *Nutrition during lactation.* Washington, DC: National Academy Press; 1991.

and weight loss, and how breastfeeding affects the mother's figure.

Exercise and Weight Loss. Mothers often ask how breastfeeding will affect their postpartum weight loss and how exercise will affect their milk production and composition. These questions are difficult to answer. Typically, clinicians promise breastfeeding mothers that they will lose their pregnancy weight faster than their counterparts who choose

to bottle-feed, based on the idea that breastfeeding burns about 500 kcal per day. Some studies report that lactating women lose weight more rapidly or are less likely to retain their pregnancy weight than those who did not lactate; other studies report no difference. Conflicting results may be explained by four main factors: (1) the definition of "breastfeeding" (full, partial, token) was not always specified; (2) some study results were based on a single

Box 5-4 MATERNAL FOODS THAT MAY BE BOTHERSOME TO INFANTS

- Broccoli
- Cabbage
- Cauliflower
- Chocolate
- Cow's milk
- Onion

These foods were identified as significantly affecting fussy behavior in infants less than 4 months. The study did not specify what percentage of these infants were newborns, so whether or not the findings can be generalized to newborns is uncertain. The authors caution that this study provides "initial evidence" that these foods are associated with fussy behavior.

This study also looked at other foods often assumed to be associated with fussy behavior, including green peppers, orange juice, brussel sprouts, and dried beans, but no significant associations were seen.

Source: Lust K, Brown J, Thomas W. *J Am Dietetic Assoc* 1996;96:47-48.

measurement, whereas others used a sequential measurement of weight loss; (3) the number of months the woman lactated was not always described; and (4) the woman's exercise and lifestyle were not always considered. The latter factor has been shown to influence the amount of weight loss among lactating women.[37] These differences in methodology help explain the differences in study results.

In 1991 an extensive literature review showed no evidence that weight loss is greater for lactating mothers.[38] Subsequent studies showed no correlation between maternal weight loss and infant feeding method.[39,40] An impressive study by Dewey and her colleagues suggests that lactating women do not lose weight sooner but that they do lose a greater total number of pounds compared with nonlactating controls.[41] The amount of weight loss between the groups was similar at 1 month and beginning to show a difference at 2 months. Thereafter, a significant difference was observed in the amount of weight lost by lactating women compared with that of the nonlactating women. At 6 months, the average weight loss was 2.8 kg (6 lb) greater, and at 12 months, the average weight loss was 3.2 kg (7 lb) greater for lactating women when compared with nonlactating women. Although this result was expressed as an absolute number, similar results were obtained when the weight loss was expressed as a percentage of prepregnancy weight.

However, other studies show that weight loss occurs sooner among lactating mothers than non-lactating mothers. Kramer and colleagues studied 24 lactating women for 6 months.[42] The women kept a log of feeding episodes and were categorized as breastfeeding only, formula-feeding only, and combining breastfeeding and formula-feeding. The outcome measures included skinfold thickness, hip circumference, weight, and physical activity. Those who were breastfeeding exclusively or those who combined breastfeeding and formula-feeding lost more weight during the first month than those who were exclusively formula-feeding only. At 6 months, breastfeeding mothers had lost their prepregnancy weight, whereas the formula-only group retained a significant amount of their prepregnancy weight. Janney and colleagues conclude that lactating women are more likely to lose all of their prepregnancy weight and to lose it faster than their nonlactating cohorts.[43] This appears to be the case even if the women breastfed for 4 months or less. In short, evidence is accumulating to suggest that the woman who breastfeeds will experience a greater weight loss than her nonlactating cohorts if she breastfeeds for several months.

Until studies are conclusive, we must give reasonable answers to women who ask about the effects of lactation on weight loss. Most women express a strong desire to lose all of the weight they gained during pregnancy. Advise them that the total amount of weight gained during pregnancy—not their lactation status—may be a better predictor of whether they will be able to shed pregnancy weight[40,44] and that short intervals between pregnancies seems to contribute to weight reten-tion.[45] Help postpartum women develop regular breakfast and lunch habits because this appears to be influential in weight loss. Discourage crash diet-ing because it contributes to irritability and inabil-ity to cope with the stresses of parenthood. (In all of the previously mentioned studies, subjects did not deliberately restrict food intake.)

Postpartum exercise among lactating mothers does not seem to affect their rate of weight loss or milk composition.[46] Recreational exercise, when compared with aerobic exercise, has not been associated with improved weight loss in exclusively breastfeeding women who are 6 to 8 weeks postpar-tum.[47] Milk composition and production are large-ly unaffected by exercise. Women with infants 9 to 24 weeks old who breastfed exclusively had no dif-ference in plasma hormones, milk energy, fat, pro-tein, or lactose content when sedentary mothers were compared with those who performed aerobic exercise. Exercising subjects tended to have higher milk volume (839 vs. 776 g/day) and energy output in milk (538 vs. 494 kcal/day).[48] Another study found no significant difference in milk volume, com-position, or infant weight gain[46] for women 6 to 8 weeks postpartum. No adverse effects on milk pro-duction or composition occur when mothers exer-cise moderately four or five times a week.[49] Moderation seems to be the key because strenuous exercise does have an adverse effect. Infants may be somewhat reluctant to suckle after the mother has exercised, presumably because of the high lactic acid concentration (and resulting sour taste) in the milk after strenuous exercise.[50,51]

Lifestyle Issues and Health Habits. Understandably, women do not want to change their lifestyle or health habits in order to breast-feed. Sometimes, believing that they will have to make dramatic lifestyle changes to breastfeed, they instead choose artificial feeding.[2] Women need in-formation about plans to combine breastfeeding and employment, using substances, and other lifestyle issues to make an informed choice about initiating and continuing to breastfeed.

Plans for Returning to Paid Employment. During the prenatal period, women commonly ask about how they will combine breastfeeding with

employment. These women need to develop a plan that fits with their particular set of circumstances; a model plan is described in Chapter 14.

Substance Use. Pregnant or lactating women need to understand the effects of substances on themselves and their fetuses or newborns. Women should also understand how cigarettes, alcohol, and illicit drugs affect lactation and the breastfeed-ing infant.

Cigarettes. Mothers who smoke have a signifi-cantly decreased volume of milk.[52] It appears that smoking has an inhibitory effect on prolactin and oxytocin levels. Smoking stimulates the release of epinephrine, which inhibits oxytocin release. Women who smoke have a 30% to 50% lower basal prolactin level on days 1 and 21, but when the infant suckles, the rise in prolactin level is not significantly different between smokers and non-smokers. The smoking subjects, however, wean their infants sooner than nonsmokers.[53,54] Smoking has also been positively correlated with the incidence of colic.[55]

Although smoking is not a contraindication for breastfeeding,[56] women who smoke should be counseled to stop. If the woman cannot stop, she should be counseled to at least decrease the num-ber of cigarettes she smokes because the adverse effects vary directly with the number of cigarettes smoked. Apart from the issue of breastfeeding, mothers should be told that cigarette smoke is harmful to all in the household, especially to young children or infants.

Alcohol. Misunderstandings about the use of alco-hol during lactation abound. Many women believe that drinking alcohol will aid in the milk-ejection reflex. Although this seems to make intuitive sense, no research supports this idea. At the other end of the spectrum, some women believe that consum-ing any alcohol is prohibited during lactation, and health care providers have often reinforced this idea. However, women in cultures outside of the United States have consumed small amounts of alcohol for centuries. Furthermore, the Institute of Medicine has clearly stated that lactating women may safely consume up to 8 oz of wine or 2 cans of beer per day.[32] However, infants aged 25 to 216 days apparently are sensitive to the odor in the

CLINICAL SCENARIO

Adolescent Mother

Jody is 17 years old. She is unmarried and gave birth to a healthy baby boy after a cesarean delivery about 36 hours ago. Her physician calls you on the postpartum unit to tell you that Jody "really wants to breastfeed but thinks she can't because her breasts are asymmetrical." You are an advocate of breastfeeding, but you have some mixed feelings; this young woman has clearly told the nursing staff she wants to bottle-feed, and the infant has been artificially fed since his birth. How can you respond to the physician, who insists that he has taken care of her since she became pregnant and "knows" she wants to breastfeed? How can you come to terms with yourself, trying to respect the patient's choice (rather than promote your own agenda)? And what, if anything, do you say to Jody?

POSSIBLE STRATEGIES

Have faith in the physician's assessment that the mother "really wants" to breastfeed. Tell him that you will talk with Jody and explore her feelings about the method of feeding she has chosen and her feelings about herself and her own body.

Ponder before you act. It is always difficult to know where to draw the fine line between supporting a patient's choice and providing more information for a truly informed choice. In Jody's case, it is likely that a 17-year-old who is grappling with her own identity and role is having difficulty integrating those concepts with her sexuality, mothering in general, and her chosen method of feeding in particular.

Establish rapport and talk with Jody about how *artificial* feeding is going. It is likely that she will have some questions or concerns. Use open-ended questions at first, then move to more closed-ended questions about any negative aspects of the feeding that she has noted. For example, "Jody, I have noticed that Danny has spit up quite a bit since the beginning of my shift. Does he do this a lot?" This gives you a chance to segue into a discussion of the many inconveniences of artificial feeding for the *mother*. Focus on things that are important to her. Then ask in a nonjudgmental way about why she did not choose breastfeeding. She will probably tell you about the asymmetrical breasts. You will have the opportunity to help her explore her feelings, and she may agree to "try" breastfeeding.

OUTCOME

Jody put Danny to her breast after our conversation. Luckily, he latched on easily and suckled well. Five months after our interaction, I received a card from Jody. She said she had done everything wrong—that she had had a baby without being married and had had a cesarean delivery, which she saw as a failure. She went on to say that breastfeeding was the only thing she had done right. Danny was still breastfeeding almost exclusively, and she was soon going to return to high school.

Years elapsed, and I continued to work in perinatal nursing, although in different hospitals and different subspecialties. On one particularly busy shift, I volunteered to act as a preceptor for a new nurse because the regular preceptor was ill. The charge nurse quickly introduced me to the new nurse and assigned us to preterm twins. I was very focused on getting my assignment under way. Just as I was right in the middle of explaining how to place the ECG leads, I suddenly stopped short. My mind raced back nearly a decade and I said to the nurse, "Do you have a baby who isn't a baby any more?" The young woman grinned and said, "I wondered how long it would take you to recognize me, because I recognized you right away." The teenaged primipara with the asymmetrical breasts had married, had a second child, and eventually obtained a degree in nursing.

milk after mothers have consumed ethanol, and they consume less milk despite more frequent suckling.[57]

Illicit Drugs. Confirmation of the woman's current use of illicit drugs is central to the question of whether breastfeeding is contraindicated. Unlike the former guidelines that strictly contraindicated breastfeeding when illicit drugs were being used,[58] the newer guidelines strongly discourage but do not identify illicit drug use as a contraindication to breastfeeding. However, if the woman is only suspected of using illicit drugs or if she has used them in the past but is not using them currently, she may breastfeed.

Benefits of and Contraindications to Breastfeeding. A discussion of the benefits of breastfeeding (see Chapter 1) can be included in prenatal education, and in some cases they are a necessary component. However, just preaching the benefits of breastfeeding is never sufficient. Women who choose artificial feeding often acknowledge that breastfeeding is better for the infant and yet they choose to bottle-feed.[59] This behavior can be explained by the concept that attitudes, which are driven by affective rather than cognitive knowledge, are the best predictors of the feeding method chosen[60] (see Chapter 3). Breastfeeding is rarely contraindicated,[61] although in some cases it may need to be temporarily interrupted. Weaning or temporary interruption of breastfeeding is always a decision that is made when the mother and all of the care providers involved have a clear understanding of the risk/benefit ratio of the decision (see Chapter 13).

Anticipatory Guidance: Common Concerns and Barriers

Although individual concerns and questions of the mother and her family should be elicited and responded to with positive, short, targeted messages, a good education program should also address concerns that have been repeatedly identified in research studies over the past 20 years. Concerns of breastfeeding mothers have been categorized as those about self (maternal concerns) or infant concerns.[62]

Concerns about Self. Throughout the literature, the worry of *not having enough milk* is the most frequently expressed concern.[26,63-70] This concern is so strong that women have reported it as the primary reason for terminating breastfeeding.[62,63,69,71] Before and after delivery, mothers need reassurance that they can easily achieve and maintain an adequate milk supply to support a healthy newborn and that effective strategies are available to overcome an insufficient milk supply should it temporarily occur.

The second most frequently reported area of concern about self is *sore breasts* and/or *sore nipples*.[63,69,70,72,73] Unfortunately, the notion that pain is an expected consequence of breastfeeding is often a deterrent to choosing or continuing to breastfeed. Women need to understand that breastfeeding should not be painful; if it is, the pain can often be alleviated with good latch-on.

Other commonly expressed concerns include fatigue and feelings of being tense and overwhelmed. If antepartum mothers express fears that they are "too nervous" to breastfeed, they should be reassured that the hormones associated with breastfeeding actually promote relaxation, as described in Chapter 4. Many times, postpartum women express feelings of being exhausted and overwhelmed and simultaneously decide to give up breastfeeding. When this occurs, reflective listening techniques are effective, followed by a gentle but clear message that these feelings are associated with the transition to parenthood and/or the many responsibilities of providing care for a new infant, as discussed in Chapter 3. In short, parenting, not breastfeeding, is associated with feelings of being exhausted and overwhelmed, and artificial feedings will not necessarily alleviate the problem.

Concerns about Infants. Mothers raise many questions about care for the newborn. Most frequently, these include physical, feeding, and behavior concerns.

Physical Concerns. Physical concerns, including those related to general wellness, growth, and development, have been reported. Some of these concerns—jaundice, stooling,[74] and similar matters—are related to breastfeeding. Mothers may be unaware of growth spurts or may be unable to anticipate or recognize when they happen. These concerns are best addressed by providing anticipatory guidance and continuing support.

Feeding Concerns. "Feeding" is the most frequently cited infant concern, and mothers report it most often during the first and second week.[62] Concerns about feeding usually relate to the frequency of feeding, the need for supplementation, and techniques for feeding.

Frequency of feeding is a common concern for mothers.[69] Mothers may feel uneasy about feeding frequency because they do not understand how to read their newborn's signs of hunger and satiety or because they expect a newborn to have longer intervals between feedings, as is characteristic of an older infant.

Mothers commonly ask whether they should supplement breastfeeding with artificial milk or water.[63] There is virtually no reason to give supplemental feedings to healthy newborns because this only upsets the natural symbiosis of supply and demand. There are few medical indications for supplementing (see Chapter 8).

Mothers often ask questions about the *technique for feeding*, usually about positioning and latch-on. Both positioning and latch-on require visual assessment and one-to-one teaching. Although pamphlets or classes might be useful for other topics or questions, nothing can substitute for personal assistance with these questions. Focus teaching efforts on what the mother *does*, not what she *knows*. This difference between doing and knowing is critical! Do not assume that a mother who *knows* can immediately *do* the technique unaided.

Behavioral Concerns. When the mother expresses worries about an insufficient milk supply, she often is asking about infant *satiety*. Mothers may have highly unrealistic expectations about how long newborns can wait before eating, and they may have difficulty determining whether the infant obtained milk or just sucked at the breast. Teach mothers to recognize signs of hunger, as well as signs of satiety (see Box 7-1).

Mothers are commonly concerned about infant *sleep* and *wakefulness*.[72,75] Concerns about sleep are often intertwined with questions and concerns about satiety. Again, new parents may have unrealistic expectations; for example, it is not realistic to think that newborns can sleep through the night. After about 1 month, if an infant's last feeding was around 11 PM and the infant wakes for the next feeding at 5 AM, the mother should consider this the longest sleeping interval she can hope for at that time.

From the beginning, parents need to be aware that infants are not simply awake or asleep. Rather, there are several different states of sleep and wakefulness. Infant states of consciousness are more fully discussed in Fig. 9-2.

In the immediate postpartum period, education of both the mother and the father is essential. One study showed that the chance of exclusive breastfeeding was 6.5 times higher at 3 months among mothers who received planned, effective postpartum education.[7] When fathers are knowledgeable about breastfeeding, the length of time for exclusive breastfeeding nearly doubles.[7] Immediate postpartum education should focus on teaching parents to interpret infant behavioral cues, giving anticipatory guidance for possible situations that might arise, and achieving good latch-on and hand expression techniques, which are described in subsequent chapters.

Behavioral Cues

Expectant families should be able to simply *list* or *describe* infant behavioral cues associated with sleep-wakefulness and hunger-satiety. During the postpartum period, however, the objective is for the parents to *interpret* and appropriately *respond* to cues their own infant is exhibiting, especially as these cues relate to feeding. To do this, the nurse will need to point out what is happening (e.g., when the newborn is showing signs of satiety) until the parents can independently recognize this and other behavioral cues.

Achieving Optimal Latch-on: Signs of Milk Transfer

The greatest priority during the hospital stay is for the mother to successfully latch her newborn on and recognize signs that milk is being transferred successfully.

Anticipatory Guidance

Anticipatory guidance should anticipate possible problems without implying that they will occur. Mothers need a general idea of what could go wrong and how to get help if the situation arises. It is difficult to know just how much information to give mothers about problems that could occur during breastfeeding. On one hand, describing all possible breastfeeding problems could scare the mother into thinking that these problems are

Table 5-4 CARE MAP FOR BREASTFEEDING

	Before 24 hr	24-48 hr	48-72 hr
Alertness	Alert sometimes	Alert most times	Alert for all feedings
Alignment	Mother correctly aligns infant in 1 or 2 positions with assistance	Mother correctly aligns infant in 1 position independently; aligns infant in 2-3 positions with help	Mother correctly aligns infant for 3 positions independently
Areolar grasp	Mother verbalizes importance of *open wide*	Mother reassured by open wide	Baby consistently opens wide
Areolar compression	Mother identifies difference in sucking patterns (nonnutritive vs. nutritive sucking)	Infant exhibits long, slow, rhythmic sucks at most feedings	Infant exhibits long, slow, rhythmic sucks at all feedings
Audible swallowing	Mother verbalizes importance of audible swallowing; presence of audible swallowing	Infant audibly swallows	Infant audibly swallows
Frequency/milk supply	Feed/stimulate q2-3h	Feed/stimulate q2-3h; mother begins to recognize hunger cues	Feed/stimulate q2-3h or mother responds to hunger cues

absolute eventualities and that breastfeeding is more trouble than it is worth. On the other hand, mothers need to recognize that problems can and do happen, but that most are transient and solvable. For example, if the issue were adequate milk supply, a list of "reassuring signs" and "worrisome signs," with clear instructions that the presence of worrisome signs requires follow-up (see Chapter 7), could be provided. General signs of worrisome situations (e.g., early signs of a plugged duct or infections) can also be put on a card for mothers.

Another issue that requires anticipatory guidance is whether the presence of disease or medications contraindicates breastfeeding or requires a temporary cessation of breastfeeding. These issues are covered in Chapter 13.

It is often difficult to streamline the new mother's education while she is in the hospital. The key is to establish clear priorities. One way to do this is through a care map, as shown in Table 5-4.

Long-Term Postpartum

A teaching/learning plan should include objectives for the long term. Undoubtedly, nurses and other

providers and educators may find it difficult to agree on the content that should be included, and who bears the primary responsibility for teaching it. Studies have not identified priorities for the content, far less the timeline for a long-term teaching plan. Using clinical experience to guide the plan, clinicians may want to include signs of impending problems, family planning issues, and when to introduce solid foods.

Signs of Impending Problems

Women can experience various problems throughout the childbearing cycle. As stated previously, it is probably *not* useful to provide all the details of every problem that might ever occur because this may only add to the idea that breastfeeding is difficult or complicated or a nuisance. The focus should be on helping the woman recognize signs of impending problems so that she can get help promptly. Some problems specific to breastfeeding, such as candidiasis or mastitis, can happen in the later postpartum period, and the woman should be prepared to recognize these (see Chapter 12).

Box 5-5 PRIORITIES FOR CARE: HELPING AN ADOLESCENT MOTHER CHOOSE BREASTFEEDING

- Recognize that an adolescent mother makes decisions based on Erikson's stage of identity versus role confusion. Use strategies that help her achieve identity and minimize role confusion, for example:
  - Emphasize that she is the only one who can "mother" if she is breastfeeding.
  - Create a new paradigm: If she thinks breastfeeding will "tie her down," focus instead on how she is the "only one who can do it" and "her mother can't take over."
- Do more listening than talking and more teaching than preaching.
- Give practical suggestions to minimize embarrassment or exposure.
- Emphasize that breastfeeding is pleasurable.
- Set short-term and realistic goals; partial breastfeeding is better than no breastfeeding, and breastfeeding until she returns

to school is better than not breastfeeding at all. Remind her that breastfeeding is not an all-or-nothing choice.
- Help her tune into Station WIIFM: "What's in it for me?"
- Present breastfeeding as "cool."
- Identify any issue the adolescent mother is committed to (e.g., saving the environment, empowering women) and show how breastfeeding promotes her stance on the issue.
- Enlist peer support/approval. Refer her to support groups for adolescent mothers who breastfeed.
- Focus on body image in a positive way; for example, tell her she is more likely to be able to zip up her jeans sooner if she breastfeeds.
- Encourage foods that are high in nutrition yet are also "social" foods.

CUSTOMIZING GOALS, OBJECTIVES, AND CONTENT

Educational programs for pregnant women, such as the one previously described, are designed to fit the needs of most American women. Some women, however, have significantly different learning needs from the majority of women that we might encounter. Educational programs must be adjusted not only in terms of the content covered but also the approach used.

Adolescents

Whether in a group or an individual setting, some challenges are specific to teaching the adolescent mother. Young women at this stage in their lives are very conscious about their body image; they have scarcely outgrown their own childhood when they find themselves raising a child. Individual discussions often work well with teens because they need an individualized plan to help them succeed. On the other hand, they may do well with a group of their peers because they will relish the opportunity to talk about their decisions and circumstances. Teens are often reluctant to attend more generic group classes

(i.e., women of all age groups, rather than teens only). Box 5-5 lists some priorities to keep in mind when counseling the adolescent mother.

In the United States, only 42.8% of mothers younger than 20 years old initiate breastfeeding.[86] This statistic comes as no surprise to those of us who have been unable to convince teens that breastfeeding is not only possible, but optimal. We are more likely to motivate them to breastfeed if we modify the standard plan used with more mature mothers. First, we need to structure the content of the information so that it includes the teen mother's developmental needs. Second, we need to use a method of delivering the content that is interactive without being threatening. Theories of psychologic development provide some clues about both content and methodology that appeal to adolescents.

In 1950, psychologist Erik Erikson identified eight developmental stages that humans experience.[87] Erikson's basic premise is that one must successfully accomplish one developmental task before moving on to the next and that one outcome is optimal (e.g., trust) and the other is undesirable (mistrust). Adolescents are struggling with the task of identity versus role confusion. As educators, we must help them engage in activities or make decisions that will minimize the possibility of role confusion and promote identity.

Breastfeeding encompasses complex issues that can serve as a catalyst for the young woman coming to grips with her own identity: body image, sexuality, independence, and social acceptance. These issues can be addressed in a positive way when trying to motivate the teen to breastfeed.

Body-Image Issues

Teens are particularly preoccupied with their body image. They are concerned about the weight they have gained during pregnancy and looking fat after giving birth. Furthermore, they often believe that breastfeeding will make their breasts sag. These young women need help recognizing that breastfeeding may be a way to improve their figures. Breastfeeding most definitely helps the uterus quickly return to its prepregnant size, so the breastfeeding mother is more likely to be able to zip up her jeans before leaving the hospital. Sagging breasts should not be a problem. Although ligaments can become overstretched during pregnancy or lactation, this problem can be prevented with a supportive bra.

Some young women—and some older women as well—do not want to breastfeed because they are afraid of embarrassment[88] or exposing their breasts. Although some exposure is likely during the early days of breastfeeding, mothers can breastfeed very discreetly during the later postpartum period. Convincing teens of this may be difficult or impossible without visual aids. Show pictures or videotapes of women who are breastfeeding discreetly, and ask the class to determine which one is cuddling and breastfeeding her infant and which one is only cuddling her infant. If the young women are comfortable with each other and with the leader, you might ask for a show of hands for which is which. If not, just ask them to write their answer on a piece paper. In either case the difficulty in making the determination may spark some lively discussion when you give the answer. Then, give some practical tips on choosing clothes that permit discreet breastfeeding.

Sexuality Issues

Here in the United States, breasts are often thought of as sexual objects, not as nurturing objects. Changing this social norm will take many decades, but in the meanwhile, the task is to help individual women recognize how breastfeeding relates to their sexuality.

First, breastfeeding should be presented within the context of how the mammary glands are organs involved in completing the reproductive cycle. When beginning classes, do not discuss breastfeeding as an add-on to previous classes. Start out by saying that classes will discuss issues about the reproductive cycle, including conception, gestation, labor, birth, and lactation.

Advise young women and their partners of how breastfeeding will affect their sexual encounters. First, emphasize that they can get pregnant while breastfeeding. Second, acknowledge that some (but not all) lactating mothers may have a lower interest in sex. This is not abnormal, but it does require some self-awareness and some candid discussion between sexual partners. Third, explain that oxytocin, the same hormone that governs orgasm during coitus and contractions during labor, governs the let-down reflex. It is therefore likely that they will experience a let-down during orgasm. The spraying of milk can be minimized if the mother feeds the infant shortly before the sexual encounter, and if it does spray, using a rubber sheet under the cloth sheets cuts down on the need to do laundry.

Delivering these short pieces of advice is fairly simple and often sparks some discussion with more mature couples. Discussion is unlikely, however, when the group is composed of adolescents. Nevertheless, it is important to help these young women gain some introspection. Individual exercises may help a young woman think about issues or feelings that she is unlikely to share with the group. Consider creating a worksheet that lists the effects of lactation on one's body image or sexuality followed by four columns: pro, con, not important to me, need more information (Box 5-6). Ask the young woman to put a check mark in the "pro" column if she sees that breastfeeding presents an advantage for that activity or a check mark in the

Box 5-6   WORKSHEET FOR VALUES CLARIFICATION: HOW BREASTFEEDING MIGHT AFFECT WHAT I WANT TO DO

Issue	Pro	Con	Not Important to Me	Need More Information
Going to parties/dances Feeding my infant on the bus Participating in school sports Wearing clothes like my friends Eating foods I like Having sex Using birth control pills (Items in this column vary)				

"con" column if she considers breastfeeding a drawback for that activity. She could also select "not important" or "need more information." Then, ask her to write her questions on an index card. After you collect anonymous cards, answer each question in front of the group. Meanwhile, communicate your willingness to discuss feelings or concerns later in a one-to-one situation without making them feel it is required.

Independence Issues

Teens are especially concerned with issues of independence, and those who choose bottle-feeding often do so because they feel it is more "convenient."[89] They are afraid that breastfeeding will "tie them down." Help them recognize that parenting—not breastfeeding—ties them down. Then, point out the reverse side of this situation. The young mother who chooses bottle-feeding quickly discovers that someone else is frequently feeding her infant. Mothers readily admit that feeding is the activity most closely associated with the mothering role, but few recognize that bottle-feeding allows another person to take over that role. For teens dealing with issues of identity versus role confusion, bottle-feeding can be a real trap because others can easily usurp the role of caregiver at feeding time. With breastfeeding, others readily recognize the mother as the caregiver who feeds the infant. This is a real source of empowerment for the young mother. I worked with one young woman who experienced multiple difficulties postpartum, but she remained unshakable in her determination to breastfeed; she insisted that

breastfeeding was the only thing in her life that her mother could not take over!

Breastfeeding looks more attractive to the adolescent if she realizes that exclusive breastfeeding after returning to school or work is only one of many choices. She may choose to wean when she returns to work or school. Alternatively, she may choose to breastfeed only when she is at home with the infant (and have the caregiver provide artificial milk other times) or she may want to pump at work or school. (A few schools now have pumping rooms.) Your job is to become aware of community resources that promote breastfeeding away from home and to present breastfeeding as a choice along a continuum, not an all-or-nothing situation. Depending on the class participants, this might be a good opportunity for a small group exercise. You could identify each option, and ask the participants to divide into small groups and discuss what they perceive as the advantages and disadvantages of that particular option. Each small group can then present those advantages and disadvantages when the large group reconvenes. You can chime in with comments that clarify or expand what they have described, but giving judgmental advice is counterproductive.

Social Acceptance/Peer Pressure Issues

Teens tend to want to do what other teens are doing—or not do what other teens are not doing—because they are seeking social acceptance. Unfortunately, few mothers have seen others breastfeed, so they assume that bottle-feeding is the social norm; this is especially true for adolescent mothers.

Peer pressure and peer support are therefore pivotal. In the prenatal period, when the aim is for the mother to choose breastfeeding, using testimonials from other adolescents who have had a happy breastfeeding experience is a very effective approach. This is best accomplished with live testimonials from other teens in the group situation. If this is not an option, however, consider using a good videotape, such as *Breastfeeding: The Natural Choice* (Volume 1: *Why Breastfeed?* InJoy Productions, 1998. See Appendix B). In the postnatal period, when the aim is to continue breastfeeding, support from peers is critical for ongoing success.

Similarly, teen mothers do not want to be "different" from their peers when it comes to common activities. For example, they want to eat what their peers are eating, and they may be worried that breastfeeding will require some special diet. Assure them that their diet should be self-selected, but at the same time, steer them toward choosing socially acceptable foods that are higher in nutrition (a vegetable pizza) rather than those with empty calories (potato chips). Reserve your list of "don'ts" for alcohol and smoking issues. Quite apart from whether or not they want to breastfeed, teenagers who smoke should be assisted to quit prenatally. The alcohol question is more difficult to address. You do not want to give the impression that if they choose to breastfeed they can never have another drink. (Research has determined that a small amount of alcohol is okay while lactating.) This will only deter them from breastfeeding. In many states, however, it is illegal for teenagers to purchase alcohol, so you do not want to say it is okay to drink either. How you handle this depends on the state's legal restrictions and your rapport with the class.

When developing and presenting content, the most important thing to remember is that preaching is ineffective. Focus on presenting the facts without being judgmental or making the young mothers feel that you have forced them into a decision they would rather not make, or that they are somehow "bad" if they do not make the "right" decision. Show your respect for them; communicate that you have confidence that they will make an informed decision and that you are there to

provide the information. Similarly, show that you are willing to be one of their sources of support postpartum and help them find many other sources of support as well.

Increasing the breastfeeding initiation and continuation among adolescents continues to be a real challenge. Although helpful studies on infant-feeding attitudes and decision making among teens have been conducted, further research is needed to determine which interventions actually make a difference.[90] A summary of some important studies is shown in Table 5-5.[90]

Cesarean Delivery

In the United States, approximately 21% of newborns are born by cesarean delivery. This statistic far exceeds the *Healthy People 2000* goal of 15%.[91] Worse still, in 1999 the rate of cesarean delivery was up for the third consecutive year. Furthermore, certain situations—prolonged labor, administration of anesthesia, and lack of adequate compression of the newborn thorax by the vaginal wall—can also contribute to the breastfeeding difficulties associated with cesarean delivery. We are good at telling mothers that they can breastfeed even if they have a cesarean birth, but we must also help them find ways to overcome potential barriers to breastfeeding after a cesarean birth. First, however, we must identify these potential barriers.

Delayed or Difficult Initiation of Breastfeeding

The first breastfeeding is often delayed because hospital policies or personnel simply do not encourage early breastfeeding, especially for cesarean-born babies. Mothers should be aware that although early breastfeeding often is not encouraged, it is not forbidden. With supervision, mothers who have had general anesthesia can and should breastfeed as soon as they are awake and alert, and those who have had regional anesthesia can breastfeed even sooner to avoid the adverse effects associated with delayed initiation of breastfeeding.

Delaying breastfeeding initiation has long been known to have adverse effects, including newborn difficulties attaching to the nipple and early discon-

Table **5-5**   OVERVIEW STUDIES RELATED TO FACTORS INFLUENCING INFANT-FEEDING DECISIONS

Study	Method, Setting, and Purpose	Sample Characteristics and Data Collection	Factors Influencing Decision
Ray, Estok[120]	Descriptive; urban Midwestern private OB practice; identify information sources and timing of decision	N = 25, ages 15-19 yr, pregnant primiparae (at least 28 wk)	Eight planned to BF (2 exclusive, 6 mix breast and bottle), 14 planned to BoF. Teens' mothers provided more feeding information than any other source. Magazines were most frequent media source of information. Prenatal classes provided more information than other health care service providers. Five teens made decision before pregnancy, 11 early in pregnancy, 6 recently, and 3 undecided.
Yoos[121]	Descriptive; University of Rochester, NY; identify infant-feeding decision factors	N = 50, ages 15-19 yr (17 breast and 33 bottle); structured interviews during postpartum hospital stay	Attitudinal factors prevailed. Teens choosing to BF identified infant-oriented advantages (health, attachment), while those choosing BoF chose more self-oriented reasons (convenience, not tied down, embarrassment, can't smoke/take "pill," school/ work, breasts as sexual organs). Older versus younger chose to BF.
Joffe, Radius[122]	Descriptive-prospective Baltimore, MD; identify factors influencing infant-feeding practices	N = 254, ages 12-19 yr (69% primiparae); pregnant inner-city teens completed written scales in prenatal clinic	51% of variance in intention to BF was explained by perceived benefits of breastfeeding, a desire for more knowledge about it, were breastfed themselves, and perceived fewer barriers.
Radius, Joffe[123]	Same as 1987 study above	Same as above	Attitudinal factors *distinguished* intended BF and BoF. Perceived barriers included BF makes you run-down, makes breasts ugly, and won't lose weight. Perceived benefits included makes girl feel important, better than formula, is natural, infants love mom more, more convenient, easier to start, get more sleep, modern, and bottle-fed infants make more mess.
Neifert et al.[124]	Descriptive, portion of a randomized clinical trial. Denver, CO; examine influence of various factors on BF incidence and duration	Part of a larger survey (N = 244); focus of this report, 60 low-income primiparous BF teens (<18 yr); initial interviews following delivery in hospital	Of the larger sample of 244, 53% BF. Increasing age associated with BF. Whites more likely to choose BF than minorities (67% vs. 31%). Of the 60 participating in the focal study, 65% of teens said they chose to BF because it was good for the infant rather than because of convenience or cost factors.

Continued

Table **5-5**   Overview Studies Related to Factors Influencing Infant-Feeding Decisions—cont'd

Study	Method, Setting, and Purpose	Sample Characteristics and Data Collection	Factors Influencing Decision
Baisch, Fox, Goldberg[125]	1. To assess BF attitudes and their relationship to demographic variables and previous exposure to BF; 2. to determine actual method and relationship of attitudes to method	N = 128, ages 13-20 yr, mostly primiparae; racially mixed; pregnant teen program participants; interviewed prenatally and followed after 0birth through WIC	Teens who had been BF had more positive attitudes than those BoF. Those planning to BF in comparison to those not or uncertain of plans also had more positive attitudes. Prenatal plans were significantly related to postnatal behaviors.
Baisch, Fox, Whitten, Pajewski[126]	Descriptive; urban inner city; compare BF attitudes and practices of low-income teens and adult women	N = 274; teen sample #1 = 127, teen sample #2 = 60, adult sample = 87, mixed parity; first data collection during pregnancy and feeding method determined at hospital 6-week postpartum or checkup	BF rates for the teen samples 7% and 32%, and 35% for adult sample. Infant feeding method significantly related to prenatal intentions. BF attitudes were significantly related to setting, race, and age. Teens in group 1 had lower attitude scores, white participants had higher scores than blacks, but did not differ from Hispanics. Higher attitude scores among white adults than black adults, no difference between white and black teens. Attitudes differed significantly among those who planned to BF, planned to BoF, and those unsure of plans. BF attitudes were more positive among those who BF. Previous exposure to BF influenced attitudes positively, as did having been BF, partners being BF, and those receiving information from family versus other sources.
Lizarraga et al.[127]	Descriptive; University of California, San Diego; assess psychosocial and economic factors in BF decision	N = 64, ages 14-18 yr; primiparae; interviewed within 48 hours of delivery in hospital	72% intended to BF and 22% intended to BoF; 58% actually BF at 48 hours after birth. BF teens significantly older than BoF. BF more often married than unmarried, were BF as infants, knew more BF women, and had seen more BF models. Spanish-speaking Hispanics, followed by English-speaking Hispanics, more likely to BF than other English-speaking groups. BoF more often in school during their pregnancy and more often planned to return to work.

Robinson et al.[128]	Descriptive; Northern Louisiana; evaluate attitudinal and other decision-making factors	$N = 84$; ages 14-19 yr; interviewed postdelivery at WIC clinic	10.5% of the sample BF. BF were older than BoF. Teen's mother or infant's father had most influence on method of feeding for 30 of the sample. Boyfriend's approval of BF was significantly associated with BF. Attitudes became more positive to BF with age. Majority agreed BF healthier and disagreed that BF was old-fashioned or made infant too close. About one third thought BF was embarrassing, will cause breast disfigurement, and did not know enough about BF.
Maehr et al.[129]	Descriptive-comparative; University of California, San Diego; compare BF reasons, timing of decision, and intended duration	$N = 48$ teen (14-18 yr) and 48 adult (23-33 yr) primiparae matched by day of birth and ethnicity; mostly Hispanic; interviewed 48 hours postdelivery	Infant health benefits and attachment were major reasons for BF, with both teens and adults reporting. Major difference was teens cited naturalness and convenience less often than did adults. Teens less likely to make decision before pregnancy. No difference in intended duration.
Ineichen et al.[130]	Descriptive; London, England; Explore attitudes, timing of decisions, and infant feeding in teens	$N = 55$ teens from teen parent centers, 36 delivered and 19 pregnant	58% BF. BF were older than BoF. 50% decided late in pregnancy to BF. Reasons for BF were related to infant health and attachment and convenience/economical. Reasons for BoF included not liking BF, fear of pain, embarrassment, and on your own. Half weaned by end of first week due to sore nipples and going back to school. Social influences were greater among BF than BoF. Among pregnant teens one third intend BF, one third intend BoF, one third unsure. Advantages and disadvantages similar to delivered teens. Most had social influence, some of it hostile toward BF.

Continued

Table 5-5 OVERVIEW STUDIES RELATED TO FACTORS INFLUENCING INFANT-FEEDING DECISIONS—CONT'D

Study	Method, Setting, and Purpose	Sample Characteristics and Data Collection	Factors Influencing Decision
Wiemann et al.[131]	Descriptive; University of Texas, Galveston; identify racial/ethnic differences in and factors influential prevalence in BF decision	$N = 696$ teens under 18 yr (274 Mexican American, 212 African-American, and 210 white); interviews conducted in postpartum ward within 48 hours of delivery	55% Mexican American (MA), 45% white (W), 15% African-American (AA) BF: Health care providers most frequent source of encouragement for BF in all groups. Role models significantly fewer among AA. Perceived benefits and educational exposure associated with BF in all groups. Many BF associated factors differed by ethnic group. MA BF factors were feeding advice and preference of partner or mother, as well as early pregnancy decision. AA BF factors were living with partner, mother who BF, feeding preference of partner or HCP, and low family support. W BF factors were HCP preference, 2+ BF role models, not in WIC, received advice, and prenatal alcohol use.
Wiemann et al.[132]	Same as Wiemann et al.[131] identify characteristics of adolescent mothers who BoF who had considered BF	Same as above	Controlling for ethnicity, in comparison with those who had not considered BF, BoF who had considered BF were more likely impoverished, delayed decision till late pregnancy, had been encouraged to BF, had BoF friends, and had low support. They cited more barriers upon return to work/school and were less likely to state BoF healthier as reasons for BoF. In comparison to those who BF, they were more likely to decide alone and later in pregnancy, had fewer BF role models, fewer encouragers of BF, 2+ encouragers of BoF, and less likely to have BF a previous child.

From Wambach KA, Cole C. J Obstet Gynecol Neonatal Nurs 2000;29:282-294.
BF, Breastfeed or breastfed; *BoF*, bottle-feed or bottle-fed; *HCP*, health care provider or professional; *WIC*, Supplemental Food Program for Women, Infants, and Children.

tinuation of breastfeeding. Like mothers who have delivered vaginally, mothers who breastfeed within 12 hours of their cesarean birth are more likely to exclusively breastfeed during hospitalization.[92]

Breastfeeding initiation may be more difficult because of the possible effects of maternal anesthesia on newborn reflexes, including suckling and swallowing. So far, study results have been conflicting, so we are not sure if there is an association, much less a cause-and-effect relationship. As much as we would like to give one simple answer about the presence or absence of adverse effects of anesthesia on newborn reflexes, we cannot. Furthermore, mothers must have anesthesia for an operative delivery, and we cannot change that. We can do some things, however. We can help mothers explore ways to minimize the risk of a cesarean delivery and identify strategies to prevent or at least minimize the possible adverse effects on breastfeeding if an operative delivery occurs. Skin-to-skin contact is a great way to help the newborn begin breastfeeding, partly because the infant's sense of smell helps him or her locate and suckle the nipple. Rooming-in, if the mother feels up to it, helps her or her partner identify the early signs of hunger, which are often subtle after the mother has had anesthesia. This improves the likelihood of a good feeding.

Increased Likelihood for Quitting Early

Some early studies suggested that mothers who had cesarean births were at risk for weaning earlier than mothers who had vaginal deliveries, but other studies have not shown this relationship. This apparent discrepancy can be better understood by looking at more recent studies that used more precise definitions and methods. Early weaning is more likely when mothers have emergency cesarean deliveries, but those with planned cesarean deliveries tend to breastfeed about as long as mothers with vaginal deliveries.[93] Furthermore, weaning before 1 month is more common for mothers who had a cesarean delivery when compared with mothers who delivered vaginally, but after 1 month, there is no difference.[94]

Interestingly, several studies have shown that professional support and the mother's confidence level are more predictive of breastfeeding continuation than the mode of delivery.[95,96] The take-home message here is fairly simple: The surrounding circumstances may be more important than the operation itself, and cesarean delivery may be a deterrent for the short term, but probably has little, if any, influence on breastfeeding over the long haul. And, once the cesarean birth has occurred, clinical management should reflect attention to the modifiable factors, such as improving the woman's comfort.

Difficulty Getting Comfortable

Getting comfortable can be a real problem for mothers who have had major surgery. Sometimes, they are in such pain that they do not feel like doing anything, far less feeding a newborn. Often, women delay initiating breastfeeding or reduce the number of times they offer the breast simply because they are in pain.[97] Delayed or reduced suckling ultimately reduces maternal milk supply and infant weight gains.

Special positioning can minimize incisional discomfort.[98] During the first day or so when the mother is usually in bed, the side-lying position works well. A modified version of the side-lying position works even better. Rather than lying on one side and then rolling over onto the other, the woman can instead use an "elevator" side-lying position (see Chapter 7). If the woman is fully alert, she can first offer the upper breast with the newborn lying on a pillow to elevate the newborn to the level of her breast. When finished on that side, she can remove the pillow and offer the newborn the lower breast (i.e., the one closest to the mattress).

In a day or two, the mother will be sitting up in either the bed or the chair, so she can use a football hold to avoid having the newborn come in contact with the suture line. (A football hold works better in the chair than in the bed.) Pressure on the suture line can be minimized when the woman flexes her knees. While she is in bed, this can be accomplished by turning a bedpan upside down and putting it under her feet. When she is seated in a chair at home, a footstool works well, or if that is not available, a laundry basket, turned upside down, can also be used.

Mothers should ask for and receive adequate pain relief. Contrary to popular myth, mothers can and should have narcotic analgesics, especially during the first 48 hours or so after their surgery. For several decades, codeine, which offers significant postoperative pain relief, has been recognized as safe for breastfeeding mothers. More recently, other narcotic or synthetic-narcotic analgesics have been prescribed for pain relief, including oxycodone (Percocet) or ketorolac (Toradol). Although there are fewer studies on the effects of these medications, it appears that they are safe during lactation. The point is that unbearable pain may be a bigger threat to breastfeeding than the medication the mother ingests. Mothers need to make informed decisions, and health care providers need to consult authoritative medical sources and use good clinical judgment.

Although the operative delivery per se may not affect milk supply, pain level has been related to milk volume. Postoperative mothers who report more intense pain on a visual analog scale also have decreased milk volume.[99] In one study, postoperative mothers who had better pain relief also had more milk volume during the first 11 days.[100] Not surprisingly, their newborns made significantly better weight gains than newborns whose mothers did not have adequate pain relief.

Risk of Insufficient Neonatal Weight Gain

Recently, some very interesting studies have suggested a relationship between cesarean delivery and the "coming-in" of milk and subsequent volume of milk, both of which are regulated by hormones.

How hormones behave during the postpartum period seems to be related to the intrapartum course. Oxytocin (which governs milk ejection) and prolactin (which governs milk production) are inhibited by stress. Typically, cesarean births are preceded by labors in which the first stage is especially long or painful. This may explain why mothers who have an unscheduled cesarean birth have a delayed "coming in" of milk, whereas mothers who have a scheduled cesarean do not seem to have this problem.[101]

Quite apart from what happens in the first stage of labor, these hormones are released differently when mothers have an operative rather than spontaneous second and third stage labor. The release of oxytocin occurs more frequently and in bigger spurts after a vaginal birth as compared with a cesarean birth.[102] Levels of prolactin surge about

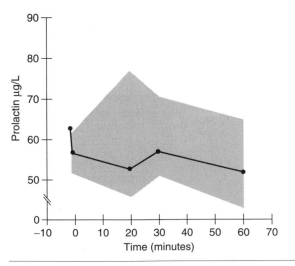
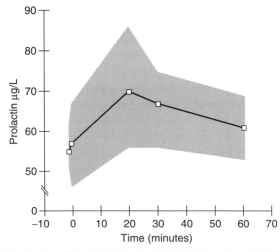

FIGURE 5-4 Levels of prolactin surge about 20 to 30 minutes after the onset of suckling when mothers have delivered spontaneously, but there is no rise after emergency cesarean delivery. The shadowed area indicates the interquartile distances (Q25-Q75). *(From Nissen E, Uvnas Moberg K, Svensson K et al. Early Hum Dev 1996;45:111.)*

20 to 30 minutes after the onset of suckling when mothers have delivered spontaneously, but the rise in prolactin levels after cesarean delivery is, by contrast, quite minimal (Fig. 5-4).

Pertinent Teaching Points

Some pertinent teaching points help mothers overcome potential breastfeeding obstacles after a cesarean birth. Tell pregnant mothers that a cesarean delivery does not preclude a successful breastfeeding experience. Emphasize how the difficulties that do arise are often more related to the time of breastfeeding initiation and the frequency of suckling. Mothers can avoid these problems by insisting on breastfeeding as soon and as often as possible.

Reassure mothers that although they may experience a delay in having their milk "come in" or have decreased milk volume for the first few days thereafter, this is not necessarily worrisome. Give parents specific directions for determining whether the infant is getting enough milk. In addition, emphasize that all mothers can improve their milk supply by holding the newborn skin-to-skin early and often.

Although not all women will choose to room-in with their newborns—particularly those who have experienced a cesarean delivery—remind them that rooming-in has clearly been linked with better breastfeeding outcomes, and urge them to at least try rooming-in, at least during the day. Emphasize that their ability to room-in and to transfer milk to the newborn will improve if they are more comfortable. Show them special positioning techniques, and encourage them to ask for medication that provides adequate pain relief.

It is especially important to note that the mother's level of confidence and commitment have consistently been related to better breastfeeding outcomes, including mothers who have had a cesarean birth. Mode of delivery is, by comparison, relatively unimportant in achieving optimal breastfeeding outcomes.

Low Literacy

The 1992 National Adult Literacy Survey (NALS) adopted the following definition of *literacy:* "Using printed and written information to function in society, to achieve one's goals, and to develop one's knowledge and potential." Literacy can be evaluated in terms of whether the person can demonstrate proficiency in prose (e.g., connected sentences), document proficiency (e.g., tables of contents, indexes, or perhaps two-dimensional graphs, simple charts), and quantitative proficiency (e.g., visual displays of quantitative information including graphs, charts, whole numbers, fractions, or percentages).

The NALS classified literacy on five levels for each of the three categories. For example, Prose literacy tasks at level 1 "require(s) the reader to locate a single piece of information that is identical to or synonymous with the information given in the question, when the text is short; or when plausible but incorrect information is either not present, or is present but located away from the correct information." Of adults in the United States, an alarming 21%, or 40 million of the 191 million, could not demonstrate proficiency beyond this category. The NALS report goes on to say, "A subgroup in this category representing roughly 4 percent of the total adult population, or about 8 million people was unable to perform even the simplest literacy tasks." More than 20% of Americans read at or below fifth-grade level. Adults who perform at or below level 1 comprise the Adult Literacy Service's primary target population—those who are sometimes referred to as *functionally illiterate.*

Approximately 19.8 million immigrants enter American communities every year, and 1.7 million of these, age 25 and older, have less than a fifth-grade education. According to the 1990 census, more than 14 million people in the United States, age 5 and older, speak English poorly or not at all. Similarly, the 1982 English Language Proficiency survey found that 37% of adults classified as illiterate do not speak English at home, and up to 86% of non-English speakers who are illiterate in English are also illiterate in their native language. These statistics suggest that a significant percentage of parents may not be able to read the printed materials they receive and that giving parents educational media written in their native language may not solve the problem.

Data from the U.S. Census Bureau[103] show that in 2000, 17.6% (44,945,452 persons) of the U.S. population spoke a language other than English at home, and 7.7% (19,526,233 persons) speak English "less than very well."[103] This information comes as no surprise to those of us who have given media to parents to augment (or even replace) teaching interactions. Furthermore, these statistics show that we can never depend solely on written instructions. The main aim for breastfeeding educators is to select or create printed materials that can be comprehended by the population who will be using them and to enhance, rather than thwart, communication efforts.

Written Materials for English-Speaking Parents

Many parents, born in the United States and able to speak English, may be unable to read the written word well enough to comprehend even the simplest of messages. Providing literature that is written at or below the fifth-grade level, a commonly used strategy, is somewhat arbitrary and will not necessarily solve the problem. Instead, create or select written materials that have fairly short sentences (prose) with relatively few tables and few, if any, decimals, fractions, or percentages. Select or create materials that use words that match the literacy levels in your community and that have been evaluated by a pilot group.

To determine literacy levels in your community, see the "State of Literacy in America," which shows the percentage of level 1 adults in each jurisdiction.[104] (A database allows you to customize the search.) Then ask a group of parents to review the materials you have chosen, and ask them simple questions about what they have just read. On an ongoing basis, evaluate if individual parents have comprehended the written materials they have received. If you ask parents if they can read the material, they may perceive your question as disrespectful, or they may be untruthful in their response because they are embarrassed. Instead, carefully watch their nonverbal behavior when they are reading the material. Those who cannot comprehend the material will have a flat affect when "reading" it, and if you ask even a simple question about

what they just read, they may be unable to answer the question or may answer only in generalities, but not specifically.

When English Is Not the Primary Spoken Language

First, we need to recognize that literacy achievements often occur with immigrants who already have a specific set of cultural values, beliefs, norms, and practices. Therefore, even if they can understand the instructions given, they will not implement instructions that are culturally unacceptable.

Especially when teaching those for whom English is not the first language, instructors need to be cautious of both the encoding and decoding of spoken messages. Although some foreign-born clients have mastered "formal" English, they may not understand colloquial phrases and slang. Similarly, instructors need to listen carefully to clients who may have strong accents that could lead to mispronunciation and cause miscommunication.

Selecting Media for Parents with Low Literacy

Perhaps one of the best strategies in using media as teaching tools is to select media that relies on images or sounds rather than on written words. Posters showing positive images of breastfeeding mothers and infants or children can be very helpful. Similarly, videotapes are helpful because they allow the viewer to rely on aural comprehension. These work only if the person has good comprehension of the spoken English language. Osborne gives some specific ideas for communication strategies for teaching adults with low literacy,[105] and the Joint Commission on Accreditation of Healthcare Organizations gives guidelines for parent education materials.

Mothers of Premature or Critically Ill Infants

Approximately 11% of infants born in the United States are born before the full term of gestation has been completed.[106] Whereas intention is the best predictor of whether women will actually breastfeed their healthy term newborns,[60] the intention to breastfeed may often be revisited when the newborn arrives early. Mothers of preterm new-borns—or those who are critically ill—need to be taught different topics, and the nurse may need to use some different approaches for teaching. The main problems for these mothers include difficulty implementing prior decisions or making new decisions, establishing lactation by mechanical means, and going home with a newborn with very special needs.

Difficulty Making and Implementing Decisions

Mothers of preterm or critically ill infants often verbalize feelings of anxiety, being overwhelmed, and being disappointed that they do not have the "perfect baby." Sometimes, mothers must integrate their feelings of joy in the birth of an infant with their feelings of grief and loss; sometimes the demise of the infant seems imminent. As a result, they often second-guess their decision to breast-feed (or other decisions) and have difficulty making even simple decisions related to infant care situations.

Use reflective listening techniques and empathize with these mothers. Be present, but not intrusive. Reassure the mother that you will support her decision and that she is in charge. Give the mother as many opportunities as possible to interact with her infant and to have updates on the infant's status when she cannot be at his bedside. Also, help the mother recognize that the preterm infant's feeding ability is, overall, a progression of events, but although the infant does sometimes "lose ground" in terms of feeding capability, these phases are normal and to be expected.[107] Emphasize to the mother (and to providers) that breast is the best method of feeding, even for the very-low-birth-weight infant[108] and that long-term breast-feeding can be accomplished.[109]

Mechanical Stimulation for Initiating and Maintaining Lactation

Establishing lactation is often a challenge for mothers if their infants cannot suckle directly at the breast. In the beginning, they find themselves able to express only a few milliliters of colostrum or milk. About 10 days after giving birth, they may find themselves expressing much, much more than the newborn could possibly consume in a day; at that point, they are likely to assume that they should not express milk so often.

While the primary purpose of mechanical stimulation is to provide milk for the newborn, an added benefit may be present. In one study, infants whose first oral feedings contained their mothers' milk tended to have a greater number of feedings; mothers also used a feeding activities calendar, which was thought to contribute to the high levels of breastfeeding among these mothers of preterm infants.[110] Mechanical stimulation is also needed to maintain lactation when the infant is unable to stimulate the mother's breast. The nurse may need to act as an advocate and a cheerleader for helping the mother keep up her efforts and to explore pharmacologic and nonpharmacologic strategies to achieve and sustain an adequate milk volume.[111]

Discharge Planning

Nurses have often espoused the idea that discharge planning should begin at admission, but somehow this idea gets lost where breastfeeding is concerned. It is not at all uncommon to find that infants have received their mother's milk through indirect means for days or weeks, when someone suddenly announces that the infant is being discharged the following day, even though he or she has never suckled at the breast. When this situation occurs, the mother receives less help with positioning and latch-on, when she actually needs more help compared with the mother of a healthy infant. A plan for transition[112] to direct feedings is found in Chapter 16, and discharge planning for the preterm infant is found in Chapter 10.

Culturally Diverse Women

Teaching programs directed at either the individual or groups must take into consideration the mother and family's cultural diversity. (See Chapters 2 and 3 that address how to assess the mother's or family's needs.) This is especially important because breastfeeding rates among minority groups in America are significantly lower than those of the mainstream majority.[86] This suggests that educational programs must be tailored to respect women in ethnic groups. Although individuals are unique, education programs should be sensitive to the beliefs, values, norms, and practices that exist in cultures other than our own.

Providing culturally sensitive care can present a true challenge for the American-born nurse who is delivering care in America, a true melting pot of ethnic, religious, and moral diversity. As products of our own culture, we therefore tend to project our own values, beliefs, norms, and practices onto others who may not embrace our culture. Perhaps the first step in providing culturally sensitive care is to become aware of our own cultural biases. We do not need to abandon our own beliefs, norms, and practices, but neither can we foist them on our clients. Instead, we need to respond in positive ways.

Before reacting or responding to parents, it is often helpful to ponder if the outcome of the cultural practice is efficacious, neutral, dysfunctional, or uncertain.[113] For example, if an Asian-American mother or family believes that eating a hot fish stew will improve her milk supply, encourage this practice. Doing so shows respect for her culture, and the outcome will be efficacious from a nutritional standpoint (she needs the fluid, high protein and minerals that the stew provides). Some situations are neutral. For example, if an African-American mother puts a paper disc onto the forehead of her newborn to stop his hiccoughs, there is no need to interfere. Although the nurse may not share in the belief that this practice is helpful, not voicing these feelings shows respect for the practice.

It becomes more difficult to react or respond appropriately to practices that are dysfunctional.

The aim of the interaction is to remain respectful but to discourage the dysfunctional practice.

Sometimes, it is difficult to respond to people who have beliefs that differ from our own or that contradict what has been proven by science. For example, many Mexican-American and Asian women believe that colostrum is dirty or bad and therefore do not begin breastfeeding at the time of birth. Preaching about the benefits of colostrum can be counterproductive because women who do not hold these beliefs may see us as the "enemy" rather than the helper in this situation. We also need to understand that the message they are trying to convey may be different from the words they are saying, as discussed in Chapter 2. In many cases the differences among members within a group are greater than the differences between groups. Therefore, when interacting with an individual mother, it is best to use the three-step process developed by Best Start. This process (Box 5-7) has been successful for over two decades with women of many ethnic backgrounds, including those who are socioeconomically disadvantaged.

It is difficult to delineate sociocultural matters from those that are psychologic or biologic. Some ethnic groups are vulnerable to health situations that have some implications for teaching. Diabetes, rickets, anemia, and lactose intolerance are common topics that may need to be included to help parents make informed choices.

The relationship between the incidence of diabetes mellitus and race is more clearly understood than the relationship between diabetes and infant feeding practices. The Native American population, however, is at especially high risk for diabetes, and the protective effect of breastfeeding against

Box 5-7 THREE-STEP PROCESS FOR INTERACTING WITH AN INDIVIDUAL MOTHER

Step 1: Ask open-ended questions. Use interviewing to elicit ideas, concerns, questions, and social norms.

Step 2: Affirm feelings. This step is the most difficult to master, particularly when the cultural feelings or biases are different from those of the interviewer.

Step 3: Educate. Education should be based on targeting the concerns uncovered in step 1, giving positive feedback, and providing small bits of information at a time.

Developed by Best Start Social Marketing, Tampa, Florida.

diabetes may be an important point to include when talking with a Native American mother about feeding methods. In Brazil, children who had been exclusively breastfed for a longer period of time were less likely to develop diabetes than children who had had a relatively early introduction to cow's milk.[114] These parents deserve to know that breastfeeding, beneficial for all infants, may be a critical factor in preventing this chronic and potentially debilitating disease from developing in their offspring.

A recent report of vitamin D deficiency among African-American infants in North Carolina involved a total of 30 breastfed infants who developed nutritional rickets.[115] (The report does not specify if these children were exclusively or partially breastfed.) The authors concluded that dark-skinned infants should be given vitamin D supplements and taken out into the sunlight more frequently. These recommendations are based on an understanding that because of the high melanin (which acts as a neutral filter and absorbs solar radiation) in their skin, dark-skinned children are at risk for vitamin D deficiency. In an accompanying editorial, Welch[116] finds it difficult to understand why there is any objection to giving vitamin

D to all children, but notes that it is currently available only in the form of drops that contain vitamins A and C as well. According to this case report and the editorial, it is likely that the American Academy of Pediatrics will soon make a recommendation about vitamin D supplementation for breastfed infants. In the meantime, it is important to realize that the case report focused only on black infants, and whether such recommendations are appropriate for other populations has not been determined.

Lactose intolerance is a health variation that may affect Asians, Africans, and Hispanics.[117] Drinking milk or consuming dairy products is not necessary for lactation, but those who abstain from consuming dairy products need to obtain calcium from alternative sources.

Diversity in Family Composition

Throughout the educational program, it is important to recognize that family composition can be widely diverse. Today's families are not necessarily made up of a woman, her husband, and their biologic children. Many women are in temporary or permanent relationships with men who may or may not be the father of their children. Stepfamilies and blended families are common, and in some

---

Box 5-8   Summary of Possible Barriers Related to Breastfeeding Attrition

(Evidence-based barriers are described in several chapters throughout this text; a condensed list of situations follows.)

INDIVIDUAL BARRIERS
- Experiencing early negative impressions of breasts or breastfeeding
- Deciding on a feeding method after the first trimester of pregnancy
- Having unresolved or ambivalent feelings/issues related to their decision
- Lacking confidence, commitment, or motivation
- Having developmental or social issues that are easily influenced by cultural norms, including adolescence

INTERPERSONAL BARRIERS
- Being unmarried and/or lacking family support

- Having a spouse or partner who has a negative attitude about breastfeeding
- Having relatives who have not breastfed or who have had a negative experience breastfeeding

SYSTEM BARRIERS
- Having little or no access to help with breastfeeding, either peer support or professional support
- Relying on help from peers, professionals, or publications that do not provide accurate information
- Giving birth in a hospital that has restrictive breastfeeding practices (e.g., delaying the first feeding)
- Living in a community (or working in an environment) that is nonsupportive of breastfeeding

RESEARCH HIGHLIGHT

No Difference in Breastfeeding Continuation Whether In-Home or Hospital-Based Follow-up

Citation: Escobar GJ, Braveman PA, Ackerson L, et al. A randomized comparison of home visits and hospital-based group follow-up visits after early postpartum discharge. *Pediatrics* 2001;108:719-727.

STUDY FOCUS

In a randomized, controlled trial, Escobar and colleagues compared home-based individual follow-up visits to hospital-based group visits in terms of clinical outcomes at 2 weeks when singleton, appropriate-for-gestational age, term newborns and their mothers, who delivered vaginally, were discharged at 48 hours after birth. A total of 1014 mother-newborn pairs were randomized into the control group (hospital-based visits, $n = 506$) or the intervention group (home-based individual visit, $n = 508$). For the 2 years preceding the study, the hospital had provided the group service where newborns and their mothers returned and a registered nurse performed an abbreviated physical examination of each infant, followed by postpartum teaching about breastfeeding and infant care issues.

RESULTS

Using data obtained from the women's report when contacted by phone at 2 weeks postpartum, investigators found no significant differences in hospital readmission, maternal depression, or continuation of breastfeeding. Maternal satisfaction and economic implications, however, were remarkably different. Significantly more mothers preferred the one-to-one contact and convenience of the in-home follow-up visit as compared with the hospital-based group follow-up. The in-home RN visit was estimated to cost $265, whereas the hospital-based RN visit cost $52 and the hospital-based pediatrician visit cost $92.

The overall breastfeeding attrition rate was 16.8% in the home-visit group, and 16.2% in the hospital-based group. Among mothers who were breastfeeding for the first time, attrition was 22% among mothers in the home-visit group and 18% in the hospital-based group. These percentages are similar to those found in previous studies.[133] Furthermore, women who had problems with breastfeeding stayed after the dismissal of the group session to ask additional questions about breastfeeding.

STRENGTHS, LIMITATION OF THE STUDY

There was no definition of breastfeeding, so it is entirely possible that women could have reported themselves as breastfeeding even if they were predominantly formula-feeding. The sample included mostly white, middle-class, well-educated women who delivered well infants by the vaginal route; therefore the results cannot be generalized to other populations. Also, women who went home substantially before 48 hours were not eligible for inclusion, so these results cannot be generalized to women who have been discharged very early.

Also, 2 weeks is a very short time, and it is possible that with a longer follow-up period, results may have differed.

CLINICAL APPLICATION

The breastfeeding attrition rate among subjects in both the control and the experimental groups signals a need for further research. In the meantime, however, nurses in clinical practice should develop programs that give mothers an opportunity to ask for and receive help to overcome their specific barriers to breastfeeding during the first 2 weeks.

cases, the infant who is being breastfed is adopted or is being breastfed by a surrogate mother. Although most Americans live with their nuclear families, others live in an extended family situation. In some families, two lesbian women are raising an infant. Any of these factors may have a direct or indirect impact on breastfeeding and should be taken into account during teaching sessions. There is no one-size-fits-all directive for how to interact with diverse families, but the main tenet of interaction is respect for the composition of the family.

EVALUATION OF EDUCATIONAL PROGRAM

Ideally, programs should be evaluated in terms of whether they have met their stated objectives. This presumes that the program has a stated objective, for example, "Cesarean delivery rate of only 15%" or "Breastfeeding initiation rate of 85%." However, it is often difficult to evaluate an *educational* program solely in terms of the program's goals because so many noneducational factors, for example, self-confidence or a supportive family, influence attainment of the goals. Unlike programs designed to achieve a specific goal for which the mother almost always consents to the provider's final decision (e.g., to deliver vaginally or by cesarean), with breastfeeding, the woman is firmly in charge of the final feeding decision. Therefore it is possible that the woman who has received excellent instruction and support decides not to initiate breastfeeding or discontinues breastfeeding early. Conversely, it is possible for a woman to receive inadequate education and support and yet breastfeed for 3 years. Perhaps a more useful evaluation is measuring whether the mother achieves *her* stated goal for breastfeeding.

Most women who initiate breastfeeding in the hospital quit before 2 weeks.[118] The reasons are many and varied, but many factors that occur during that time can make the woman vulnerable to defeat. Evidence-based barriers are described in several chapters throughout this text, but a condensed list of situations that might alert the nurse to possible barriers is in Box 5-8.

The barriers mentioned here are not necessarily all-inclusive. This list is meant to help the nurse

develop educational strategies that will include short, positive, targeted messages that address some of these potential barriers. Education for the mother and her family, although vitally important, does not completely explain her final decision to initiate or continue breastfeeding. So although it may be helpful to measure breastfeeding initiation and continuation rates, this is only one outcome that should be measured, and results might be interpreted in terms of "benchmarking" (better initiation and continuation rates this year, compared with last) rather than cause and effect.

Evaluation of programs should include other outcomes.[119] A major part of the program that requires evaluation is participant satisfaction. For example, I ask parents if the schedule for classes was convenient, if the handouts were useful, or if the content of the instruction matched the parent's perceived needs. It is critical to evaluate whether the program met the stated learning objectives.

SUMMARY

Breastfeeding education must occur within a positive, participative environment. Multiple short, positive, targeted messages throughout the perinatal cycle are more effective in helping the woman to initiate and continue breastfeeding. Whether delivered in one-to-one or group situations, optimal educational programs include a variety of formats and resources. Formal educational programs, augmented by support in the community, are best implemented when specific goals and learning objectives are established for the mother and her family. Content to support these goals and objectives during the antepartum, intrapartum and postpartum period generally includes common issues, questions, and concerns but should also include individual concerns. A customized educational program should be designed for special target audiences such as adolescent mothers, mothers who have experienced cesarean birth, mothers of preterm or critically ill infants, mothers with low literacy levels, and culturally diverse mothers and families. Evaluation of the educational program, although often elusive, is essential.

REFERENCES

1. United States Department of Health and Human Services. *Report of the Surgeon General's workshop on breastfeeding and human lactation.* Rockville, MD: Health Resources and Services Administration; 1984.

2. Gabriel A, Gabriel KR, Lawrence RA. Cultural values and biomedical knowledge: choices in infant feeding. Analysis of a survey. *Soc Sci Med* 1986;23:501-509.

3. Bryant CA, Coreil J, D'Angelo SL et al. A strategy for promoting breastfeeding among economically disadvantaged women and adolescents. *NAACOGS Clin Iss Perinat Womens Health Nurs* 1992;3:723-730.

4. Moore ML, Givens SR. *Window of opportunity.* White Plains, NY: March of Dimes Foundation; 1994.

5. Sciacca JP, Dube DA, Phipps BL et al. A breast feeding education and promotion program: effects on knowledge, attitudes, and support for breast feeding. *J Community Health* 1995;20:473-490.

6. Smith LJ. *Coach's notebook: Games and strategies for lactation education.* Boston, MA: Jones & Bartlett; 2002.

7. Susin LR, Giugliani ER, Kummer SC et al. Does parental breastfeeding knowledge increase breastfeeding rates? *Birth* 1999;26:149-156.

8. Ryan K, Beresford RA. The power of support groups: influence on infant feeding trends in New Zealand. *J Hum Lact* 1997;13:183-190.

9. Shaw E, Kaczorowski J. The effect of a peer counseling program on breastfeeding initiation and longevity in a low-income rural population. *J Hum Lact* 1999;15:19-25.

10. Schafer E, Vogel MK, Viegas S et al. Volunteer peer counselors increase breastfeeding duration among rural low-income women. *Birth* 1998;25:101-106.

11. Raisler J. Against the odds: breastfeeding experiences of low income mothers. *J Midwifery Womens Health* 2000;45:253-263.

12. Kistin N, Abramson R, Dublin P. Effect of peer counselors on breastfeeding initiation, exclusivity, and duration among low-income urban women. *J Hum Lact* 1994;10:11-15.

13. Ahluwalia IB, Tessaro I, Grummer-Strawn LM et al. Georgia's breastfeeding promotion program for low-income women. *Pediatrics* 2000;105:E85.

14. Humphreys AS, Thompson NJ, Miner KR. Intention to breastfeed in low-income pregnant women: the role of social support and previous experience. *Birth* 1998;25:169-174.

15. Arlotti JP, Cottrell BH, Lee SH et al. Breastfeeding among low-income women with and without peer support. *J Community Health Nurs* 1998;15:163-178.

16. Caulfield LE, Gross SM, Bentley ME et al. WIC-based interventions to promote breastfeeding among African-American Women in Baltimore: effects on breastfeeding initiation and continuation. *J Hum Lact* 1998;14:15-22.

17. Morrow AL, Guerrero ML, Shults J et al. Efficacy of home-based peer counselling to promote exclusive breastfeeding: a randomised controlled trial. *Lancet* 1999;353:1226-1231.

18. Biancuzzo M. Breastfeeding education for early discharge: a three-tiered approach. *J Perinat Neonatal Nurs* 1997;11:10-22.

19. Ekwo EE, Dusdieker LB, Booth BM. Factors influencing initiation of breast-feeding. *Am J Dis Child* 1983;137:375-377.

20. Hoyer S, Pokorn D. The influence of various factors on breast-feeding in Slovenia. *J Adv Nurs* 1998;27:1250-1256.

21. Mackey S, Fried PA. Infant breast and bottle feeding practices: some related factors and attitudes. *Can J Public Health* 1981;72:312-318.

22. Rousseau EH, Lescop JN, Fontaine S et al. Influence of cultural and environmental factors on breast-feeding. *Can Med Assoc J* 1982;127:701-704.

23. Hally MR, Bond J, Crawley J et al. Factors influencing the feeding of first-born infants. *Acta Paediatr Scand* 1984;73:33-39.

24. Shepherd CK, Power KG, Carter H. Examining the correspondence of breastfeeding and bottle-feeding couples' infant feeding attitudes. *J Adv Nurs* 2000;31:651-660.

25. Hally MR, Bond J, Crawley J et al. What influences a mother's choice of infant feeding method? *Nurs Times* 1984;80:65-68.

26. Holt GM, Wolkind SN. Early abandonment of breast feeding: causes and effects. *Child Care Health Dev* 1983;9:349-355.

27. Hartley BM, O'Connor ME. Evaluation of the 'Best Start' breast-feeding education program. *Arch Pediatr Adolesc Med* 1996;150:868-871.

28. Bryant CA. The impact of kin, friend and neighbor networks on infant feeding practices. Cuban, Puerto Rican and Anglo families in Florida. *Soc Sci Med* 1982;16:1757-1765.

29. Dusdieker LB, Booth BM, Stumbo PJ et al. Effect of supplemental fluids on human milk production. *J Pediatr* 1985;106:207-211.

30. Dusdieker LB, Stumbo PJ, Booth BM et al. Prolonged maternal fluid supplementation in breast-feeding. *Pediatrics* 1990;86:737-740.

31. Morse JM, Ewing G, Gamble D et al. The effect of maternal fluid intake on breast milk supply: a pilot study. *Can J Public Health* 1992;83:213-216.

32. Institute of Medicine. *Nutrition during lactation.* Washington, DC: National Academy Press; 1991.

33. Worthington-Roberts B, Williams SR. *Nutrition in pregnancy and lactation.* 6th ed. Madison, WI: Brown Benchmark; 1997.

34. Mennella JA, Beauchamp GK. Maternal diet alters the sensory qualities of human milk and the nursling's behavior. *Pediatrics* 1991;88:737-744.

35. Lust KD, Brown JE, Thomas W. Maternal intake of cruciferous vegetables and other foods and colic symptoms in exclusively breast-fed infants. *J Am Diet Assoc* 1996;96:46-48.

36. Frank L, Marian A, Visser M et al. Exposure to peanuts in utero and in infancy and the development of sensitization to peanut allergens in young children. *Pediatr Allergy Immunol* 1999;10:27-32.

37. Ohlin A, Rossner S. Factors related to body weight changes during and after pregnancy: the Stockholm pregnancy and weight development study. *Obes Res* 1996;4:271-276.

38. Johnston EM. Weight changes during pregnancy and the postpartum period. *Prog Food Nutr Sci* 1991;15:117-157.

39. Potter S, Hannum S, McFarlin B et al. Does infant feeding method influence maternal postpartum weight loss? *J Am Diet Assoc* 1991;91:441-446.

40. Schauberger CW, Rooney BL, Brimer LM. Factors that influence weight loss in the puerperium. *Obstet Gynecol* 1992;79:424-429.

41. Dewey KG, Heinig MJ, Nommsen LA. Maternal weight-loss patterns during prolonged lactation. *Am J Clin Nutr* 1993;58:162-166.

42. Kramer FM, Stunkard AJ, Marshall KA et al. Breast-feeding reduces maternal lower-body fat. *J Am Diet Assoc* 1993;93:429-433.

43. Janney CA, Zhang D, Sowers M. Lactation and weight retention. *Am J Clin Nutr* 1997;66:1116-1124.

44. Ohlin A, Rossner S. Maternal body weight development after pregnancy. *Int J Obes* 1990;14:159-173.

45. Sowers M, Zhang D, Janney CA. Interpregnancy weight retention patterning in women who breastfed. *J Matern Fetal Med* 1998;7:89-94.

46. Prentice A. Should lactating women exercise? *Nutr Rev* 1994;52:358-360.

47. Lovelady CA, Nommsen-Rivers LA, McCrory MA et al. Effects of exercise on plasma lipids and metabolism of lactating women. *Med Sci Sports Exerc* 1995;27:22-28.

48. Lovelady CA, Lonnerdal B, Dewey KG. Lactation performance of exercising women. *Am J Clin Nutr* 1990;52:103-109.

49. Dewey KG, Lovelady CA, Nommsen-Rivers LA et al. A randomized study of the effects of aerobic exercise by lactating women on breast-milk volume and composition. *N Engl J Med* 1994;330:449-453.

50. Wallace JP, Inbar G, Ernsthausen K. Infant acceptance of postexercise breast milk. *Pediatrics* 1992;89:1245-1247.

51. Dewey KG, Lovelady C. Exercise and breast-feeding: a different experience. *Pediatrics* 1993;91:514-515 (letter).

52. Vio F, Salazar G, Infante C. Smoking during pregnancy and lactation and its effects on breast-milk volume. *Am J Clin Nutr* 1991;54:1011-1016.

53. Andersen AN, Lund-Andersen C, Larsen JF et al. Suppressed prolactin but normal neurophysin levels in cigarette smoking breast-feeding women. *Clin Endocrinol Oxf* 1982;17:363-368.

54. Hill PD, Aldag JC. Smoking and breastfeeding status. *Res Nurs Health* 1996;19:125-132.

55. Matheson I, Rivrud GN. The effect of smoking on lactation and infantile colic. *JAMA* 1989;261:42-43.

56. American Academy of Pediatrics Committee on Drugs. Transfer of drugs and other chemicals into human milk. *Pediatrics* 2001;108:776-789.

57. Mennella JA, Beauchamp GK. The transfer of alcohol to human milk. Effects on flavor and the infant's behavior. *N Engl J Med* 1991;325:981-985.

58. American Academy of Pediatrics Committee on Drugs. The transfer of drugs and other chemicals into human milk. *Pediatrics* 1994;93:137-150.

59. Dix DN. Why women decide not to breastfeed. *Birth* 1991;18:222-225.

60. Losch M, Dungy CI, Russell D et al. Impact of attitudes on maternal decisions regarding infant feeding. *J Pediatr* 1995;126:507-514.

61. Lawrence RA. *A review of the medical benefits and contraindications to breastfeeding in the United States (maternal and child health technical information bulletin)*. Arlington, VA: National Center for Education in Maternal and Child Health; 1997.

62. Graef P, McGhee K, Rozycki J et al. Postpartum concerns of breastfeeding mothers. *J Nurse Midwifery* 1988;33:62-66.

63. Mogan J. A study of mothers' breastfeeding concerns. *Birth* 1986;13:104-108.

64. Bevan ML, Mosley D, Solimano GR. Factors influencing breast feeding in an urban WIC program. *J Am Diet Assoc* 1984;84:563-567.

65. Gunn TR. The incidence of breast feeding and reasons for weaning. *N Z Med J* 1984;97:360-363.

66. Hill PD. Effects of education on breastfeeding success. *Matern Child Nurs J* 1987;16:145-156.

67. Hill PD, Humenick SS. Insufficient milk supply. *Image J Nurs Sch* 1989;21:145-148.

68. Quickfall J. Can the duration of breast feeding be extended. *Health Visit* 1979;52:223-225.

69. Chapman JJ, Macey MJ, Keegan M et al. Concerns of breast-feeding mothers from birth to 4 months. *Nurs Res* 1985;34:374-377.

70. Bergman V, Larsson S, Lomberg H et al. A survey of Swedish mothers' view on breastfeeding and experiences of social and professional support. *Scand J Caring Sci* 1993;7:47-52.

71. Quinn AO, Koepsell D, Haller S. Breastfeeding incidence after early discharge and factors influencing breastfeeding cessation. *J Obstet Gynecol Neonatal Nurs* 1997;26:289-294.

72. Beske EJ, Garvis MS. Important factors in breast-feeding success. *MCN Am J Matern Child Nurs* 1982;7:174-179.

73. Graffy JP. Mothers' attitudes to and experience of breast feeding: a primary care study. *Br J Gen Pract* 1992;42:61-64.

74. Morley R, Abbott RA, Lucas A. Infant feeding and maternal concerns about stool hardness. *Child Care Health Dev* 1997;23:475-478.

75. Knopp RH, Walden CE, Wahl PW et al. Effect of postpartum lactation on lipoprotein lipids and apoproteins. *J Clin Endocrinol Metab* 1985;60:542-547.

76. American College of Obstetricians and Gynecologists. *ACOG educational bulletin #258 breastfeeding: maternal and infant aspects*. Washington, DC: American College of Obstetricians and Gynecologists; 2000.

77. Labbok MH, Stallings RY, Shah F et al. Ovulation method use during breastfeeding: is there increased risk of unplanned pregnancy? *Am J Obstet Gynecol* 1991; 165:2031-2036.

78. Perez A, Labbok MH, Queenan JT. Clinical study of the lactational amenorrhoea method for family planning. *Lancet* 1992;339:968-970.

79. Anonymous. Breastfeeding as a family planning method. *Lancet* 1988;2:1204-1205.

80. Labbok MH, Hight-Laukaran V, Peterson AE et al. Multicenter study of the lactational amenorrhea method (LAM): I. Efficacy, duration, and implications for clinical application. *Contraception* 1997;55:327-336.

81. The World Health Organization Multinational Study of Breast-feeding and Lactational Amenorrhea. II. Factors associated with the length of amenorrhea. World Health Organization Task Force on Methods for the Natural Regulation of Fertility. *Fertil Steril* 1998;70:461-471.

82. The World Health Organization Multinational Study of Breast-feeding and Lactational Amenorrhea. III. Pregnancy during breast-feeding. World Health Organization Task Force on Methods for the Natural Regulation of Fertility. *Fertil Steril* 1999;72:431-440.

83. Hight-Laukaran V, Labbok MH, Peterson AE et al. Multicenter study of the lactational amenorrhea method (LAM): II. Acceptability, utility, and policy implications. *Contraception* 1997;55:337-346.

84. Peterson AE, Perez-Escamilla R, Labbok MH et al. Multicenter study of the lactational amenorrhea method (LAM): III. effectiveness, duration, and satisfaction with reduced client-provider contact. *Contraception* 2000; 62:221-230.

85. World Health Organization: Acceptable medical reasons for supplementation. Baby-Friendly Hospital Initiative: Part II: Hospital-level implementation. *Promoting breastfeeding in health facilities a short course for administrators and policy-makers*, Geneva: World Health Organization; 1996.

86. Ryan AS. The resurgence of breastfeeding in the United States. *Pediatrics* 1997;99:E12.

87. Erikson EH. Eight ages of man. *Childhood and society*. New York: Norton; 1969.

88. Hannon PR, Willis SK, Bishop-Townsend V et al. African-American and Latina adolescent mothers' infant feeding decisions and breastfeeding practices: a qualitative study. *J Adolesc Health* 2000;26:399-407.

89. Wiemann CM, DuBois JC, Berenson AB. Strategies to promote breast-feeding among adolescent mothers. *Arch Pediatr Adolesc Med* 1998;152:862-869.

90. Wambach KA, Cole C. Breastfeeding and adolescents. *J Obstet Gynecol Neonatal Nurs* 2000;29:282-294.

91. United States Department of Health and Human Services. *Healthy people 2000: national health promotion and disease prevention objectives*. Washington, DC: Government Printing Office; 1991.

92. Mathur GP, Pandey PK, Mathur S et al. Breastfeeding in babies delivered by cesarean section. *Indian Pediatr* 1993;30:1285-1290.

93. Victora CG, Huttly SR, Barros FC et al. Caesarean section and duration of breast feeding among Brazilians. *Arch Dis Child* 1990;65:632-634.

94. Perez-Escamilla R, Maulen Radovan I, Dewey KG. The association between cesarean delivery and breast-feeding outcomes among Mexican women. *Am J Public Health* 1996;86:832-836.

95. Kearney MH, Cronenwett LR, Reinhardt R. Cesarean delivery and breastfeeding outcomes. *Birth* 1990;17:97-103.

96. Tamminen T, Verronen P, Saarikoski S et al. The influence of perinatal factors on breast feeding. *Acta Paediatr Scand* 1983;72:9-12.

97. Kapil U, Kaul S, Vohra G et al. Breast feeding practices amongst mothers having undergone cesarean section. *Indian Pediatr* 1992;29:222-224.

98. Frantz KB, Kalmen BA. Breastfeeding works for cesareans, too. *RN* 1979;42:39-47.

99. Hirose M, Hara Y, Hosokawa T et al. The effect of postoperative analgesia with continuous epidural bupivacaine after cesarean section on the amount of breast feeding and infant weight gain. *Anesth-Analg* 1996;82:1166-1169.

100. Hirose M, Hosokawa T, Tanaka Y. Extradural buprenorphine suppresses breast feeding after caesarean section. *Br J Anaesth* 1997;79:120-121.

101. Chapman DJ, Perez-Escamilla R. Identification of risk factors for delayed onset of lactation. *J Am Diet Assoc* 1999;99:450-454.

102. Nissen E, Uvnas Moberg K, Svensson K et al. Different patterns of oxytocin, prolactin but not cortisol release during breastfeeding in women delivered by caesarean section or by the vaginal route. *Early Hum Dev* 1996;45:103-118.

103. United States Census Bureau. 2001. Available at http://factfinder.census.gov.

104. National Institute for Literacy. The state of literacy in America. Estimates at the local, state and national levels. Washington, DC: National Institute for Literacy; 1998. Available at http://www.nifl.gov.

105. Osborne H. *Overcoming communication barriers in patient education*. Gaithersburg MD: Aspen; 2001.

106. March of Dimes, 2000. Available at http://www.modimes.org/HealthLibrary2/InfantHealthStatistics/stats.htm#Prematurity and Low Birthweight.

107. Wheeler JL, Johnson M, Collie L et al. Promoting breastfeeding in the neonatal intensive care unit. *Breastfeed Rev* 1999;7:15-18.

108. Lawrence RA. Breastfeeding support benefits very low-birth-weight infants. *Arch Pediatr Adolesc Med* 2001;155:543-544.

109. Pinelli J, Atkinson SA, Saigal S. Randomized trial of breastfeeding support in very low-birth-weight infants. *Arch Pediatr Adolesc Med* 2001;155:548-553.

110. Wheeler J, Chapman C, Johnson M et al. Feeding outcomes and influences within the neonatal unit. *Int J Nurs Pract* 2000;6:196-206.

111. Meier PP. Breastfeeding in the special care nursery. Prematures and infants with medical problems. *Pediatr Clin North Am* 2001;48:425-442.

112. Bell EH, Geyer J, Jones L. A structured intervention improves breastfeeding success for ill or preterm infants. *MCN Am J Matern Child Nurs* 1995;20:309-314.

113. Giger JN, Davidhizar RE. *Transcultural nursing*. 3rd ed. St. Louis: Mosby; 1999.

114. Gimeno SG, de Souza JM. IDDM and milk consumption. A case-control study in Sao Paulo, Brazil. *Diabetes Care* 1997;20:1256-1260.

115. Kreiter SR, Schwartz RP, Kirkman HN et al. Nutritional rickets in African American breast-fed infants. *J Pediatr* 2000;137:153-157.

116. Welch TR, Bergstrom WH, Tsang RC. Vitamin D-deficient rickets: the reemergence of a once-conquered disease. *J Pediatr* 2000;137:143-145.

117. Scrimshaw NS, Murray EB. The acceptability of milk and milk products in populations with a high prevalence of lactose intolerance. *Am J Clin Nutr* 1988;48:1079-1159.

118. Ertem IO, Votto N, Leventhal JM. The timing and predictors of the early termination of breastfeeding. *Pediatrics* 2001;107:543-548.

119. Biancuzzo M. Developing a poster about a clinical innovation. Part I: Ideas and abstract. *Clin Nurse Spec* 1994;8:153-155, 172.

120. Ray DV, Estok PJ. Infant feeding choice and the adolescent mother. *JOGN Nurs* 1984;13:115-118.

121. Yoos L. Developmental issues and the choice of feeding method of adolescent mothers. *J Obstet Gynecol Neonatal Nurs* 1985;14:68-72.

122. Joffe A, Radius SM. Breast versus bottle: correlates of adolescent mothers' infant-feeding practices. *Pediatrics* 1987;79:689-695.

123. Radius SM, Joffe A. Understanding adolescent mothers' feelings about breast-feeding. A study of perceived benefits and barriers. *J Adolesc Health Care* 1988;9:156-160.

124. Neifert M, Gray J, Gary N et al. Effect of two types of hospital feeding gift packs on duration of breast-feeding among adolescent mothers. *J Adolesc Health Care* 1988;9:411-413.

125. Baisch MJ, Fox RA, Goldberg BD. Breast-feeding attitudes and practices among adolescents. *J Adolesc Health Care* 1989;10:41-45.

126. Baisch MJ, Fox RA, Whitten E et al. Comparison of breast-feeding attitudes and practices: low-income adolescents and adult women. *Matern Child Nurs J* 1989;18:61-71.

127. Lizarraga JL, Maehr JC, Wingard DL et al. Psychosocial and economic factors associated with infant feeding intentions of adolescent mothers. *J Adolesc Health* 1992;13:676-681.

128. Robinson JB, Hunt AE, Pope J et al. Attitudes toward infant feeding among adolescent mothers from a WIC population in northern Louisiana. *J Am Diet Assoc* 1993;93:1311-1313.

129. Maehr JC, Lizarraga JL, Wingard DL et al. A comparative study of adolescent and adult mothers who intend to breastfeed. *J Adolesc Health* 1993;14:453-457.

130. Ineichen B, Pierce M, Lawrenson R. Teenage mothers as breastfeeders: attitudes and behaviour. *J Adolesc* 1997;20:505-509.

131. Wiemann CM, DuBois JC, Berenson AB. Racial/ethnic differences in the decision to breastfeed among adolescent mothers. *Pediatrics* 1998a;101:E11.

132. Wiemann CM, DuBois JC, Berenson AB. Strategies to promote breast-feeding among adolescent mothers. *Arch Pediatr Adolesc Med* 1998b;152:862-869.

133. Lieu TA, Wikler C, Capra AM et al. Clinical outcomes and maternal perceptions of an updated model of perinatal care. *Pediatrics* 1998;102:1437-1444.

CHAPTER 6

Maternal Physical Assessment and Counseling

The need for physical assessment and counseling, while ongoing throughout the childbearing cycle, should be initiated during the prenatal period. Although the techniques of inspection and palpation of the breast are the same for all women, the hormonal changes that occur with pregnancy and lactation require the nurse to more precisely delineate normal from abnormal data. Similarly, although the basic interview skills described in Chapter 5 can be used with all women, carefully developed questions specific to breastfeeding and lactation must be used to obtain meaningful data prenatally and throughout the intrapartum and postpartum periods.

The aim of this chapter is to help the nurse delineate normal from abnormal data (through either the physical examination or history) and to use that data as a basis for developing clinical strategies that will optimize breastfeeding initiation and continuation.

NORMAL PARAMETERS
Brief Review of Breast Structure

The breast consists of glandular, muscular, connective, and adipose tissue. The glandular tissue has 15 to 20 lobes, 20 to 24 lobules, and a complete ductal system. The breasts lie over the pectoral muscles (pectoralis major and pectoralis minor muscles) and other muscles (serratus anterior, latissimus dorsi, subscapularis, external oblique, and rectus abdominus muscles). The mammary artery and lateral thoracic artery provide most of the breast's vascular supply. Nerve supply is cutaneous (from the supraclavicular branches of the cervical plexus and the lateral perforating branches of the second,

third, fourth, and fifth intercostal nerves) and deep (from branches of the fourth, fifth, and sixth intercostal nerves). The breasts are generally discussed according to quadrants (upper outer, upper inner, lower outer, and lower inner); the tail of Spence is an extension of the upper outer quadrant, as shown in Fig. 6-1.

Brief Review of Five Stages of Mammary Function

The breast undergoes five stages of mammary function: embryogenesis, pubertal development, lactogenesis, lactation, and involution.[1] This brief review aims to provide background for the physical assessment of the breast during lactogenesis. (See Chapter 4 for a more complete discussion.)

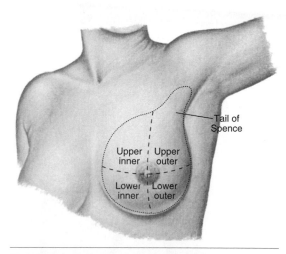

FIGURE **6-1** Quadrants of the left breast and axillary tail of Spence. (*From Seidel HM, Ball JW, Dains JE, Benedict GW.* Mosby's guide to physical examination. *4th ed. St. Louis: Mosby; 1999.*)

The mammary gland can be identified in a developing embryo by 6 weeks postfertilization, when a line, called the *mammary line* (or *mammary ridge*) of ectodermal cells, can be seen from the base of the embryonic forelimb (axillary) to the region of the hindlimb (inguinal). From this milk line, as shown in Fig. 6-2, the nipple and areola eventually arise.

Shortly after conception and throughout the woman's life cycle, the breast undergoes changes in structure and function. Changes in the glandular, muscular, connective, and adipose tissue can be observed, especially at puberty, during preg-

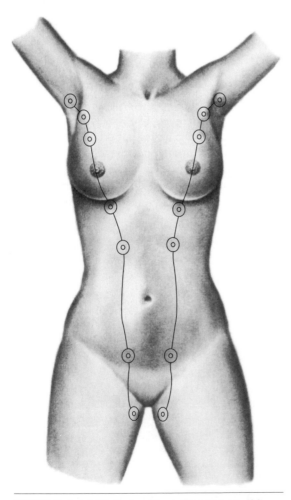

FIGURE **6-2** Milk lines. *(From Thompson JM, McFarland GK, Hirsch JE et al. Mosby's clinical nursing. 5th ed. St. Louis: Mosby; 2002.)*

nancy, and after delivery. During the physical assessment or interview, the woman is likely to describe these changes in terms of their associated discomforts. Talking with the woman provides an opportunity to reassure her of how these normal changes enable her to provide nourishment for her infant.

Assessment of the Breasts and Nipples

The discussion in this chapter is limited to those points that are most pertinent to the breast during pregnancy or lactation. It should be understood, however, that anything that can happen to a nongravid or nonlactating woman can also happen during pregnancy and lactation. Therefore do not dismiss potentially pathologic findings as a harmless change associated with lactation. Help the woman become aware of how her breasts feel before lactation—and preferably before pregnancy—so that she can better identify pathologic clues later. Teach or reinforce the technique for performing breast self-examination because the hormones associated with pregnancy increase the risk for proliferation of malignant cells. Refer the woman to her physician or primary care provider for any suspicious findings.

Assessment of Corpus Mammae

Early in the first trimester, hormones cause the ductular and lobular structures to begin proliferating, and the gravida may report swelling and tenderness in her breasts. As lactogenesis progresses internally, the external changes that were subtle at the beginning of the pregnancy gradually become more visible. Because the upper outer quadrant has the greatest amount of glandular tissue, enlargement in this area is especially noticeable. After delivery, changes occur in the size and contour of the breast. The breasts normally become engorged (i.e., the mammary tissue becomes distended). Physiologic engorgement, described in Chapter 4 is a normal and reassuring sign; absence of physiologic engorgement during lactogenesis is a nonreassuring sign. Fig. 6-3 shows how the breast undergoes changes during lactogenesis. These changes in size, shape, and symmetry are normal and reassuring.

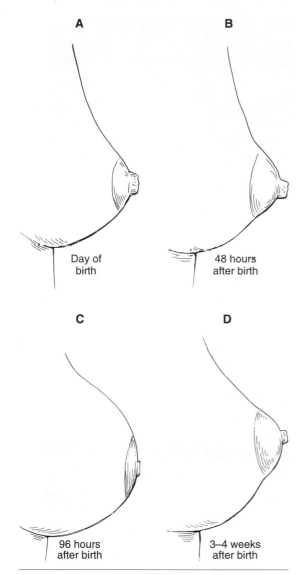

A, Day of birth

B, 48 hours after birth

C, 96 hours after birth

D, 3–4 weeks after birth

FIGURE **6-3** Breast and nipple changes as lactation is established. **A,** Day of birth. **B,** 48 hours after birth. **C,** 96 hours after birth. Note shortening of nipple areola caused by engorgement. **D,** 3 to 4 weeks after birth.

Size. During pregnancy the glandular tissue is influenced by the presence of luteal and placental hormones. These hormones stimulate proliferation of the lactiferous ducts and the alveoli, which can cause the breasts to increase significantly beyond their normal size. The glandular tissue usually displaces the connective tissue, which becomes softer and looser, especially in large-breasted women. Cooper's ligaments, which suspend the breast, may therefore become overstretched, causing large breasts to sag. A supportive bra is helpful in minimizing this problem.

The size of the breasts has nothing to do with their ability to synthesize milk. However, the size of a woman's breast may influence her self-image and her decision to breastfeed. If a woman has especially small or especially large breasts, open a dialogue with her about her feelings or anxieties. Reassure the small-breasted woman that breastfeeding is possible and that she may be delighted to finally have cleavage! Similarly, invite the well-endowed woman to discuss how she feels about her breasts, recommend a supportive bra, and plan to teach specific positioning techniques after delivery of the newborn.

Shape. Breasts can be described as having one of four different contours: conical, convex, pendulous, or large pendulous. These shapes remain largely unchanged during pregnancy and lactation, and the shape of the breast usually has no impact on the ability to breastfeed. These shapes are shown in Fig. 6-4. The "tubular" breasts are a more extreme variation of conical breasts. Women with tubular breasts may be unable to fully lactate.[2]

Symmetry. The breasts should be more or less symmetric, although the left breast is often slightly larger than the right. During pregnancy, however, note any marked asymmetry because this may indicate that the glandular tissue is not proliferating properly. Refer the woman to her physician, but reassure her that even if one breast is not capable of fully lactating, unilateral breastfeeding may be an option. Breasts that are symmetric during pregnancy but somewhat asymmetric during lactation suggest that the infant suckles more frequently or more efficiently on one side than on the other. This is usually harmless, assuming that the infant is getting enough milk.

Assessment of General Skin

Assessment of the skin includes observations about the appearance, color, and pigmentation; the texture and tautness; and the presence of any lesions on the breast.

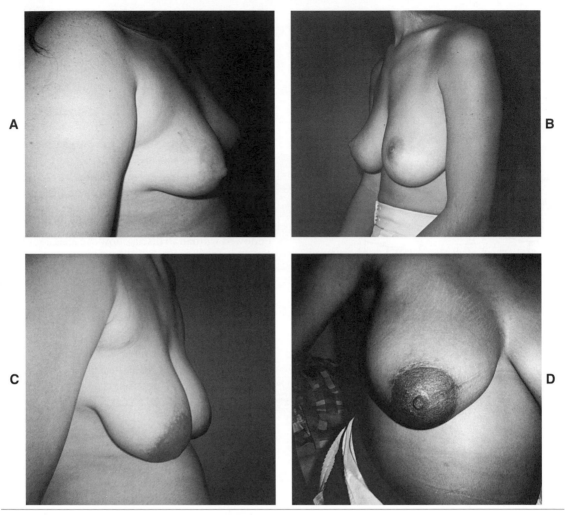

FIGURE **6-4** Variations in breast size and contour. **A,** Conical. **B,** Convex. **C,** Pendulous. **D,** Large pendulous. *(From Seidel HM, Ball JW, Dains JE, Benedict GW. Mosby's guide to physical examination. 4th ed. St. Louis: Mosby; 1999.)*

Appearance, Color, and Pigmentation. The skin should appear smooth, soft, and intact. During pregnancy, striae gravidarum (stretch marks) appear in various places throughout the body and may be especially noticeable at the outer aspects of the breasts. These marks are the result of stretching of the tissue and may be unsightly, but they have no effect on breastfeeding. Lack of smoothness in the skin or any extraneous structures, such as supernumerary nipples, as shown in Fig. 6-5, should be noted. Supernumerary nipples appear as raised bumps anywhere along the milk line. They

may secrete milk during lactation but do not interfere with breastfeeding. Upon palpation, the skin of the lactating breast should feel warm but not hot and somewhat firm but not hard.

The skin should appear about the same color as the rest of the torso, and the color of the two breasts should be the same. During the postpartum period, any red streaking is a sign of infection and requires follow-up. Discoloration—usually ecchymotic areas—is the result of bruising.

Antepartally, note any scarring around the areolae and determine the extent and origin of the

Historical Highlight

Postpartum Engorgement of the Breast

Citation: Newton M, Newton NR. Postpartum engorgement of the breast. *Am J Obstet Gynecol* 1951;61:664.

A study was conducted on 47 women at the Hospital of Pennsylvania. The women were first seen within 24 hours of delivery, then seen again to determine the amount of engorgement at a mean of 67 hours (range, 38 to 100 hours) after delivery. The engorgement was rated as 0, +1, +2, +3, or +4; a rating of 0 was given if there was no engorgement, and +4 was given to describe very hard, lumpy, tense breast tissue.

The researchers measured the amount of milk obtained in these women by weighing the infant before and after feeding and by measuring the amount of milk obtained by the pump. Today, we know these measures would have been somewhat inaccurate because pumps were not as efficient then as now, and test-weighing on the balance scales—which were used at that time—would have been an inaccurate measure of milk obtained from the breast.

However, the authors draw some important conclusions that have implications for today's care. They state: "Our conception of engorgement is that it begins with retention of milk in the alveoli. The alveoli become distended and compress surrounding milk ducts. This leads to obstruction of the outflow of milk, further distention of the alveoli, and increased obstruction. If unrelieved this may lead to secondary vascular lymphatic stasis. Increasing pressure in the obstructed portion of the breast gradually causes cessation of secretion [of milk] and eventually it is probable that milk is reabsorbed" (p. 666). To date, no research has refuted this statement.

The authors emphasize that milk is retained in the alveoli for three main reasons: (1) failure of the milk-ejection reflex, (2) mothers' allowing insufficient suckling, and similarly (3) hospital protocols' not allowing for sufficient infant suckling in terms of frequency of feedings or duration at the breast.

---

scar. It is fairly common for women of childbearing age to have had previous cosmetic breast surgery (augmentation or reduction), but prior surgery does not necessarily preclude breastfeeding. Question the gravida about her history and, if needed, retrieve previous medical records. Scars on the breast and/or nipple indicate prior trauma, and require further questioning. Surgery and trauma are discussed further later in the chapter.

Texture and Tautness. During the antepartum period, note the skin for texture and tautness. Inelastic skin, more likely to be noted in the primigravida, is tight and not easily picked up by the examiner's fingers. Elastic breast tissue is looser and is more common in the multigravida because of stretching from the previous pregnancy. If the breast tissue is inelastic antepartally, the woman is at greater risk for postpartum pathologic engorgement.[3] During the postpartum period, palpate for

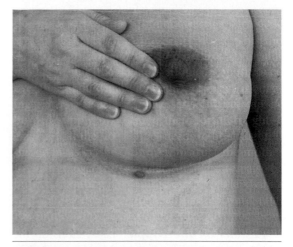

FIGURE **6-5** Supernumerary nipple. *(From Seidel HM, Ball JW, Dains JE et al. Mosby's guide to physical examination. 4th ed. St. Louis: Mosby; 1999.)*

tautness also. Very taut and shiny skin suggests pathologic engorgement or infection. Other signs and symptoms of engorgement and infection are described in Chapter 12.

Vascularity. Vascular changes during pregnancy are significant. During a singleton pregnancy, total body blood volume increases by about 45%, and the richer supply available to the breasts dilates the vessels beneath the skin. Venous congestion may be more obvious in primigravidae. As pregnancy progresses, the general skin appears very thin and veins are quite visible just beneath the skin.

Lesions. Generally, lesions should not be present on the breast. Perhaps the most important data are the time of onset of the lesion and whether a similar lesion is present on other parts of the body (see Chapter 12). For example, psoriasis found on the breast tissue is usually present elsewhere, often the skin over the elbow.

Assessment of the Nipple and Nipple Skin

Assessment of the nipple and nipple skin includes observations about appearance, color, and pigmentation; size and shape of the nipple; symmetry; discharge or secretions; and protractility. These general data-gathering points are presented in the following sections; specific deviations and their management are discussed in Chapter 12.

Appearance, Color, and Pigmentation. During pregnancy and lactation, nipples become more erectile because of the influence of hormones. Sebaceous glands keep the nipple lubricated, and the protective oils should therefore be preserved. Soap, alcohol, or other products have a drying effect on the areolar and nipple tissue. Rinsing the nipples in the shower suffices for hygiene.

The nipple should be only slightly darker than the areola, and it should be even in color. In the breastfeeding woman, a white stripe, either vertical or horizontal, signals a poor latch-on.

Lesions on the Nipple. Like lesions on the breast, lesions on the nipple should be noted in terms of their onset and whether the lesion has occurred elsewhere on the body. During lactation, however, lesions on the nipples—blisters, fissures,

ulcers, and other lesions—are usually the result of incorrect latch-on, but pathologic conditions can also be present.

Symmetry. The nipple should be located in the center of the areola. Occasionally, it is not, but this is unlikely to hamper breastfeeding efforts. It does require a little more care in helping the infant latch on because the visual illusion may tempt the mother to center the areola, not the nipple. The nipple should always be centered in the infant's mouth during breastfeeding.

Protractility. Visual inspection of the nipple is not enough to determine adequacy for breastfeeding; palpation is essential. To properly palpate, compress the nipple/areola between the thumb and forefinger. This should be done at least twice, once in the first trimester and once in the third trimester.

Normally, nipples should be well everted, which means that when the base of the nipple is compressed between the thumb and forefinger, the nipple protrudes, as shown in Fig. 6-6, *A*. With inspection only, some nipples may appear everted, but compression may reveal that the nipples will retract; these are inverted nipples, as shown in Fig. 6-6, *B*. Inverted nipples (those that do not evert with gentle compression) are sometimes identified during the pregnancy, but they disappear later in pregnancy. No special treatment is required in the early part of the pregnancy. If the inverted nipples persist until later, further follow-up may be indicated.

Size and Shape. Several nipple variations exist. These variations include especially small nipples, large or elongated nipples, flat nipples, or other variations. Note and document these observations in the record, but remain optimistic that these variations will require little or no special management techniques postpartally.

Small or Flat Nipples. Flat nipples are neither well everted nor inverted. During the antepartum period, no treatment is required. Postpartally, the infant is likely to exert enough negative pressure so that the nipple is everted in his mouth and so that the nipple can be elongated and a teat formed when suckling. Sometimes, it may be helpful to suggest the scissors hold because this does help the

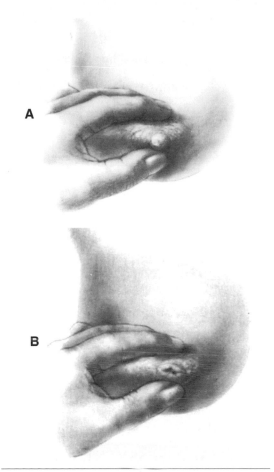

FIGURE 6-6 **A,** Normal nipple everts with gentle pressure. **B,** Inverted or tied nipple inverts with gentle pressure. *(From Lawrence RA, Lawrence RM: Breastfeeding: a guide for the medical profession. 5th ed. St. Louis: Mosby; 1999.)*

nipple protrude somewhat. Manual expression of a few drops may help the nipple become more prominent. (If these simple actions do not correct the problem, consider using the devices described in Chapter 12.) Small nipples can be managed using the same techniques described for flat nipples, and the woman may breastfeed without any real problems.

Large or Elongated Nipples. Like small or flat nipples, large or elongated nipples pose little or no problem for breastfeeding. Occasionally, a mother with very large or long nipples tries to suckle an infant with a very small mouth, and the infant may

be somewhat overwhelmed by the amount of tissue. This is best managed by enticing the infant to open wide before latching on. Otherwise, he may be tempted to latch on to the nipple only.

Discharge and Secretions. There is a clear difference between "nipple discharge" and "nipple secretions." Lawrence states, "A discharge from the nipple is defined as fluid that escapes spontaneously. A secretion, on the other hand, is fluid present in the ducts that must be collected by nipple aspiration or by other means such as conventional breast pump or gentle massage and expression from the ducts"[3] (p. 540).

Discharges can be milky (e.g., galactorrhea), multicolored and sticky, purulent, watery, serous, or serosanguineous.[3] Galactorrhea is a condition in which milk escapes from the nipples in a non-lactating woman. Some nipple discharges may be harmless, whereas others are worrisome and require follow-up. For example, during pregnancy and lactation, there may be a bloody discharge from the nipple, which usually is harmless. In some cases, however, immediate medical follow-up is indicated. Table 6-1 shows pertinent assessment points to distinguish when the patient can be watched and reassured and when immediate medical attention is indicated. A bloody discharge in the postpartum period can occur if the nipple skin has been broken.

During pregnancy, *precolostrum,* a thin, clear, viscous fluid, is present as early as the first trimester, although it may not be evident upon inspection. As the pregnancy progresses, the fluid thickens and becomes yellowish white. *Colostrum* can be expressed during the second and third trimesters or may spontaneously leak in the multigravida. Production of colostrum continues until it is gradually replaced by transitional milk during the first week postpartum.

Occasionally, mothers secrete milk with various tints. Milk will sometimes have a red-orange tint. The reason for this so-called rusty-pipe milk is unclear, but it appears to be the result of the increased vascularity and is harmless. Milk can have a green tint after the mother has consumed a large amount of green vegetables. In one reported case, milk was black, presumably because of the patient's

Table **6-1**   Bloody Discharge during Pregnancy and Lactation

Physical Assessment Finding	Possible Explanation/Alteration during Pregnancy and/or Lactation	Clinical Implications
Bloody nipple discharge	During pregnancy, may be due to increased vascularity and epithelial proliferation; typically bilateral and not confined to a single duct	Ominous when woman is not pregnant or lactating; may be physiologic during pregnancy and lactation
		Reassure mother that bloody discharge is not harmful to the infant
	During lactation, may be due to poor latch-on; typically accompanied by visible signs of trauma to the nipples; this typically resolves within the week	Persistent bloody nipple discharge, especially if from a single duct, requires further evaluation
Bloody nipple discharge and a breast mass	When both are present, this is an ominous sign	Prepare woman for mammography
		Galactography, used to localize the abnormality to assist with excision, has not been used during pregnancy and lactation

Source: Berens P, Newton ER. *ABM News and Views* 1997;3:4-6.

minocycline therapy. The various tints that have been identified in milk are harmless. Infants probably consume this colored milk more often than we realize, but it is most evident when the mother is expressing and saving her milk.

Assessment of Areola and Areolar Skin

Appearance, Color, and Pigmentation. The areola should be centered on the breast. Hair on the areola is normal and harmless; absence of hair suggests that the mother may have been pulling it out, and this is a potential infection hazard.

The color of the areola varies according to the color of the woman's skin. Normally, however, the areola is somewhat lighter in color than the nipple, and it becomes more pigmented during pregnancy and lactation. During the postpartum period, the color of the areola should be only slightly lighter than the color of the nipple; a more noticeable difference may signal a fungal infection.

Size, Shape, and Symmetry. The areolae surround the nipples, and each should be the same in size and symmetry. During pregnancy, the areola increases in diameter from about 34 to

50 mm. The Montgomery's glands also become more prominent during pregnancy. A summary of points for physical assessment of the breasts is provided in Table 6-2.

PRENATAL ASSESSMENT AND COUNSELING

The aim of prenatal physical assessment is to establish that the pregnancy is progressing optimally and to identify any factors that might compromise the fetus or newborn. Because the breasts are designed to nourish the neonate, any prenatal assessment that excludes physical assessment of the breasts is negligent. The antenatal assessment of the breasts has an added benefit: It gives the mother confidence that she can breastfeed if the examiner says she can.[4] More specifically, the prenatal breast examination should focus on the adequacy of the breasts for breastfeeding. Physical assessment—inspection and palpation of the breasts—should be performed at least twice: once at the first prenatal visit and again during the third trimester.

Breastfeeding is not a topic that is separate from other prenatal teaching. Present breastfeeding as the completion of the reproductive cycle. For

Table 6-2 ASSESSMENT OF THE BREASTS AND AXILLAE

	Observations	Deviations and Clinical Implications
Inspect Both Breasts While the Patient's Arms Are Hanging Loosely at Her Sides, and Compare the Following		
Size	Breasts may be small, moderate, or large but should enlarge during pregnancy and lactation	Size of breasts before pregnancy does not affect ability to produce milk or to breastfeed; the key is for both breasts to enlarge from their prepregnant state
Symmetry	Breasts and nipples should be symmetric	Asymmetric breasts may be due to the following: • Inadequate glandular tissue and failure to enlarge during pregnancy; determine whether mother can completely lactate from that breast • Uneven stimulation of breasts; infant has preferred side, or mother is suckling multiple infants with differing needs • Pathologic condition
Contour	Describe as follows: • Conical • Convex • Pendulous • Large pendulous	Women with various contours are able to successfully breastfeed
Retractions or dimpling	Retraction or dimpling is abnormal	Retraction or dimpling of the breast skin indicates pathology; refer to physician
Skin color, texture, and general appearance	Skin should not appear shiny	• Skin may appear stretched if engorged but should not appear shiny • Presence of red streaking is pathologic and requires referral • Peau d'orange is pathologic and requires immediate referral
Venous patterns	Striae may be present during pregnancy and lactation Dilated subcutaneous veins during pregnancy and lactation are readily visible	These are harmless

Continued

Table **6-2**   ASSESSMENT OF THE BREASTS AND AXILLAE—CONT'D

	Observations	Deviations and Clinical Implications
Lesions	Any number of lesions may be present on the breast; these may be unremarkable or may be pathologic	Common lesions include eczema, herpes, and various others; unlike eczema, which does not preclude breastfeeding and is bilateral, Paget's disease appears as a crusty lesion on the breast, but it is unilateral; except for herpes lesions, breastfeeding can continue uninterrupted when lesions are covered
Supernumerary nipples	These may be found anywhere along the milk line, before or during lactation	These do not preclude breastfeeding, but they may "drip" while the infant is being fed
Inspect Both Areolae and Nipples While the Patient's Arms Are Hanging Loosely at Her Sides, and Compare the Following		
Size, shape, and symmetry	Nipples and areola should look the same	Unilateral deviation usually suggests presence of pathology
Location	Nipples should be centered on the areola	Slightly off-center nipple not problematic but requires mother to be more careful about centering the infant on the areola
Color	Areola will darken during pregnancy and lactation. Color should appear even	Darkening is normal • Horizontal white stripes • Vertical white stripes
Intactness	Nipple/areola skin should be intact	• Cracking • Bleeding • Fissures
Size	Varies	Varies
Protractility	Most nipples are everted	• Inverted • Flat • Dimpled
Discharge	• Delineate *secretion* from *discharge* (see text) • Describe characteristics of discharge	Most nipple discharges are benign in nature but should be referred to physician because they may be malignant

example, while listening to the fetal heart tones, point out the sound of the placenta and explain its function in nourishing the fetus. This becomes an excellent segue for examining the breasts as the next part of the physical assessment. It is easy for the nurse to comment, "Oh, your breasts are enlarging. This is a good sign! Your breasts are getting ready to take over the job of nourishing the baby after he is born." In this way breastfeeding is presented as a normal, physiologic process, which helps the woman gain confidence that her body is already becoming capable of this task. (Chapters 3 and 5 more fully address the reasons underlying the feeding decision and the educational and interview approach to positively influence the woman's feeding decision.) During the prenatal period, the goal is to help the woman make an informed choice about a feeding method, and counseling should include a clear discussion about contraindications to breastfeeding (as described in Chapter 13), if those contraindications are identified.

If the woman has already decided to breastfeed, providing anticipatory guidance is a critical role for the nurse. Apart from providing information to help the woman make an informed choice, however, the nurse must help the woman recognize any and all factors that may affect breastfeeding and lactation—positively or negative—and help her develop a plan that will optimize her experience. Much of this is accomplished by taking a careful history and performing a thorough physical assessment.

Physical Assessment

Physical assessment of the breast in the first and last trimesters of pregnancy should aim to determine the adequacy of the breasts for breastfeeding. Changes in breast tissue (or lack thereof) and the eversion of the nipple are key assessment points and may require further follow-up. Physical assessment of the breasts should also occur immediately after the birth of the infant because intravenous fluids are often given during labor, and the nipple/aveolar tissue can become edematous. In the postpartum period, the main aim of assessment is to ensure that lactogenesis is progressing normally and that the woman is free of breast problems. Interpretation of the physical assessment depends on a clear understanding of normal parameters for the pregnant or lactating woman.

Health History

The health history, initiated during the prenatal period, continues throughout the postpartum course. The social, obstetric, medical, and surgical histories can all influence the woman's breastfeeding experience. The aim is to anticipate any possible problems and develop strategies for optimizing the breastfeeding experience.

Social History

A social history is critical when providing care for pregnant women. Generally, the forms that are commercially available help identify and record social problems and lifestyle issues, but the nurse will need to use good interviewing skills to gain specific information about the woman's family situation, feeding choice, and other relevant data. Questions about smoking are especially pertinent to breastfeeding because smoking can interfere with milk supply, as described in other chapters.

Obstetric History

Most of the standard history forms that are completed for obstetric patients are useful in identifying basic information, such as gravity, parity, and other pertinent facts. These forms, however, often lend little structure for obtaining a history of the woman's breastfeeding and lactation experience. Some open-ended questions (often as simple, "How'd it go?") can be useful, along with some specific, closed-ended questions such as "How long did you breastfeed?" At the end of the prenatal period, a summary form, such as that found in Box 6-1, helps summarize data for other health care providers.

Obstetric history includes the history of past reproductive experiences, as well as the history of the current pregnancy and delivery. Therefore the obstetric "history" is really an ongoing effort from the first prenatal visit until the infant is weaned.

Although there is a widespread belief that a history of infertility is a risk factor for insufficient milk supply, no data substantiate this claim. Such data are unlikely to be forthcoming because the

Box 6-1   Antepartum Breastfeeding Assessment Form

Name_____ Age_____ Date of first visit_____

Term_____ Preterm_____ Abortion_____ Live_____ Reexamined_____

The Gravida
❏ Verbalizes feelings about breastfeeding, including prior breastfeeding experience, myths she has heard about breastfeeding, etc.
❏ Acknowledges benefits of breastfeeding for _____ self _____ infant
❏ Has not made decision about feeding method (date _____)
❏ Made decision to initiate _____ breastfeeding _____ artificial feeding
❏ Identified resources/support persons for feeding method chosen

Subjective and Objective Data
❏ Well-everted nipples
❏ Flat or inverted nipples (circle one)
❏ Adequate nutritional intake
❏ Breast tenderness and enlargement
❏ Symmetric breasts
❏ Cultural/dietary values _____

Recommendations
❏ Referred to breastfeeding class
❏ Received written materials
❏ Recommended breast shells
❏ Other

woman who has hormonal levels sufficient to support a pregnancy should indeed have the hormonal levels needed to successfully lactate.

Medical and Surgical History

Medical and surgical history and examination should focus on data about maternal infections, endocrine dysfunction, breast pathology, and breast surgery. In most cases the benefits of breastfeeding outweigh the possible risks. Special considerations for lactating women with significant medical or surgical history are listed in Box 6-2.

Maternal Infections. Infection can occur any time, including before pregnancy. It is important to identify infections in the prenatal period and to develop a plan to eradicate them or, if that is not possible, to achieve an optimal feeding experience. Often, infectious diseases do not contraindicate breastfeeding. However, in the interest of informed consent, women should be told of infectious diseases that place the breastfed infant at risk. A further discussion of infections as they relate to

breastfeeding is found in Chapter 13. As a general consideration, infections that are accompanied by fever generally require more fluids, and this is even more important for the lactating mother. Strict handwashing precautions should also be implemented.

Alterations in Endocrine and Metabolic Function. Hormones play a significant role during both pregnancy and lactation. Dramatic hormonal fluctuations normally affect the mammary gland, but undesirable alterations in endocrine and metabolic function can also become more evident during those times.

Diabetes Mellitus. Diabetes mellitus does not preclude breastfeeding. Although breastfeeding is usually initiated because of its benefits to the infant, this is an excellent example of how it also is beneficial to the mother. Prolactin maintains mammary gland insulin receptors to ensure anabolism— metabolism that converts simple substances into more complex compounds. Apparently, this hormone enhances the anabolic processes to bring about better diabetic control during lactation.

Box 6-2 Considerations for Lactating Women with Significant Medical or Surgical History

- Is breastfeeding contraindicated, or might it need to be temporarily interrupted?
- Is the identified pathologic condition likely to be resolved before the infant is born?
- What special precautions (e.g., vaccines, isolation), if any, are required?
- What general precautions might be helpful? (Handwashing is always a helpful precaution.)
- Are medications used to treat the maternal pathologic condition safe for the newborn, and what side effects might result? Should the mother have blood drawn to determine whether a therapeutic level of

the medication has been achieved before putting the infant to breast?
- What, if any, is the risk for decreased milk supply?
- Will the maternal medical management differ during lactation (e.g., insulin administration in the diabetic mother)?
- Will maternal pathology affect the mother's basic food and fluid needs during lactation?
- Does a pathologic condition limit the lactating woman's contraceptive choices?
- If the woman is expressing and storing her milk when an infection is present, are any special precautions needed?

Studies have shown that breastfeeding is beneficial for both insulin-dependent diabetic mothers (type 1) and gestational diabetic mothers. (Note that gestational diabetes occurs only during pregnancy and is classified neither as type 1 nor as type 2.) Insulin-dependent diabetic mothers who breastfeed exclusively have lower fasting glucose levels at 6 weeks postpartum (82 ± 40 mg/dl) than do women who began but later stopped breastfeeding (145 ± 37 mg/dl) or type 1 mothers who initially chose to bottle-feed (120 ± 30 mg/dl).[5] Gestational diabetics have improved glucose metabolism while breastfeeding (during the 4- to 12-week period), and fasting blood glucose levels are significantly lowered (93 ± 13 vs. 98 ± 17 mg/dl; $p = .0001$).[6] It appears, too, that insulin production (β-cell function) during lactation is better utilized at the cellular level regardless of adiposity.[7] Furthermore, breastfeeding helps reduce or delay the onset of diabetes in subsequent pregnancies.[6]

As with other mothers, milk production and composition in mothers with type 1 diabetes are altered by many factors, including method of delivery, feeding frequency, fetal condition, gestational age, mastitis incidence, metabolic control, and maternal dietary intake.[8] There are minor differences in milk composition in mothers with type 1 diabetes, but this does not preclude breastfeed-

ing. Good control of the woman's glucose status is important not only for her general well-being but also for lactation. It appears that poor metabolic control results in a delay of lactogenesis.[9] Generally, oral hypoglycemic agents are safe for lactating mothers, although this should be verified in individual cases.

Breastfeeding mothers who had recent gestational diabetes should be counseled about the possible adverse effects of progestin-only oral contraceptives (OCs). The progestin-only pills have been associated with increased risk of diabetes in lactating Latino women who experienced gestational diabetes. It is therefore unlikely that a recent gestational diabetic woman will have a prescription for these, so she may need some help in exploring other alternative methods of birth control.[10] However, "Long-term use of low-dose *combination* OCs did not increase the risk of type 2 (non–insulin-dependent) diabetes compared with use of nonhormonal contraception."[10]

Thyroid Disease. Women with hypothyroid disease may breastfeed. If the woman is receiving thyroid-replacement therapy, she should have no trouble producing plenty of milk. Insufficient milk, however, can sometimes be an early sign of a hypothyroid condition, so if other reasons for insufficient milk have been ruled out, this possibility should be explored.

Women with hyperthyroid disease can breast-feed if the infant is monitored biochemically while the mother is taking thyroid preparations. Pro-pylthiouracil (PTU; trade name Propyl-Thyracil) is the drug of choice for women with hyperthyroid disease. A minimal amount of PTU reaches the milk because it is ionized and protein bound.[11] Therefore encourage breastfeeding but monitor the infant's thyroxine (T_4) and thyroid-stimulating hormone (TSH) levels.

Pituitary Dysfunction. Sheehan's syndrome can occur after severe postpartum hemorrhage. The hemorrhage causes necrosis of the pituitary and hypopituitarism. The pituitary gland, which secretes hormones associated with lactation, including prolactin, is particularly vulnerable to decreased vascular flow, and this results in mam-mary involution and lactation failure. Sheehan's syndrome occurs in about 0.01% to 0.02% of post-partum women and results in lactation failure.[3] Retained placental fragments can lead to an insuf-ficient milk supply even before postpartum hem-orrhage occurs, as explained in Chapter 7. A clear, collaborative plan includes assessing milk output, checking newborn weight on a consistent basis, and if medically indicated, explaining to the mother why artificial supplementation might be required.

As previously mentioned, *galactorrhea* refers to lactation not associated with childbirth or breast-feeding. The condition is sometimes a symptom of a pituitary gland dysfunction. It can also occur after reduction mammaplasty.[12]

Other Conditions. Eclampsia does not preclude breastfeeding; however, breastfeeding is generally not initiated when seizure precautions are in effect (if the woman can have complete supervision, this restriction could be modified). Also, breastfeeding is not initiated when the maternal dose of pheno-barbital is greater than 360 mg/day or until the case is reviewed by the physician. The mother may express her milk during this time. Whether the milk should be saved and given to the infant or discarded depends on the dosage of drugs that the mother is receiving and the discretion of the physician.

Maternal diarrhea does not require cessation of breastfeeding. Breastfeeding may continue unin-terrupted, but the mother will experience very high thirst and need plenty of fluids.

Pathology of the Breast. Pathology related to the breast often does not preclude breastfeeding. Women with fibrocystic disease or suspicious lumps or those who have had prior radiation ther-apy may breastfeed, but they require ongoing assessment and evaluation.

Fibrocystic Disease. Fibrocystic disease is a benign condition in which cysts form within enlarged ducts. Typically, the woman reports ten-derness that increases just before menses. On physi-cal examination, multiple, round, mobile nodules can be palpated bilaterally; borders are well defined, and the consistency is soft to firm.[13] These nodules may become somewhat more tender and noticeable during lactation, but they do not pre-clude breastfeeding. Although the nodules make it more difficult for women to interpret their find-ings of breast self-examination, they should under-stand that breast changes are the key to successful interpretation.

Suspicious Lumps. No woman should wait for her routine medical examination to discover a lump. Lumps are usually apparent to women themselves or to their partners. The American Cancer Society and all health care providers con-tinually emphasize to women the importance of performing breast self-examination to promote early detection. The woman who has never per-formed breast self-examination, however, will find it more difficult to learn during lactation because of the presence of multiple nodules, normally asso-ciated with lactation, and she may be unable to dif-ferentiate normal from worrisome signs until she learns the landscape of her nonlactating breasts.

Throughout her life, the woman must lose no time in identifying any suspicious lump and seek-ing prompt follow-up. However, women are espe-cially vulnerable to delaying follow-up during pregnancy and lactation.[14] In an attempt to attrib-ute the problem to their lactation status, serious problems can be overlooked.

Abruptly refusing to suckle a previously accepted breast is a worrisome sign. Known as *Goldsmith's sign,* this can be an early sign of breast cancer.[15]

Prior Radiation Therapy. Women who require radiation while lactating should wean. Occasionally, however, women have undergone treatment for radiation before childbearing. The radiation therapy causes fibrosis and massive destruction of the lobules.[2] The effects of radiation on lactation have not been well documented, so it is difficult to provide these women with any realistic expectation of what will happen in relation to future breastfeeding experiences.

There are a few cases in which lactation after radiation therapy was successful, but this is not typical. Unfortunately, nearly all published reports lack a definition of "successful" lactation and are anecdotal, so it is difficult to reach any substantive conclusions.

Two cases were reported by Rodger and colleagues. In the first case, the woman lactated from both the irradiated and the untreated breast; in the other case, the woman lactated only from the untreated breast.[16] Higgins did a retrospective chart review and interviews and observed that most patients did not lactate from the treated breast, and only one woman "successfully" suckled her infant from the treated breast for 4 months, although others breastfed using only the untreated breast.[17] Tralins reported that lactation occurred on the affected side in only about 25% of cases in which women had received conservative treatment.[18] Varsos reports that one woman produced only small amounts of colostrum and milk from the previously irradiated breast for about 2 months, while the untreated breast lactated normally.[19] Guix reports that a nullipara with a periareolar incision for lumpectomy had delayed milk secretion in the treated breast, and the treated breast did not show characteristic changes in size as the untreated breast did; hence, marked asymmetry was noted. Nonetheless, she was able to lactate from both breasts and "successfully" suckle her infant from both breasts for 6 weeks.[20] Ulmer describes a case in which the treated breast showed no characteristic changes in size and did not lactate.[21] The effects of radiation are poorly understood. One expert has suggested that success or failure of lactation may be dose related.[22]

Breast Trauma. Breast trauma can occur either before pregnancy or during lactation. Multiple causes, including physical abuse or accidents, may affect the woman's decision to breastfeed, or perhaps, her ability to lactate successfully.

Scars caused by burns of the breast are a concern, as much from a psychologic standpoint as from a milk synthesis standpoint. Even if the woman has come to terms with her body image, her self-confidence related to breastfeeding may be diminished. Reassure her that breastfeeding is possible after third-degree burns because the damage most often affects only the skin, not the glandular tissue beneath it (see the Clinical Scenario box).

Unusual accidents can and do occur; I am aware of one situation in which a woman's breast had been bitten some years earlier by a horse. This, along with other situations, does not automatically preclude breastfeeding; careful assessment and follow-up are essential. In most cases the critical question about milk production relates to the extent of the trauma and whether the structures of the breast—most notably the fourth intercostal nerve and the ducts—remain intact. Therefore breastfeeding can go reasonably well.[23,24]

Breast Surgery. In many respects, caring for the woman who is undergoing breast surgery is similar to caring for any other person undergoing surgery. Preoperative management should focus on advocating for informed consent, providing options and anticipatory guidance, carrying out actions that maintain homeostasis during the immediate recovery period, and implementing a teaching plan designed to optimize full physical and psychologic recovery. In this sense an operation on the mammary gland bears many similarities to an operation on the thyroid gland. There are, however, some unique aspects to caring for the woman who is undergoing breast surgery. In American culture the breast is more than a mammary gland; in some way it helps the woman define herself as a woman and a mother. The nurse bears much responsibility for helping the woman to mobilize her emotional resources to deal with this procedure, which invades not only her body but

CLINICAL SCENARIO

Mother with Third-Degree Burns

Mrs. X., age 28, gravida 1, para 1, had a spontaneous delivery of a term, appropriate-for-gestational age male. She was about 36 hours postpartum when I first encountered her. It was nighttime, but she was wide awake and appeared uneasy. I established rapport with her and asked what was keeping her awake.

She said that she longed to breastfeed but felt this was not a realistic option for her. When she was 7 years old, she had suffered third-degree burns from her neck to her knees. She had had multiple skin grafts over the years. Despite the extensive trauma, she seemed to have a positive self-image, and she displayed self-confidence.

She had put the infant to the breast several times, but nothing seemed to happen. She felt discouraged and was more or less resigned to the fact that this was just one more loss she would have to experience. We talked for a while about her feelings about breastfeeding, her feelings about her breasts, her relationship with her husband, and her newborn's natural urge to suckle. I promised her nothing but asked to see her breasts.

The skin had the course, irregular appearance that typically follows severe burns. The nipples were small, but present and slightly everted. Upon palpation, it appeared that her breasts were beginning to fill with milk. We waited until the newborn was hungry, and put him to the breast. Happily, the greatest impediment to breastfeeding was that she had not been taught how to latch the infant onto the breast. We were able to quickly overcome this problem, and the newborn suckled until he was content. We could hear him swallowing. She was thrilled with the progress.

I had the great pleasure of caring for this woman a few years later when she delivered her second child. She reported that she had fed the first infant for more than 6 months and felt confident that she could nurse the new one as well.

also her privacy and her self-concept. However, this text does not intend to replicate the comprehensive directives for breast surgery outlined in more general textbooks.

Nowadays, it is not uncommon for women of childbearing age to have had prior therapeutic or cosmetic breast surgery. Often, however, women receive little encouragement or practical information from their surgeons about the implications for lactation. Two situations may emerge. In one, the woman wants to breastfeed long after the time when the surgery was performed; in this case the surgery may have been performed for either therapeutic or cosmetic reasons. In the other situation the woman needs breast surgery while she is lactating; this is a less common occurrence, but for therapeutic reasons it does occasionally arise. Either situation has clear implications for those providing care, with less clear indications for how lactation will actually progress.

Surgery before Initiation of Lactation. Surgery that is performed on the breast before lactation may or may not have a significant effect on lactation.

Multiple factors influence the woman's ability to lactate after surgery, but generally speaking, her success or failure is related to whether and to what degree the following structures were affected: (1) tissue— the amount of tissue removed, and the extent and character of resulting scar tissue or contractures, and the interruption of the nipple/areolar complex; (2) ducts—whether the lactiferous ducts are intact after the surgical procedure; (3) blood supply— whether it is interrupted; and (4) nerves—whether they are intact. Simply stated, the more intact the structures, the better the chances for successful lactation, which depends largely on the procedure performed and the type of incision the surgeon used.

Generally, five different incisions can be used when performing breast surgery. These include periareolar, infrasubmammary, axillary, pedicle (transposition), and free nipple (autotransplantation). Upon inspection, it is fairly easy to determine which type of incision was performed. Fig. 6-7 shows the location of the incisions.

Types of Incisions. The *periareolar* incision is a half circle around the lower border of the areola.

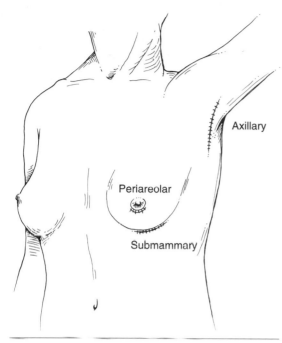

FIGURE 6-7 Types of incisions used for breast surgery.

The advantage of this type of incision is that it is less visible. It carries several disadvantages, however, including possible loss of sensation. This incision, compared with other types, may make the woman more vulnerable to lactation failure.[25,26] Damage to the lactiferous ducts is likely with a periareolar incision, and although engorgement may uniformly occur, milk production and emptying occur only in the areas where the ducts are intact.[2] Usually, the periareolar technique is used for biopsies or for augmentation mammaplasty.

The *infrasubmammary* incision is located mostly beneath the mammary gland. An advantage to this type of incision is that breastfeeding is possible. A disadvantage, however, is that the incision is located close to the edge of the bra, which may interfere with wound healing in the beginning or cause irritation later on. Another possible disadvantage is that the scar tissue is visible. This technique is used for augmentation.

The *axillary* incision is located at the axilla. It provides a clear advantage because it is practically invisible, unless the woman raises her arm.

Relatively little has been written about this type of incision, but it appears that lactation is likely to be successful when this type of incision has been used. Disadvantages include the possibility for contractures of the skin and later difficulty detecting breast cancer. This technique can be used for augmentation or, occasionally, biopsy.

With the *pedicle,* or *transposition,* technique, the nipple/areola complex remains attached to the underlying parenchyma; this "stem" of tissue remains intact, while wedges of excess tissue are excised from the sides and undersides of the stem. This type of incision is commonly used and enables the surgeon to leave the skin of the nipple/areola complex, lactiferous ducts, blood supply, and some nerves intact.

The *free nipple* technique is seldom used today. Usually, it is indicated when the woman has extremely large breasts. Because this technique disrupts the nipple/areola complex and severs lactiferous ducts, subsequent lactation is unlikely. Also, women with this type of incision tend to have decreased nipple sensation.[27]

Surgical Procedure. Aside from the type of incision used, multiple factors affect breastfeeding and lactation. As for all mothers, breastfeeding is more likely to be successful if the mother receives accurate information and ongoing support for her decision. The information she receives before the procedure will result in her realistic or unrealistic expectations of how breastfeeding is likely to proceed; receiving information before and during the breastfeeding experience helps her consider some alternatives, including unilateral breastfeeding. The woman's self-image and her feelings of comfort or guilt about having the surgery should be considered. The procedure used, the indication for the surgery in the first place, and the use of prostheses are all factors that contribute to the breastfeeding experience.

Four central questions should be explored when the mother has had prior breast surgery: (1) Are there reassuring signs of milk production? (2) Is there evidence of milk ejection and drainage? (3) What are the woman's concerns, anxieties, and goals? and (4) What is the effect on the infant (i.e., is the infant making adequate weight gains)?

Answers vary, depending on the individual woman and on the surgery performed. Overall, women with prior breast surgery are more likely to have decreased milk supply than those who have not had surgery.[26]

Breast Reduction. Women may elect to have their breasts reduced for various physical and psychologic reasons. Especially large breasts, called *macromastia*, can cause a variety of physical discomforts: posture problems, "back trouble," and other discomforts. Such large breasts, which tend to be familial, also interfere with the woman's self-image; her breasts are usually disproportionate to the rest of her body, and she may feel very self-conscious. Typically, women who seek reduction surgery are very young—often in their late teens. They may not value breastfeeding as something they would later wish to do or may not recognize how the surgery could limit their feeding options. Complications, including infections and galactorrhea, have been reported,[28,29] in addition to the impact on milk supply as described earlier.

The pedicle technique is typically used for reduction mammaplasty, as shown in Fig. 6-8. Because most of the ducts, blood supply, and nerves remain intact, breastfeeding is usually possible after this type of surgery. Unfortunately, women who have had had a pedicle reduction mammaplasty have often been dissuaded from breastfeeding,[24] and many have regretted that they did not receive adequate preoperative counseling for this procedure.[30] As many as 72% of patients who have had this incision are able to lactate.[31]

Most women who have undergone reduction using this technique have reportedly experienced "normal lactation and breastfeeding," but the authors had no objective criteria by which to measure "normal."[32] One study defined *successful breastfeeding* as "the ability to feed for a duration equal to or greater than 2 weeks."[24] Authors who conclude that mothers have "sufficient milk," often make no mention of measure of milk yield or infant test-weighings.[33] In one study, only 35% of women who had had surgery using the pedicle technique initiated and continued breastfeeding, but again, there was little evidence of how "successful" the experience was.[34]

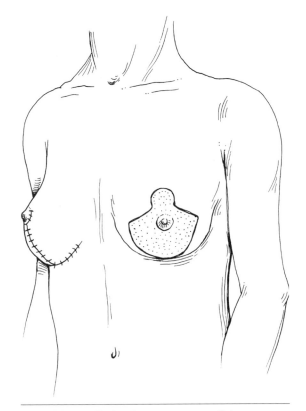

FIGURE **6-8** Reduction surgery: pedicle technique.

As with all mothers, the nurse will need to observe for the reassuring presence of physiologic engorgement and subsequent milk production. One case report describes a mother who had only one breast reduced, using the pedicle technique. Both breasts became fully engorged by 84 hours postpartum, but milk yield from the reduced breast was noticeably less than that from the other breast.[35] Other patients have reported a slight delay in engorgement.[36] Neifert reports that she has encountered women who can produce and deliver a full supply of milk after reduction surgery using the pedicle technique, but she cautions that in most cases supplementation with artificial milk is required for the infant to make adequate weight gains.[26]

Reduction surgery is also occasionally accomplished through the free nipple (autotransplantation) technique. If the woman is unable to lactate successfully afterward, she is likely to blame herself for seeking reduction surgery. In the real world, whether or not the surgery ruined her chances of lactating is a moot point; the surgery has been done and cannot be undone. She may find it comforting to know that some women with macromastia are never able to fully lactate because the extraordinary amount of adipose tissue crowds the lactiferous ducts, rendering them less functional.

Breast Augmentation. Breast augmentation is usually done using the periareolar technique, which clearly carries a risk of lactation failure. Lactation has reportedly occurred after breast augmentation.[37] However, there is no acknowledgment of quantity of milk or the infant's well-being as a yardstick for success. In controlled studies, lactation insufficiency is more likely in augmented than in nonaugmented breasts; more specifically, the periareolar approach was most significantly associated with lactation insufficiency.[25,26]

The implants used for augmentation raise another issue. Even if lactation is possible, the question becomes, Is breastfeeding safe? Two types of implants are used for augmentation: saline and silicone. Many women raise questions about the safety of the silicone, fearing that it will "leak" into their milk. The silicone itself is inert, and it does not break down; it also is found in over-the-counter products such as Di-Gel. Other products in the implant do break down, but whether they present a safety hazard is not well understood. The other products are toluenediisocyanate (TDI) and toluenediaminene (TDA), which have been implicated as carcinogenic in industry (e.g., in seat covers), but their safety has not been described in the lactation literature. It is possible, however, to test a pregnant women's urine for breakdown products; if they are present, it is likely that they also will be present in the milk postpartum.* Further discussion is found in Chapter 13.

Surgical Biopsy. If a simple biopsy procedure is used, there apparently is no effect on subsequent lactation. However, if a periareolar incision is used, lactation may be seriously hampered. One woman, who had successfully breastfed her first infant before the biopsy, was later unable to successfully lactate from the affected breast for a second infant. The woman experienced bilateral engorgement, but normal milk flow from the affected breast was impeded. She tried the usual interventions to increase stimulation and enhance the milk-ejection reflex—applying warm packs, using oxytocin nasal spray, and starting the feeding on the affected side—but after 6 weeks she realized that her efforts had failed to produce any meaningful change. However, she was able to produce enough milk with the unaffected breast; the infant soon ceased suckling on the affected side, and the breast involuted.[38]

Mastopexy. A mastopexy is a breast "lift." The skin from the submammary area is involved, and the resulting scar looks similar to that after reduction surgery. Lactation is likely to be unaffected because only the skin is involved, but this has not been studied.

Lumpectomy. A lumpectomy is performed to remove a lump in the breast. Lumpectomies may be performed during lactation, or the woman may be required to wean her infant before surgery because the lactating breast is very vascular. The effects on lactation are not well described. One woman who had a lumpectomy, axillary node dissection, and whole-breast external radiation therapy produced only drops of milk from the treated breast, but she breastfed successfully from the untreated breast.[39]

Mastectomy. A mastectomy is the surgical removal of the breast. If a woman has had only one breast removed, it is entirely possible to breastfeed using the other breast.

Breast Surgery While Lactating. Elective surgery involving the breast should be postponed as long as possible. Even a short delay would provide her with more options such as time to collect and store milk if she chooses to do so. In nonelective situations, however, it is entirely possible that the need for the surgery outweighs the infant's need to breastfeed. A few guiding principles help organize care for this woman.

Preoperative Nursing Care of the Lactating Woman. Ask, or suggest that the mother ask, when breastfeeding can resume. This is undoubtedly a question that is on her mind, so it is best to address it

*The testing can be done by the National Medical Services (800-522-6671).

before the surgery rather than after. If it is anticipated that breastfeeding cannot resume for a very long time, the woman should be so informed; she may choose to wean. However, the definition of "too long" should be her definition; the health care team should not discourage her from maintaining lactation until the infant can return to the breast, unless that is contraindicated.

The location of the woman's incision may determine whether she can continue breastfeeding. The infant's mouth, which generally harbors bacteria, should not touch a new incision. Where the mother is hospitalized may present some logistic problems with breastfeeding. If she is admitted to the general surgical floor, which is likely, there may be restrictions on the presence of infants. Some hospitals are more relaxed about this and permit the infant to room-in if the mother accepts full responsibility for his care. Depending on the extent of her surgery, she may or may not be able to do this. She may need help gathering objective information so that she can choose options that best fit her needs and those of her infant.

Identify any equipment or resources that the mother may need during her period of separation from the infant. Also review the anticipated length of separation and her financial and emotional resources to cope with prolonged milk expression. Suggest that she consider expressing and saving her milk unless her physician determines that the milk is unsafe for consumption. If her milk is only temporarily unsafe, instruct her to "pump and dump" until the circumstances change.

Postoperative Care of the Lactating Woman. Postoperative care of the lactating woman is in many ways similar to postoperative care for a non-lactating woman. However, some specific areas need to be addressed.

Nursing Assessments and Actions. Check the mother's breasts. It is likely that a separation from the infant, even for a short time, will result in milk stasis. At a minimum, this is uncomfortable. At worst, it can trigger a host of other problems associated with lack of drainage, including extreme engorgement, which would impede wound healing. Ideally, bring the infant for suckling. If this is not possible, encourage the mother to express milk from her breasts. Offer comfort measures, such as ice to the breasts, and a mild analgesic as ordered.

Perform the usual assessments for a postoperative patient, with some additions. Note the location and extent of the incision; reevaluate whether the infant should go to the breast if his mouth will be on or very near to the incision, because the infant's mouth has bacteria that would impede wound healing. Check the incision for drainage, and note the color of the drainage. Note the woman's intake and output; be sure to count suckled or expressed milk as output.

Safe Medication Administration. Administer medication with the realization that it must be safe for both the mother and the infant. However, do not hesitate to offer analgesics in the prescribed dosages, because women often delay initiating breastfeeding or reduce the number of times that they offer the breast simply because they are in pain,[40] and a cascade of adverse effects may result.

Optimize Breastfeeding and Lactation Efforts. Be creative in finding ways to optimize the breastfeeding experience. For example, if breastfeeding from the operative breast is contraindicated, suggest that the woman feed from the unaffected side until the affected side is ready for breastfeeding again. Even if she is using both breasts, the stress and separation may diminish her milk supply. Help her understand that supply can be reestablished relatively quickly, assuming that the separation is minimal and that she is making an uneventful recovery.

Help the mother deal with her sense of loss and separation. She may feel that she is depriving the infant of her milk, or she may feel guilty that she does not feel well enough to feed the infant. Reassure her that she must take care of herself before she can take care of her infant. If expressed milk is unavailable, providing artificial milk for the infant is not a disaster, particularly when lactation has already been well established.

Infants who are separated from their mothers for a substantial length of time are vulnerable to dehydration or failure to thrive. Collaboration with the pediatrician and thorough follow-up are essential to ensure adequate food and fluids for these infants.

Box 6-3   RED FLAGS FOR BREASTFEEDING PROBLEMS

- *Lack of a clear commitment from the mother:* A mother who says she is going to "try" breastfeeding, or breastfeed "for a few weeks," or who gives "they" messages about breastfeeding rather than "I" messages needs multiple, positive, targeted messages and a strong network of breastfeeding supporters throughout the perinatal period.
- *Neutral or negative messages about breastfeeding:* Such messages from individual family members, health care providers, or the community where the mother lives or works do not provide the positive support needed to successfully breastfeed.
- *Social history:* A social history that includes things that are known to decrease milk supply (e.g., smoking), past difficulties breastfeeding, or having a relative or close friend who did not have a positive breastfeeding experience all indicate a need for strong support for her decision.

- *Physical assessment:* A physical assessment should include looking for alterations in breast anatomy, which may be conditions that a woman was born with or that were acquired through surgery, therapy, or accident. Alterations that affect the woman's body image, her ability to secrete an adequate supply of milk, and her ability to successfully latch her infant onto her breast require ongoing assessment and evaluation and much interaction and collaboration among health care providers.
- *Breast changes:* No changes in the breast during pregnancy (or asymmetric changes) should be noted.
- *Obstetric factors:* These include challenges such as multiple gestation and more serious problems, such as Sheehan's syndrome.
- *Medical history:* Infections or chronic disease may be problematic.
- *Delay or interruption in breastfeeding:* A delay in the initial breastfeeding experience or any later interruption in the breastfeeding relationship may cause problems.

Copyright 2001 Marie Biancuzzo.

"Red Flags" for Breastfeeding Problems

In many cases the pathology or less-than-optimal situation can be identified in the prenatal period. In-depth and ongoing assessment is needed to help the woman have a positive breastfeeding experience. Most of these problems do not simply go away, but rather persist into the postpartum period unless they are adequate addressed. With sensitive care and counseling and adequate follow-up, however, most can be overcome. To combine some of the assessment data discussed in this chapter and others, Box 6-3 lists "red flags" that require vigorous follow-up in the prenatal period, so as to avoid major problems in the postnatal period.

SUMMARY

Assessment of the mother's physical well-being is essential for good breastfeeding management. Preexisting problems affecting either the breast itself or the woman's overall health can influence the breastfeeding experience. Problems can also develop while the woman is lactating. In either case special strategies can be used to help the woman breastfeed for as along as she wishes. Breastfeeding is contraindicated in very few situations. In most cases, then, the nurse can provide sensitive counseling and special strategies to help the woman attain her goals related to breastfeeding.

REFERENCES

1. Neville MC. Anatomy and physiology of lactation. *Pediatr Clin North Am* 2001;48:13-34.
2. Neifert M. Breastfeeding after breast surgical procedure or breast cancer. *NAACOGS Clin Iss Perinat Womens Health Nurs* 1992;3:673-682.
3. Lawrence RA, Lawrence RM. *Breastfeeding: a guide for the medical profession.* 5th ed. St. Louis: Mosby; 1999.
4. Barnes GR, Lethin AN, Jackson EB et al. Management of breastfeeding. *JAMA* 1953;151:192-199.
5. Ferris AM, Dalidowitz CK, Ingardia CM et al. Lactation outcome in insulin-dependent diabetic women. *J Am Diet Assoc* 1988;88:317-322.

6. Kjos SL, Henry O, Lee RM et al. The effect of lactation on glucose and lipid metabolism in women with recent gestational diabetes. *Obstet Gynecol* 1993;82:451-455.

7. McManus RM, Cunningham I, Watson A et al. Beta-cell function and visceral fat in lactating women with a history of gestational diabetes. *Metabolism* 2001;50:715-719.

8. Neubauer SH. Lactation in insulin-dependent diabetes. *Prog Food Nutr Sci* 1990;14:333-370.

9. Neubauer SH, Ferris AM, Chase CG et al. Delayed lactogenesis in women with insulin-dependent diabetes mellitus. *Am J Clin Nutr* 1993;58:54-60.

10. Kjos SL, Peters RK, Xiang A et al. Contraception and the risk of type 2 diabetes mellitus in Latina women with prior gestational diabetes mellitus. *JAMA* 1998;280:533-538.

11. Kampmann JP, Johansen K, Hansen JM et al. Propylthiouracil in human milk. Revision of a dogma. *Lancet* 1980;1:736-737.

12. Bruck JC. Galactorrhea: a rare complication following reduction mammaplasty. *Ann Plast Surg* 1987;19:384-385.

13. Seidel HM, Ball JW, Dains JE et al. Mosby's guide to physical examination. 4th ed. St. Louis: Mosby; 1999.

14. Canter JW, Oliver GC, Zaloudek CJ. Surgical diseases of the breast during pregnancy. *Clin Obstet Gynecol* 1983;26: 853-864.

15. Goldsmith HS. Milk-rejection sign of breast cancer. *Am J Surg* 1974;127:280-281.

16. Rodger A, Corbett PJ, Chetty U. Lactation after breast conserving therapy, including radiation therapy, for early breast cancer. *Radiother Oncol* 1989;15:243-244.

17. Higgins S, Haffty BG. Pregnancy and lactation after breast-conserving therapy for early stage breast cancer. *Cancer* 1994;73:2175-2180.

18. Tralins AH. Lactation after conservative breast surgery combined with radiation therapy. *Am J Clin Oncol* 1995;18:40-43.

19. Varsos G, Yahalom J. Lactation following conservation surgery and radiotherapy for breast cancer. *J Surg Oncol* 1991;46:141-144.

20. Guix B, Tello JI, Finestres F et al. Lactation after conservative treatment for breast cancer. *Int J Radiat Oncol Biol Phys* 2000;46:515-516.

21. Ulmer HU. Lactation after conserving therapy of breast cancer? *Int J Radiat Oncol Biol Phys* 1988;15:512-513.

22. Rostom AY. Failure of lactation following radiotherapy for breast cancer. *Int J Radiat Oncol Biol Phys* 1988; 15:511.

23. Akpuaka FC, Jiburum BC. Reduction mammaplasty by the inferior pedicle technique: experience with moderate to severe breast enlargement. *West Afr J Med* 1998;17: 199-201.

24. Brzozowski D, Niessen M, Evans HB et al. Breast-feeding after inferior pedicle reduction mammaplasty. *Plast Reconstr Surg* 2000;105:530-534.

25. Hurst NM. Lactation after augmentation mammoplasty. *Obstet Gynecol* 1996;87:30-34.

26. Neifert M, DeMarzo S, Seacat J et al. The influence of breast surgery, breast appearance, and pregnancy-induced breast changes on lactation sufficiency as measured by infant weight gain. *Birth* 1990;17:31-38.

27. Townsend PL. Nipple sensation following breast reduction and free nipple transplantation. *Br J Plast Surg* 1974;27:308-310.

28. DeCholnoky T. Augmentation mammaplasty. Survey of complications in 10,941 patients by 265 surgeons. *Plast Reconstr Surg* 1970;45:573-577.

29. Song IC, Hunter JG. Galactorrhea after reduction mammaplasty [letter; comment]. *Plast Reconstr Surg* 1989;84:857.

30. Engstrom BL, Fridlund B. Women's views of counselling received in connection with breast-feeding after reduction mammaplasty. *J Adv Nurs* 2000;32:1143-1151.

31. Mandrekas AD, Zambacos GJ, Anastasopoulos A et al. Reduction mammaplasty with the inferior pedicle technique: early and late complications in 371 patients. *Br J Plast Surg* 1996;49:442-446.

32. Aboudib JH, de Castro CC, Coelho RS et al. Analysis of late results in postpregnancy mammoplasty. *Ann Plast Surg* 1991;26:111-116.

33. Hatton M, Keleher KC. Breastfeeding after breast reduction mammaplasty. *J Nurse Midwifery* 1983;28:19-22.

34. Harris L, Morris SF, Freiberg A. Is breast feeding possible after reduction mammaplasty? *Plast Reconstr Surg* 1992;89:836-839.

35. Schoch RM. Breast feeding after reduction mammoplasty. *J Nurse Midwifery* 1985;30:240.

36. Hughes V, Owen J. Is breast-feeding possible after breast surgery? *MCN Am J Matern Child Nurs* 1993; 18:213-217.

37. Hugill JV. Lactation following breast augmentation: a third case. *Plast Reconstr Surg* 1991;87:806-807.

38. Day TW. Unilateral failure of lactation after breast biopsy. *J Fam Pract* 1986;23:161-162.

39. Findlay PA, Gorrell CR, d'Angelo T et al. Lactation after breast radiation. *Int J Radiat Oncol Biol Phys* 1988;15: 511-512.

40. Kapil U, Kaul S, Vohra G et al. Breast feeding practices amongst mothers having undergone cesarean section. *Indian Pediatr* 1992;29:222-224.

Breastfeeding is not a task that is completed in isolation. Rather, it is an ongoing, reciprocal process whereby the mother and the infant are in harmony with one another. Although this process may seem instinctive, it may not be for mothers in cultures such as ours, where breastfeeding is not the cultural norm. It is not unusual for mothers to express uncertainty about how to make enough milk, whether they have experienced a "let-down," and whether the infant has obtained enough milk. *All* nurses have a fundamental responsibility to help mothers with these and related questions. The purpose of this chapter is to help the nurse facilitate and evaluate optimal milk production, ejection, and transfer and to generate corrective strategies when needed.

MECHANISMS OF MILK PRODUCTION

Human milk is produced through two main mechanisms: endocrine function and autocrine function. As described in Chapter 4, neurohormonal mechanisms, including the triggering of oxytocin and prolactin and other hormones, control the initiation of milk production as soon as the placenta is delivered. However, milk will not continue to be produced unless suckling is initiated and maintained. Continuation of milk production is controlled by autocrine mechanisms. That is, for milk production to continue, milk must be continually and effectively *removed*.[1] Effective milk removal depends on the frequency, duration, and efficiency of infant suckling (or maternal expression of milk).

Frequency of Suckling

Klaus has pointed out that "increasing the frequency of feeding decreases nipple pain and breast tenderness, significantly increases milk output and infant weight gain, decreases the peak serum bilirubin levels, and ... decreases ovulation, markedly improving the contraceptive effect of breastfeeding."[2] Most of these benefits are discussed in Chapter 8; the focus of discussion here is milk production and subsequent infant weight gain.

Effect of Frequency on Milk Production

Frequency of suckling is important because it provides stimulation to the maternal breasts and a source of food for the infant. Ideally, then, infants should suckle immediately after birth and frequently thereafter.

Milk production increases as the frequency of stimulation increases *during the first month of life*.[3,4] Thereafter, when the mother's milk supply is well established, milk synthesis does *not* correlate with feeding frequency.[5-7] Similarly, milk volume is also influenced by of the age of the infant. Breastfeeding is not considered "well established" until around 3 or 4 weeks after birth. If frequency has a great influence on milk synthesis during the first few weeks but little influence thereafter, increased milk volume may be explained by infants' ability to self-regulate their intake; they may indeed empty the breast more completely during the first few weeks and during "growth spurts." This concept forms the basis for recommendations about early contact, a dwindling milk supply, and so-called growth spurts.

Frequency of suckling, however, is not enough; the milk must actually be *removed*. Effective milk removal, whether through suckling or through expression of milk, increases milk volume. For example, when the mother expresses "extra" milk for 2 weeks, milk production increases by more than 73 g per day over baseline.[8]

The number of times an infant feeds during a 24-hour period, or the intervals at which he or she exhibits hunger cues, is highly variable. During the first 60 hours of life, time between feeds is 3.36 ± 0.17 hours, for an average of 7 to 8 feedings per 24 hours.[9] However, in the early days, feeding 10 to 15 times in a 24-hour period is not unusual.[10] It also appears that infants exhibit hunger cues more frequently on the second day of life and thereafter compared with the first day.[11] Furthermore, the time elapsed from one feeding to the next appears to influence consumption. When there is a greater period of time before a feeding, infants (ages 2, 4, 6, and 8 weeks) tend to take a greater volume of milk.[12]

Determinants of Feeding Intervals

Several factors determine how often newborns are suckled. Ideally, feedings are offered as frequently as they are physiologically needed, but parenting behaviors or hospital practices can sometimes increase the interval between feedings or decrease the number of feedings in a 24-hour period.

States of Consciousness. Feeding can be accomplished any time the infant is awake. However, infants are not simply asleep or awake; Fig. 7-1 shows the sleep-wake continuum. Ideally, term infants should be offered the breast when they are in the quiet alert state. A simple concept governs breastfeeding management here: It is difficult to get a hungry infant to sleep, and it is difficult to get a sleepy infant to eat. Keeping the infant unwrapped can sometimes help keep him

awake. It also allows him to maintain temperature through skin-to-skin contact with his mother.

Cue-Based Feedings. In contrast to scheduled feedings, cue-based feedings occur spontaneously, whenever the infant exhibits hunger cues, and the mother responds.

Ideally, feedings should be offered when the infant exhibits early hunger cues, as shown in Box 7-1. Parents should be taught to recognize early hunger cues and should understand that crying is a *late* sign of hunger. Early hunger cues, for example, hands-to-mouth activity, results in the newborn opening his mouth,[13] and mothers can capitalize on this by offering the breast when they notice this and other early signs of hunger. Parents should also understand that these cues may be transient (i.e., may not persist very long) or subtle. In general, however, healthy, term infants who have not experi-

Box 7-1   SIGNS OF HUNGER AND SATIETY

SIGNS OF HUNGER

- Rooting
- Suckling motions
- Motor activity: hands-to-mouth, flexion of arms, legs moving as though riding a bicycle
- Posture/affect: tense; clenched fists
- Crying: note that this is the *last* sign of hunger

SIGNS OF SATIETY

- Audible swallowing during feeding
- Cessation of audible swallowing; increased nonnutritive sucking and longer pauses between sucking bursts
- Infant takes himself off from the breast, rather than being taken off
- Disappearance of hunger cues
- Posture/affect: arms and legs relaxed, drowsy
- Sleeping

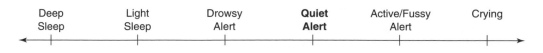

| Deep Sleep | Light Sleep | Drowsy Alert | **Quiet Alert** | Active/Fussy Alert | Crying |

FIGURE **7-1** The sleep-wake continuum. The quiet alert state is optimal for breastfeeding.

enced intrapartum medications exhibit feeding cues about every 3 hours, or even more frequently. Newborns who have been exposed to intrapartum analgesia exhibit subtle feeding cues.[14]

Newborns who are offered cue-based feedings do eat more frequently than their schedule-fed cohorts,[3] but infants appear to self-regulate their intake.[8,15] That is, they do not overeat. Other benefits of cue-based feeding, including the increased probability of continuation of breastfeeding,[16] are described in Chapter 8.

Newborn's Gastrointestinal Capabilities and Limitations. During fetal life, the infant has had continuous feedings. It makes sense, then, that immediately after birth, the newborn's anatomy and physiology are designed to have something close to continuous feedings (i.e., very frequent feedings). Frequent feedings are needed because the newborn has a limited stomach capacity. The newborn's stomach is about the size of a golf ball and has both an anatomic and a physiologic capacity.[17] The *anatomic* capacity of the stomach is what the stomach can actually accommodate when it is "stuffed." (Artificially fed infants tend to "stuff" themselves because of the volume available in the bottle.) The *physiologic* capacity of the stomach is reached when the infant feels satiated. The physiologic stomach capacity of a 2- to 4-kg newborn on day 1 is about 7 ml per feeding (about the amount of colostrum the mother produces), whereas the anatomic capacity is about 30 to 35 ml on day 1, which is the volume that is often consumed by the artificially fed newborn. Because of a low ratio of casein to whey, human milk is more easily digested than artificial milk and gastric emptying time is about 90 minutes.

Night Feedings. Breastfeeding at night might be considered optional by hospital staff and a chore by mothers after they return home. This negative view is based more on cultural perceptions than on the known biologic benefits of night feedings and the normal physiology of the mother and newborn.

Skipping night feedings in the hospital is a deterrent to establishing a good milk supply; efforts to "let mothers sleep" in the hospital only delay problems until they return home. The result-

ing difficulties, including initial engorgement and later insufficient milk supply, are direct consequences of skipped or infrequent feedings. Efforts to let mothers sleep should be aimed at helping them to sleep undisturbed during the day; women who give birth in hospitals are more frequently awakened on the first postpartum day by nurses and visitors than by the newborn.[18] Reexamining protocols that awaken mothers for "routine" vital signs, clustering care, and limiting visitors would be infinitely more beneficial than limiting or discouraging night feedings.

Once at home, parents frequently want to skip night feedings in an effort to get a good night's rest. This is understandable, but it is unrealistic during the newborn period, and for several months thereafter. Night feedings may be more tolerable for tired parents when they understand normal newborn sleep cycles and work with nature, rather than against it.

Newborn sleep cycles are highly individualized, but at least once during a 24-hour period, they have a "long stretch" (4 to 6 hours) when they sleep.[19] If the mother offers multiple feedings during her waking hours, the infant will be more likely to have his "long stretch" of sleep at night. Infants who consume more milk in the morning can be socialized to sleep for substantial periods during the night at around 8 weeks, although not during the hospital stay.[20]

Infants may be more likely to sleep at night when they ingest the higher-fat milk during the evening. The fat content of milk peaks in the evening,[21,22] which may help the infant consume more calories and therefore feel more satiated. It appears that offering a "focal feeding" in the evening helps infants sleep through the night beginning around 8 weeks of age.[23]

Omitting night feedings decreases both the frequency and the overall number of feedings that occur in a 24-hour period; consequently, milk production and infant intake can be diminished. In older infants it may also decrease their overall intake; infants can ingest anywhere from 77 to 344 g of milk during the night.[24] Such a volume of milk, although negligible for some, may be critical for others.

Duration of Suckling

Mothers often ask how long to allow the newborn to suckle. The best answer is, "Watch the baby, not the clock." What the infant is doing at the breast is a good indicator of milk transfer, whereas the time spent at the breast gives little information about the milk actually obtained. Ideally, feedings should be terminated when the infant spontaneously detaches and ends the feeding. As Uvnas-Moberg points out, all nonaggressive social behavior has an approach phase, an interactive phase, and a termination phase,[25] and unless such termination is initiated by the infant, he is probably not satiated. It is likely that cholecystokinin (a hormone that stimulates contraction of the gallbladder and secretion

of pancreatic enzymes) may be a satiety factor that helps infants regulate their intake (and quit feeding),[26] especially during the first 4 days.[27]

It is seldom helpful to make determinations about milk transfer by looking at the clock. Different infants exhibit different characteristics when they go to the breast; some take more time than others. Early researchers identified five basic styles of sucking and used the terms *barracuda, excited ineffective, procrastinator, gourmet,* and *rester* to describe the associated characteristics (Box 7-2).[28] It is helpful for the mother to recognize her newborn's feeding style—not the associated term—so that she can better understand how variations in style make clock-watching mean-

---

Box 7-2   NEWBORN SUCKING STYLES

BARRACUDAS

Barracudas promptly grasp the nipple and suckle with energy and vigor for 10 to 20 minutes. The barracuda is likely to exert unrelieved negative pressure on the nipple, making the mother's nipple sore for a few days.

EXCITED INEFFECTIVES

The excited ineffective infant alternately grasps and loses the nipple, then starts screaming. This behavior usually makes the mother tense and can greatly interfere with her milk-ejection reflex. It is sometimes helpful to remove the infant from the breast, soothe him until he becomes quieter, and then try again.

PROCRASTINATORS

Procrastinators put off for tomorrow what they could have done today. With early discharge, nurses and mothers worry about these infants. Prodding them, however, does little to speed up the process. They will breastfeed when they are ready. In the meantime, watch for signs of hypoglycemia and hypothermia. The term newborn who has no risk factors may be fine; those with other health problems may require medical referral and supplementation.

GOURMETS (OR MOUTHERS)

Typically, the gourmet tastes the milk and may even smack his lips before starting to suckle.

Hurrying or prodding the gourmet often results in his screaming. Allow the infant to try a taste, and in a few minutes he will usually settle down.

RESTERS OR SNACKERS

Resters suckle a few minutes and then rest a few minutes. Mothers are often inclined to jiggle these infants, but that is not helpful. Advise the mother that breastfeeding may take a little longer, but these infants usually do just fine when they are unhurried. The rester is the extreme opposite of the barracuda; for this reason, the number of minutes spent at the breast provides little information about how the infant breastfed; the rester might suckle every bit as effectively as the barracuda, but the time it takes to do so differs significantly.

The behavior of the rester or snacker can be better understood by realizing that the fetus is fed continuously via the umbilical cord. In some cultures the infant is continually at the mother's breast, allowing him to "snack" in a way that mimics the continuous feeding that occurred via the umbilical cord before birth.

OTHERS

There are a variety of other sucking styles, but they are usually some combination of those described here.

ingless. Recognizing sucking styles may be the mother's first opportunity to learn and respect that her child's pace may be different from her other children's pace or different from the style or pace that she might prefer.

The duration of suckling varies significantly. In one study, mean duration was 17.3 minutes, ±3.1 minutes with a range of 7 to 30 minutes among newborns who were 5 to 7 days old.[29] The real question is how long it takes infants to "empty" the breasts. Some infants can get most of the milk within the first 10 minutes.[30,31] However, newborns with different sucking styles take different amounts of time to empty the breast.

Duration of the feeding may be related to infant consumption but not maternal production of milk. The duration of a suckling episode is less influential in the volume of milk produced than the overall time spent suckling during a 24-hour period.[4] Parity is a more significant predictor of milk output, however.[32] It is likely that the feeding duration, as well as interval, affects weight gain. Interrupting the infant before he spontaneously detaches is likely to result in the infant not getting the rich hindmilk and will therefore result in poor weight gains.[33]

In the past it has been commonly believed that limiting time at the breast minimizes or prevents sore nipples. This notion is not supported by research, however.[34] Furthermore, it appears that the opposite is true; restricted breastfeeding has been associated with an increase in sore nipples.[35] Sore nipples are almost always the result of poor latch-on[36] (see Chapter 12 for a discussion of sore nipples). Quoting Chloe Fisher, one source says, "Unlimited sucking time + no nipple trauma = no pain, no damage. Any length of sucking + nipple trauma = nipple pain, nipple damage."[37]

Effectiveness of Suckling

Effective suckling results in removal of milk from the breast.[38] Removal of the milk, not just mouth-to-nipple contact, is also an accurate predictor of intake.[4] Infants suckle effectively when they achieve milk transfer, as described in the next section. Although healthy newborns suckle frequently and effectively, ineffective suckling can happen

under some circumstances. These circumstances may be nonpathologic or pathologic.

Nonpathologic Causes of Ineffective Suckling

Most times, ineffective suckling at the breast is the result of poor latch-on related to inexperience of the infant, the mother, or both. Perhaps the most telling visual cue is the pistonlike motion (jaws move up and down in a choppy motion rather than a smooth, undulating motion), gumming the nipple or areola. In all of these cases the tongue is positioned behind the gum line rather than over the lower alveolar ridge. Clicking or smacking can sometimes be heard as well.[39] The most telling auditory cue is lack of swallowing; if audible swallowing is present, milk transfer is occurring.

In a healthy term newborn, most of these problems can be swiftly resolved with some simple interventions. Signs of ineffective suckling are listed in Table 7-1. Most frequently, *the root of the problem is that the infant has not opened wide*. This can be overcome by eliciting a wide-open mouth before latching the infant onto the breast. If the tongue is indeed over the lower alveolar ridge during latch-on, the position of the tongue is not the problem. Introducing a little glucose water or milk via a syringe at the corner of the mouth while the infant is at the breast can be helpful. This bolus of fluid helps initiate the suck/swallow reflex and encourages the infant to use the tongue in an undulating motion. Stimulating the palms of the newborn's hands can also help him to open wide.

In the past decade or so, anecdotal reports have described "suck training," a deliberate manipulation of the newborn's oral cavity, to alleviate the problems associated with suckling during the early days.[40] However, no controlled studies have shown that suck training is effective. With a few simple interventions, such as those just described, and a little time and experience, ineffective suckling often disappears.

Pathologic Causes of Ineffective Suckling

Ineffective suckling is sometimes the result of more generalized problems. The data the nurse gathers

Table 7-1 Evaluating the Effectiveness of Latch-on and Suck

Proper Alignment

- Helps keep nipple and areola in infant's mouth
- Reduces traction on mother's nipples
- Facilitates swallowing

Proper Alignment	Improper Alignment	Nursing Interventions
Infant flexed and relaxed	Muscular rigidity	Comfort and calm the infant Try a football hold to get flexion
Head and body at breast level	Head and body sagging; baby "reaching" for the breast	Provide pillows to facilitate baby's head and body at breast level
Head squarely facing breast	Head turned: • Laterally • Hyperextended • Hyperflexed • Trunk facing the ceiling instead of skin-to-skin with mother • This results in poor compression of the sinuses and obstructed swallowing	Help mother to adjust her hold Do not force baby's head against the nipple; instead, help mother to move arm to align infant Hold "tummy-to-tummy"
Infant's body aligned from shoulder to iliac crest		

Areolar Grasp

Peristaltic motions of tongue result in effective areolar compression (i.e., compression of the lactiferous sinuses)

Proper Areolar Grasp	Improper Areolar Grasp	Nursing Interventions
Infant's mouth opens widely to cover lactiferous sinuses	Pursed lips indicate that mouth is not open wide enough	Tickle lips with nipple or finger Move mother's arm quickly toward breast when baby finally opens wide (see text)
Lips flanged outward	Lips pursed: lip(s) curled under	As above
Complete seal formed around areola; strong vacuum	Incomplete seal; baby can be easily pulled away from nipple	Hook your finger (or have mother hook her finger) under infant's chin
Approximately 1.5 inches of in areolar tissue is centered infant's mouth	Only nipple is in mouth, or nipple is not centered	Break suction and reposition
Tongue is troughed and extends over lower alveolar ridge	Tongue partially inside mouth Nurse has "biting" sensation if she inserts her finger in infant's mouth Results in sore nipples and diminished milk supply Likely to happen if infant does not open wide	Break suction and reposition

Note: Data in left column expanded from Shrago L, Bocar D. *J Obstet Gynecol Neonatal Nurs* 1990;19:209-215. Table from Biancuzzo M. *Breastfeeding the healthy newborn.* 1994:31-32. Copyright 1994 by March of Dimes Birth Defects Foundation. Reprinted by permission.

Table **7-1**   EVALUATING THE EFFECTIVENESS OF LATCH-ON AND SUCK—CONT'D

Areolar Compression
Removes milk from breast

Proper Areolar Compression	Improper Areolar Compression	Nursing Interventions
Mandible moves in a rhythmic motion	Mandible moves in tiny motions up and down; appears more like "chewing" instead of gliding	Break suction and reposition
If indicated, a digital suck assessment reveals a wavelike motion of the tongue from the anterior mouth toward the oropharynx; tongue is cupped or "troughed"	Incorrect tongue motions include the following: • Side-to-side movement • Deviation of the tongue to one side • Peristaltic movement from the posterior region to the anterior region of the tongue • Frank tongue thrusting (actively pushing the finger out of the mouth with the tongue) • Diminished negative pressure • Absence of seal around lips • Tongue not troughed	Digital suck assessment is not routinely performed Break suction and reposition Suck training has been advocated[40] but has not been proven effective in well-controlled, scientific studies Sucking is a reflex, and deviations in reflexes should be followed up with a complete neurologic assessment
Cheeks full and rounded when sucking	Cheeks dimple when sucking	Break suction and reposition

Audible Swallowing
(Most reliable indicator of milk intake)

Proper	Improper	Nursing Interventions
Audible swallowing present	Lack of audible swallowing	Reevaluate alignment, areolar grasp, areolar compression
Quiet sound of swallowing is heard	No swallowing is heard	Break suction; take baby off breast and try again; be sure to get baby to open wide, which frequently solves the problem
May be preceded by several sucking motions, especially in first few days	Even after many rapid sucks, infant does not display rhythmic sucking motion and swallowing is not heard	Reevaluate latch-on Evaluate milk supply Evaluate milk-ejection reflex
May increase in frequency and consistency after milk-ejection reflex occurs	No change in observable pattern after milk ejection occurs; flutter-sucking more common	Reevaluate latch-on Evaluate milk supply Evaluate milk-ejection reflex

can assist in determining whether this observation is a breastfeeding problem or a symptom of a pathologic condition. For example, a newborn with a neurologic deficit will have poor rooting and other reflexes and may not be able to exert enough negative pressure to hold the nipple/areola in place. Infants with these types of problems are discussed in Chapter 10.

ACHIEVING SUCCESSFUL MILK TRANSFER

Transfer of milk—often referred to as the infant "emptying" the breast—is critical to milk synthesis and volume during the first month or so. (The lactating breast is never completely empty, but the term is meant to convey the idea that the milk has been successfully transferred.)

Often, mothers who express concerns about not having enough milk are instructed to suckle their infants more frequently. Frequent suckling provides stimulation, which is good, but often, this does not solve the problem. The frequency of suckling at the breast does not determine milk volume unless the milk is actually *removed from the breast and transferred* to the newborn.[41] It is critical to remember that increasing *the suckling frequency will not increase the supply unless milk transfer is successfully occurring;* the best reassurance of milk transfer in the term infant is *audible swallowing.* As explained earlier, milk transfer from the breast to the newborn is a major factor in helping the mother generate a supply of milk that meets her infant's needs. Good positioning and latch-on are prerequisites for milk transfer. When latched on properly, as shown in Fig. 7-2, the healthy newborn successfully obtains a quantity of milk that is adequate to meet his needs and the mother has few, if any, problems.

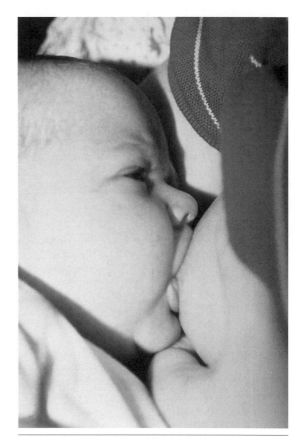

FIGURE 7-2 Excellent latch-on. *(Copyright Debi Bocar, Lactation Consultant Services, Oklahoma City, OK.)*

Preparing for Latch-on

The mother who is preparing to latch her infant on will need some helpful tips. First, tell her that the nipple should be centered in her newborn's mouth. Help her visualize this as a nose-to-nipple idea; if the infant's nose is directly in line with the mother's nipple, he is centered. Instruct the mother to use her fingers to tilt her nipple upward. The infant should be ready to go to the breast chin first, and as soon as he has adequately grasped the nipple, the mother should stop tilting the nipple upward.

Show the mother how to stimulate the newborn with her nipple by allowing him to search and make progressively more active movements to grasp the nipple. Explain that she may need to alternately offer and withdraw the nipple before he

opens wide. It is imperative, however, to wait until the jaw is completely extended, as shown in Fig. 7-3. This open-wide concept is central to achieving effective latch-on. The tongue should be troughed, or scoop-shaped. If the infant latches on before his mouth is gaping open, show the mother how to insert her finger between the mouth and her nipple to break the suction (to prevent sore nipples).

When the infant is ready—nipple centered, mouth gaping open, tongue troughed—quickly move the mother's arm to bring the infant onto the nipple/areola complex. Note that the directive here is to move the mother's arm, not to push the newborn's head onto the breast. Pushing the head stimulates the reflex to hyperextend the neck, which is not desirable. Also, swiftly moving the mother's arm gives her the kinesthetic feeling of

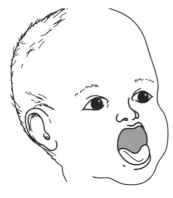

A. Correct

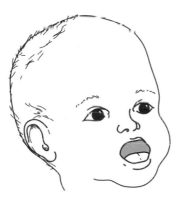

B. Incorrect

FIGURE **7-3** Wait until the infant's mouth is opened wide before he grasps the breast. **A,** The mouth should be gaping with tongue troughed and extended over the lower alveolar ridge and lower lip. **B,** The mouth is not completely gaping, with a flat tongue, resulting in poor latch-on.

how to accomplish latch-on, and in the absence of the nurse, she will not feel a need for an extra hand.

Show the mother how to bring the infant onto the breast chin first. Although we often preach that the infant should "take as much of the areola as possible," this might not be the best advice. One experienced clinician points out that this advice causes women to bring the infant's mouth farther *up* onto the breast, rather than having the chin indent the breast *below* the nipple.[42] If properly positioned, the chin should slightly indent the breast as shown in early x-ray films.[43] Remember that at first the mother relies on visualization

because she cannot see the underside of her breast. Bringing the infant on chin first increases the likelihood that his gums will compress the lactiferous sinuses properly, as shown in Fig. 7-4.

Positioning

Good positioning is paramount to achieving good latch-on and effective suckling. Furthermore, good positioning promotes comfort for both mother and infant.

Basic Positions for Mother
Body Position

Good positioning starts with good maternal posture. It is best for the mother to be in a chair, rather than in bed, because the chair facilitates good posture. Some simple items help with good alignment. If the woman's feet do not touch the floor, a footstool beneath her feet will help maintain good posture. Pillows, especially during the very early days, should be positioned beneath the woman's arms so that her neck, arm, shoulder, and back muscles do not need to support the weight of the infant. A pillow can also be placed beneath the infant so that he is not "reaching" for the breast. The idea is to bring the infant to the breast, not the breast to the infant,

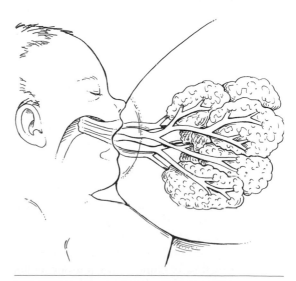

FIGURE **7-4** Lateral view of breast (with anatomy) and position of infant's mouth.

and pillows help raise the infant to the height of the breast in some circumstances. Women with especially large breasts may need to use a rolled-up cloth diaper between their breast and torso so that the weight of the breast does not rest on the infant's chin.

Unfortunately, the first breastfeeding experience usually takes place in the bed, and achieving good posture there is a challenge at best. When the mother leans back—as in a semi-Fowler's position in bed—her nipples point upward; this may be acceptable in a special circumstance, but it usually makes it more difficult for the infant to grasp as much of the nipple/areola complex as he otherwise might. Hunching forward—bringing the breast to the infant rather than the infant to the breast—results in the nipples pointing downward. When the woman's back is straight, the nipples are in a position where the newborn can best achieve good latch-on.

Some simple actions and observations help to get breastfeeding off to a good start. Remind the mother to relax her shoulders—otherwise, she will soon become uncomfortable. Note the mother who hunches over when breastfeeding; instruct her to sit erect and bring the infant to the breast, not the breast to the infant. An important part of positioning is making sure that the infant's skin is touching the mother's skin. Unswaddling the newborn promotes skin-to-skin contact, which helps maintain or improve thermoregulation and highlights the chest-to-chest idea. Unswaddling also allows the infant to use his hands to stroke the breast, which has been shown to increase oxytocin in the mother.[44]

If the woman has had a cesarean delivery, comfort and good positioning are essential. Administer ordered analgesics to the mother who needs them; if the woman is miserable, depriving her of medication will not enhance the breastfeeding experience. Before suggesting a position for breastfeeding, determine the woman's level of comfort and mobility. The mother who has had a cesarean delivery may find that sitting is difficult and puts pressure on her suture line. To reduce pressure on the suture line using this position, the woman's knees should be flexed and feet flat. A bedpan, turned upside down in the bed, can serve as a "footstool" for this purpose. Or she may wish to use the side-lying position (see Fig. 7-10). An older article written by a master clinician still offers many practical hints for positioning the mother and infant for breastfeeding after a cesarean delivery.[45]

Hand Positions

There are few rules about the mother's hand position or body posture. Some techniques are better for some mothers, and it may not be possible to immediately identify the best one. The guiding light about hand position is *fit*. The position used should not allow the fingers to occlude the lactiferous sinuses. The hand position used by a woman with a small hand and a large breast will usually not work well for a woman with a large hand and a small breast. Encourage the woman to experiment to find which hold works best; eventually at least one of them will become second nature.

Either of two hand positions can be used to support the breast while breastfeeding: (1) the *palmar grasp*, also called the *C-hold* (Fig. 7-5, *A,* shows how the mother's thumb is on top and her fingers below) and (2) the *scissors hold*, also called the *V-hold* or *cigarette hold* (Fig. 7-5, *B,* shows how the mother supports the breast using the index finger on top and third finger below the breast). Either position is acceptable, although several years ago the scissors hold fell out of favor. Some breastfeeding advocates have claimed that this position was wrong, but to date no research has shown that this position is less effective than the palmar grasp. The important thing to remember regardless of the position used is that the mother's fingers should not obstruct the lactiferous sinuses. In general, the palmar grasp works better for women with larger breasts, probably because their fingers are not large enough to grasp the breast without obstructing the lactiferous sinuses. Contrary to popular advice, the mother should not use her finger to push the breast tissue out of the way of the infant's nose. Sometimes this technique is suggested as a way to "allow the baby to breathe." Rather than pushing the breast tissue with her finger, which can interfere with good latch-on, the mother should use her other hand to bring the infant's buttocks in closer.

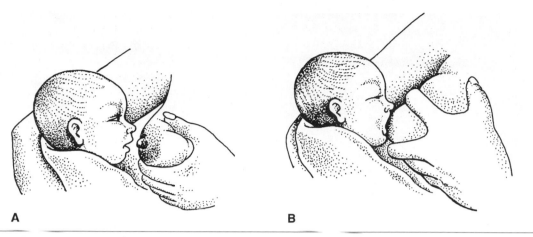

FIGURE 7-5 Supporting the breast using palmar grasp **(A)**; scissors hold **(B).** Thumb and fingers are outside the areola. *(From Spangler A. Amy Spangler's breastfeeding: a parent's guide. 7th ed. Atlanta: Author; 1999.)*

This should alleviate the problem, and the infant will be able to breathe freely.

For the first week or so, the mother will need to hold her breast in place during the feeding. After that time, she should be able to get the feeding started and then let go, unless her breasts are unusually large. Certainly, the large breast should not at any time rest on the infant's chin. The infant who requires continuous breast support throughout the feeding after week 1 may need further evaluation.

Basic Positions for the Newborn

Three basic positions can be used when breastfeeding: (1) *cradle hold* (sometimes called *Madonna hold*), (2) *side-lying hold* (sometimes called *parallel hold*), and (3) *football hold* (sometimes called *clutch hold*). Regardless of which position is used, the infant's ventral surface should always be skin-to-skin with the mother's ventral surface; this is generally referred to as *tummy-to-tummy* or *chest-to-chest.* This technique permits the newborn's head and neck to be in good alignment; if the infant is not chest-to-chest, he will need to turn his head to breastfeed, which interferes with swallowing. Teach the mother to recognize the difference between chest-to-chest, as shown in Fig. 7-6, and chest-to-ceiling, as shown in Fig. 7-7. When the infant is not chest-to-chest, point it out to the mother. Help her visualize a camera that is hanging from the ceiling; if the camera would "see" the infant's skin between his nipples and umbilicus, he is not chest-to-chest.

Cradle Position. The cradle position, shown in Fig. 7-8, is used most frequently and works well for most mothers. Mothers generally identify this position first because it is similar to the position they have seen used by bottle-feeding mothers, but it is only one option and sometimes not the best option for the circumstances. A few important points about the cradle position that are often overlooked include the following:

- Make sure mother and newborn are chest-to-chest.
- Discourage the mother from holding her newborn above the level of the nipple; the milk would need to overcome gravity to be transferred to the infant.
- Alert the mother not to hold the newborn below the level of the nipple; this will cause a "drag" on the nipple and subsequent bruising.
- Point out that the infant's head should not be directly in the antecubital fossa, as bottle-fed infants are held. Rather, the infant should rest slightly lower on the mother's forearm to ensure better alignment.

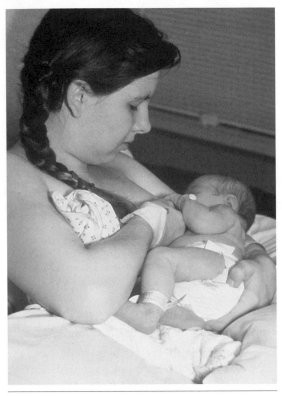

FIGURE 7-6 Cradle hold, with **correct** chest-to-chest positioning and no space between the mother's body and newborn's body. This adolescent mother is supporting her newborn's buttocks close to her body, holding him skin-to-skin. *(Copyright Debi Bocar, Lactation Consultant Services, Oklahoma City, OK.)*

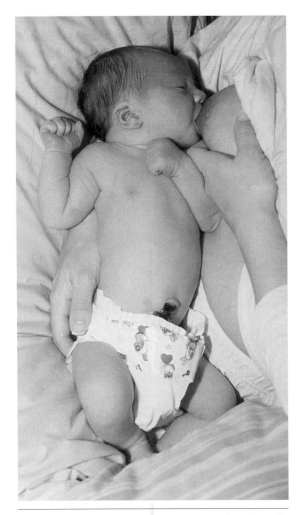

FIGURE 7-7 Cradle hold, **incorrect.** Newborn is mostly on his back, making it necessary for him to turn his head to the breast. *(Copyright Debi Bocar, Lactation Consultant Services, Oklahoma City, OK.)*

- Encourage the mother to hold the newborn at the base of the neck, not on the crown of the head. This usually occurs when her fingers are pointing toward the ears, rather than toward the crown, as shown in Fig. 7-9.
- Instruct the mother to avoid pushing the newborn's head onto the breast or holding it there. The newborn needs the freedom to adjust, if necessary.
- Facilitate flexion of the infant's knees and hips; flexion enables him to maintain postural control.

Side-Lying Position. The side-lying position, shown in Fig. 7-10, works well for nighttime

feeding, when the mother does not want to get up and sit in a chair, or after a vaginal birth when the mother is trying to avoid sitting on her "sore bottom." It also works for mothers who have had cesarean deliveries. Furthermore, the mother who has had a cesarean delivery may be able to use both breasts without rolling over. Instruct the woman to feed first from the bottom breast (the one nearest the mattress); then, when the infant has finished on that side, she can "tuck" the first breast under

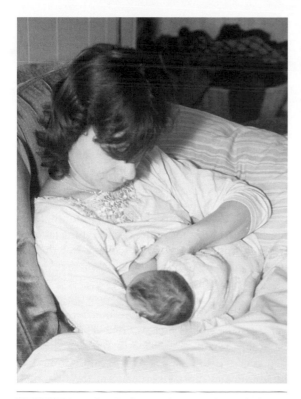

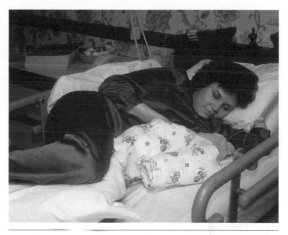

FIGURE **7-10** Side-lying hold. *(Copyright Debi Bocar, Lactation Consultant Services, Oklahoma City, OK.)*

FIGURE **7-8** Cradle hold. Newborn is curled around mother's abdomen in cradle hold with pillow support. Mother supports breast with palmar grasp. *(Copyright Debi Bocar, Lactation Consultant Services, Oklahoma City, OK.)*

her torso and offer the upper breast. This "elevator position" works reasonably well for mothers who have average-sized breasts. (It works less well if the mother has especially small or especially large breasts.) Use a rolled-up receiving blanket behind the newborn to maintain his position and a pillow tucked behind the mother's back to maintain her position and comfort.

Football Position. The football hold, shown in Fig. 7-11, is useful for mothers who have had a cesarean delivery because it eliminates the fear that the infant will kick the mother's incision. The football hold is also useful if the mother needs better visualization of the latch-on process. It can also be used when the mother wishes to offer a second breast without moving her own position; she can move the infant from a cradle position on the left breast to the football position on the right breast.

These common positions should work well under most circumstances. Special circumstances, such as when the infant has any sort of hypotonia or craniofacial abnormality, however, require other techniques, discussed in Chapter 11.

Any of the basic positions can be used (regardless of whether the woman had a vaginal or cesarean birth), but the mother should be encouraged to find the one that is most comfortable for her, given her set of circumstances. A summary of

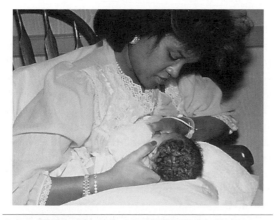

FIGURE **7-9** Mother grasps infant so that he can readjust his head if he needs to. (Pointing fingers toward his ears.) *(Copyright Debi Bocar, Lactation Consultant Services, Oklahoma City, OK.)*

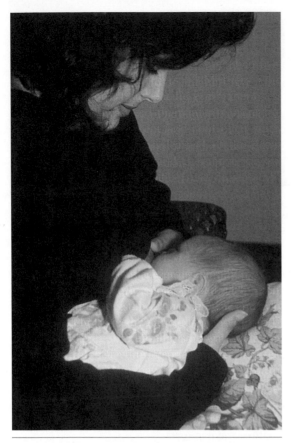

FIGURE **7-11** Football hold. *(Copyright Debi Bocar, Lactation Consultant Services, Oklahoma City, OK.)*

advantages, disadvantages, and important tips is provided in Table 7-2.

Feeding-Related Questions

Mothers raise numerous questions to which nurses must respond. The most important guideline to answering questions is this: Keep it simple! Creating too many "rules" for breastfeeding only dissuades women from continuing. The following are some common questions.

One Side or Two? Presuming that the infant is still awake and not showing signs of satiation, the mother should offer the second breast. It is ideal for the infant to stimulate both breasts, particularly during the first month, but it is not imperative. Sometimes, removing the newborn from the first breast for the sole purpose of stimulating the second breast may deprive him of the hindmilk that, left to his own efforts, he would have happily suckled. When interrupted before finishing, preterm newborns may "forget" what they were doing when offered the second breast.

Suckling only one side at a feeding appears to have little if any effect—positive or negative—on infant well-being. Infants exhibit no differences in restlessness, crying, frequency of feedings, wet diapers, or loose stools when fed from one rather than two breasts.[46] In infants older than 1 month, feeding on one side or both sides can affect the fat concentration in one particular feeding, but the net intake over a 24-hour period suggests that "baby-led" feeding is preferable.[47]

Alternating sides is done to provide more or less equal stimulation for the mother's breasts. Whether the infant suckles one side at a feeding or both, the aim should be to start on the side that received the least (or no) stimulation. The infant suckles most vigorously on the first side, so feeding should start on the side where the newborn left off last time, or if he suckled only one side, the feeding should start with the side that he did not suckle at the last feeding. It is easiest for mothers to remember this if they attach a pin to the bra on the side where they wish to begin next time.

Starting on the side where she left off might not always be practical, however. If, for example, the mother has an intravenous (IV) site in a location that would make breastfeeding awkward, it would do no harm to start on the side where she is most comfortable until after the IV is removed. This strategy increases her chances for feeling successful and increases the likelihood of successful milk transfer to the infant. If the mother has a sore breast, correct the root of the problem, but meanwhile start on the least sore side first because the infant suckles more vigorously on the first side.

Mothers often comment that the infant has a "favorite" side. In reality, the mother probably is more comfortable holding the infant on one side—usually the left side, regardless of which

Table 7-2   ADVANTAGES AND LIMITATIONS OF BASIC POSITIONS

Position	Advantages	Limitations	Pertinent Points
Cradle hold	• Women are most likely to have seen this position used • Works best for most situations	• Difficult to achieve good sitting position in hospital bed; use chair if possible • Requires sitting; cesarean incision or hemorrhoids may make sitting a less desirable position	• Be sure that infant is chest-to-chest rather than chest-to-ceiling • Infant should be at the level of the nipple
Side-lying hold	• Helpful after cesarean birth • Great for nighttime feedings	• Difficult to visualize latch-on	• Be sure that infant is chest-to-chest rather than chest-to-ceiling • Use folded receiving blanket behind infant to maintain chest-to-chest position • Mother's body should be at a slight angle to the mattress, leaning backward just a bit against a pillow
Football hold	• Helpful after cesarean birth • Helpful for women with especially large breasts • Provides better visualization of latch-on process	• Often difficult to do sitting up in hospital bed	• Be sure that infant is chest-to-chest rather than chest-to-ceiling

hand is dominant. Mothers may ask what will happen if the infant feeds more often or more vigorously at the same side over a period of time. Reassure the mother that nothing "bad" happens; the uneven stimulation may result in one breast being slightly larger than the other, but the infant experiences no negative effects.

Rotating Positions. Mothers are commonly told that they must always alternate the position they use—cradle hold this time, side-lying next time, and football hold the next time. This advice is based on the idea that pressure from the infant's mouth will cause soreness to the mother's nipple. This advice is not necessarily bad, but it usually is superfluous. First, it requires the mother to learn several positions when she may be struggling to learn just one. Second, poor latch-on, in any position, is usually the cause for sore nipples; rotating the position will not prevent sore nipples if this

is the root of the problem. However, rotating positions may be useful if the infant has a barracuda style of sucking.

Burping and Sleep Positions. Typically, mothers think that infants should be positioned over their shoulder and patted vigorously for burping. This is usually unnecessary. Infants can be burped simply by keeping their torso straight—explain that the "food pipe" needs to be straight. If the infant is crying, however, instruct the mother to put him over the shoulder. An infant can also be burped by sitting him on the caregiver's lap with a hand on his chest, leaning the infant forward a bit. Recommend to mothers that they give the newborn the opportunity to burp after suckling one breast, but if the infant does not burp, reassure mothers that they do not need to worry about it; some infants do not take in much air and will not need to burp. Signs that the infant needs to burp include arching the back, throwing out the legs, and pulling away from the breast.

MECHANISMS OF INFANT SUCKLING

The Sucking Sequence

Several studies have shown the movements associated with feeding. Ardran and colleagues performed two landmark studies, the first on artificially fed infants[48] and the second on breast-fed infants.[43] Movements of the nipple, jaw, and tongue were clearly seen. Later, using ultrasound, Woolridge visualized the movements involved in suckling the breast and had an artist create drawings to replicate the ultrasound image of the suck cycle.[49] Fig. 7-12 shows the sucking cycle and gives a description. A few points are especially notable.

Nipple

The nipple and areola are drawn into the mouth, and a teat is formed that is approximately three times the length of the resting nipple. Despite technology's attempts to manufacture a teat to mimic the human nipple, no artificial nipple lengthens like the human nipple.[50]

Jaw

The jaw should move up and down in a rhythmic motion when milk transfer is occurring. The observer will also see the infant's ears wiggling. The cheeks should be full and rounded, not sucked in.

Lips

Both upper and lower lip should be flanged, although not too far. Sometimes, particularly in preterm or hypotonic infants, the lower lip folds inward, resulting in a sucking blister for the infant and sore nipples for the mother.

Tongue

The tongue should be troughed—cup-shaped or scoop-shaped—and should begin movement at the bottom of the mouth, extending over the lower alveolar ridge. When the lateral aspects of the tongue are troughed in this way, the tongue can correctly draw in the nipple, press it against the hard palate, and form a teat. The tip of the tongue does not create friction along the teat (like fingers squeezing the length of a nearly empty tube of toothpaste). Rather, the tongue humps up from back to front in an undulating movement when milk is transferred.

Reflexes

Reflexes are important factors in milk transfer. Rooting, sucking, and swallowing help initiate and sustain milk transfer.

Rooting

The rooting reflex, usually defined as a one-component operation, is more accurately described by Woolridge as having two components: "(1) tactile stimulation of the skin around the mouth causes the infant to turn his head towards that source of stimulation, and (2) his mouth gapes in preparation to accept the nipple."[49] This second component is called the *oral searching reflex* by Righard and Alade.[51] The term used for this action is unimportant; what is important is that the newborn exhibits the gaping, open-wide behavior before attaching to the breast.

Sucking

The sucking reflex is elicited by tactile or chemical stimulation of the *palate*, not the tongue.[49] Although we are tempted to assume that the sweet taste of the milk stimulates sucking, Woolridge emphasizes that the lower jaw and tongue are the motive force for milk expulsion; therefore the palate, situated above the jaw and tongue, provides a target for stimulation by the nipple.

The sucking reflex is often misunderstood. The word *suck* conjures up a notion of negative pressure, for example, sucking through a straw creates suction (i.e., negative pressure). When the infant suckles the breast, the suction (i.e., *negative* pressure) created is only related in small part to milk transfer; transfer of milk is accomplished mostly by the *positive* pressure of the jaw and tongue in an undulating motion compressing the teat against the hard palate.

A landmark study of infants using artificial teats showed that they were not able to fully compress the rubber teat.[48] Admittedly, today's rubber

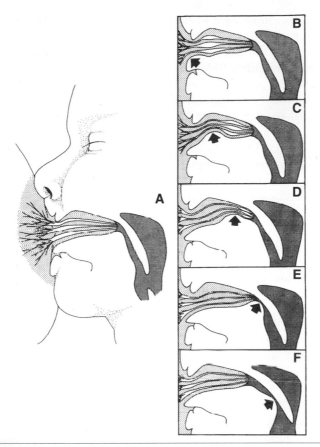

FIGURE 7-12 A complete suck cycle; the baby is shown in median section. The baby exhibits good feeding technique with the nipple drawn well into the mouth, extending back to the junction of the hard and soft palate (the lactiferous sinuses are depicted within the teat although these cannot be visualized on scans). **A,** Teat is formed from the nipple and much of the areola, with the lacteal sinuses, which lie behind the nipple, being drawn into the mouth with the breast tissue. The soft palate is relaxed and the nasopharynx is open for breathing. The shape of the tongue at the back represents its position at rest, cupped around the tip of the nipple. **B,** The suck cycle is initiated by a welling up of the anterior tip of the tongue. At the same time, the lower jaw, which had been momentarily relaxed (not shown), is raised to constrict the base of the nipple, thereby pinching off milk within the ducts of the teat (these movements are inferred because they lie outside the sector viewed in ultrasound scans). **C,** The wave of compression by the tongue moves along the underside of the nipple in a posterior direction, pushing against the hard palate. This rollerlike action squeezes milk from the nipple. The posterior portion of the tongue may be depressed as milk collects in the oropharynx. **D** and **E,** The wave of compression passes back past the tip of the nipple and pushes against the soft palate. As the tongue impinges on the soft palate, the levator muscles of the palate contract, raising it to seal off the nasal cavity. Milk is pushed into the oropharynx and is swallowed if a sufficient amount has collected. **F,** The cycle of compression continues and ends at the posterior base of the tongue. Depression of the back portion of the tongue creates negative pressure, drawing the nipple and its milk contents once more into the mouth. This is accompanied by a lowering of the jaw, which allows milk to flow back into the nipple. In ultrasound scans it appears that compression by the tongue and negative pressure within the mouth maintain the tongue in close conformation to the nipple and palate. Events are portrayed here more loosely to aid clarity. *(From Woolridge MW.* Midwifery *1986;2:164-171.)*

nipples are more pliable than those used in the study, but the infant using an artificial teat still obtains milk transfer primarily through negative pressure. An example may help illustrate this concept of negative and mechanical pressure. Assume that the plastic-liner type of bottle is being used. If the infant could exert enough negative pressure, he could presumably use only this method to obtain milk from the container. If he could not, an adult could use her cupped hand to alternately compress and release the plastic bag—exerting mechanical pressure only—and the milk would shoot out; with either type of pressure, milk would be transferred from one place to another.

During breastfeeding, mechanical pressure is the primary method of obtaining milk; the infant's jaws and tongue are beneath the breast's lactiferous sinuses, compressing them (much as the adult's hand would compress the bag in the preceding example). The negative pressure that the infant exerts is used primarily to hold the nipple and the areola in place, resulting in a good seal, but contributes only minimally to obtaining milk.

Lawrence and Lawrence[52] differentiate between *suckling* and *sucking.* Suckling means "to take nourishment at the breast and specifically refers to breastfeeding in all species. Sucking, on the other hand, means to draw into the mouth by means of a partial vacuum, which is the process employed during bottle feeding. Sucking also means to consume by licking."[52] Here and in most other texts, the terms are used somewhat interchangeably. There must be a clear understanding, however, that milk transfer while breastfeeding is dependent on mechanical, not negative, pressure. The terminology helps delineate the two feeding modes, nutritive and nonnutritive, used by the infant.

Wolff[53] first identified two different modes of sucking: nutritive and nonnutritive. Although his classic study was conducted with artificially fed infants, he defined *nonnutritive sucking* as that which occurs in the absence of fluid. At the beginning of a feeding session, the infant exhibits nonnutritive sucking characterized by a pattern of short bursts of fast sucking (rate of about two per second). Wolff concerned himself with two basic premises: presence or absence of palatable fluid

and the rate of sucking in relation to the presence or absence of fluid.

As soon as palatable fluid enters the mouth, nutritive sucking begins for the artificially fed infant. Wolff's study showed that nutritive sucking occurs at a slower, more continuous rate of about one per second with the presence of fluid, and later studies confirmed that this initial nutritive sucking and faster sucking rate occur in breastfed infants as well.

Similarly, breastfed infants begin with a faster, two-per-second type of suck, which helps the mother achieve a milk-ejection reflex (MER). At this time, the infant is exerting only negative pressure, and in the absence of fluid in the oral cavity, the negative pressure will be highest (and therefore pressure on the mother's nipple greatest). When the mother has an MER, nutritive suckling begins. This is exhibited by a slow, rhythmic suck of about one per second, with no pauses in the early stages. After the MER, there is a decreased need for negative pressure because of fluid in the oral cavity, and hence maternal discomfort disappears.

As the feeding progresses, however, some differences between the breastfed and artificially fed infant are notable. Artificially fed infants show a distinct difference between nonnutritive and nutritive sucking, eventually returning to the faster suck exhibited at the beginning of the feed. Unlike artificially fed infants, breastfed infants have a less clear distinction between the nutritive and nonnutritive modes after the feeding has progressed for a while. The change in sucking rate varies inversely with milk flow; the higher the milk flow, the slower the rate.[54] As the milk flow decreases toward the end of the feed on each breast, the sucking rate within sucking bursts increases, but there are more and longer rests between bursts.[55] For this reason, the observer or mother can see when the milk starts to flow, as the infant's suckling rate slows down when the mother experiences an MER. Similarly, suckling returns to a more rapid rate as milk becomes less abundant and flow diminishes. Suckling terminates with sleep (in infants younger than 12 weeks). Both the behavior (satiation ending with sleep) and age (younger than 12 weeks) are important factors in determining whether the feeding has been successful. Infants younger than 12 weeks who continue to suckle and do not terminate the feeding with sleep should be evaluated carefully; these infants are probably not latched on well and not achieving milk transfer.

Swallowing

Swallowing is really a continuation of the sucking reflex; that is, sucking can occur apart from swallowing, but swallowing cannot occur apart from sucking. The up-and-down movements of the larynx are associated with swallowing and have been used to identify swallowing in studies.

During the first 5 to 9 days, breastfed newborns consume a relatively small volume even when supply is plentiful, with a mean volume of 34.2 g on the first breast and 26.2 g on the second breast at each feeding. Each suck yields 0.14 ml at the beginning of the feed and 0.01 ml by the end.[56] Important clinical implications emerge from this data: (1) Newborns consume more milk from the first breast than from the second, and (2) newborns obtain more milk per suck at the beginning of a feeding but continue to suck even when intake is negligible.

Coordination of Sucking, Swallowing, and Breathing

Although the rooting, sucking, and swallowing reflexes are somewhat easier to describe, the coordination of the reflexes, together with breathing, is more difficult to explain. One study[57] gave particular attention to this coordination.

Coordination of Sucking and Swallowing. In the first 2 to 3 days after birth, breastfed newborns may need to suck several times before they swallow. For this reason, it is sometimes difficult to hear swallowing because the nurse or mother may need to observe several sucks—perhaps as many as 20—before the infant obtains a volume of fluid great enough to stimulate the swallowing reflex. Furthermore, because of the low volume of fluid, the swallowing is generally very quiet. It is critical to note, however, that swallowing can be heard long before the mother's milk "comes in," although it is easier to hear after her milk becomes abundant. At 4 days and thereafter, the newborn will

generally swallow with every nutritive suck in the beginning of the feeding and will have about two sucks for every swallow toward the end of the feeding.

Coordination of Swallowing and Breathing. Newborns must pause to swallow. However, the pause is different for the newborns at 2 days of age than for those at 4 days of age. Weber and colleagues[57] showed that 2-day-olds paused, held their breath, and swallowed. Those who were 4 days old paused but swallowed at the end-expiratory pause (the pause between expiration and inspiration).

Coordination of Sucking and Breathing. Similarly, in this same study, 2- and 3-day-old newborns breathed in a somewhat more uncoordinated rhythm, whereas 4- or 5-day-olds had a smoother pattern of breathing and sucking.[57] The newborn's breathing was faster when it occurred in the presence of sucking only (no swallow component) and slower when the suck-swallow occurred. Recognizing these behaviors helps the observer determine that milk transfer is taking place.

EVALUATION OF BREASTFEEDING

Determining the effectiveness of breastfeeding is the nurse's responsibility and shifting this responsibility to anyone else is negligence. As with the adult patient, for whom the nurse is responsible for observing, recording intake and output, and intervening if the intake or output is inadequate, so, too, the nurse has a responsibility to assess the intake (breastfeeding) of the newborn. Similarly, the nurse is responsible for assessing many other parameters of the newborn's physical well-being.

Effective latch-on is easy to achieve with only a small amount of practice. When infants are latched on incorrectly, multiple problems result. If the problems are left uncorrected, women whose infants have ineffective suckling techniques are more likely to wean early than those who receive help.[51] Effective latch-on prevents most of the problems associated with sore nipples. Furthermore, mothers who experience problems with breastfeeding and use compensatory strategies (including supplementation) to overcome them are more likely to discontinue breastfeeding.[58,59]

Data Gathering to Evaluate Effective Milk Transfer

There is no substitute for direct observation of the breastfeeding process. Every mother—primipara or multipara—should have a registered nurse evaluate the effectiveness of milk transfer. Visual cues that indicate successful milk transfer are shown in Table 7-1. However, visual assessment of breastfeeding is often inadequate. That is, the infant may appear to be latched on well, but sometimes, he is not. Therefore confirmation can be obtained by using auditory and kinesthetic indicators.

Mothers should report that breastfeeding is comfortable, and with the exception of perhaps some tenderness when the newborn first latches on, pain should not occur. With a little prompting, mothers are able to report the sensation of gentle "pulling and tugging."[60]

Audible cues are often more reliable indicators of milk transfer than visual cues. The infant's mouth on the mother's breast does not guarantee milk transfer; audible swallowing signals milk transfer. Swallowing can occur at the very first breastfeeding episode moments after birth, but it may be difficult to hear. First, it does not happen very often because it takes many, many sucks to yield a sufficient volume of fluid required to trigger the swallowing reflex. Second, when it does happen, it is not very loud, so it helps to have an ear very close to the newborn. If the newborn is latched on correctly, most parents can hear swallowing during the first few hours if it is pointed out to them. During the first 24 hours or so, the infant may be sleepy and have few sustained periods of audible swallowing, so it may be difficult to hear swallowing even when it is present. *Audible swallowing is one of the most important evaluation criteria.* The presence of swallowing may not guarantee that all is well, but the absence of swallowing is a sure sign that something is wrong. Audible swallowing is evidence that milk is being removed from the breast; without this removal, more milk will not be produced.

Documenting Appraisal of Breastfeeding Efforts

Traditionally, documentation of the breastfed infant's intake has been grossly inadequate. Most hospitals use a subjective good-fair-poor rating or rely on the reporting of the number of minutes of breastfeeding. Good-fair-poor descriptions work well if the observer is well trained in breastfeeding management and actually present when suckling occurs. Documenting the number of minutes is virtually meaningless. First, asking mothers how many minutes the infant suckled after telling them that they should "watch the baby, not the clock" delivers a mixed message. In addition, because it is a self-report system, the mother's reporting is accurate only if she uses a watch, which again defeats the "watch the baby, not the clock" directive. Finally, the number of minutes the newborn was at the breast may be completely irrelevant. Resters will take longer than barracudas, for example. More important, however, if no milk transfer occurred, any amount of time spent at the breast does not help determine adequacy of intake.

A more objective method of determining intake is therefore needed. If the newborn has a clinical condition that requires close monitoring, test-weighing, described in the next section, is one way to quantify intake. Under most circumstances, however, it is best to use a tool that simply documents the observation of the feeding. Numerous tools for evaluating and documenting the term infant's breastfeeding efforts have been developed to overcome the subjectivity of good-fair-poor descriptions and the meaningless reporting of minutes at the breast. Each of the following documentation tools was designed to provide some objective data, and most require direct observation, rather than relying on self-report. Table 7-3 compares four tools.

To be clinically useful, however, the following tools must be valid (the extent to which the tool measures what it says it measures) and clinically reliable (consistently measuring the concept or behavior they intend to). So far in their development, the Infant Breastfeeding Assessment Tool (IBFAT) and Mother-Baby Assessment (MBA)

Table **7-3** Comparison of Breastfeeding Assessment Tools

Characteristic	IBFAT	MBA	LATCH	SAIB
Focus on	Infant	Infant and mother	Infant and mother	Infant and mother
Scored by	Mother or nurse	Nurse	Mother or nurse	Nurse
Time frame	Progressive: beginning to ending	Progressive: beginning to ending	Static	Any point in the feeding
Analysis of sequential scores	Use mean of scores	Use best of scores	Expect increase in scores	Does not apply; this is a yes-no tool
Measures	Signaling Rooting Suckling	Readiness Position Latch-on; milk transfer Outcome	Latch-on Audible swallowing Type of nipple Comfort Help needed with positioning	Alignment Areolar grasp Areolar compression Audible swallowing

Modified from Riordan JM, Koehn M. *J Obstet Gynecol Neonatal Nurs* 1997;26:183.
IBFAT, Infant Breastfeeding Assessment Tool; *MBA*, Mother-Baby Assessment; *SAIB*, Systematic Assessment of the Infant at Breast.

tools described in the following sections have been shown to be neither valid nor reliable according to one study.[61] The LATCH tool has had mixed reviews in terms of its reliability[62,63] but appears to be reliable.[63] Furthermore, although maternal satisfaction has been reported[62] to correlate with the LATCH tool,[63,64] a careful reading of the studies shows that such correlation was not shown with the *original* tool, or was not statistically significant.[64] The Systematic Assessment of the Infant at Breast (SAIB) has not been studied for reliability and validity. Further studies are needed.

Systematic Assessment of the Infant at Breast

Shrago and Bocar developed the SAIB.[65] They have identified criteria for evaluating the effectiveness of infant's breastfeeding behavior: alignment, areolar grasp, areolar compression, and audible swallowing. This tool's underlying principle is that when alignment, areolar grasp, areolar compression, and audible swallowing are present, breastfeeding is usually going well. The strengths of this tool are that it is simple and straightforward to use and it captures the most important points that the nurse should be observing in the breastfeeding couplet. The original criteria are found in the first column

of Table 7-1; the other columns describe signs and symptoms of incorrect technique. Recommendations for correcting the problems associated with incorrect technique have been added to help the reader implement corrective strategies. A limitation is that, unlike the others, this tool has not been studied for reliability or validity.

Infant Breastfeeding Assessment Tool

Matthews developed the IBFAT,[66] a system that assigns a score of 0, 1, 2, or 3 to behaviors such as readiness, rooting, fixing (latching on), and sucking. The tool as written in the original text may be cumbersome to use; Table 7-4 summarizes the text that describes the scoring system. The tool's greatest strength is that one of the criteria is readiness to feed—the display of alertness and rooting behavior before the infant gets to the breast. A strong limitation of the system, however, is that the criteria do not address swallowing. If used, this tool should be modified to include information about the infant's swallowing.

LATCH

Jensen and colleagues developed the LATCH system.[67] This system assigns a score of 0, 1, or 2 to key elements, including latch-on, audible swallowing, type of nipple, comfort of the mother, and help the mother needs. Table 7-5 describes

Table 7-4   Infant Breastfeeding Assessment Tool*

	3	2	1	0
Readiness to feed	Baby starts to feed readily without effort (alert)	Needs mild stimulation to start feeding	Needs more stimulation to rouse and start feeding	Cannot be roused
Rooting	Roots effectively immediately	Needs some coaxing, prompting, or encouragement to root	Roots poorly, even with coaxing	Did not try to root
Fixing ("latch-on")	Starts to feed immediately	Takes 3-10 minutes to start	Takes more than 10 minutes to start	Did not feed
Sucking pattern	Sucks well on one or both breasts	Sucks on and off, but needs encouragement	Weak suck, suck on and off for short periods	Did not suck

Data derived from Matthews MK. *Midwifery* 1988;4:154-165. Table adaptation reprinted from Biancuzzo M. *Breastfeeding the healthy newborn: a nursing perspective*. White Plains, NY: March of Dimes Birth Defect Foundation; 1994.
*Maximum possible score is 12.

Table 7-5   The LATCH Scoring System*

	0	1	2
Latch	• Too sleepy or reluctant • No latch achieved	• Repeated attempts • Hold nipple in mouth • Stimulate to suck	• Grasps breast • Tongue down • Lips flanged • Rhythmic sucking
Audible swallowing	• None	• A few with stimulation	• Spontaneous and intermittent, 24 hours old • Spontaneous and frequent >24 hours old
Type of nipple	• Inverted	• Flat	• Everted (after stimulation)
Comfort (breast/nipple)	• Engorged • Cracked, bleeding, large blisters, or bruises	• Filling • Reddened/small blisters or bruises • Mild/moderate discomfort	• Soft • Tender
Hold (positioning)	• Full assist (staff holds infant at breast)	• Minimal assist (i.e., elevate head of bed; place pillows for support) • Teach one side; mother does other • Staff holds and then mother takes over	• No assist from staff • Mother able to position/hold infant

From Jensen D, Wallace S, Kelsay P. *J Obstet Gynecol Neonatal Nurs* 1994;23:29.
*Maximum possible score is 10.

the scoring. This documentation tool has some merits, including identification of key criteria and simplicity. Limitations are that the tool may overemphasize how much assistance the mother needs and may minimize the actual observations of whether the infant is correctly latched on.

Mother-Baby Assessment

Mulford has devised the MBA,[68] as described in Table 7-6, to evaluate and document the infant's breastfeeding efforts using a score fashioned after the Apgar score. A strength of this tool is that it evaluates maternal recognition of and response to feeding cues, as well as how the

Table 7-6 USING THE MBA SCORING SYSTEM*

Steps	Points	What to Look For/Criteria
1. Signaling	1	Mother watches and listens for baby's cues. She may hold, stroke, rock, talk to baby. She stimulates baby if he is sleepy, calms baby if he is fussy.
	1	Baby gives readiness cues: stirring, alertness, rooting, sucking, hand-to-mouth, vocal cues, cry.
2. Positioning	1	Mother holds baby in good alignment within latch-on range of nipple. Baby's body is slightly flexed, entire ventral surface facing mother's body. Baby's head and shoulders are supported.
	1	Baby roots well at breast, opens mouth wide, tongue cupped and covering lower gum.
3. Fixing	1	Mother holds her breast to assist baby as needed, brings baby in close when his mouth is wide open. She may express drops of milk.
	1	Baby latches on, takes all of nipple and about 2 cm (1-inch) of areola into mouth, then suckles, demonstrating a recurrent burst-pause sucking pattern.
4. Milk transfer	1	Mother reports feeling any of the following: thirst, uterine cramps, increased lochia, breast ache or tingling, relaxation, sleepiness. Milk leaks from opposite breast.
	1	Baby swallows audibly; milk is observed in baby's mouth, baby may spit up milk when burping. Rapid "call-up sucking" rate (two sucks/second) changes to "nutritive sucking" rate of about one suck/second.
5. Ending	1	Mother's breasts are comfortable; she lets baby suckle until he is finished. After nursing, her breasts feel softer; she has no lumps, engorgement, or nipple soreness.
	1	Baby releases breast spontaneously, appears satiated. Baby does not root when stimulated. Baby's face, arms, and hands are relaxed; baby may fall asleep.

This is an assessment method for rating the progress of a mother and baby who are *learning* to breast-feed.
For every step, each person—both mother and baby—should receive a "+" before either one can be scored on the following step. If the observer does not observe any of the designated indicators, score "0" for that person on that step.
If help is needed at any step for either the mother or the baby, check "Help" for that step. This notation will not change the total score for mother and baby.

From Mulford C. *J Hum Lact* 1992;8:82.
*Maximum possible score is 10.

feeding ends. A limitation is that, like the others, it has not been shown to be reliable or valid.

Parameters Beyond the Breastfeeding Interaction

There is no substitute for direct observation of the breastfeeding interaction. To more completely evaluate milk transfer and correct unmet needs, however, other parameters such as weighing and growth spurts should be monitored.

Output

Just as nurses are responsible for observing and recording intake, so, too, they are responsible for output. The relationship of intake to output is a critical assessment because this is one way to determine whether intake is adequate to meet the newborn's need for maintenance and growth. If the output is not appropriate, the nurse needs to begin to devise strategies to overcome problems related to intake. Box 7-3 describes appropriate output assessments for the first week.

Urine Output. During the first few days, two or three wet diapers per day is probably sufficient because the mother's milk has not become abundant and the infant is therefore ingesting little volume. If the mother has had a particularly long

---

Box 7-3 OUTPUT FOR BREASTFED BABIES

WITHIN 24 HOURS

- Meconium stools are composed of amniotic fluid and related constituents. It is black or dark green, and very sticky.
- Colostrum acts as a laxative on the gut, and meconium (along with bilirubin) should be excreted within the first 24 hours. Otherwise, follow-up is required.
- Stools should not continue to be dark brown/black for more than 3 to 4 days.
- At least 1 void should occur within the first 24 hours. If the newborn does not void within the first 24 hours, a reasonable explanation for the delay and/or follow-up is required.
- Easy to remember: By 1 day of age, the newborn should have had at least one stool and one void

BY 2 TO 3 DAYS AFTER INITIATION OF FEEDING

- Transitional stools, comprised of meconium and milk curds, are greenish brown to yellowish brown, pasty, and less sticky than meconium.
- Stools should not continue to be brown after 3 days, presuming mother's milk is in.
- At least two to three voids should occur; urine should be a straw-colored yellow and should not smell "strong."
- Easy to remember: By 3 days of age, the newborn should be having at least 3 stools and 3 voids per 24 hours.

BY 4 TO 7 DAYS AFTER INITIATION OF FEEDING

- Milk stools are composed of milk curds ingested by the newborn. The mother should have an abundant supply of milk by the fourth day. Presuming she does, the newborn should have milk stools by the fourth day. If she or the newborn does not, follow-up is required.
- Milk stools from exclusively breastfed infants are yellow (look like cottage cheese and mustard mixed together).
- If an exclusively breastfed newborn does not have yellow stools by the fourth day, follow-up is required. Color is important! If the newborn has had an ounce or more of formula, however, color is not such a good indicator.
- Ultraabsorbent diapers make it difficult to count voids. Putting a piece of toilet paper or 4 × 4 gauze pad inside the diaper helps quickly identify a void.
- What counts as a stool? For most, a smudge does not count. Unless it is at least the size of a quarter, it probably should not count.
- If stools are *not* yellow by the fourth day, medical follow-up is required.
- Easy to remember: By 4 days, and until 4 weeks, the newborn should have 3 to 4 stools and at least 6 to 8 voids per 24 hours.

---

labor, multiple episodes of vomiting during labor, or other factors that would cause her to be somewhat dehydrated, the infant is likely to have diminished urine output during those first few days. After the first 4 to 7 days and for the remainder of the first month, the infant should have at least six wet diapers, with one really soaked (eight wet diapers per day would be preferable); any smaller output should be reported.

Stool Output. There is no clear evidence to identify the "normal" number of stools excreted by a breastfed newborn. The newborn has a strong gastrocolic reflex, however, and usually produces stools with each feeding. The number of stools varies markedly. At minimum, however, the newborn should have at least three stools per day beginning after the third or fourth day of life and continuing thereafter during the first month of life. The stool should be fairly loose and non-malodorous.[52]

Stool color is important when assessing the newborn. The time it takes for meconium to be passed is indicative of gastrointestinal activity in the newborn.[69] Gastrointestinal activity is an important consideration because bilirubin is excreted primarily in the stool. Differences in stool color are related to the newborn's daily weight loss. Maximum weight loss occurs 2 days after delivery, and newborns can regain their birth weight as early as the fifth day of life.[70]

Consistency of stools is an important assessment parameter. After about the third day, stools from breastfed infants are soft and look like cottage cheese and mustard mixed together. Stools from formula-fed infants are harder than those from breastfed infants,[71] and their mothers are more likely to have concerns about stool hardness.[72]

Noting and recording the number, color, and consistency of the stools is especially important for the hospital nurse, but parents also need to observe stool patterns. Tell the mother that if during the first month the newborn does not have at least three stools per day that look like cottage cheese and mustard, she should call the pediatrician. During the newborn period, lack of at least one stool per day is a marker for inadequate weight

gain. Reassure the mother, however, that *after* the first month of life, it is not at all uncommon for breastfed infants to go several days without stooling.

Test-Weighing

Routine test-weighing—weighing before and after a feeding—should be reserved for the infant who is not healthy. Otherwise, the procedure may erode the mother's confidence by emphasizing the outcome rather than the process of breastfeeding. If test-weighing is indicated, it is acceptable to use electronic scales because they are more accurate than other methods.[73] Before the 1980s, objections to test-weighing prevailed, and these objections had a sound rationale. In those days, test-weighing was accomplished using the balance scales, which did not have the accuracy that modern-day electronic scales now provide.[74] Test-weighing is not an infallible measure of intake, however. For example, if defecation occurs during feeding—which it often does—then it is difficult to interpret the results of the test weights.

Weight Gain/Loss

A parent or professional often asks, "How much weight did he gain?" This question is a good one, but it sometimes implies that weight gain is the sole means of quantifying infant well-being or breastfeeding success; it is a factor, but not the sole indicator. It also does not imply maternal failure or success; mothers commonly worry that they "don't have enough milk." These two issues are certainly related, but problems with weight gain are not necessarily caused by an insufficient milk supply. Determining the adequacy of infant weight gain involves more than simply putting the infant on the scales. Observing the infant at the breast and noting other clinical parameters, such as weight, length, and head circumference, help form a broader picture of the infant's intake and overall well-being.

Weight from Birth to 1 Week. Most healthy, term newborns weigh between 2250 and 3900 g at birth. It is not at all uncommon for newborns to lose weight during the first few days because they are born with extra fluids "on board" to compensate for the fact that the mother's rich colostrum

Historical Highlight

Milk-Ejection Reflex and the Mother-Baby Connection

Citation: Newton NR, Newton MN. The let-down relex in human lactation. *Pediatrics* 1950;5:726-733.

A descriptive study was undertaken in 1949 at the Hospital of the University of Pennsylvania to determine whether the milk-ejection reflex influenced exclusive breastfeeding past 4 days postpartum. A total of 127 breastfeeding women were recruited for the study and were asked about their signs of milk ejection during the first 4 days. The investigator looked for both objective and subjective signs of the milk-ejection reflex. Objective signs included (1) uterine cramps, (2) contralateral dripping, (3) dripping when the infant was not suckling, and (4) cessation of nipple pain after the infant had sucked for a few seconds. The objective sign was the test-weighing of the infant to determine milk intake. Those with more signs and symptoms of milk-ejection reflex were more likely to be exclusively breastfeeding by the fourth day postpartum.

This study raises many questions for today's nurse, who may be seeing mothers immediately postpartum or following up later in a home visit, clinic visit, or telephone assessment. When we see infants with inappropriate weight gains, do we ask about signs of milk ejection? Do we routinely ask mothers about the presence of uterine cramping while breastfeeding, contralateral dripping, dripping at times other than breastfeeding, or cessation of nipple pain after the infant has suckled? Where on our flow sheet can we record these signs and symptoms of milk ejection? We often become focused on objective and subjective indicators associated with other bodily processes or diseases, but we are less aware of the signs and symptoms of milk ejection. It is important to keep in mind that "the [milk-ejection reflex] is a psychosomatic mechanism which influences the expulsion of milk which has already been secreted," (p. 726). Even if milk is secreted, without milk ejection, there can be no transfer. The nurse often has the opportunity to reduce environmental factors that interfere with the milk-ejection reflex, such as stress or distraction, or to enhance factors that promote the reflex, such as relaxation.

does not provide much fluid. Assuming that the infant suckles frequently during the first couple of days, a volume of milk will be available before the third day.

Although multiple studies have described the "normal" weight gains or losses in older infants, little data are available to describe these parameters in newborns. Marchini and colleagues noted that newborns who had cue-based feedings had steady weight loss up to 2 days of age, with a maximal decrease of 5.8 ± 2.1% from the birth and began to gain weight on day 3.[11]

During the first week or so of life, a 5% weight loss is acceptable, if all is going well. However, any maternal or newborn factors that signal trouble need prompt medical follow-up. A 10% weight loss is usually considered the outside limit of what is acceptable. By 7 to 10 days the newborn should start to "turn the corner," gradually gaining a little weight.

Weight from 7 to 28 Days. By 2 weeks, the newborn should have completely regained his birth weight. In general, a weight gain of at least 0.5 ounce per day (average) during the first month is appropriate.[52] Infants who gain less than this amount require medical follow-up.

Continued Weight Gains. It has often been assumed that unless breastfed infants gained weight according to the standard growth charts, they were underfed. Breastfed infants do not gain weight at the same rate as bottle-fed infants. For this reason, breastfed infants sometimes receive supplemental feedings because they are not gaining weight as rapidly as their bottle-fed cohorts. Until 1999, the growth charts used to determine adequacy of weight gain were based on studies conducted during the 1950s, when most infants were bottle-fed. More recent studies that focus on the difference between breastfeeding and bottle-feeding show that breastfed infants gain weight more rapidly during the first 2 months and less rapidly from month 3 to 12 than bottle-fed infants.[75] The new growth charts are downloadable from http://www.cdc.gov/growthcharts/. Box 7-4 contains helpful information for determining intake and needs in relation to weight gain.

Growth Spurts. Unlike in the teenage boy who visibly grows out of his trousers, "growth spurts" in newborns—usually around 2 weeks, 6 weeks, and 3 months—reflect the infant's need for increased calories. This situation is best handled by forewarning the mother that it will occur. Advise her to suckle her infant as often as he is hungry; usually her supply will meet the infant's need within about 72 hours.

ALTERATIONS IN MILK PRODUCTION OR EJECTION

Sometimes, a woman may have less-than-optimal milk production or ejection. These situations, which are often preventable, can be managed.

Alterations in Optimal Let-Down

"Let-down" or the milk-ejection reflex (MER), described in Chapter 4, is governed primarily by the hormone oxytocin. When the mother's nipple is stimulated, smooth muscles surrounding the alveoli contract and milk is then ejected. More than one MER can and often does occur during one feeding. Sometimes, mothers report that they do not have an MER. Under some circumstances, an MER might not occur, but in most cases the woman is simply unaware that that she has experienced an MER. Box 7-5 describes the localized and systemic objective and subjective indicators that

---

Box 7-4 HELPFUL POINTS FOR THE FIRST MONTH OF LIFE

INFANT WEIGHT GAIN
- Baby may lose 5% to 10% of birth weight the first week. By 7 to 10 days, baby should "turn the corner" and start to gain.
- Baby will gain approximately 0.5 to 1 oz per day after that, during the first month.

HOW MUCH IS ENOUGH?
Maintaining Weight
100 kcal/kg/day
Gaining Weight
120 kcal/kg/day

MOTHER'S MILK
Calories
- Colostrum = 20 kcal/oz
- Mature milk = 22 kcal/oz

Pumping Time
If pumping, mother should achieve a total pumping time of 90 to 100 minutes per day.

Total Volume
Mother will produce about 750 g of milk per day by 1 month. (This, of course, varies with the number of times per day that the breast is stimulated.)

CALCULATING WEIGHT LOSS FROM BIRTH
- Identify birth weight.
- Subtract present weight from birth weight; this will give you the difference.
- Multiply the *difference* by 100, and divide by the birth weight. This will give you the *percentage* of weight lost.

APPROXIMATE EQUIVALENTS
28 g = 1 oz (approximately)
1 kg = 2.2 lb

CONVERSIONS
To convert baby's weight to metric:
- Multiply the number of pounds by 16 so that you have the total *ounces* that the baby weighs.
- Multiply that by 28. This will be the approximate number of grams that the baby weighs.

Example: Baby weighs 8 lb, 4 oz
Calculation:
8 lb × 16 = 128 oz. Add 4 oz. Baby weighs a total of 132 oz.
(132 × 28) = 3584 g

Box 7-5   Signs and Symptoms of Milk-Ejection Reflex

INFANT-CENTERED OBSERVATIONS
- Change in rate of infant suckling, such as infant changing from more frequent, "little" sucks to a pattern of longer, slower, more rhythmic sucks followed by swallowing
- Infant gastrocolic reflex

MATERNAL-CENTERED OBSERVATIONS
- Breast tingling, often described as a "pins-and-needles" sensation
- Contralateral dripping
- Maternal uterine contractions that are more perceptible than before suckling began
- Sense of calm and tranquility, relaxation, even drowsiness
- Thirst[127]

occur in either the mother or infant when an MER has occurred. Anecdotally, one might observe that mothers are less likely to be aware of their MER until the onset of lactogenesis stage II, and often, multiparae seem to be more aware than primiparae. All seem to be more aware of an MER when their breasts are fuller.

Certainly, MER can be inhibited by various factors. The most common reasons could be described in terms of psychologic and biologic factors and pain.

Psychologic Reasons

Extreme stress or anxiety inhibits the MER. When someone becomes especially stressed or anxious, the body produces more epinephrine, a substance that interferes with the release of oxytocin. Stress, anxiety, and embarrassment are common in the early days of breastfeeding, and the woman is unlikely to have ideas for how to overcome the difficulty. More than a half-century ago, Newton showed that stress can inhibit the MER.[76] More recently, stress and anxiety levels, such as that which occurs with noise or mental computations, also inhibit MER.[77] (Presumably, this is because of the accompanying increased serum epinephrine levels, which cause vasoconstriction and subsequent reduction of the amount of circulating oxytocin.) Mothers who are especially at risk include those with circumstances noted by Newton[76] and identified previously. More specifically, mothers who have infants who are critically ill and unable to

suckle are also at risk. Strategies to help any of these women elicit an MER are listed in Box 7-6.

Although fatigue is a common problem, it is often overlooked as a possible reason for why mothers cannot let down their milk. Why fatigue is such an inhibitor of let-down is not entirely understood. However, the hypothalamus is the major relay station between the emotions and changed bodily functions; that is, the hypothalamus governs psychosomatic phenomena. Furthermore, the hypothalamus plays an essential role in maintaining the waking state. Given these facts, it is not surprising that release of oxytocin from the brain is somehow inhibited when the woman is fatigued.

Biologic Reasons

Ice, commonly recommended to help nipples become erect for easy latch-on, inhibits milk ejection. Cold temperatures reduce the size of the involved blood vessels, which in turn reduces the amount of blood flow. Reduced blood flow therefore causes less oxytocin to be at the site, so milk is not ejected. Ice is sometimes used to reduce the discomforts of engorgement because it also reduces tissue swelling. The message here is simple: Ice may be applied to the breasts *after* the feeding as a comfort measure, but it should never be applied to the nipples *before* the feeding.

Folklore has often asserted that beer consumption improves a mother's MER, but this has never been proven.[78] To the contrary, alcohol interferes with release of oxytocin (and hence milk ejection)

Box 7-6   STRATEGIES FOR INCREASING MILK-EJECTION REFLEX

THERMAL METHODS

- Drink warm liquids.
- Use warm, moist heat directly on the breasts. This may be accomplished by applying warm packs (2-3 minutes), taking warm showers, or leaning over and immersing breasts into warm basin of water.
- Warm the flange of the breast pump before applying it to the breasts.

PSYCHOLOGIC METHODS

- Touch: Suckle or express milk in a warm, quiet, private environment, free of noise and interruptions.
- Visual: Look at the baby, a picture of the baby, or even a picture of an older sibling (if the mother is separated from the newborn).
- Visualize milk flowing from the breasts.
- Auditory: Use relaxing music.[128]
- Use relaxation and breathing techniques (psychoprophylaxis used for labor is one example).

OTHER

- Stroke the nipple.
- Use the fingertips to massage the breasts toward the nipple to raise oxytocin levels.[129]
- Consider the possible use of exogenous oxytocin (Pitocin) (nasal formulation is not currently available in the United States).[130]

Copyright 2001 Marie Biancuzzo.

in laboratory animals. Research suggests, however, that a diminished MER is dose-related in humans and that decreased secretion—not just let-down—is a possible short-term effect of alcohol consumption. In addition, alcohol changes the flavor of the milk,[79] and infants do not suckle as well at a feeding immediately after the mother's consumption of a drink.[79,80]

Nicotine, long thought to adversely affect oxytocin levels, has been examined in only one study over the last several years and such adverse effects cannot be confirmed.[81] Likewise, anecdotal reports have suggested that caffeine has an effect on MER,[82] but this has not been confirmed in randomized clinical studies. Smoking should still be considered as a possible reason for inhibition of the MER, however, because nicotine causes vasoconstriction and therefore less oxytocin-rich blood circulates.

Pain

Pain can interfere with the MER. This can be pain that is unrelated to the breasts, for example, inci-

sional pain from a cesarean birth. More commonly, however, the pain is related to severe engorgement or sore nipples. The problem with engorgement can be cyclical. The more difficulty the woman has letting down, the more engorged she becomes; the more engorged she becomes, the more pain she has and hence the less able she is to have a good MER. Just before engorgement, another problem is that the mother is frequently asked if she has experienced a let-down, with an implicit message that if she has not, she should. This is nearly impossible, however. During the first 3 to 5 days—before her milk becomes abundant—she will deny the "tingling" and other localized sensations that are present after, but not before, she has a full supply. This does not mean that her MER is absent, but rather that the internal milk ducts are not distended with enough milk to create much, if any, sensation.

Overactive MER

Some women experience an overactive, or "forceful," MER. Often, these are women who have an especially great volume of milk (e.g., mothers of multiples). These women experience a forceful milk ejection when their infant suckles, and they can experience leaking throughout the day as well. Or, women with a "normal" milk supply may notice these sensations in the morning when, typically, most women have more milk.

Leaking appears to be a very common problem. During the first few weeks, more than 90% of women experience copious leaking.[83] In some women, leaking continues until 6 months postpartum.[84] Simple strategies to help women with this include suggesting wearing clothing that does not show the splotches (e.g., printed rather than plain blouses) and using commercial products designed to absorb or reduce the leakage. A new product called the Breast Leakage Inhibitor System (BLIS)* has been designed to reduce leakage. Breast pads can help absorb leakage.

Forceful milk flow, like leaking, most often happens in the morning, when milk volume is greatest. It also happens when infants are somewhat beneath the breast and milk is then propelled more forcefully by gravity. When a forceful "spray" comes very fast, it can stimulate the soft palate and the infant may cough and gag. To overcome the problems with forceful MER, first position the infant so that the force of gravity is minimized. The Australian hold (Fig. 7-13) or the

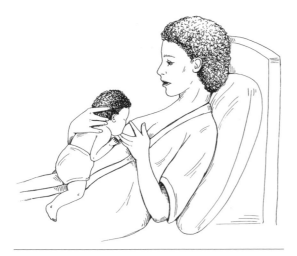

FIGURE **7-13** Modified Australian hold.

*Prolac Inc., 888-410-2547.

football hold (see Fig. 7-11) works well. If the infant starts coughing, it is helpful to briefly detach him from the breast until the milk flow diminishes. (Otherwise, they get a face full of milk before even beginning to suckle.) A little hand expression before suckling the infant can also be helpful.

Problems with Milk Production

This text uses the term *lactation failure* in sharp contrast to *insufficient milk supply*. The former term is used to describe a situation whereby lactation is not possible because of some serious usually irreversible factor. The latter is used to describe some situation in which, with better breastfeeding management, milk supply could improve.

Primary Lactation Failure

Insufficient glandular development is one possibility for lactation failure.[85] This condition, however, is thought to be extremely rare. It may be predicted by the absence of prenatal breast changes or the absence of postpartum engorgement. Either or both of these findings warrant further investigation. If this diagnosis is made, the woman needs a clear message that the inability to lactate is not her "fault." The focus of discussion should be on the mammary gland, not breastfeeding. Counseling should reflect an understanding that certain deficiencies occur in certain individuals—just as one woman may be born without a fully functioning pancreas, another can be born without a fully functioning mammary gland.

Placental retention is another cause of lactation failure. From early in their education, nurses are taught to observe for hemorrhage as a sign of placental retention. However, in some cases hemorrhage may not be the first sign of placental retention. Neifert and colleagues[86] showed that the first sign of retained placenta was related to lactation status. In the three cases reported, women did not experience breast engorgement or leaking of milk. I once took care of a 15-year-old primipara who had had a cesarean delivery for cephalopelvic disproportion. She had chosen not to breastfeed, so no one was paying much attention to her lactation status. On the third day postpartum, she passed a piece of placenta about the size of a small lemon. Retained placenta had occurred without the presence of hemorrhage. In both the documented and the anecdotal cases, there is a clear lesson to be learned: Do not assume that hemorrhage is the only or first indicator of retained placenta. Include the woman's breasts as part of the overall assessment regardless of whether she is breastfeeding; such assessment may provide useful information about the mother's overall well-being.

Some other primary causes of lactation failure may exist. The effect of anemia on lactation is poorly understood, but some data suggest an association between anemia and milk supply.[87] Similarly, the role of sodium content in the milk is incompletely understood, but it appears that when elevated levels of sodium persist, lactogenesis is impaired and the risk of failure is high.[88] Unilateral lactation failure after breast biopsy has been reported.[89]

Insufficient Milk Supply

The phenomenon of insufficient milk supply is difficult to understand. Experts have generated frameworks based largely on the premise that physiologic or emotional conditions or events contribute to insufficient milk supply.[52,90,91] These frameworks, although well researched and technically correct, have limited usefulness for the practicing nurse who continually hears mothers say that they "don't have enough milk." It is easy to take the mother's comment at face value, but this may or may not be the case. In clinical practice it has become readily apparent that sometimes there is an *actual* insufficient milk supply (i.e., production of milk is insufficient) or the MER is not functioning optimally. In most cases, however, mothers have a *perceived* insufficient milk supply; that is, lack of maternal motivation or understanding of basic lactation physiology leads them to believe that their supply is inadequate.[90]

The academic literature offers little to illuminate the clues that distinguish actual insufficient milk supply from perceived insufficient milk supply. This is an important distinction for the clinical nurse who is gathering both subjective and objective data from the mother. Clinical experience and research studies consistently substantiate that "not enough milk" is the primary concern of primiparae[92] and the reason for discontinuing breastfeeding.[93-98]

Actual and perceived insufficient milk supply are certainly interrelated. For purposes of clarity, however, this text discusses them separately.

Insufficient Milk Supply: Actual. Hill and Humenick[91] describe insufficient milk supply in terms of potential determinants and indicators. They use the word *determinants* to mean a factor that is likely to lead to insufficient milk supply and the word *indicators* to mean those factors that can be observed and quantified. Potential determinants include both indirect and direct influences on milk production. Indicators include such factors as decreased infant weight gain and the need for increased supplementation. The framework, shown in Fig. 7-14, reflects inadequate milk production, while a suboptimal MER is vaguely implied. Mothers are especially at risk for insufficient milk supply when they have low-birth weight infants.[99]

Insufficient Milk Supply: Perceived. Two teams have delineated some important concepts about women's perceptions of having insufficient milk. Segura-Millan and colleagues compiled several potential risk factors for perceived insufficient milk.[90] Theirs is a useful list, but many of the factors listed, such as hormonal contraceptives, are not necessarily limited to a perceived situation; these can indeed result in *actual* poor production.

Refining their earlier work, Hill and Aldag[100] described both determinant factors and potential indicator factors for "reported" insufficient milk supply. Although the authors do not specify the possibility of perception, it is apparent that at least three of five "determinants" in their study are closely linked to perceptions that mothers might have. Potential determinant factors were identified as maternal confidence, paternal support, maternal health, mother-in-law disapproval, and infant birth weight. Potential indicators included infant behavior factors (e.g., fussy, refused, poor feeder, poor weight gain), solid food factors, and formula factors (whether or not artificial milk was used and, if so, the pattern—"topping off" a feeding

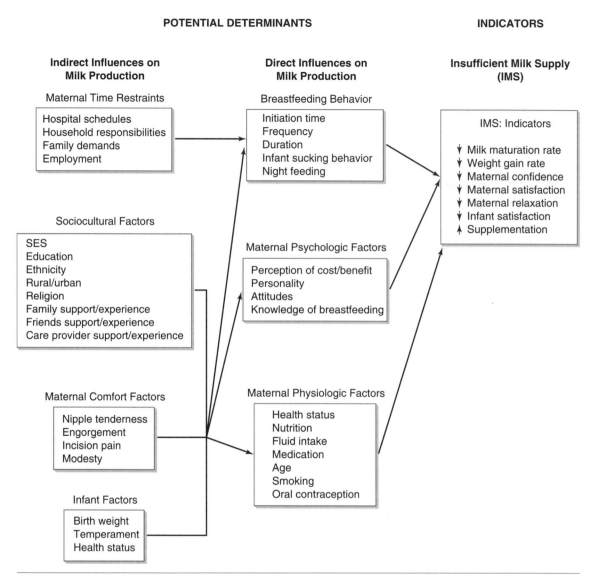

FIGURE 7-14 Insufficient milk supply: potential determinants and indicators. *(From Hill PD, Humenick SS.* Image J Nurs Sch *1989;21:145-148.)*

or completely replacing a feeding with artificial milk).

Management Strategies: Actual or Perceived. Unfortunately, insufficient milk supply that is at first only perceived can rapidly turn into a real insufficient milk supply. This happens because mothers interpret their infants' behaviors (short sleep times or fussiness after eating) as a sign that they need more milk. To compensate,

they introduce artificial milk. (Some mothers introduce solids before 8 weeks as well.) When the infant has artificial milk, he will suckle less frequently at the mother's breast and, according to the law of supply and demand, her milk will indeed become insufficient.

Priorities for care are listed in Box 7-7. It is difficult to prioritize these because the order of priority differs depending on whether the problem is

Box 7-7   PRIORITIES FOR CARE:
INSUFFICIENT MILK SUPPLY

- Instill confidence in the mother.
- Determine whether problem is real or perceived.
- Identify associated nonreassuring signs.
- Initiate strategies to increase milk production.
- Enhance milk-ejection reflex, if indicated.
- Correct mismanagement of breastfeeding.
- Verify or initiate measures to achieve audible swallowing.
- Develop plan to overcome deviations noted on physical assessment.
- Note pathologic conditions and refer the woman for medical help as appropriate.
- Help mother develop realistic expectations about infant's needs and behavior.
- Set a target date; contract with mother to continue breastfeeding until that date.
- Identify multiple sources of support.
- Counter negative messages.

actual or perceived. Furthermore, how each mother reacts to the situation will also determine the priority order.

- First, aim to instill confidence in the mother. In one study, 80% of the mothers expressed concern that they had an insufficient supply of milk.[90] Also, mothers are more likely to have perceived insufficient milk supply if they have ambivalent feelings about breastfeeding.[93] Provide continuous, positive feedback to the woman about reassuring, objective signs that lactation is going well when it is. If it is not going well, reassure her that she has done the right thing by coming for help and that most breastfeeding problems are transient and solvable.
- Determine whether the problem is actual or perceived. Having an actual problem means that physiologic factors such as inadequate production, inadequate ejection, or ineffective milk transfer are present. An "actual" insufficient milk supply is either physiologic or functional. *Physiologic* means that the infant's needs are greater than the amount of milk syn-

thesized by the mammary gland; this is rare. *Functional* problems are usually related to milk transfer; the amount of milk synthesized would be adequate for the infant's needs, but it is not being transferred. Then, identify the *exact* root of the problem before intervening.

- Identify reassuring and nonreassuring signs, and help the mother to do so (Box 7-8). If the supply is truly insufficient, it will be accompanied by signs of insufficient production or suboptimal milk ejection.
- Initiate strategies to increase milk production; these are many and varied, depending on the cause. Mothers whose infants have a weak or inadequate suck may need to express milk after feedings to adequately empty their breasts. Offering the breast more frequently may or may not help increase supply. It will help only if the infant is swallowing; that is, if milk is not transferred, the mere presence of the infant is insufficient. Sometimes, mothers of multiples will have a low milk supply because one or more infants are not suckling at the breast for all feedings. The best strategy in this case is to get all of the infants to the breast for each feeding. If this is not possible, the mother should increase the frequency of hand or pump expression. Supply often dwindles when the infant is ill and unable to suckle vigorously. To establish and maintain a full supply, the mother needs to express her breasts as often as the infant would suckle, or a total of about 100 minutes per day.[101]
- Use strategies to enhance the MER, as noted in Box 7-6. Very often, these simple strategies work quickly.
- Correct mismanagement of breastfeeding. Various forms of mismanagement have contributed to insufficient milk supply. For the newborn, feeding intervals of greater than 2 or 3 hours, taking the infant off the breast before he has completely finished, switch-nursing (rapid switching from one breast to the other during one feeding), and using nipple shields are prime contributors to the problem. The absence of audible swallowing and skipping night feedings are among the most

Box **7-8** Getting Enough Milk: Reassuring and Worrisome Signs

REASSURING SIGNS

- Mother experiences prenatal breast enlargement.
- Mother experiences postpartum engorgement.
- Mother has milk dripping from opposite breast when infant suckles.
- Parents can hear the swallowing; less consistent the first 1-2 days; thereafter, at least 10 minutes of sustained swallowing is noted at each feeding.
- Newborn begins regaining birth weight by about 7-10 days after birth.
- Newborn has at least 6-8 wet diapers per day, with at least 1 really soaked.
- Newborn has at least 3 soft stools per day, at least the size of a quarter (first month).
- Parents respond quickly to early hunger cues and infant suckles well.
- Newborn ends feeding and appears satiated afterward.

- Mother can list at least 3 sources of support for breastfeeding.

WORRISOME SIGNS

- Two or more reassuring signs are not present.
- Audible swallowing is lacking.
- Newborn loses more than 5% of birth weight.
- Newborn has medical condition that requires special breastfeeding management.
- Mother has past or present medical or surgical condition that interferes with lactation.
- Baby is fussy after feedings; hands and feet usually are chilly; baby does not exhibit hunger cues before feeding.
- Baby has mottled, wrinkled, or "tented" skin.
- Baby has dry eyes or gums.
- Baby has sunken eyes or fontanelles.
- Mother is unable to list 3 sources of support for breastfeeding.

Copyright 1999 Marie Biancuzzo.

common mismanagement occurrences. Mismanagement also occurs when health care providers give erroneous advice to "improve" milk production. The most common recommendation is to drink more fluids. However, merely increasing maternal fluids does not increase milk volume (see Fig. 5-1).[102,103]

- Verify or initiate measures to achieve audible swallowing. Hearing the infant swallow is an objective, reassuring sign that milk is being produced, ejected, and transferred into the infant's digestive tract. Not being able to verify audible swallowing is always a worrisome sign; the woman has or will have an insufficient milk supply. (The converse is not true, however. The mother may be synthesizing plenty of milk, her MER may be vigorous, and the infant may be swallowing milk, but if he has a high need, the mother's supply may indeed be insufficient to meet his need.)
- Develop a plan to overcome deviations or poor health habits. While performing physical assess-

ment of the breasts, note problems that may impede breastfeeding success, for example, flat nipples. These are discussed at length in Chapter 6. Similarly, help the woman modify her health habits. Eating foods high in iron is helpful if she has been diagnosed with anemia because anemia has been implicated as a possible cause of insufficient milk supply.[87] Increased stress, fatigue, and infection are possible causes. Smoking also decreases milk supply, and smokers are more likely to report an insufficient supply of milk than nonsmokers.[104,105]

- Help mothers develop realistic expectations. Often, mothers cite infant fussiness as the reason they think they do not have enough milk or as the reason they introduce artificial milk or even solids. Review the normal sleep-wake cycles, the infant's stomach capacity, and the signs and symptoms of hunger and satiety.
- Set a target date. It is often helpful to refocus the mother so that she can see the proverbial light at the end of the tunnel. Many mothers

cannot see themselves reaching their 6-month goal. Therefore I often suggest that they circle a day on the calendar about 2 or 3 weeks from the time they call, and we agree to stay in touch until that date.

- Identify multiple sources of support, and help mothers counter negative messages from others. If she cannot identify at least three support persons, help her to do so (more is better). Similarly, help her fend off well-meaning relatives who may undermine her confidence to breastfeed her infant.

- Beware of the swift and overuse of galactagogues. A variety of galactagogues—substances thought to increase milk supply, such as beer or brewer's yeast—may help (Box 7-9). Galactagogues should not be presumed to be harmless, however, and research studies have not shown them to be effective in promoting a better milk supply. More important, galactagogues are sometimes used on the presumption that they will solve the problem, and the real root of the problem often goes undetected and uncorrected.

Oversupply of Milk

Occasionally, mothers can have an oversupply of milk.[106] Although this would be a happy situation for most, some mothers seem baffled by it. The mother with an oversupply of milk is particularly vulnerable to milk stasis. Therefore observe her for signs and symptoms of inflammation or infection. Advise her to breastfeed with the infant somewhat above the nipple because this slows a quick flow of milk. Refer her to a donor milk bank if she wishes to donate unused milk (see Chapter 14).

Relactation/Induced Lactation

Relactation is the "reestablishment of a milk supply and nursing after the cessation of nursing for a variable period."[107] Although most mothers commence breastfeeding immediately after giving birth, occasionally women decide to bottle-feed initially and later decide to breastfeed. In other cases, such as when an infant cannot suckle vigorously and the mother gives up breastfeeding, she might want to make another attempt to breastfeed when the infant can suckle more vigorously. Mothers might wish to relactate for various reasons,[108] including the infant's negative reaction to weaning.[109]

Induced lactation means "establishing a milk supply in a woman who has never been pregnant."[107] In most cases this is a woman who has adopted an infant. Whether relactating or having lactation induced, clinical management needs to reflect an assessment of the mother's motivation, a plan for physical and psychologic preparation, supportive implementation, and ongoing evaluation of the infant's milk intake.

Assessment

Open a dialogue with the woman about why she wants to breastfeed. Asking the "why" question, however, must be done in such a way that the woman does not feel she needs to defend her posi-

---

Box 7-9 COMMON GALACTAGOGUES*

PRESCRIBED MEDICATIONS

Domperidone (Motilium)†
Metoclopramide (Reglan)
Oxytocin nasal spray (Syntocin)‡
Sulpiride
Thyrotrophin-releasing hormone

HERBAL PREPARATIONS§

Milk thistle (*Silybum mariarnum*)
Fennel seed (*Foeniculum vulgare*)
Fenugreek seed (*Trigonella foenum-graecum*)
Caraway seed (*Carum carvi*)
Lemon balm herb (*Melissa officinales*)
Chaste tree berry (*Vitex agnus castus*)

OTHER SUBSTANCES

Beer and wine[126]
Brewer's yeast

---

*Evidence for effectiveness may be lacking.
†Not approved by the FDA for use in the United States.
‡Not commercially available in the United States as a nasal spray; however, it can be prepared extemporaneously with normal saline if the pharmacy has the appropriate compounding resources.
§Based in part on handout supplied by Tieraona Low Dog, MD. Presentation: The Use of Herbal Medicine During Lactation. ILCA Annual Conference, 1999, Scottsdale, AZ.

tion. It would be more useful to say, "You seem excited about adopting a baby, and just as excited about the possibility of breastfeeding. Tell me a little about how you heard about breastfeeding adopted babies and what you found most appealing about it." Or, if the woman gave birth but did not initiate breastfeeding immediately thereafter, one approach might be: "I'm delighted to hear you've decided to breastfeed Sara. It would be helpful to me if you could tell me a little about how she was fed right after birth, and how you felt about that." In this way, it is easier to determine whether breastfeeding was started and stopped or whether it was never started at all. If it was never started, in recounting the details of what happened, the woman will give some indications about whether the infant was not breastfed because she chose not to do so or because circumstances were such that she was unable to.

Help the woman identify her goals for breastfeeding. Although her motive reflects why she wants to breastfeed (i.e., a reflection of her decision-making *process*), her goal is the *outcome* she hopes to obtain from the decision. Women who focus on the relationship, rather than on the volume of milk produced, are more likely to evaluate their experience positively.[110] Women who wish to feed their infants nothing except their milk—for whatever reason—may be in for a disappointment.

Inquire about the how the woman's family has reacted to her decision. More than other women, this woman's family must provide strong support for her decision to breastfeed. The entire health care team must support her decision as well. The nurse is in an ideal position to coordinate these efforts. Not everyone will agree with the mother's decision or her rationale; they may need some help in realizing that feeding is part of mothering and that this value in some way drives the woman's desire to breastfeed.

Collect data on the history of the mother and infant. The nullipara is less likely to be successful than the woman who has lactated before.[111] The mother who can devote a fair amount of time to stimulating her breasts, either with suckling the infant or using the electric breast pump (or both), is more likely to be successful than one who has time constraints. In general, the younger the infant

is, the more willing he will be to suckle the breast.[108,110-112] On the other hand, some mothers whose children are 12 to 48 months old have successfully relactated.[113]

Preparation and Interventions

Preparation for induced lactation or relactation begins with the woman's understanding of normal lactation. She also needs to initiate strategies to increase her milk supply. The strategies listed in Box 7-7 should be helpful. Also, the mother needs a list of reassuring and nonreassuring signs. The infant who is breastfed under these circumstances is vulnerable to dehydration and failure to thrive.

The existing literature is unclear about what interventions should be used and the specifics of using such interventions. Nipple stimulation is generally begun up to 2 months before the arrival of the infant is anticipated.[52] Once the infant does suckle, use of the Lact-Aid or Supplemental Nurser System (see Chapter 16) helps provide maternal nipple stimulation while delivering supplemental milk to the infant.

In some reports, women were able to produce an adequate supply of milk for their infants with suckling only.[114] The use of metoclopramide, often assumed to be a key intervention for relactation or induced lactation, may be unnecessary. In a randomized controlled study, galactagogues were not shown to offer any benefit.[115] Furthermore, there is no evidence-based protocol for timing and dosage for metoclopramide use. Other drugs, including domperidone,[116] thyrotrophin-releasing hormone,[117] sulpiride,[118] and chlorpromazine,[119,120] have also been used to induce or augment lactation. Oxytocin nasal spray, no longer available in the United States, appears to work best when it is combined with nipple stimulation.[111]

Several papers report nipple stimulation as a primary means of achieving induced lactation or relactation.[110,111,121-123] Presumably, the basis for this intervention is that oxytocin levels increase with the mechanical pump.[121]

Evaluation of Relactation/Induced Lactation

As noted earlier, the closeness of the mother-infant relationship is, in itself, a measure of success for relactation or induced lactation. Some possible physiologic outcomes are also important. The time of appearance of first milk is difficult to predict because it has not been clearly defined. In one study, milk was produced 3 to 8 days after attempting to induce lactation.[124] However, in another case 4 months elapsed before a mother had a measurable amount of milk.[123] Maximum levels of milk production can occur anywhere from 8 to 58 days.[108]

The extent to which mothers can completely or partially lactate varies considerably. In many published reports, mothers are unable to breastfeed exclusively. However, breastfeeding is a realistic goal. In one study, 89% of the women who had not given birth to the infant they were breastfeeding were successful.[120] In one report the intended mother of a surrogate pregnancy was able to successfully lactate for her infant.[125] Success, however, is often attributed to strong maternal motivation and strong provider support and encouragement.

Pattern of weight gain is perhaps the most important parameter. Infant weight gains have been deemed adequate with induced lactation or those who are relactating.[114,115] These reports simply report satisfactory weight gains for the subjects, but this cannot be interpreted to mean that all infants will make adequate weight gains without the use of supplementation. These infants require careful follow-up, with frequent weight checks.

In the case of induced lactation or relactation, dehydration and failure to thrive are real threats. Ongoing evaluation is crucial. The mother should be taught signs of adequate intake (see Box 7-8), and the provider should arrange for frequent assessment of infant weight gain. If the mother cannot provide sufficient milk, encourage her to continue to suckle the infant, even though she may require the help of banked donor milk or artificial milk as a supplement.

SUMMARY

Breastfeeding is truly a reciprocal process. Mothers produce and eject milk, and the milk is transferred to the newborn when he suckles effectively. Maternal milk supply best meets the newborn's demands when breastfeeding is initiated early and

is not restricted in any way. Achieving good positioning and latch-on is critical, and the nurse has a responsibility to assist the mother with these efforts. Immediate evaluation of the breastfeeding interaction is best accomplished through direct observation, but ongoing evaluation is also needed. Some special situations that affect milk production, ejection, and transfer can usually be overcome by using targeted clinical strategies.

REFERENCES

1. Wilde CJ, Addey CV, Bryson JM et al. Autocrine regulation of milk secretion. *Biochem Soc Symp* 1998;63:81-90.
2. Klaus MH. The frequency of suckling. A neglected but essential ingredient of breast-feeding. *Obstet Gynecol Clin North Am* 1987;14:623-633.
3. DeCarvalho M, Robertson S, Friedman A et al. Effect of frequent breast-feeding on early milk production and infant weight gain. *Pediatrics* 1983;72:307-311.
4. Drewett RF, Woolridge MW, Jackson DA et al. Relationships between nursing patterns, supplementary food intake and breast-milk intake in a rural Thai population. *Early Hum Dev* 1989;20:13-23.
5. Dewey KG, Heinig MJ, Nommsen LA et al. Maternal versus infant factors related to breast milk intake and residual milk volume: the DARLING study. *Pediatrics* 1991;87:829-837.
6. Butte NF, Garza C, Smith EO et al. Human milk intake and growth in exclusively breast-fed infants. *J Pediatr* 1984;104:187-195.
7. Butte NF, Wills C, Jean CA et al. Feeding patterns of exclusively breast-fed infants during the first four months of life. *Early Hum Dev* 1985;12:291-300.
8. Dewey KG, Lonnerdal B. Infant self-regulation of breast milk intake. *Acta Paediatr Scand* 1986;75:893-898.
9. Benson S. What is normal? A study of normal breastfeeding dyads during the first sixty hours of life. *Breastfeed Rev* 2001;9:27-32.
10. Diaz S, Herreros C, Aravena R et al. Breast-feeding duration and growth of fully breast-fed infants in a poor urban Chilean population. *Am J Clin Nutr* 1995;62:371-376.
11. Marchini G, Persson B, Berggren V et al. Hunger behaviour contributes to early nutritional homeostasis. *Acta Paediatr* 1998;87:671-675.
12. Matheny RJ, Birch LL, Picciano MF. Control of intake by human-milk-fed infants: relationships between feeding size and interval. *Dev Psychobiol* 1990;23:511-518.
13. Lew AR, Butterworth G. The effects of hunger on hand-mouth coordination in newborn infants. *Dev Psychol* 1995;31:456-463.
14. Ransjo-Arvidson AB, Matthiesen AS, Lilja G et al. Maternal analgesia during labor disturbs newborn

behavior: effects on breastfeeding, temperature, and crying. *Birth* 2001;28: 5-12.

15. Daly SE, Kent JC, Huynh DQ et al. The determination of short-term breast volume changes and the rate of synthesis of human milk using computerized breast measurement. *Exp Physiol* 1992;77:79-87.

16. Salariya EM, Easton PM, Cater JI. Duration of breastfeeding after early initiation and frequent feeding. *Lancet* 1978;2:1141-1143.

17. Scammon RD, Doyle LO. Observations on the capacity of the stomach in the first ten days of postnatal life. *Am J Dis Child* 1920;20:516-538.

18. Lentz MJ, Killien MG. Are you sleeping? Sleep patterns during postpartum hospitalization. *J Perinatal Neonatal Nurs* 1991;4:30-38.

19. Emde RN, Swedberg J, Suzuki B. Human wakefulness and biological rhythms after birth. *Arch Gen Psychiatry* 1975;32:780-783.

20. Pinilla T, Birch LL. Help me make it through the night: behavioral entrainment of breast-fed infants' sleep patterns. *Pediatrics* 1993;91:436-444.

21. Jackson DA, Imong SM, Silprasert A et al. Circadian variation in fat concentration of breast-milk in a rural northern Thai population. *Br J Nutr* 1988;59:349-363.

22. Stafford J, Villalpando S, Urquieta et al. Circadian variation and changes after a meal in volume and lipid production of human milk from rural Mexican women. *Ann Nutr Metab* 1994;38:232-237.

23. Renfrew MJ, Lang S, Martin L, et al. Interventions for influencing sleep patterns in exclusively breastfed infants. *Cochrane Database Syst Rev* 2000:CD000113.

24. Imong SM, Jackson DA, Woolridge MW et al. Indirect test weighing: a new method for measuring overnight breast milk intakes in the field. *J Pediatr Gastroenterol Nutr* 1988;7:699-706.

25. Uvnas-Moberg K. Physiological and endocrine effects of social contact. *Ann NY Acad Sci* 1997:807:146-163.

26. Marchini G, Linden A. Cholecystokinin, a satiety signal in newborn infants? *J Dev Physiol* 1992;17:215-219.

27. Uvnas-Moberg K, Marchini G, Winberg J. Plasma cholecystokinin concentrations after breast feeding in healthy 4 day old infants. *Arch Dis Child* 1993;68:46-48.

28. Barnes GR, Lethin AN, Jackson EB et al. Management of breastfeeding. *JAMA* 1953;151:192-199.

29. Howie PW, Houston MJ, Cook A et al. How long should a breast feed last? *Early Hum Dev* 1981;5:71-77.

30. Lucas A, Lucas PJ, Baum JD. Pattern of milk flow in breastfed infants. *Lancet* 1979;2:57-58.

31. Lucas A, Lucas PJ, Baum JD. Differences in the pattern of milk intake between breast and bottle fed infants. *Early Hum Dev* 1981;5:195-199.

32. Ingram JC, Woolridge MW, Greenwood RJ et al. Maternal predictors of early breast milk output. *Acta Paediatr* 1999;88:493-499.

33. Drewett R, Amatayakul K, Wongsawasdii L et al. Nursing frequency and the energy intake from breast milk and supplementary food in a rural Thai population: a longitudinal study. *Eur J Clin Nutr* 1993;47:880-891.

34. L'Esperance C, Frantz K. Time limitation for early breastfeeding. *J Obstet Gynecol Neonatal Nurs* 1985;14:114-118.

35. Renfrew MJ, Lang S, Martin L et al. Feeding schedules in hospitals for newborn infants. *Cochrane Database Syst Rev* 2000:CD000090.

36. Righard L. Are breastfeeding problems related to incorrect breastfeeding technique and the use of pacifiers and bottles? *Birth* 1998;25:40-44.

37. Woolridge MW. The 'anatomy' of infant sucking. *Midwifery* 1986;2:164-171.

38. Daly SE, Owens RA, Hartmann PE. The short-term synthesis and infant-regulated removal of milk in lactating women. *Exp Physiol* 1993;78:209-220.

39. Widstrom AM, Thingstrom-Paulsson J. The position of the tongue during rooting reflexes elicited in newborn infants before the first suckle. *Acta Paediatr* 1993;82:281-283.

40. Marmet C, Shell E. Training neonates to suck correctly. *MCN Am J Matern Child Nurs* 1984;9:401-407.

41. Daly SE, Hartmann PE. Infant demand and milk supply. Part 2: the short-term control of milk synthesis in lactating women. *J Hum Lact* 1995;11:27-37.

42. Minchin MK. Positioning for breastfeeding. *Birth* 1989;16:67-73.

43. Ardran GM, Kemp FH, Lind J. A cineradiographic study of breast feeding. *Br J Radiol* 1958;31:156-162.

44. Matthiesen AS, Ransjo-Arvidson AB, Nissen E et al. Postpartum maternal oxytocin release by newborns: effects of infant hand massage and sucking. *Birth* 2001;28:13-19.

45. Frantz KB, Kalmen BA. Breastfeeding works for cesareans, too. *RN* 1979;42:39-47.

46. Righard L, Flodmark CE, Lothe L et al. Breastfeeding patterns: comparing the effects on infant behavior and maternal satisfaction of using one or two breasts. *Birth* 1993;20:182-185.

47. Woolridge MW, Ingram JC, Baum JD. Do changes in pattern of breast usage alter the baby's nutrient intake? *Lancet* 1990;336:395-397.

48. Ardran GM, Kemp FH, Lind J. A cineradiographic study of bottle feeding. *Br J Radiol* 1956;31:11-22.

49. Woolridge MW. Aetiology of sore nipples. *Midwifery* 1986;2:172-176.

50. Nowak AJ, Smith WL, Erenberg A. Imaging evaluation of artificial nipples during bottle feeding. *Arch Pediatr Adolesc Med* 1994;148:40-42.

51. Righard L, Alade MO. Sucking technique and its effect on success of breastfeeding. *Birth* 1992;19:185-189.

52. Lawrence RA, Lawrence RM. *Breastfeeding: A guide for the medical profession.* 5th ed. St. Louis: Mosby; 1999.

53. Wolff PH. The serial organization of sucking in the young infant. *Pediatrics* 1968;42:943-956.

54. Bowen-Jones A, Thompson C, Drewett RF. Milk flow and sucking rates during breast-feeding. *Dev Med Child Neurol* 1982;24:626-633.

55. Drewett RF, Woolridge M. Sucking patterns of human babies on the breast. *Early Hum Dev* 1979;3:315-321.

56. Woolridge MW, Baum JD, Drewett RF. Does a change in the composition of human milk affect sucking patterns and milk intake? *Lancet* 1980;2:1292-1293.

57. Weber F, Woolridge MW, Baum JD. An ultrasonographic study of the organisation of sucking and swallowing by newborn infants. *Dev Med Child Neurol* 1986;28:19-24.

58. Blomquist HK, Jonsbo F, Serenius F et al. Supplementary feeding in the maternity ward shortens the duration of breast feeding. *Acta Paediatr* 1994;83:1122-1126.

59. DiGirolamo AM, Grummer-Strawn LM, Fein S. Maternity care practices: implications for breastfeeding. *Birth* 2001;28:94-100.

60. Stancil J. Personal communication, 2001.

61. Riordan JM, Koehn M. Reliability and validity testing of three breastfeeding assessment tools. *J Obstet Gynecol Neonatal Nurs* 1997;26:181 187.

62. Riordan J, Bibb D, Miller M et al. Predicting breastfeeding duration using the LATCH breastfeeding assessment tool. *J Hum Lact* 2001;17:20-23.

63. Adams D, Hewell S. Maternal and professional assessment of breastfeeding. *J Hum Lact* 1997;13:279-283.

64. Schlomer JA, Kemmerer J, Twiss JJ. Evaluating the association of two breastfeeding assessment tools with breastfeeding problems and breastfeeding satisfaction. *J Hum Lact* 1999;15:35-39.

65. Shrago L, Bocar D. The infant's contribution to breastfeeding. *J Obstet Gynecol Neonatal Nurs* 1990;19:209-215.

66. Matthews MK. Assessments and suggested interventions to assist newborn breastfeeding behavior. *J Hum Lact* 1993;9:243-248.

67. Jensen D, Wallace S, Kelsay P. LATCH: a breastfeeding charting system and documentation tool. *J Obstet Gynecol Neonatal Nurs* 1994;23:27-32.

68. Mulford C. The Mother-Baby Assessment (MBA): an "Apgar score" for breastfeeding. *J Hum Lact* 1992;8:79-82.

69. Salariya EM, Robertson CM. The development of a neonatal stool colour comparator. *Midwifery* 1993;9:35-40.

70. Salariya EM, Robertson CM. Relationships between baby feeding types and patterns, gut transit time of meconium and the incidence of neonatal jaundice. *Midwifery* 1993;9:235-242.

71. Quinlan PT, Lockton S, Irwin J et al. The relationship between stool hardness and stool composition in breast- and formula-fed infants. *J Pediatr Gastroenterol Nutr* 1995;20:81-90.

72. Morley R, Abbott RA, Lucas A. Infant feeding and maternal concerns about stool hardness. *Child Care Health Dev* 1997;23:475-478.

73. Butte NF, Garza C, Smith EO et al. Evaluation of the deuterium dilution technique against the test-weighing procedure for the determination of breast milk intake. *Am J Clin Nutr* 1983;37:996-1003.

74. Drewett RF, Woolridge MW, Greasley V et al. Evaluating breast-milk intake by test weighing: a portable electronic balance suitable for community and field studies. *Early Hum Dev* 1984;10:123-126.

75. Dewey KG, Peerson JM, Brown KH et al. Growth of breast-fed infants deviates from current reference data: a pooled analysis of US, Canadian, and European data sets. World Health Organization Working Group on Infant Growth. *Pediatrics* 1995;96:495-503.

76. Newton M, Newton NR. The let-down reflex in human lactation. *Journal of Pediatrics.* 1948;33:698-704.

77. Ueda T, Yokoyama Y, Irahara M et al. Influence of psychological stress on suckling-induced pulsatile oxytocin release. *Obstet Gynecol* 1994;84:259-262.

78. Mennella JA, Beauchamp GK. Beer, breast feeding, and folklore. *Dev Psychobiol* 1993;26:459-466.

79. Mennella JA. Infants' suckling responses to the flavor of alcohol in mothers' milk. *Alcohol Clin Exp Res* 1997;21:581-585.

80. Mennella JA. Regulation of milk intake after exposure to alcohol in mothers' milk. *Alcohol Clin Exp Res* 2001;25:590-593.

81. Amir LH. Maternal smoking and reduced duration of breastfeeding: a review of possible mechanisms. *Early Hum Dev* 2001;64:45-67.

82. Liston J. Breastfeeding and the use of recreational drugs—alcohol, caffeine, nicotine and marijuana. *Breastfeed Rev* 1998;6:27-30.

83. Griffiths RJ. Breast pads: their effectiveness and use by lactating women. *J Hum Lact* 1993;9:19-26.

84. Morse JM, Bottorff JL. Leaking: a problem of lactation. *J Nurse Midwifery* 1989;34:15-20.

85. Neifert MR, Seacat JM, Jobe WE. Lactation failure due to insufficient glandular development of the breast. *Pediatrics* 1985;76:823-828.

86. Neifert MR, McDonough SL, Neville MC. Failure of lactogenesis associated with placental retention. *Am J Obstet Gynecol* 1981;140:477-478.

87. Henly SJ, Anderson CM, Avery MD et al. Anemia and insufficient milk in first-time mothers. *Birth* 1995;22:86-92.

88. Morton JA. The clinical usefulness of breast milk sodium in the assessment of lactogenesis. *Pediatrics* 1994;93:802-806.

89. Day TW. Unilateral failure of lactation after breast biopsy. *J Fam Pract* 1986;23:161-162.

90. Segura-Millan S, Dewey KG, Perez-Escamilla R. Factors associated with perceived insufficient milk in a low-income urban population in Mexico. *J Nutr* 1994;124:202-212.

91. Hill PD, Humenick SS. Insufficient milk supply. *Image J Nurs Sch* 1989;21:145-148.

92. Mogan J. A study of mothers' breastfeeding concerns. *Birth* 1986;13:104-108.

93. Hillervik-Lindquist C. Studies on perceived breast milk insufficiency. A prospective study in a group of Swedish women. *Acta Paediatr Scand Suppl* 1991;376:1-27.

94. Bevan ML, Mosley D, Solimano GR. Factors influencing breast feeding in an urban WIC program. *J Am Diet Assoc* 1984;84:563-567.

95. Gunn TR. The incidence of breast feeding and reasons for weaning. *N Z Med J* 1984;97:360-363.

96. Hawkins LM, Nichols FH, Tanner JL. Predictors of the duration of breastfeeding in low-income women. *Birth* 1987;14:204-209.

97. Hill PD. Effects of education on breastfeeding success. *Matern Child Nurs J* 1987;16:145-156.

98. Holt GM, Wolkind SN. Early abandonment of breast feeding: causes and effects. *Child Care Health Dev* 1983;9:349-355.

99. Hill PD, Hanson KS, Mefford AL. Mothers of low birthweight infants: breastfeeding patterns and problems. *J Hum Lact* 1994;10:169-176.

100. Hill PD, Aldag J. Potential indicators of insufficient milk supply syndrome. *Res Nurs Health* 1991;14:11-19.

101. Hopkinson JM, Schanler RJ, Garza C. Milk production by mothers of premature infants. *Pediatrics* 1988;81:815-820.

102. Dusdieker LB, Booth BM, Stumbo PJ et al. Effect of supplemental fluids on human milk production. *J Pediatr* 1985;106:207-211.

103. Dusdieker LB, Stumbo PJ, Booth BM et al. Prolonged maternal fluid supplementation in breast-feeding. *Pediatrics* 1990;86:737-740.

104. Vio F, Salazar G, Infante C. Smoking during pregnancy and lactation and its effects on breast-milk volume. *Am J Clin Nutr* 1991;54:1011-1016.

105. Hill PD, Aldag JC. Smoking and breastfeeding status. *Res Nurs Health* 1996;19:125-132.

106. Livingstone V. Too much of a good thing. Maternal and infant hyperlactation syndromes. *Can Fam Physician* 1996;42:89-99.

107. Waletzky LR, Herman EC. Relactation. *Am Fam Physician* 1976;14:69-74.

108. Bose CL, D'Ercole AJ, Lester AG et al. Relactation by mothers of sick and premature infants. *Pediatrics* 1981;67:565-569.

109. Marquis GS, Diaz J, Bartolini R et al. Recognizing the reversible nature of child-feeding decisions: breastfeeding, weaning, and relactation patterns in a shanty town community of Lima, Peru. *Soc Sci Med* 1998;47:645-656.

110. Auerbach KG, Avery JL. Relactation: a study of 366 cases. *Pediatrics* 1980;65:236-242.

111. Auerbach KG, Avery JL. Induced lactation. A study of adoptive nursing by 240 women. *Am J Dis Child* 1981;135:340-343.

112. Rogers IS. Relactation. *Early Hum Dev* 1997;49(Suppl):S75-S81.

113. Phillips V. Relactation in mothers of children over 12 months. *J Trop Pediatr* 1993;39:45-48.

114. Abejide OR, Tadese MA, Babajide DE et al. Non-puerperal induced lactation in a Nigerian community: case reports. *Ann Trop Paediatr* 1997;17:109-114.

115. Seema, Patwari AK, Satyanarayana L. Relactation: An effective intervention to promote exclusive breastfeeding. *J Trop Pediatr* 1997;43:213-216.

116. Petraglia F, De Leo V, Sardelli S et al. Domperidone in defective and insufficient lactation. *Eur J Obstet Gynecol Reprod Biol* 1985;19:281-287.

117. Peters F, Schulze Tollert J, Schuth W. Thyrotrophin-releasing hormone—a lactation-promoting agent? *Br J Obstet Gynaecol* 1991;98:880-885.

118. Hallbauer U. Sulpiride (Eglonyl)—use to stimulate lactation. *S Afr Med J* 1997;87:774-775.

119. Brown RE. Relactation: an overview. *Pediatrics* 1977;60:116-120.

120. Nemba K. Induced lactation: a study of 37 non-puerperal mothers. *J Trop Pediatr* 1994;40:240-242.

121. Amico JA, Finley BE. Breast stimulation in cycling women, pregnant women and a woman with induced lactation: pattern of release of oxytocin, prolactin and luteinizing hormone. *Clin Endocrinol Oxf* 1986;25:97-106.

122. Auerbach KG. Extraordinary breast feeding: relactation/induced lactation. *J Trop Pediatr* 1981;27:52-55.

123. Cheales-Siebenaler NJ. Induced lactation in an adoptive mother. *J Hum Lact* 1999;15:41-43.

124. Banapurmath CR, Banapurmath S, Kesaree N. Successful induced non-puerperal lactation in surrogate mothers. *Indian J Pediatr* 1993;60:639-643.

125. Biervliet FP, Maguiness SD, Hay DM et al. Induction of lactation in the intended mother of a surrogate pregnancy: case report. *Hum Reprod* 2001;16:581-583.

126. Carlson HE, Wasser HL, Reidelberger RD. Beer-induced prolactin secretion: a clinical and laboratory study of the role of salsolinol. *J Clin Endocrinol Metab* 1985;60:673-677.

127. James RJ, Irons DW, Holmes C et al. Thirst induced by a suckling episode during breast feeding and relation with plasma vasopressin, oxytocin and osmoregulation. *Clin Endocrinol Oxf* 1995;43:277-282.

128. Feher SD, Berger LR, Johnson JD et al. Increasing breast milk production for premature infants with a relaxation/imagery audiotape. *Pediatrics* 1989;83:57-60.

129. Yokoyama Y, Ueda T, Irahara M et al. Releases of oxytocin and prolactin during breast massage and suckling in puerperal women. *Eur J Obstet Gynecol Reprod Biol* 1994;53:17-20.

130. Newton N, Egli GE. The effect of intranasal administration of oxytocin on the let-down of milk in lactating women. *Am J Obstet Gynaecol* 1958:103.

Hospital Practices to Support Successful Breastfeeding

During the latter part of the twentieth century, well over 90% of births in the United States took place in hospitals. The hospital environment ushered in an era when birth practices followed a medical model. Routine supplementation, separation of mothers and newborns through central nurseries, water supplementation, and rigid feeding schedules became common, and these practices became barriers to breastfeeding initiation and continuation. Some of these practices persist, but the Baby-Friendly™ Hospital Initiative (BFHI) discussed in Chapter 1, has done much to abolish "routine" practices through its "Ten Steps to Successful Breastfeeding" (Box 8-1). The BFHI is a global initiative that grew out of the work of the World Health Assembly in 1989 and was later formalized by the World Health Organization (WHO) in 1991. It is a voluntary program, recognized with an award, not an accreditation. (The application process and related documents are found in Appendix D.) Hospitals are awarded the Baby-Friendly designation after they have implemented protocol and practice standards to promote, protect, and support breastfeeding.

The Ten Steps to Successful Breastfeeding were designed to overcome the barriers to breastfeeding that had become prevalent in hospitals throughout the world. Since 1991, more than 16,000 hospitals in the world have successfully completed the Ten Steps and earned the Baby-Friendly award, but to date, only 33 others have earned the award in the United States. (Visit http://www.babyfriendlyusa.org for updates.) In the United States the BFHI is spearheaded by Baby-Friendly USA.

Barriers to breastfeeding still exist in American hospitals. As the current president of Baby-Friendly USA, I often talk with many health care providers who claim to be committed to evidence-based practice but who are unaware of the evidence that supports the BFHI. The aim of this chapter is to review the evidence to support the Ten Steps and to generate strategies that foster an environment that favors breastfeeding initiation and continuation. (Other chapters address the clinical management of issues discussed here.)

STEP 1: Have a Written Breastfeeding Policy That Is Routinely Communicated to All Health Care Staff

POLICIES

WHO gives a clear directive that facilities offering maternity services should write a breastfeeding policy that is routinely communicated to all health care staff.[1] In the United States, however, we have a range of situations, from hospitals that have no policy at all to those that have strong, formal policies that are routinely communicated and implemented.

Lack of a formal, written policy is an old and ongoing problem. In the early 1980s, Winikoff and colleagues[2] showed that the lack of a written policy resulted in lip service that "breast is best" while practices that undermined breastfeeding initiation and continuation pervaded in an urban American hospital. Winikoff further observed that staff assumed that parents did *not* want the practices that would have promoted exclusive

Box 8-1   The Ten Steps to Successful Breastfeeding

The Baby-Friendly Hospital Initiative promotes, protects, and supports breastfeeding through The Ten Steps to Successful Breastfeeding for Hospitals as outlined by UNICEF and WHO. The steps for the United States are as follows:

1. Have a written breastfeeding policy that is routinely communicated to all health care staff.
2. Train all health care staff in skills necessary to implement this policy.
3. Inform all pregnant women about the benefits and management of breastfeeding.
4. Help mothers initiate breastfeeding within an hour of birth.*

5. Show mothers how to breastfeed and how to maintain lactation even if they should be separated from their infants.
6. Give newborn infants no food or drink other than breast milk, unless medically indicated.
7. Practice "rooming-in" by allowing mothers and infants to remain together 24 hours a day.
8. Encourage breastfeeding on demand.
9. Give no artificial teats, pacifiers, dummies, or soothers to breastfeeding infants.
10. Foster the establishment of breastfeeding support groups and refer mothers to them on discharge from the hospital or birthing center.

From WHO and UNICEF. *Protecting, promoting, and supporting breastfeeding. The special role of maternity services.* Geneva: World Health Organization; 1989.
*When written in 1989, this step required breastfeeding initiation within the first *half*-hour. Research in the 1990s showed that the natural sequence of behavior is for suckling to occur within the first hour. Therefore this step was modified for United States hospitals by BFHI.

breastfeeding; her interviews with parents, however, showed that they *did* want such practices.

A decade ago, it was recognized that having a breastfeeding policy can strongly influence breastfeeding initiation and continuation.[3] However, many hospitals that offer maternity services are still lacking a formal, written policy that is communicated to all staff. For example, a survey of 76 hospitals in Missouri showed that only 28% of the hospitals had a written policy that was communicated to all staff.[4] Some of the most ignored policy topics include breastfeeding education for health care providers, breastfeeding initiation, and support of the breastfeeding mother, particularly in the postdischarge stage.[5]

The mere existence of a written policy will not result in better practices. In the United States we know from experience, as well as from the literature, that unless administrative personnel support the policy and issue reprimands for noncompliance, practice will change little.[6]

Sometimes, a formal, written policy is lacking, but a breastfeeding "policy" may be informally but clearly understood and communicated to staff. The resulting effects of these unwritten "policies" are not reported in the published literature because it

is difficult or impossible to study something that exists only in verbal form or as an implicit understanding among staff members. In my clinical experience, however, such "policies" are strongly entrenched in the system, and they encourage staff to restrict breastfeeding based on tradition rather than on evidence. Fortunately, some women are so motivated and supported that they will initiate and persist in breastfeeding despite the obstacles in the birth environment.

Effects of Weak or Incomplete Policies

In other cases, although a written breastfeeding policy exists, it is weak or incomplete. Weak or incomplete policies are likely to negatively influence either the initiation of breastfeeding, the continuation of breastfeeding, or both. For example, although a supportive policy existed in one university hospital in the United States, 66% of mothers who delivered there initially expressed an intention to breastfeed, but only 23% of them were actually breastfeeding at 2 weeks of age.[7] The policy, although supportive of breastfeeding in general, did not limit the use of supplements, and at least one bottle of ready-to-feed formula was given to all newborns in the nursery. Similar situations have been encountered in England[8] and Jamaica.[9] A descriptive study in Canada showed that although 58% of the surveyed hospitals reported having a written policy on breastfeeding, only 1.3% reported restricting free samples of formula for mothers at discharge.[10]

Effects of Strong Policies

Strong breastfeeding policies include directives for staff training and maternal education and promote, rather than restrict, breastfeeding. The effects of such policies in countries other than the United States have been studied and shown to be effective in increasing the incidence[11,12] and the duration[13,14] of breastfeeding, or both.[15]

Nearly all of the existing quasi-experimental studies of effective hospital policies have been conducted outside of the United States. However, one comparative study conducted in the United States showed that the incidence of breastfeeding was significantly increased in the facility that had strong staff education, user-tested patient education materials, and a strong policy, compared with a control site that did not. The incidence of breastfeeding increased from 15% to 56% at the intervention site, and exclusive breastfeeding for more than three fourths of feedings increased from 0% to 15%.[16] In addition, although the BFHI program was designed for hospitals only, a U.S. study showed that the principles of the BFHI program improved breastfeeding outcomes when the principles were implemented in offices.[17]

In the United States, when at least five of the Ten Steps are implemented, mothers are significantly more likely to continue breastfeeding until at least 6 weeks. To date, however, the most compelling study is one conducted by Kramer and colleagues in Canada.[18] In this study, having a strong breastfeeding policy and implementing it increased both the overall breastfeeding at 12 months and the rates of exclusive breastfeeding at 3 months (Research Highlight box).

Creating a Policy

Creating the policy requires one to first pursue the definition and elements of a policy. Policies cover "everything from physical and environmental issues to philosophical and administrative issues."[19] The Ten Steps focus primarily on environmental issues but certainly deal with philosophic and administrative issues as well.

Unlike other standards, for example, protocols, policies are deliberately inflexible. A real-life example is a restaurant's smoking policy or a department store's return policy. When you see "This is a smoke-free restaurant," you know that smoking is prohibited by all patrons at all times. Similarly, you know the exact conditions under which you can receive your money back when you see, "Cash refunds will be allowed for unworn merchandise that is returned within 30 days of purchase and accompanied by the original sales receipt; otherwise store credit will be given." Likewise, a breastfeeding policy should spell out the hospital's rules and philosophy about breastfeeding.

Creating a policy also begs the questions of what elements of the policy are essential. Following is a verbatim quote from WHO, articulating elements of a breastfeeding policy[20]:

- General section on aims and objectives
- Any national or international guidelines which provide the basis of the hospital policy
- National and local data such as breastfeeding rates
- The Ten Steps to Successful Breastfeeding[1] and relevant provisions of the Code[21]
- Details of practice related to the local situation for each step and the Code
- Technical information and references

WHO urges that policies be written according to local custom. Unless a hospital has an accepted, unchangeable format that has been previously established, I recommend using Smith-Marker's model.[19] She encourages brevity, thoroughness, organization, approval/review, and consistency. In my experience, policies that exceed one printed page are useless. Lengthy policies are usually difficult for those who are trying to send, as well as those trying to receive, the policy's main message. Ideally, staff members should be able to state, in their own words, the essence of the policy's content.

Creating a breastfeeding policy is not merely a task to be completed. Rather, it is an integral part of the change process that occurs when stake-holders

RESEARCH HIGHLIGHT

BFHI Principles Work!

Citation: Kramer MS. Promotion of breastfeeding intervention trial (PROBIT): a randomized trial in the republic of Belarus. *JAMA* 2001;285: 413-420.

Kramer and his colleagues have conducted the first prospective, randomized trial describing the impact of a breastfeeding promotion program modeled after the Baby-Friendly Hospital Initiative (BFHI). The study was conducted in 31 hospitals and polyclinics in the Republic of Belarus. Mothers who expressed an interest in breastfeeding were eligible to participate in the study. A total of 17,406 healthy singleton infants and their healthy mothers participated in the study; only 3.3% were lost to follow-up during the first year.

All physicians and registered nurses in the experimental group (16 hospitals and polyclinics) participated in the UNICEF 18-hour Breastfeeding and Management Promotion course and then implemented the course's supportive strategies to help mothers initiate and maintain breastfeeding. The control group (15 hospitals and polyclinics) simply continued to give routine care and breastfeeding advice as they have always done.

Results were astounding. Compared with the mother-infant couplets who got "routine" care, those in the promotional program were 7 times more likely to be exclusively breastfeeding at 3 months, and 12 times more likely to be breastfeeding exclusively at 6 months ($p < .001$). Furthermore, early weaning was significantly greater among infants in the routine care group than those in the experimental group. Risk for morbidity was greater in the control group: Compared with 9% of the subjects in the experimental group, 13% of the subjects in the control group had intestinal infections during the first year of life. Similarly, 3% of the subjects who were born at hospitals participating in the breastfeeding promotion program had episodes of eczema during the first year, whereas 6% of the subjects in the control group had such episodes in this same time frame. There was no significant difference in respiratory infection between the groups.

In an accompanying editorial,[247] Dr. Ruth Lawrence calls this a "masterful study," and indeed it is. Subjects were remarkably similar. The double randomization dramatically reduced the possibility of sampling error. The huge sample size gives the study enormous statistical power, and the 1-year follow-up design is also impressive. A clear definition of "breastfeeding" (exclusive or predominant) makes the outcomes more understandable.

Although Dr. Lawrence points out that "the statistical model they used meets or exceeds the usual criticism of such studies"[247] the investigators themselves point out a few limitations. It is difficult to generalize the findings to other cultures because the experimental group rigorously implemented the promotional program. In the United States and in other cultures where health care is not a centralized system, it may be difficult or impossible to achieve the same outcomes. The typical maternity stay of 6 to 7 days in Belarus is far different from the very brief stays here. The obligatory 3-year maternity leave in Belarus is unlike our system where women go back to work early and put their children in day care with all of the concomitant problems of that environment.

The Belarus setting brings some distinct advantages to the study, however. Maternity care there is similar to care that was given in the United States about 20 years ago, before there was much influence from the Baby-Friendly Hospital Initiative. Yet, unlike third-world nations, Belarus is a region where health services and clean water are readily available, so these similarities to the United States health care system are striking. This may be the most convincing breastfeeding study of the year.

From Biancuzzo M. *Breastfeeding Outlook* 2001;3:3.

work collaboratively. At one hospital, a breastfeeding advocate tried to change policies and practices between 1990 and 1993 without the participation of the obstetrics department. Although it was a strong policy in terms of promoting breastfeeding, it did not address the restrictive practices—notably distribution of discharge packs—which continued.[22]

Over many years of clinical practice, people have often asked to *borrow* my hospital's breastfeeding policy, and I generally refuse. To be actually implemented, policies and in-hospital programs must be *owned* by the staff and administration.[23] This ownership comes from a multidisciplinary group that works together over time. Having one person create the policy—or worse still, borrowing it from a neighboring hospital and foisting it on the staff—is unlikely to be implemented when supervisors are absent. It is helpful, however, to review a model policy before writing new ones. One model policy, originally developed by Naylor and Wester in 1977, was remarkably unchanged in its content when it was updated and reprinted in 1994.[24] Reviewing this strong policy may serve to jump-start interdisciplinary groups who are creating their own policy.

In summary, a written policy that is clearly communicated to all staff is the cornerstone for establishing and maintaining an environment that fosters breastfeeding. Weak or incomplete policies or those that have been created without the input and support of multiple disciplines are likely to be ineffective. WHO has suggested components of a policy, but the exact content and format must be determined by the facility itself. By incorporating the main ideas from the Ten Steps to Successful Breastfeeding, the facility can better move forward with educating their staff and establishing evidence-based practices for care.

STEP 2: Train All Health Care Staff in Skills Necessary to Implement This Policy

STAFF EDUCATION

A general lack of education among health professionals about breastfeeding and lactation management, originally reported in the follow-up to the Surgeon General's Workshop,[25] continues as an ongoing barrier. Although lack of education among other health care providers is likely, most studies documenting the lack of knowledge have focused on nurses and physicians.

The majority of nurses have obtained most of their information about breastfeeding through clinical experience.[26] Although most nursing schools have not integrated breastfeeding management into their curricula, sometimes nurses have relied on the limited information that was available during their basic education. In one study[27] approximately half of the nurses surveyed identified nursing school as their main source of information about breastfeeding, yet they were unable to give accurate information on such basic matters as the let-down reflex. Admittedly, this is an old study, but those who attended nursing school during the time of the study are likely to be practicing today. Another study showed that entry-level nursing education correlated negatively with nurses' knowledge of breastfeeding[28] or did not correlate with their total score on the researcher's questionnaire.[26] Limited knowledge continues to be a problem.[26,29]

Closely aligned to lack of knowledge is a negative attitude. The effect of the health care provider's attitude on the individual's decision to initiate or continue breastfeeding is discussed in Chapter 3, but this negative attitude also affects the discipline as a whole. The common perception that nurses are not supportive of breastfeeding appears to be based in reality. Nutritionists, dietitians, and physicians express more positive beliefs about breastfeeding than nurses,[30] and dietitians show greater knowledge about breastfeeding issues than hospital nurses.[31] Those who have breastfed their own children tend to have a positive attitude about breastfeeding and are more likely to recommend it to mothers.[32,33]

Physician education—both basic and continuing education—has improved since the days of the Surgeon General's Workshop, but it is still inadequate. Physicians themselves report that they did not have adequate education in breastfeeding management.[34] In the past, medical school curricula have had little, if any, content about breastfeeding management issues. In a national survey, more than half of the pediatricians queried rated their residency training in breastfeeding as inadequate, and not surprisingly, their recommendations and medical interventions reflected their lack of knowledge.[35] More than half of pediatricians were unable to choose appropriate management strategies for jaundice or breast abscesses,[35] and only 64% of practitioners and 52% of residents knew that supplementing during the first few weeks of life interferes with successful lactation. A more recent study indicated that almost all pediatric residents were unaware that breastfed infants grow at slower rates after 4 months of age than bottle-fed infants.[36]

Although the problem originates with basic medical education, continuing medical education is also inadequate for physicians. Schanler and colleagues conducted a survey among members of the American Academy of Pediatrics (AAP) and found that most American pediatricians had not attended a presentation on breastfeeding management in the previous 3 years.[37] This may help explain why physicians often erroneously assume that breastfeeding is contraindicated or why they choose inappropriate treatment strategies.

In Schanler and colleagues' study, American pediatricians did not encourage breastfeeding for conditions (and treatments) that do not contraindicate breastfeeding.[37] Similarly, a report in the Philippines that described the knowledge, attitudes, and practices of midwives, nurses, physicians, and community health workers showed that even those who had generally positive attitudes often had little knowledge about what did or did not constitute a contraindication to breastfeeding.[38] Physicians are more likely to encourage women to initiate breastfeeding if they believe in the immune properties of human milk and if they are confident in their own ability to counsel the breastfeeding mother.[39]

Although curricula for nurses, physicians, and those educated in other health care disciplines have improved, the consequences of inadequate basic education will remain because those who were educated a few decades ago are likely to continue to give inadequate advice as a result of their lack of knowledge. Inaccurate advice, absence of advice, or inconsistent advice can be discouraging and confusing to consumers. Similarly, inaccurate, incomplete, or inappropriate advice for the circumstances can undermine breastfeeding initiation and continuation.

Improving nursing education about breastfeeding management has been an ongoing effort. Fortunately, the national registered nurse licensure examination now includes questions about breastfeeding; this was a giant step forward in advancing nurses' awareness and competence in basic breastfeeding management. It is not only optimal but also possible to successfully integrate lactation management into health care curricula.[40] Today's textbooks have more (and more accurate) information about lactation and breastfeeding management than did textbooks a decade ago, but colleges of nursing have been slow to incorporate lectures on breastfeeding into student curricula at either the undergraduate or the graduate level (Clinical Scenario box).

Training Program

WHO has recommended that "training in breastfeeding and lactation management should be given to various types of staff including new employees, it should be at least 18 hours in total with a minimum of 3 hours of supervised clinical experience and cover at least 8 steps."[41] The practicality of the situation begs three questions: (1) Who, exactly, are these employees? (2) Is 18 hours really needed or realistic? and (3) Are educational programs for professionals effective?

Who Needs the Training?

Those of us who carry a heavy responsibility for staff development usually know who *does* need training; the more perplexing question is who *does not* need training. Quite obviously, nurses and licensed personnel who provide direct care on the maternity unit need the full training program.

WHO makes it clear that *all* staff must be trained, but the extent of the training required for ancillary personnel who work on the maternity units (e.g., housekeepers or laboratory technicians) or nurses who work on nonmaternity units (e.g., the emergency room) is deliberately vague.

CLINICAL SCENARIO

Integrating Breastfeeding into College Curricula

After many years of practice in the hospital, you accept a part-time position as a clinical instructor at a school of nursing. In the hospital where you and your students are assigned, you see that breastfeeding practices are less than optimal. You note breastfeeding is not mentioned in the maternal-child curricula. What might you do?

I did some hands-on teaching with the students and some casual "hallway" education of the staff when the opportunity arose. After talking with the course coordinator several times, I was unable to persuade her that breastfeeding was an integral part of student education. Meanwhile, I whet the appetites of the students in my own clinical group and suggested that they ask the course coordinator why the topic was not included in the classroom lectures.

Eventually, the course coordinator agreed to give me 45 minutes of class time to talk about breastfeeding. So, although she did not value my suggestion, she did respond when the students themselves asked for the information.

I carefully thought through how to use that short amount of time to maximize the students' knowledge of breastfeeding management. I focused on the detrimental effects of restricting breastfeeding (e.g., long intervals between feeds, supplementation) and how to achieve optimal positioning for milk transfer. I hoped that eventually the course coordinator would give me more than 45 minutes to cover my topic, but that never happened. I offered students in my own clinical group the opportunity to do a project on breastfeeding for extra credit, which several of them undertook.

Each country or even each facility must determine for themselves the extent of the training for personnel who do not provide direct care, with a strong rationale for their interpretations. A condensed training program can be designed to help staff fulfill their responsibilities in a way that promotes breastfeeding. For example, training emergency room nurses should focus on the management of common postdischarge situations and the relatively *few* situations for which breastfeeding should be interrupted or discontinued. Training for ancillary staff members should focus on how they might support breastfeeding mothers, rather than disturbing or negatively reacting to a woman who is breastfeeding when they enter the room, and this could simply be included in their unit orientation.

How Much Training Is Needed?

WHO's recommendation for 18 hours of training is often a significant obstacle for U.S. hospitals. Substantial planning and skill are essential to convince administrative personnel for the need to mandate 18 hours of training for breastfeeding when staff training for other perinatal issues (e.g., perinatal grief and loss or electronic fetal monitor-

ing) is nonexistent or considerably shorter. In addition, if the in-service education is not mandated by managers, it is unlikely to be attended and will therefore be unsuccessful.[16,42] The aim, therefore, is to get the education in place and mandated by administration, but starting by asking for 18 hours of training may put a damper on any support from the administration.

As the change process begins in a hospital, it is often advantageous to create a shorter training program that tackles some of the greatest barriers relative to the specific practice setting. I created a 5-year educational plan that began with very short, focused sessions in the first years and methodically expanded thereafter. As staff became more knowledgeable, administration became more supportive because they saw the desire to learn more from within the ranks. It is also imperative to create and analyze the effectiveness of short programs because these evaluations set the stage for future, more intense learning programs. Having the participant complete a "satisfaction" form at the end of the learning experience, however, is inadequate. Instead, the person responsible for staff education should collaborate with the person who is in charge of quality assurance on the unit, thereby establishing a link between improved staff knowledge and better clinical outcomes. If the hospital has multiple maternity units, this can become a competitive project, or even a game.

Are Educational Programs Effective?

Many interdisciplinary educational programs have been conducted in various hospitals throughout the world. However, few have published their findings about the effects of staff education on practice recommendations or the incidence or continuation of breastfeeding. None of the published studies addressing that question have been conducted in the United States.

Training programs can be effective. In a small survey in Ireland, the knowledge level of the professionals on the unit correlated with an increase in breastfeeding initiation.[43] In Brazil, participants from eight hospitals completed a 3-week course, and investigators gave a pretest and posttest to measure the participants' attitudes and knowledge. Analysis of the pretest and posttest results suggested that the knowledge and attitudes of most participants improved substantially after participating in the course.[44] The same authors conducted a later study in Brazil to determine the effect of staff education on the continuation of breastfeeding.[45] Those infants who were born in hospitals with trained personnel had longer continuation of exclusive and full breastfeeding. In Kenya, researchers aimed to measure the effect of the course on providers' recommendations 6 years after they took the course.[13] Course participants were more likely to recommend exclusive breastfeeding and rooming-in and to discourage prelacteal feeds. In Brazil, those who participated in a 40-hour training course were better able to give breastfeeding counseling than controls who did not participate in the course.[46]

Research showing a direct cause- and effect relationship between staff education and clinical outcomes is unlikely to be forthcoming. Information alone is not always sufficient to change the practices or recommendations of the nurses who attend the educational sessions.[42,47] Often, educational programs are designed with many cognitive objectives and few, if any, affective objectives. Moreover, it is fairly fast and easy to raise a learner's cognitive grasp of new information, but it takes a long-term plan and patience to change attitudes, beliefs, and values that have been ingrained for many years.

Barriers to and Strategies for Staff Education

Although education is highly valued in American society, staff education about breastfeeding is often placed on a back burner. Once a policy for breastfeeding has been established, however, it is imperative that both initial and ongoing education be provided for the staff. There are several perceived barriers, but most of them can be overcome. Often, the most significant barrier is perceived lack of funding for staff education.

The traditional lecture method, often assumed to be the only alternative, is likely to be the most expensive. Other alternatives may be just as professionally enriching and more cost effective. Furthermore, a combination of methods may be used to achieve the main goal of enabling staff to correctly implement the breastfeeding policy. For example, a 3-day course that used various teaching methods in Chile improved participants' knowledge and practices.[48] Following are some teaching strategies that offer an economy of financial resources and flexible scheduling.

Grand Rounds

The format for grand rounds varies widely from hospital to hospital. However, in most cases, grand rounds involve a learning environment in which both veteran and inexperienced personnel have an opportunity to discuss real-life situations and look at outcomes in relation to clinical management strategies. Grand rounds can be very focused and limited with very in-depth discussions among colleagues in the same discipline or, ideally, with colleagues from many disciplines who share differing perspectives.

Self-Study Programs

Self-study programs are ideal when staffing patterns do not allow for many people to attend a lecture at the same time. These programs, sometimes called *self-learning modules, independent-study modules,* or *self-learning packages,* are designed to help the participant learn at his or her own pace and on "down" time or off-duty time. A word of caution about self-learning programs: The best ones are those designed as self-learning programs, rather than those that use existing media and, in retrospect, provide a test for that media. Such "retro-fitted" programs have limited usefulness for learners. Some good self-learning modules are noted in Appendix C.

Posters

Posters are a great way to give small pieces of information over a long period. The most effective strategy is to plan a series of posters, each with a single message. Post each for perhaps a week or two (depending on staffing patterns) along with a set of questions and offer a reward for the person(s) who submit the greatest number of right answers. Rewards are not necessarily monetary; working closely with the nurse manager, I have arranged for the reward to be an extra weekend off during the time-block. (You must have clear discussions with the nurse manager to generate ideas for rewards; the rewards must be feasible.) Some of the special elements in this book (e.g., Table 9-8) originally started out as posters at my hospital. Posters are a great way to put messages in front of staff who would resist or refuse going to a lecture on the topic. A great side effect is that the poster generates discussion among colleagues. Furthermore, if the hospital implements a successful breastfeeding project, a poster is a great way to educate the community—professionals and parents—about your program.[49-51]

Games

Games are a fun and cost-effective way for staff to learn. Games can be done either as an independent or group activity. Those who have a strong background in educational presentations and methods may feel ambitious enough to create their own games. However, it is more cost effective and time efficient to purchase a game that has already been created, user-tested, and peer-reviewed. Games that have strong, evidence-based answers and carry continuing education credit have been developed by Games Nurses Play.[*]

Videotaping (or Audio Taping)

If staff cannot go to a "live" lecture, it may be permissible for one person to attend the lecture and purchase a videotape or audio tape of the lecture for use by other staff members. To be effective, however, all learners, whether hearing the live lecture or the tape, need to have accompanying lecture handouts. Tapes have the advantage of being reasonably accessible, and staff members can use them on their down time. A clear disadvantage, however, is that those who are listening to or viewing the tape are participating in a very passive learning activity, and this type of learning is less effective than more active learning methods.

In summary, initiation and continuation of breastfeeding have been linked to effective staff education. Staff education programs are likely to be effective if they are mandated by administration and designed using creative learning strategies that reflect principles of adult education. A strong staff development program, although not the only solution to improving practice, is a vital component of improving the birth environment to foster breastfeeding. Staff who are knowledgeable are more able to teach mothers and implement best practices.

STEP 3: Inform All Pregnant Women about the Benefits and Management of Breastfeeding

TEACHING PREGNANT WOMEN BENEFITS AND MANAGEMENT OF BREASTFEEDING

Although WHO has included the directive to teach pregnant women the benefits and management of breastfeeding, the evidence for this step is considerably weaker than that for the other steps. Interestingly, in citing existing studies to support

*Contact GamesNurse@aol.com or P.O. Box 25273, Winston-Salem, NC 27114.

this step when they published in 1998,[20] WHO identified only four quasi-experimental studies[52-55] showing better outcomes when pregnant women are taught the benefits of breastfeeding. (They did, however, identify some descriptive studies as well, including those that involved community-based lay counselors,[56-59] which were combined with postnatal care and are described further under Step 10.) These four studies also have some distinct limitations.

Effects of Teaching Breastfeeding Benefits to Pregnant Women

One well-controlled quasi-experimental study conducted in the United States showed that providing a series of five pamphlets (at appropriate reading levels) increased 44 pregnant mothers' awareness of breastfeeding but did not affect their attitudes or the number of months that they continued breastfeeding.[52] Another U.S. study looked at breastfeeding among 20 primiparae who had attended a group class in comparison to 20 who had not.[53] Those in the intervention group reported that breastfeeding was more successful at 1 month, but "breastfeeding" and "successful" were not defined. In Chicago, low-income, inner-city subjects (total $N = 130$) who attended antenatal workshops were more likely to continue breastfeeding at 8 to 12 weeks compared with control subjects who did not.[54] In Chile, women (total $N = 735$) who had prenatal breastfeeding education—especially primiparae—were more likely to be fully breastfeeding at 6 months in comparison with a group who did not.[55] An extensive MEDLINE search uncovered one more recent study that was conducted by the same author and concluded that mothers who received prenatal teaching were more likely to exclusively breastfeed for 6 months, even if they returned to work.[60] A descriptive study suggested that teaching pregnant women the benefits of breastfeeding is associated with the continuation of breastfeeding.[61] It is important to interpret these studies with the understanding that the instructional content was not always specified in the study, and the teaching methods differed.

Since the advent of 48-hour maternity stays, some breastfeeding educators have shifted what used to be the postpartum teaching content into the prenatal period. This strategy violates principles of adult education, which favor aligning the material with the time frame when learners can use it to increase knowledge retention. Also, there is no evidence that early discharge is a deterrent to breastfeeding.[62,63]

WHO also gives a clear directive that teaching about the *benefits* of breastfeeding is not sufficient; pregnant women also need to have information about the *management* of breastfeeding. WHO says that women need to be able to discuss at least two of the following four topics:

- Importance of rooming-in
- Importance of feeding on cue
- How to ensure enough milk
- Positioning and attachment of the newborn at the breast

WHO is silent on what the content of postpartum instruction should be. Specific objectives are found in Chapter 5, along with evidence of the effectiveness of postpartum education programs.

Barriers to and Strategies for Teaching Pregnant Women

Some barriers to teaching women, including suboptimal communication techniques, inappropriate reading levels in education materials, and other factors, are discussed in Chapter 5. In a more global way, however, other barriers impede prenatal education about breastfeeding.

In the early 1980s, women often lacked access to health care professionals trained in lactation management. This barrier is decreasing as several schools of nursing and medicine have included breastfeeding management as part of the curricula. Furthermore, several continuing education programs have strengthened the knowledge and skills of professionals whose basic education curriculum did not include breastfeeding management (see Appendix C). Some organizations now offer certificates for those who have demonstrated competence in breastfeeding management. The most notable certification program is the International Board of Lactation Consultant Examiners. With so many seeking and obtaining better education and certification status, more and more mothers have access to accurate breastfeeding and lactation advice.

Lack of funds for teaching are sometimes identified as a barrier to teaching pregnant women about breastfeeding. However, instruction does not necessarily need to take place in a formal classroom. Omission of instruction about breastfeeding raises the question of legal and ethical responsibility; lack of funding does not thwart other topics such as the importance of immunizations for the infant. Omission of breastfeeding instruction reflects the low priority that health care providers assign to this topic.[64]

A major potential barrier to teaching women about the benefits of breastfeeding is that it may be difficult to identify pregnant women who especially need the information. In my experience, socially or financially disadvantaged women living in urban settings often delay seeking prenatal care until the second or third trimester; some have had no prenatal care. Therefore it is likely that these late registrants have already made up their minds about feeding before they enter the health care system. Certainly, it is always worth a try to talk to the woman about breastfeeding as soon as she delivers, but encouraging words may fall on deaf ears. It is often more useful to try using more community-based techniques to arouse interest in breastfeeding among pregnant women. In one city where I worked, I urged the local task force to begin efforts to post promotional posters on the city buses. The idea of meeting women literally "where they're at" is likely to be more influential than preaching to women in the postpartum period.

In summary, a few controlled studies show weak evidence to support the efficacy of teaching pregnant women the benefits of breastfeeding, and conclusions are limited mostly to primiparae. There is certainly no reason not to teach these benefits, and in the Ten Steps, WHO requires that women be told the benefits; however, simply listing the benefits is not *sufficient*. If women know the benefits of breastfeeding, they may be better able to convince their partner or families of the superiority of breastfeeding and human milk.

STEP 4: Help Mothers Initiate Breastfeeding within 1 Hour of Birth

THE FIRST HOUR

As originally written in 1989, WHO stated, "Help mothers initiate breastfeeding within a half-hour of birth."[1] More specifically, WHO spelled out that the help would be done with maternal-infant skin-to-skin contact. "Mothers ... who have had normal vaginal deliveries should confirm that within a half-hour of birth, they were given their babies to hold with skin contact, for at least 30 minutes, and offered help by a staff member to initiate breastfeeding."[41]

When the BFHI gained popularity in the United States, the criteria here was changed to "within 1 hour." This modification was made because subsequent to the Ten Steps, published in 1989, newer research[65] indicated that human infants follow a sequence of familiarization at the breast that culminates in infant-initiated latch-on around 1 hour postpartum. Furthermore, this fits the long-established knowledge about periods of reactivity during the first few hours of life; infants are more alert during that period (Fig. 8-1). During this time, newborns and their mothers are alert and display a heightened sensitivity to one another, whereby the attachment and bonding process is intensified and enhances interactions.[66] The aim, of course, is to provide newborns with the opportunity to suckle when they are in a most optimal state for the suckling experience. Ideally, newborns should have the opportunity to suckle immediately after birth.

The directive for early breastfeeding was given to deter the practice of separating mothers and infants for days until the mother's milk "came in," or even shorter time periods. Mothers and newborns are commonly separated for brief periods (i.e., to perform "admission" procedures for the newborn) or for fairly lengthy times. A more subtle variation of separation is bundling an infant in a crib or placing him under a radiant warmer. Of course, a newborn cannot suckle when he is several feet away from his mother or, worse, housed in a completely separate unit of the maternity service.

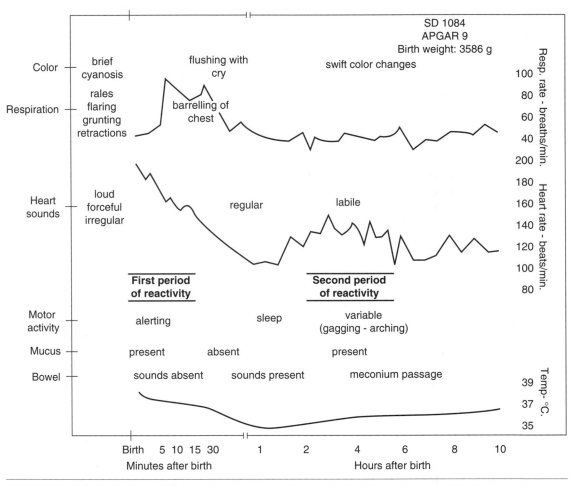

FIGURE **8-1** Periods of reactivity during the first 10 hours of life. *(From Desmond M, Rudolph A, Phitakspharaiwan P. Pediatr Clin North Am 1966;13:656.)*

It is important to note that WHO does not stipulate that the newborn actually suckle. Rather, the focus is on creating a situation in which suckling is likely to occur, that is, having the newborn skin-to-skin with his mother and having assistance with latch-on. Interestingly, some published studies use the terms *suckling* and *skin-to-skin contact* as interchangeable or synonymous, whereas other studies[65,67,68] make a clear distinction between contact and suckling. This distinction or lack thereof should be kept in mind when interpreting studies that describe "contact."

Mothers who experience a cesarean delivery should be given the opportunity to be skin-to-skin with and suckle their newborns as soon as possible. If the mother has had general anesthesia, breastfeeding may begin as soon as she regains consciousness.[69] Mothers who have had other types of anesthesia (e.g., epidural anesthesia) can probably have contact even sooner. In the United States the aim is for mothers to be given the opportunity to hold their infants and have skin-to-skin contact within the first *half*-hour of when they are able to respond to them. Assistance with breastfeeding should be offered within the first hour of when the mother is able to respond to her infant.[70]

Effect of Early Contact on Continuation of Breastfeeding

Several studies have identified the benefits of early contact on breastfeeding. Benefits include the ability to suckle more effectively, longer continuation of breastfeeding, and other benefits not directly related to breastfeeding.

Healthy newborns who experience early contact are significantly ($p < .001$) more likely to suckle correctly than cohorts who have been separated for even a short time.[68] Presumably, infants who are allowed to use their natural abilities to find and locate food are able to "imprint" on the human nipple more effectively.

Whether early contact is associated with longer continuation of breastfeeding has been a topic of much debate. One study[71] showed that early contact had no significant effect on continuation of breastfeeding. Another showed that early contact was associated with breastfeeding continuation at 1 week, but not thereafter.[72] At 2 months, skin-to-skin contact by itself did not affect breastfeeding duration unless suckling also occurred.[73]

Most of the controlled research, however, has shown that a primary benefit of early contact is continuation of breastfeeding. Early contact has been associated with continuation of breastfeeding at 2 to 3 months[74-76] and up to 8 months.[67] A meta-analysis of the quasi-experimental studies concluded that continuation of breastfeeding was more likely at 2 months when the infants had early contact compared with those who did not.[77] Descriptive studies in the United States have shown similar results. A descriptive study of 726 women in Washington, D.C., showed a strong correlation between the time that the newborn first suckled and the time that artificial milk was first introduced.[78] A mail survey showed that delayed suckling was among the greatest risk factors (along with supplementation) for early breastfeeding attrition.[79]

Other Benefits of Early Contact

Apart from improved breastfeeding initiation or continuation, early breastfeeding is beneficial for several other biologic and behavioral maternal and infant tasks. Although it has long been known that suckling creates uterine contractions in the postpartum woman, recent research has confirmed that early suckling reduces the risk for postpartum hemorrhage.[80] Early contact—including nuzzling, licking, and suckling the nipple (with or without swallowing)—provides stimulation to the nipples, which enhances lactogenesis. Having the infant touch the mother's areola seems to positively influence early mother-infant relationship.[65]

Benefits abound for the infant who is making the biologic transition from intrauterine to extrauterine life. Colostrum has a laxative effect on the gut, thereby promoting excretion of bilirubin and reducing the risk for newborn jaundice. Thermoregulation is also affected by maternal contact. Newborns who have skin-to-skin contact have significantly higher axillary skin temperatures, higher blood glucose levels at 90 minutes, and a more rapid return toward zero of the negative base excess.[81]

Infant behavior is also influenced by early breastfeeding. Crying appears to be decreased in newborns who have early contact.[81] Those who are separated emit a "separation distress call" with a quality similar to what other mammals emit when they are separated from their mothers."[82] Decreased crying among infants who have skin-to-skin contact might be explained by the soothing effect of amniotic fluid. The total postnatal crying time from 31 to 90 minutes was registered on tapes in 47 healthy term newborns, and those exposed to amniotic fluid cried significantly less than those who were not.[83] Additional benefits of early breastfeeding are listed in Box 8-2.

Barriers to and Strategies for Promoting Early Contact

Armed with results of a very early study,[92] I began helping mothers initiate early contact with their newborns in the late 1970s and early 1980s, only to find staunch opposition from my colleagues, superiors, and medical staff. They cited multiple events and responsibilities that needed to be completed before breastfeeding or skin-to-skin contact, including waiting until the episiotomy was repaired,

Box 8-2   Benefits of Early Breastfeeding

Exclusive breastfeeding during the first few days provides many benefits for the mother, which may include the following:

- Sooner onset of lactogenesis stage II[84]
- Decreased severity of engorgement[85]
- Supply of milk that is more likely to meet infant's demand[86,87]
- Reduced risk for early breastfeeding attrition[79]
- Improved uterine involution and reduced postpartum hemorrhage[80]
- Enhanced bonding[66,88,89] and maternal confidence
- Opportunity for mother to learn breastfeeding in the presence of the health care provider

Early exclusive breastfeeding includes the following benefits for the infant:

- Colostrum acts as a laxative on the gut, thereby minimizing the risk of jaundice.[90]
- Colostrum, richer in immunoglobulins than mature milk, especially Ig A,[90,91] is the first "immunization" and thereby reduces the threat of infection.
- Suckling[67,73] and early skin-to-skin contact have been associated with longer continuation of breastfeeding.[72,74-76]
- The opportunity for imprinting on an artificial nipple is reduced.

performing postpartum fundal checks, evaluating the threat of newborn hypothermia, and completing newborn admissions procedures. Unfortunately, I still hear nurses citing these and similar reasons for delaying early contact between the mother and newborn. Worse still, sometimes the perception is that early contact has occurred when in reality it has not; staff members truly do not recognize delays. With a greater number of studies and more convincing studies, we should be able to simply cite evidence substantiating the benefits of early breastfeeding and thereby change clinical practices. However, the reality of the situation is that scientific data are often less influential than empiric data. Over the years, I identified a few strategies that helped change practice.

- Role model by providing an opportunity for early contact to newly delivered mothers. When other staff members can see that early contact does not preclude performing fundal checks, they are more likely to follow your example and do fundal checks when the infant is on the mother's abdomen. Similarly, seeing newborns suckle spontaneously and vigorously often helps some staff members change their minds about whether newborns can actually accomplish that task. In short, role modeling is often a powerful and underused change strategy; staff who read or hear

about the benefits of early contact may be unconvinced, but seeing is believing.

- Enhance situations that foster newborn interest in the breast. Staff are unlikely to deny newborns the opportunity to suckle when they are crawling and rooting and literally begging to suckle the breast. However, some "routine admissions" procedures thwart the newborn's natural instincts to locate and ingest food. Noxious stimuli are deterrents to breastfeeding; for example, routine gastric suctioning is unnecessary[93] and interferes with the newborn's natural ability to suckle.[94] Similarly, bright lights interfere with eye-to-eye contact. (Keep the light on the perineum if the obstetrician is repairing the episiotomy, but turn the overhead lights down.) Even short delays for eye prophylaxis or weight checks can interfere with the newborn's ability to establish contact with his mother.

- Collaborate with the quality-assurance (QA) coordinator to conduct a short QA study. This is most easily accomplished when there is a designated spot on the medical record to document the time that contact and/or suckling first occurred. Audits of the medical record can be done to determine how many infants experienced early contact within the first hour of life. Furthermore, this sort of study is most impressive when it is correlated with other data such as the number of infants who did or did not experience hyperbilirubinemia.

In summary, over the past two decades, mounting evidence has shown that during the first hour of life, skin-to-skin contact, including breastfeeding, is related to better initiation of breastfeeding, longer continuation of breastfeeding, and numerous other biologic and behavioral benefits for both the mother and the newborn. Although some staff members still harbor perceived barriers to this, some simple strategies are often helpful in overcoming those barriers.

STEP 5: Show Mothers How to Breastfeed and How to Maintain Lactation, Even if They Are Separated from Their Infants

TEACHING MOTHERS HOW TO BREASTFEED, EVEN WHEN SEPARATED

So many times, people say, "But why do you have to teach women how to breastfeed? Isn't it instinctive?" It is likely that the infant has instincts to help him find and ingest food. However, the mother is a product of her culture, and many, especially primiparae, need to be shown how to breastfeed.

Separation of the mother and newborn can happen for any number of reasons. A common situation that creates separation is cesarean delivery.[95] However, operative deliveries do not preclude breastfeeding. (Chapters 5 and 7 explain care and teaching implications.)

Effects of Postpartum Teaching Programs

It is widely assumed that some sort of teaching or guidance will improve the initiation or continuation of breastfeeding. This assumption is not necessarily inaccurate, but there are relatively few controlled, comparative studies that support the positive effects, and most of them have been conducted in countries outside of the United States. In Sweden, where breastfeeding rates are relatively high, studies showed that mothers,[96] especially primiparae,[92] who had help breastfeeding in the

hospital continued significantly longer than mothers who did not. Similar results have been found in the United Kingdom,[97] Nicaragua,[72] Mexico,[98] and Africa.[99] An extensive search of MEDLINE showed only one U.S. study, and in that study, teaching was not associated with longer continuation of breastfeeding.[100]

Barriers to and Strategies for Teaching Mothers

Barriers for teaching mothers how to breastfeed abound, but none are insurmountable. Strategies to help mothers who are separated from their infants are described in detail in Chapter 14, along with Table 14-3, which outlines a logical approach for teaching these mothers.

In summary, breastfeeding initiation often may depend on having the nurse teach the woman how to breastfeed because some new mothers have never even seen an infant suckling a mother's breast. The influence of staff teaching on the continuation of breastfeeding has been demonstrated abroad, but not in the United States. (See Chapter 5 for strategies to teach mothers.)

STEP 6: Give Newborn Infants No Food or Drink Other Than Breast Milk, Unless Medically Indicated

SUPPLEMENTATION

The directive to give "no food or drink" other than human milk begs the question of how, exactly, to define "breastfeeding." Multiple definitions are found throughout the published literature, but perhaps the most useful and widely recognized definition is that put forth by Labbok and Krasovec,[101] which was later adopted by WHO and is described in Chapter 1. Giving a newborn any kind of food or drink, either before the first suckling experience, as a replacement for any feeding, or in addition to a feeding, could be roughly described as supplementation.

Prelacteal Feedings

Over the years, it has been assumed that newborns need something other than human colostrum or human milk. So-called prelacteal feedings—feedings before the first suckling experience—are generally done for cultural reasons or for misguided "medical" reasons. In some cultures, prelacteal feedings are initiated by the family because colostrum is culturally unacceptable.[102] Until recently in the United States, however, so-called prelacteal feedings were routinely given to ensure that the infant could successfully swallow. The rationale for the prelacteal feeding—usually sterile water—was to prevent aspiration of artificial milk into the newborn's lungs if an unidentified anatomic defect was present. Although that rationale may be useful for the artificially fed newborn, human milk is more physiologic, and aspiration of human milk, although undesirable, is harmless.[90]

Most American hospitals have given up offering water as a prelacteal feed. This practice still occurs in some hospitals[103] and in anecdotal reports, however. There is an assumption that prelacteal feeds are harmless. However, prelacteal feedings, of either artificial milk or water, have been associated with less breastfeeding.[104] Furthermore, even a few prelacteal feeds of artificial milk can result in the development of cow's milk intolerance or allergy, with symptoms appearing later in infancy.[105]

After the initial feeding, whatever it may be, the practice of supplementing newborns with water or artificial milk is not uncommon in many American hospitals. Although multiple organizations and documents have declared that supplementation is unnecessary for most healthy term newborns, the practice continues.

Reasons Why Supplements Are Given

Most reasons given for supplementation are unproven. Several clinical situations were thought to be helped by giving glucose water, including dehydration, jaundice, and hypoglycemia.

Dehydration is unlikely to occur among healthy infants, unless milk production and transfer are thwarted. Infants get plenty of water through breastfeeding because about 87% of human milk is water. Even in hot, dry climates, infants generally do not need supplementary water.[106-108]

Giving water or glucose water, long-assumed to be effective in reducing hyperbilirubinemia, was

first proven ineffective more than two decades ago.[109,110] Subsequent research has confirmed that this is ineffective.[111]

Newborns who are at risk for hypoglycemia are sometimes given glucose water. The rationale is that the 5% or 10% glucose water will prevent or at least minimize the hypoglycemia because of the rapid administration of calories. This reasoning has not been proven in the scientific literature, however. In a randomized study, newborns did not have clinical signs of hypoglycemia during the first 48 hours whether they were fed glucose water or not.[112] Furthermore, if infants *do* become hypoglycemic and they are given glucose water to correct the condition, they generally experience a "sugar high" and then a "sugar crash" because absorption of this simple sugar occurs so quickly. Nursery protocols should avoid using glucose water and instead favor the use of human or artificial milk,[113] which contains protein and therefore maintains normoglycemia over a longer period.

A decade or so ago, glucose water was routinely given to healthy term newborns either to replace a feeding—typically a night feeding—or to "top off" a breastfeeding. In these situations, newborns are given glucose water with the rationale that they need the calories from the glucose water. This reasoning is faulty, however. If the newborn needs the calories, he would obtain more calories by consuming human or artificial milk, as shown in Fig. 8-2. The explanation for this is simple: 5% glucose water contains 5 kcal per ounce, and 10% glucose water provides 10 kcal per ounce. Human or artificial milk provides about 20 to 24 kcal per ounce, depending on human milk maturity or the commercial formula provided. Therefore the newborn would need to consume at least twice as much volume to obtain the same amount of calories from the glucose water as from the milk.

Even though no evidence supports it, the practice of giving glucose water to newborns still exists in the twenty-first century in developing countries,[114] in Europe,[115] and in the United States.[116] As previously shown, the administration of glucose water has no positive effects on jaundice, hypoglycemia, or other conditions. For a while, however, it was believed to be harmless. Recent studies

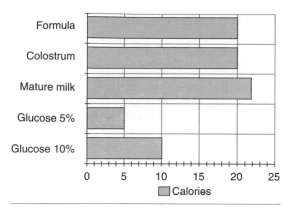

FIGURE 8-2 Calories in human milk, artificial milk, and glucose water.

have shown otherwise. In a prospective study, 80% of newborns who did not receive glucose water continued to be exclusively breastfed during the first month of life, whereas only 65% of those fed glucose water were unsupplemented at that time.[112]

The reasons given for using glucose water are not evidence based, and mounting research shows that giving glucose water confers no advantages but does pose potential disadvantages. Citing other sources,[106,117-119] the AAP[120] recommends against the use of glucose water.

Effects of Early Supplementation

Early supplementation thwarts successful breastfeeding because of its effect on milk supply and its association with early weaning. The main problem with supplementation is that it interferes with the natural process of maternal supply and infant demand.[121]

One of the most well-proven but underpublicized effects of artificial milk supplementation is its effect on the continuation of breastfeeding. WHO[20] identified five quasi-experimental studies addressing the relationship between supplementation and early weaning. Although one study in Europe[122] showed no difference in breastfeeding continuation either early (5 days) or later (6 months), several others have consistently and convincingly shown an association between early supplementation and early weaning. In Sweden, newborns who were exclusively breastfed were

more likely to continue breastfeeding, whereas newborns who got routine supplementation were more likely to be weaned at 2 weeks.[92] The mean duration of breastfeeding was 95 days for the breastfeeding-only groups, but 42 days in the supplemented group ($p < .0005$). In Canada, infants who had supplementation in the hospital were less likely to be breastfeeding at 4 or 9 weeks of age.[123] In Norway, the average duration of breastfeeding among 203 unsupplemented newborns was 4.5 months, compared with only 3.5 months in the supplemented group ($p < .001$).[111] A more recent descriptive study also showed an association between the giving of supplements and early termination of breastfeeding.[124]

Several prospective descriptive studies have also shown the same association. In Chicago a study of 166 newborns showed that those who received a minimal number of supplemental feedings in the hospital were more likely to be breastfeeding at 4 months.[125] Similar to Nylander's study in Norway,[111] a study in Sweden has shown that 521 infants given supplementary feedings in the first few days after birth have an almost fourfold increased risk of being weaned before they are 3 months old.[126] A descriptive study of more than 2000 mothers in Spain showed that formula supplementation during hospitalization was associated with significantly shorter duration of exclusive breastfeeding ($p = .03$).[127]

When Supplements Are Indicated

In most cases the healthy term newborn does not need supplementation. WHO spells out a few medically acceptable reasons for supplementation (Box 8-3). In most cases, however, supplementation is unnecessary. Supplemental feedings, both regular and occasional, may be indicated in some special circumstances, such as when an infant is born much before term or the mother has had previous breast surgery or trauma. (Supplementation for these infants is described in Chapters 15 and 16.)

Barriers to and Strategies for Achieving Unsupplemented Breastfeeding

Supplementing without a medically indicated reason continues to occur in U.S. hospitals. It is likely

Box 8-3   Acceptable Medical Reasons for Supplementation

A few medical indications in a maternity facility may require that individual infants be given fluids or food in addition to, or in place of, breast milk.

It is assumed that severely ill babies, babies in need of surgery, and very low-birth-weight infants will be in a special care unit. Their feeding will be individually decided, given their particular nutritional requirements and functional capabilities, although breast milk is recommended whenever possible. These infants in special care are likely to include:

- Infants with very low-birth-weight (less than 1500 g) or who are born before 32 weeks gestational age
- Infants with severe dysmaturity with potentially severe hypoglycemia, or who require therapy for hypoglycemia, and who do not improve through increased breastfeeding or by being given breast milk

For infants who are well enough to be with their mothers on the maternity ward, there are very few indications for supplements. In order to assess whether a facility is inappropriately using fluids or breast-milk substitutes, any infants receiving additional supplements must have been diagnosed as:

- Infants whose mothers have severe maternal illness (e.g., psychosis, eclampsia, or shock)
- Infants with inborn errors of metabolism (e.g., galactosemia, phenylketonuria, maple syrup urine disease)
- Infants with acute water loss, for example, during phototherapy for jaundice, whenever increased breastfeeding or use of expressed breast-milk cannot provide adequate hydration
- Infants whose mothers require medication that is contraindicated when breastfeeding (e.g., cytotoxic drugs, radioactive drugs, and antithyroid drugs other than propylthiouracil)

When breastfeeding has to be temporarily delayed, interrupted, or supplemented, mothers should be helped to establish or maintain lactation, for example, through manual or hand-pump expression of milk, in preparation for the moment when full breastfeeding may be begun or resumed. If the interruption is due to problems with the infant, milk can be expressed, stored if necessary, and provided to the infant as soon as medically advisable. If it is due to a maternal medication or disease that negatively affects the quality of milk, the milk should be pumped and discarded.

From World Health Organization. Acceptable medical reasons for supplementation. Baby-Friendly Hospital Initiative: Part II: Hospital-Level Implementation. Promoting Breast-Feeding in Health Facilities. A Short Course for Administrators and Policy-makers. Geneva: WHO; 1996.

that staff will continue to generate all sorts of seemingly plausible reasons why infants should receive supplements until the real barriers are identified and overcome. The main barriers to unsupplemented breastfeeding probably revolve around the concept that both medical and nursing personnel place a lower value on unsupplemented breastfeeding than on their anxieties about completing tasks and possible sequelae if the newborn is underfed.

One of the biggest problems is that staff get busy. Personnel recognize that helping mothers with breastfeeding takes time. Especially if the mother is tired, inexperienced, or uncertain of herself, or if the newborn is a reluctant nurser, the

nurse needs to spend a substantial amount of time at the bedside, facilitating latch-on, giving positive feedback to the mother, and evaluating whether milk transfer occurred.

I admit that helping a breastfeeding couplet sometimes seems time consuming when I feel pressured by multiple other responsibilities. That feeling is always present when my assignment is especially heavy, or if I feel pulled toward another patient who is at high risk for some potentially critical problem, such as a respiratory problem. I have occasionally been tempted to get the bottle; it would be faster. Therefore, when staff supplement newborns, I try to talk with them a little about what is happening on the unit and what their assignment is like. I try to empathize and admit that I find it challenging to achieve the ideal care for a normal, healthy couplet when another patient has a seemingly more threatening condition to deal with or when we all are working at top speed. But I try to gently remind them that upholding the agency standards is never optional. This soft-sell approach to changing attitudes is often helpful.

Advertising

WHO's International Code of Marketing of Breast-milk Substitutes aims to protect parents and

---

CLINICAL SCENARIO

Unnecessary Supplementation

You work on the mother-baby unit of your hospital. Often, you have noticed that infants who are delivered by cesarean birth are given first feedings of formula. Despite your best efforts to educate the labor/delivery staff about the importance of the first feeding being at the breast and the unlikely need for formula supplementation, this practice continues. Staff insist that the baby is or will become hypoglycemic, so they routinely do a heelstick to check glucose levels. Usually, a bottle of formula is then given. (You note that in one case, the reagent strip results were recorded as 65!) The father says, "Oh, by the way, my wife wants to breastfeed" and the nurse responds, "Oh fine, that's okay, but right now, she's too sick, so we'll just have to give the baby a bottle." How would you handle this situation?

This is one of the more frustrating scenarios that I have encountered in clinical practice. The problem is multifocused. One component is a lack of staff knowledge and another is the staff's belief that some harm will befall this baby—and they will be held liable—if some measurable amount of formula is not given. Still another component is that the administration does not have appropriate standards in place for breastfeeding, hypoglycemia, or cesarean delivery. Perhaps the most distressing component is that the mother's wishes have been violated, and in addition to a public relations issue, there's the ethical issue of what the staff should or should not be doing without her consent.

How I have handled this has depended on my role; I can usually do more when I am functioning in the clinical nurse specialist role than when I am functioning in the staff nurse role, but I do tackle this, regardless of my role.

Educating the staff is one possible strategy for fixing this problem, but I have never been very successful with that. Instead, I have tried to look at the existing hospital standards, or lack thereof. The existing hospital standards need to be consistent with and refer to statements from national standards (e.g., the American Academy of Pediatrics states that "Universal neonatal screening of blood glucose for hypoglycemia is not warranted in most nurseries").[93] Standards of care for the cesarean delivery should include directives on feeding the newborn. A hypoglycemia protocol for all infants—not just breastfeeding infants—should be in place. If all of these standards existed in my hospital, and if staff were not compliant, I would then be doubting if an interdisciplinary team had created the standards and wondering if they are consistently enforced by the administration.

To some extent, I have sometimes been successful by confronting staff, directly or indirectly, about actions that are contrary to mothers' wishes. I have done this in various ways, such as through grand rounds, forums set up to discuss ethical issues, and the hospital's consumer satisfaction department. (Getting this included on the questionnaire that is given to patients at discharge is a terrific strategy for changing this situation.) I have also talked with individual staff people and helped them recognize when mothers have felt disempowered or violated, and we have talked about the meaning of informed consent and the possible consequences when staff do not honor parents' wishes. Overall, I try to take this problem out of the context of breastfeeding and frame it in terms of the larger issues. I also try to remember that even when I am successful in solving this and similar problems, the system-level change has come very slowly.

health care providers from pressure to buy or endorse artificial milk products.[21] Later, in their Global Criteria for the BFHI, WHO specified, "No promotion for infants foods or drinks other than breastmilk should be displayed or distributed to mothers, staff, or the facility."[41] WHO, as well as medical organizations and published studies, recognizes that advertising can have deleterious effects.

The history and ongoing status of advertising in the United States has not always reflected the aims of the Code. In 1932, companies that manufactured artificial milk made an agreement with the medical community that they would not advertise formula directly to parents. However, in 1988, the year the "Goals for the Nation" were drafted (but not yet published), these companies broke their pact with the medical community and marketed directly to consumers, a move the AAP swiftly and staunchly opposed.[128] This advertising persists, and the Code continues to be violated. A study conducted in the late 1980s in Virginia showed that all hospitals in the survey were receiving free formula samples, which were being distributed to 95% of the breastfeeding mothers in those hospitals, and sometimes in direct contrast to physicians' wishes.[129] Indeed, the physician has often become the advertiser for a product that they understand discourages breastfeeding.[130]

Getting a product's name out where consumers can see it and providing a means for consumers to try the product are effective marketing strategies. Brand-level advertising directly relates to preferences for adult nutritional supplements[131] and increases sales of brand-name alcohol, although the overall market for alcohol does not expand.[132] Advertisements by artificial milk companies *work;* if the company did not realize greater profits, it would change its marketing strategies. The artificial milk business generates well over a billion U.S. dollars each year.

Makers of artificial milk want to get visibility for their product early and often. Pregnant women and those who have just given birth are the target audience for manufacturers of artificial milk, who recognize that it is easy to reach these women by distributing literature and formula samples through the prenatal office or clinic and the hospital. One marketing strategy is to advertise during the antepartum period; another involves distributing free formula to hospitals and free "gift packs" to women when they are discharged from the hospital.

Free "Formula" Samples and Other Items

During the antepartum period, manufacturers send free samples and coupons to prenatal patients and their health care providers. Howard and colleagues showed that 90% of pregnant women received free formula from their prenatal health care providers.[133] Fortunately, it appears that these free samples do not deter women from choosing to breastfeed, but women who quit breastfeeding during the first 2 weeks after delivery are more likely to have received commercial advertising materials than those who continue to breastfeed beyond that time.[134]

For many decades, makers of artificial milk have provided hospitals with free artificial milk; most hospitals do not purchase these ready-to-feed bottles. Along with these free samples, mothers are given videos, pamphlets, or infant items provided by the artificial milk company. These promotional materials are designed to encourage the mother to later purchase the brand with which they are most familiar. Not surprisingly, these efforts work. When mothers are not offered artificial milk, either as a supplement or as a gift pack, they are much less likely to recognize the "house brand."[7]

Hospital Discharge Gift Packs

Over the last several decades, manufacturers of artificial milk have routinely provided hospitals with "discharge packs" that may contain artificial milk, infant items, or coupons. In the past, these packs have been routinely and indiscriminately distributed in hospitals for breastfeeding mothers, sometimes with the approval of the physician.[129] Multiple studies have been conducted to determine whether these discharge packs have sabotaged breastfeeding efforts. At first glance, it may be tempting to dismiss these studies entirely because conflicting results have been reported. On closer look, however, it becomes apparent that studies that have shown no detrimental effects have had poor methodologies.[135-137] Studies that have had control groups, clear definitions of breastfeeding, or otherwise better methodology have shown that these gift packs do indeed thwart continuation of breastfeeding.[125,138,139] A meta-analysis[77] of six controlled studies[125,135,138-141] showed that exclusive breastfeeding at 1 month and any breastfeeding at 4 months were significantly less among mothers who had received commercial discharge packs. The authors concluded that these discharge samples were associated mostly with breastfeeding attrition in primiparae and low-income women in developing countries.

Overwhelming evidence has shown that supplementation is detrimental to the continuation of breastfeeding. Supplements of artificial milk or water are unnecessary in most cases, yet they continue to be advertised and distributed in prenatal and birth facilities. Despite the detrimental effects of supplements and concomitant advertising, artificial milk is not the only "problem" underlying breastfeeding initiation and continuation rates. No single factor can be blamed.

Barriers to and Strategies for Reducing or Eliminating Commercial Products

Routine supplementation with artificial milk has become the cultural norm in most hospitals. Similarly, accepting commercial pamphlets, videotapes, and advertisements that accompany them is also the cultural norm. There are really two barriers to overcome. The first barrier is the indiscriminate distribution of artificial milk, either as a way for staff to "top off" or replace breastfeedings during hospitalization or as free "gift pack." The second barrier is that hospitals accept free artificial milk supplements from the companies that make it.

Chapter 1 shows the benefits of breastfeeding, and this chapter shows the detrimental effects of artificial milk supplementation. Some staff or parents, persuaded by the evidence that supplementation undermines successful breastfeeding, may be eager to simply stop using it. For most, however, it is likely that a new hospital "culture" will need to be established to reduce or eliminate supplemental

feedings. A few strategies to deal with the routine and indiscriminate use of artificial milk supplementation are found in Box 8-4.

The *last* step in breastfeeding promotion is to eliminate the practice of accepting free or subsidized formula. It cannot be overemphasized how efforts to eliminate free or subsidized formula can be accomplished only after the facility has established *all other activities* to promote the initiation and continuation of breastfeeding.

The BFHI program requires facilities to purchase formula, rather than accepting "free" formula. The aim is to eliminate formula samples that are free, subsidized, or highly discounted because this practice violates the WHO Code.[21] The question of how, exactly, to eliminate the acceptance of free formula differs from facility to facility. Two reports in the literature describe U.S. hospitals that wanted to eliminate free formula in their quest to achieve the BFHI award. In one, the move to eliminate free commercial supplements was readily accomplished without much ado.[142] In the another hospital, purchasing of formula had begun some years earlier, was temporarily reinstated, and then was once again purchased when the BFHI program was undertaken.[143] These situations are atypical of most American hospitals, however.

Eliminating free formula first requires that everyone involved favors this arrangement. This means those involved at the unit level (e.g., the nurse manager or other) and at the hospital level (e.g., the chief financial officer and the purchasing supervisor) must interact frequently. In these conversations it is important for breastfeeding advocates to remember that those who look out for the hospital's financial welfare or purchasing power are not concerned with arguments of how supplementation affects breastfeeding success. Rather, they are concerned with the hospital's fiscal "bottom line," and hence, the clinical people will need to present clear arguments for how much formula is needed (which can be obtained through the logs) and the ethics of purchasing formula. Conversations about purchase of formula, however, should seek to describe the formula that is actually used, not necessarily the number of bottles of formula that are delivered to hospitals.

Box **8-4**   Strategies for Reducing or Eliminating Supplemental Feedings in the Hospital

- Develop a strong breastfeeding policy with collaboration from multiple licensed personnel in more than one discipline. This policy should explicitly say that exclusive breastfeeding is preferable, unless there is a medical indication for supplements.
- Get all staff "on board" with the idea that artificial supplementation should be used only when medically indicated. This involves both cognitive and affective learning. How this is accomplished differs from facility to facility, depending on the philosophy, educational level, and past "baggage" of the staff. Unless this strategy is successfully accomplished, however, the suggestions that follow are meaningless.
- Muster support for peer pressure to conform to the policy. Peer pressure may be the one most important strategy in gaining staff compliance. When it is no longer acceptable to indiscriminately distribute supplements, the practice is likely to stop.
- Incorporate medically indicated reasons for supplementation into existing protocols or other standards, or write new ones, if needed. Such standards should stipulate that supplements may not be given without a medical indication. The medical indications for supplements should be based on the reasons identified by WHO and UNICEF, and found in Box 8-3.
- Require parents to sign a form showing that they have received information about the potential adverse effects of formula supplementation. This should not be a "scare tactic" but rather, an instructive, science-based tool that documents parents' awareness of the potential adverse effects.
- Be alert for health care providers who frequently write orders for supplementation of healthy newborns. Recognize that although clinical management strategies may need to be individualized, frequent or recurrent orders that override a collaboratively developed policy or protocol signal lack of "buy-in" from the person writing the orders. In this case, follow up with the individual, or revisit the breastfeeding policy.
- Log the number of bottles of formula that are delivered to the maternity unit. This can be accomplished in a way similar to how controlled substances are accounted for when they arrive on the unit.
- Limit access to the supplements. Rather than storing artificial milk supplements in a cupboard that is accessible to all staff, put the supplements into a locked area that can be accessed only by the nurse manager or his or her designee.
- "Sign out" bottles of artificial milk. The sign-out sheet, similar to a sign-out sheet for narcotics, should include information about the indication for giving the supplement and the date, time, and signature of the registered nurse (RN) who is signing out the supplement. (This could also be done through electronic means, although paper logs would probably be easier.) If "wasted," supplements should be signed for by two RNs.
- Make some simple, descriptive inferences about information gathered on the sign-out sheet. Note trends and identify possible reasons for these trends. For example, if the supplements are usually given at night, confine corrective strategies to issues or practices that would logically be associated with that trend. Or, if one nurse seems to frequently be "wasting" bottles of artificial milk, she should be confronted directly.
- Tie the log to a quality-assurance study. Even for medically acceptable reasons, there should be relatively few situations for which supplementation is required. If there are several, or a trend develops, a QI study could uncover the underlying reason for the clinical condition.
- Impose consequences on staff who violate the breastfeeding policies and protocols, congruent with the way that consequences are given for violations of other polices and protocols. This is tricky because consequences that are delivered before the program is well established or consequences that are too frequent or too severe are likely to erode staff morale. Consequences might include anything from a verbal follow-up

Box **8-4** Strategies for Reducing or Eliminating Supplemental Feedings in the Hospital—cont'd

("Mrs. L. says that baby Diane got a supplement, and I'm wondering why, since I couldn't identify a medically indicated reason for it") to noting it on the employee's annual performance appraisal. The key is to make these consequences congruent with other consequences for policy/protocol noncompliance. More severe consequences—such as writing an incident report or including the violation on the nurse's annual performance appraisal—should rarely need to occur, and if they do, unit leaders should revisit the question of whether the staff "buy into" the policies.

- Avoid the temptation to "reward" those who comply with the policy as a replacement for establishing consequences. Frequently, the "carrot in front" strategy is presumed to be better than the "stick from behind" strategy. Although the "carrot" strategy is usually preferable, it is not helpful here. Employees should not be given a reward for doing their jobs according to the established standard. Worse still, a reward system might foster the withholding of supplements when they are medically indicated, which would be deplorable.

Copyright 2001 Marie Biancuzzo.

Purchasing formula requires one to estimate not only how many bottles would be used but also the fair market price and the budget for these. One facility determined that 20 cents per ready-to-feed bottle was an acceptable price to pay for the formula. Using that figure, they were able to calculate that with 1800 births per year, they would need to be prepared to purchase approximately $20,000 worth of formula annually,[144] when their breastfeeding rate was approximately 33%. (This figure differs from facility to facility, and Baby-Friendly USA has developed a mathematical formula for estimating the cost of infant formula and can give guidance to hospitals who are enrolled in the BFHI program.)

Aside from the financial concerns, however, are the ethical concerns. Likely as not, administrative personnel will be asking, "Why should we buy formula when we can get it for free?" This question, although seemingly logical, really is not. Box 8-5 asks, Why has formula been granted a most-favored status in American hospitals?

In summary, exclusive breastfeeding, especially during the neonatal period, has been shown to be advantageous in most clinical situations. The indiscriminate distribution of formula—either as in-hospital supplements to "top-off" or replace a breastfeeding or as part of a discharge gift—is counterproductive to the initiation and continuation of breastfeeding. Strategies to reduce formula use, and eventually eliminate acceptance of free formula, can be undertaken after other breastfeeding promotional activities are completely espoused by staff.

STEP 7: Practice Rooming-in; Allow Mothers and Infants to Remain Together 24 Hours a Day

ROOMING-IN

The idea of "rooming-in," although it has gained much attention in this decade, is not a new concept. The first "rooming-in" project in the United States was begun in the 1940s,[145] as shown in the Historical Highlight box. Although prominent pediatricians, such as John Kennell and Marshall Klaus,[146] have been advocating rooming-in since the late 1970s, the concept has been slow to be accepted in American hospitals. Today in the United States, rooming-in has become more popular with the advent of the BFHI, but most hospitals have only daytime rooming-in and are struggling to implement 24-hour rooming-in as stated in the BFHI criteria.

Box 8-5   Wake up and Smell the Formula

Scores of health care professionals have told me that they'd like to get rid of free formula in their hospitals, but they can't. They say, "No one here understands why we would want to buy our formula when we can get it for free." I would pose a different question: Why has formula been granted a most-favored status in the hospital?

What other newborn products do we accept or expect to be provided for free? In 20 years of practice, I've never heard someone say, "Let's get the diaper companies to give us some disposable diapers so that we don't have to buy them." Of course, in every hospital where I've worked, the hospital has never paid for disposable diapers—they are charged to patients, the same as bulb syringes or sterile gloves. The parents, or the insurance companies, bear the cost for this item. So apparently hospitals happily charge for what goes on one end of the baby, but don't charge for what goes in the other end of the baby. Tell me this makes sense!

Conversely, what other *free* product do we distribute—on the maternity service or elsewhere in the hospital—which clearly bears the product's brand name? True, we give away tissues, but they don't say "Kleenex™" on the box. Disposable diapers do come packaged in boxes with the trade name clearly shown, but there's a critical difference between this product and the tissues: The diapers are *charged* to the client; they are not given for free. Unfortunately, those pesky gift packs that are given at hospital discharge do contain brand-name items, but that's a one-shot deal. (The whole idea of discharge packs is, in my opinion, unethical anyway.) Clearly, formula enjoys a most-favored status. Why is formula the one and only name-brand item that is repeatedly distributed during the patient's hospitalization without charge?

Hospital administrators who argue for accepting and distributing this "free" formula need to be hospitalized for a while to realize that they're promoting an inconsistent model. Have you ever been a patient? Have you looked at your hospital bill? Were you charged $7 for one aspirin? Do you think that the hospital paid $7 for the tablet? Of course not! The charge reflects the freight costs to have the medication delivered, the labor of the guy working at the receiving dock, the hourly wage of the nurse who brings it to you, the price of the recycling bin that holds the discarded packaging, and so forth. Similarly, the "free" formula is actually costing the hospital money, but again, formula enjoys a most-favored status because the hospital willingly absorbs the extra costs to distribute this particular product.

Finally, by stocking only the bottled, ready-to-feed formula do we shirk our professional and ethical responsibility? Few, if any, of us have ever had the powdered or concentrate formula available in the hospital. How then, can we show parents the correct way to mix it? With only the bottled, ready-to-feed formula on hand, we have no evidence that bottle-feeding parents have mastered a skill that could literally be a life-and-death matter. We apparently have no compunctions about sending parents home without having mastered these skills, yet we know that the bottled ready-to-feed preparations are not widely available in the pharmacies or grocery stores of many of the communities where parents live. (Admittedly, they could be special-ordered.) Let's gain some control here. Let's stop accepting what we're given and instead buy the "inconvenient" formula preparations so that we can show parents how to mix formula. We can then observe and document the parents' return demonstration proving their ability to safely and independently perform this task. This might have the side effect of helping the breastfeeding agnostics—both parents and staff—to see first-hand that bottle-feeding is a not a convenience, but a nuisance.

The time has come to stop asking why we would purchase the formula if we could get it for free. It's time to start asking why this is the only product that we've been peddling samples of for more than half of a century. It's time to ask why we're using hospital money to absorb the costs associated with this "free" product. It's time to question why we've let thousands of parents go home without demonstrating that they can capably mix the formula that they're likely to buy. When we ask and answer these questions, maybe we'll wake up and smell the formula—and stop being unpaid shills for the formula companies.

From Biancuzzo M. *Breastfeeding Outlook* 2001;3:1-2, 7.

Historical Highlight

A Hospital Rooming-in Unit for Newborn Infants and Their Mothers

Citation: Jackson EB, Olmsted RW, Foord A et al. A hospital rooming-in unit for four newborn infants and their mothers: descriptive account of background, development and procedures with a few preliminary observations. *Pediatrics* 1948;1:28-43.

A brief survey conducted in 1937 at the New Haven Hospital showed that mothers did not feel adequately prepared to care for their infants after their discharge from the hospital. In response to this survey and the demands of mothers, a rooming-in arrangement, whereby the mother had her newborn in a crib by her bedside whenever she wished, was begun in New Haven, Connecticut, in 1946. Mothers who met the criteria (having a healthy, term newborn and similar criteria) were offered the opportunity to have rooming-in.

When breastfeeding women were offered this choice, their reactions in 1946 were similar to the responses of women today, but in different proportions than we might expect to see now. In those days, the majority of women considered rooming-in a privilege, and a typical response, quoted from the article, was, "Of course, after waiting so long, I would want to keep my baby with me!" A small minority declined the rooming-in arrangement, saying they believed they would get less rest in the rooming-in unit. Multiparas who participated in rooming-in, however, unanimously agreed that they felt they did not get less rest than during their previous hospitalizations and said that their previous experience was more unsettling because they continually worried about what was happening to their babies in the nurseries.

After the rooming-in project was implemented, mothers who roomed-in were almost unanimous in spontaneously expressing confidence in taking care of their newborns after discharge, whereas the mothers who were separated from their infants did not express this confidence.

It is noteworthy that the typical hospital stay was 8 days in 1946, and also that mothers were more likely to be in closer proximity to their own families. If these mothers lacked confidence, it is difficult to imagine how contemporary women, who are hospitalized for a much shorter time and often live hundreds of miles away from family members, can gain the skills and confidence they need to care for their newborns when they are separated from them.

Effects of Rooming-in

Studies conducted to determine the effects of rooming-in are limited, and results are mixed. A descriptive study conducted in Georgia looked at predictive factors for breastfeeding attrition before 7 days; rooming-in was one of four variables determined to be strongly predictive.[147] A descriptive study in the United States showed a correlation between rooming-in and longer breastfeeding continuation.[22] To date, however, only six quasi-experimental studies have addressed the effects of rooming-in on breastfeeding.[72,98,148-151] Most of these studies have been conducted outside of the United States.

Brazilian mothers who had rooming-in were more likely to express a desire to continue breastfeeding after hospital discharge than those whose newborns had been assigned to standard nursery care ($p < .001$).[148] Compared with those who were separated from their newborns, Swedish mothers of newborns undergoing phototherapy were significantly more likely to be breastfeeding at 4 weeks ($p < .05$) and somewhat more likely to be breastfeeding at 12 weeks.[149] Nicaraguan primiparae who roomed-in and got positive breastfeeding messages were more likely to report full breastfeeding at 1 week ($p < .001$) and any breastfeeding at 4 months ($p < .05$) when compared with non–rooming-in cohorts.[72] Mexican women, both multiparae and primiparae, were studied for the effects of rooming-in and special guidance on the continuation of breastfeeding (full or partial). Among primiparae who were rooming-in, full breastfeeding was significantly more prevalent at 1 month compared with primiparae in the non–rooming-in group.[98] Indonesian women appeared to have an earlier onset of mature milk when they roomed-in, presumably because of more infant suckling, than those whose newborns remained in the nursery.[150] In that same study, the incidence of clinical jaundice was significantly different; 26% of those housed in the nursery were diagnosed with clinical jaundice, compared with only 13% of those who roomed-in.[150] In Japan, newborns who roomed-in with their mothers breastfed more frequently and showed larger weight gains during the immediate postpartum period.[151]

Barriers to 24-Hour Rooming-in

In the hospital setting, barriers to 24-hour rooming-in or daytime rooming-in can present a significant but not insurmountable barrier to breastfeeding. The resistance to rooming-in stems from either staff or parents who object.

Often, staff try to justify nighttime nursery care by arguing that mothers are tired and need their sleep. To this end, they often devise a variety of ways to keep the newborn in the nursery. Among Swedish mothers, nighttime rooming-in affected neither the total number of hours the mother slept nor their daytime alertness, even though they breastfed more frequently at night.[152] One U.S. investigator conducted two compelling studies, one dealing with the newborn aspect and one dealing with the maternal aspect of sleep patterns of rooming-in versus non–rooming-in subjects. Newborns who slept in the nursery or in the mothers' rooms were monitored for 2 consecutive nights. Newborns who slept in the nursery had more crying episodes with less caregiver response than those who roomed-in.[153] The maternal aspect of sleeping was also favorable for the rooming-in situation. Comparing the nighttime sleep patterns of mothers who roomed-in 24 hours a day with those who roomed-in only from 7 AM until 10 PM, the total number of hours slept was the same in both groups.[154] (Interestingly, 7 of the 10 mothers in the nursery group took medication to help them sleep at night, yet they did not sleep longer than mothers in the rooming-in group who took none at all.) Furthermore, newborns who roomed-in spent 33% of the time in the quiet-sleep state compared with only 25% in the nursery group ($p < .05$). In short, the results of these studies suggest

that newborns who room-in achieve a better sleep pattern and cry less than those in the nursery and that the mothers' sleep patterns are not worse— and may be better—than those whose newborns are in the nursery.

Quite apart from the effects of rooming-in on breastfeeding, rooming-in seems to offer other advantages. In one developing country, rooming-in reduced maternal complications and costs.[69] Abandonment is reduced among mothers who have experienced rooming-in.[155,156] This behavior may be explained by the finding that women who room-in with their newborns have higher attachment scores.[157] The environment seems to foster more frequent interactions: Compared with those who do not, mothers who room-in look at, talk to, and touch their newborns more often, and they watch less television and talk on the phone less than mothers whose newborns are in the nursery.[158]

In the United States, however, parents often perceive rooming-in as more of a penalty than a privilege. It is not uncommon for a mother to request that the newborn go to the central nursery for the night so that she can "get her rest," and health care personnel not only support but often encourage this request. Worse still, well-intentioned health care providers frequently plant the seed for this request.

Mothers sometimes resist or openly refuse to room-in; sometimes they refuse any rooming-in, but more often, their objection centers around nighttime rooming-in. In my clinical experience, as well as in the scant literature that is available, those who are willing or eager to room-in are usually primiparae, those who have attended positive prenatal classes, and those who are breastfeeding.[159] Multiparae seem especially negative about rooming-in at night; they say that they want to get their rest before they return home to their other children.

Strategies to Implement Rooming-in

A few strategies that may facilitate rooming-in emerge from the available research and my clinical experience. The first step, however, is to determine whether the resistance stems mostly from the mother's beliefs and preferences or those of the staff.

Reducing Staff Resistance

Some staff members are willing to read and accept the results of research studies, but many are not. Those who are not are encumbered by their own biases and attitudes that rooming-in is a bad thing or a nuisance. Because they focus on the negatives of rooming-in, I usually focus on the negatives of nursery care. I suggest that the rooming-in arrangement is generally less work for the nurse, in terms of performing tasks. (It is more work in terms of monitoring the couplet, stocking the bassinets, and so forth.) Sometimes, the nonbelievers can be persuaded in the better outcomes of rooming-in by conducting or contributing to a small quality-improvement (QI) project. For example, it would be easy to design a study that looked at the incidence of clinical jaundice among rooming-in versus non–rooming-in newborns.[160] Cross-infection may also decrease with rooming-in; this also might provide a topic for a QI study.

Sometimes, reducing negative behaviors can be accomplished by pointing out to staff members that their verbal and/or and nonverbal messages have been observed. Having worked many nights, I remember a nurse who worked evenings and would shake her head "no" and say to the mother, "You don't want to have your baby in your room tonight, do you?" As a colleague, I could let her know that I had observed this or that the mother had reported it. I could also point out that the mother's choice was different from what she felt too intimidated to request. Had I been the nurse's boss, I would have confronted her and conveyed that this sort of biased persuasion is unacceptable.

In some hospitals the problem with nighttime rooming-in is unintentional. I am aware of one hospital where the infants were all weighed in the evening shift. As a result, the newborns were simply never returned to their mothers' rooms. Staff nurses who advocate 24-hour rooming-in need to be aware of this and similar situations in which the infant goes to the nursery and then is stuck there. Although I am a great advocate of rooming-in, breastfeeding, and so forth, when I have an assign-ment of 10 newborns, I find it difficult, if not impossible, to provide an optimal environment for all of them. So, the main strategy here is to reduce the possibility of the newborn being indefinitely "stuck" in the nursery.

Reducing Maternal Resistance

Parents may express or perceive that rooming-in is a negative thing, so they may resist it. Information is the key to changing that perception. In one study, when mothers were given information about rooming-in, they considered it as a feasible and safe alternative to the traditional nursery care.[161] Furthermore, rooming-in can be successfully accomplished, even if the mother has had a cesarean delivery.[162]

During pregnancy, it is critical to discuss rooming-in with mothers and their families. Otherwise, they may arrive at the labor and delivery suite expecting to have their newborn housed in a separate nursery, and they are less open to an alternative plan at that point. Teaching individual parents, or teaching group classes, is only one strategy for educating parents about the benefits of rooming-in. Consider other alternatives as well. For example, try a newspaper campaign in the community. If your church has a mother's group that meets once a month, offer to give a short presentation. Using a more community-based approach helps raise awareness and change the social norm in the community, and rooming-in may eventually be something that the parents request rather than resist.

I like to help parents to see the "down" side of central nurseries and the more subtle advantages of rooming-in. For example, if a mother is eager to see her milk "come in," I warn her it is less likely to happen during the hospital stay without a rooming-in arrangement. Similarly, rooming-in provides a way for mothers and their newborns to be mutual caregivers[163]; I like to talk to mothers about how they might be depriving themselves of that experience if they opt for the central nursery.

In summary, multiple studies have shown the benefits of rooming-in for breastfeeding couplets. Barriers emanating from parents or professionals are often due to lack of information, but also reflect a cultural bias. Multiple strategies aimed at changing the knowledge level of attitudes of individuals, or strategies that are more community focused, can be successful.

STEP 8: Encourage Breastfeeding on Demand

CUE-BASED FEEDINGS

WHO says, "Mothers of normal babies (including cesareans) who are breastfeeding should have no restrictions placed on the frequency or length of their babies' breastfeeds. They should be advised to breastfeed their babies whenever they are hungry or as often as the baby wants and they should wake their babies for breastfeeding if babies sleep too long or the mother's breasts are overfull."[41] Few

facilities that offer maternity services in the United States today perfectly fulfill the directive for "no restriction" of breastfeeding.

Restrictions are many and varied but include such practices as delayed first feedings, limited frequency or duration of suckling, supplementation with artificial milk (including "topping off" a breastfeeding), and the use of pacifiers. Even if these restrictions are not imposed, however, the lack of 24-hour rooming-in restricts breastfeeding, for WHO says, "truly unrestricted feeding is only possible for 24-hour rooming-in which enables the mother to respond when her infant shows readiness to feed."[20] The opposite of restricted feeding is unrestricted feedings, sometimes called *on-demand, demand, baby-led,* or *cue-based feedings.* In this text the term *cue-based feeding* is used

Historical Highlight

Cue-Based Feedings Improve Weight Gains and Continuation of Breastfeeding

Citation: Illingworth RS, Stone DGH, Jowett GH et al. Self-demand feeding in a maternity unit. *Lancet* 1952;1:683-687.

Illingworth and colleagues studied 237 healthy newborns from birth until 1 month of age. There were 106 newborns in the rigid-schedule feeding group ("scheduled" group), and they were fed 6 times per 24 hours. There were 131 in the self-demand group ("cue-based" group), and they were allowed to suckle as often as they showed interest. All infants were in the same hospital, and managed by the same physicians and nursing staff before they were discharged on the ninth day postpartum.

Investigators noted that the infants who were offered cue-based feedings suckled most frequently between the fourth and seventh days, and the majority took more than 6 feedings per 24 hours. Weight gains were better among the cue-based subjects. By the ninth day, 49.1% of the cue-based subjects had regained

their birth weight, compared with 36.1% of those in the scheduled groups. There was a strong positive correlation between the weight gain and the amount of milk consumed, as determined by test-weighing. The incidence of pathologic engorgement and nipple soreness was more than doubled among the mothers in the scheduled group compared with those in the cue-based group. Although not statistically significant, continuation of breastfeeding was also greater in the cue-based group: At discharge, 88% of the scheduled group were fully breastfeeding, compared with 94% of the cue-based subjects. At 1 month of age, 80% of the cue-based subjects were still breastfeeding, compared with only 65% of the scheduled subjects ($p < .01$).

Subsequent research has confirmed these results, particularly that cue-based feedings are related to continuation of breastfeeding throughout the neonatal period and beyond.

because it reflects the idea of symbiosis. The infant gives cues, and the mother responds to those cues.

Feedings that restrict the frequency or duration of suckling are generally called *scheduled feedings*. Scheduled feedings usually limit newborns to six, possibly eight feedings per day, but this is not the physiologic norm. In the absence of restrictions, and left to their own instincts, mothers and infants will have wide variations in the frequency and length of breastfeeding. Length of each feeding at 5 to 7 days postpartum can be between 7 and 30 minutes.[164] The frequency and number of feedings, when unrestricted, are substantially higher than what is allowed with scheduled feedings. In the early days, feeding 10 to 15 times in a 24-hour period is not unusual during the first month.[165] In the United States, mothers offer 6.5 to 16.5 feeds per 24 hours during the first 2 weeks and from 5 to 11 feedings per 24 hours at 1 month.[166]

Effects of Unrestricted Breastfeeding

Unrestricted breastfeeding has effects on both the mother and the infant. For the infant, the most notable effects are on total milk intake and weight gain/loss and serum bilirubin levels. For the mother, the most notable effects are on engorgement and nipple soreness, and for both mother and infant, the continuation of breastfeeding.

Effects on Milk Intake and Weight Gain/Loss

As early as 1952, evidence for unrestricted breastfeeding started accumulating. A quasi-experimental study, comparing infants who were given six feedings per day to those who were fully breastfeeding without restrictions showed that 49% of unrestricted infants regained their birth weight by 9 days of age compared with only 36% of those in the scheduled group.[167] In later studies, greater weight gain and milk intake were correlated with higher feeding frequencies at days 3 and 5[168] and day 15[169] but not at day 35.[169] It appears that feeding frequency during the neonatal period, but not thereafter, is the key to intake and weight gain; this fits with the fact that during that same period, maternal milk is produced in response to the removal of the milk that is in the breast.[170]

Effects on Serum Bilirubin Levels

Nearly two decades ago, DeCarvalho showed that there was a significant association between the frequency of breastfeeding (more than eight times per 24 hours) during the first few days of life and lower serum bilirubin levels on day 3.[171] A prospective study a decade later showed a strong correlation between the number of feedings on the first day of life and lower serum bilirubin levels on day 6.[168]

Effects on Engorgement and Nipple Soreness

With low stimulation of the nipples, the onset of an abundant milk supply is delayed. The breasts therefore become engorged and the nipples shorter and more difficult to grasp. This, in turn, leads to a frustrated infant who has difficulty attaching to the engorged areola and short nipple, and a cascade of deleterious events is likely to follow.

It has long been believed that severe restriction of suckling duration prevents sore nipples. This notion, however, is yet unproven. When compared with women who offered scheduled feedings, women who offered unrestricted feedings experienced no difference in engorgement or sore nipples, meaning "no worse" than that experienced by mothers who offer scheduled feedings.[172,173] A more recent analysis has shown that severely restricted breastfeeding is associated with *increased* incidence of sore nipples, engorgement, and the need to give additional formula supplementation when compared with scheduled feedings.[174]

Effects on Continuation of Breastfeeding

Studies have shown a correlation between unrestricted breastfeeding and delayed weaning. At 1 month, 80% of infants who had unrestricted breastfeeding were still breastfeeding, compared with only 65% of those who had scheduled feedings[167] (Fig. 8-3). Similarly, at 6 months, a strong correlation exists between unrestricted breastfeeding and delayed weaning ($p < .0005$).[173] A prospective descriptive study in Brazil showed that infants who had more than six feedings during their hospital stay and during the first month at home were more likely to be breastfeeding at 3 and 6 months.[175]

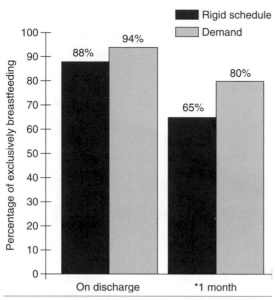

FIGURE **8-3** Proportion of infants fully breast-feeding on discharge and at 1 month of age. *(Data from Illingworth RS, Leeds MD, Stone DGH. Lancet 1952;1:683-687.)*

Barriers to and Strategies for Cue-Based Feedings

A notable barrier to cue-based feedings is that the parent or the provider may not recognize early signs of hunger. Education for both parents and providers helps overcome this problem. Videotapes showing footage of the early hunger cues are especially helpful (see Appendix B). Similarly, some parents can recognize the early signs of hunger when those signs are fairly blatant, but subtle signs, such as those that occur after the infant has had some exposure to analgesia, anesthesia, or magnesium sulfate, often go unrecognized. Finally, to state the obvious, parents will not recognize early signs of hunger when the infant is housed several hundred yards away in a central nursery. Rooming-in facilitates cue-based feedings.

A similar but more subtle barrier to cue-based feedings is that people sometimes think in terms of minutes and hours. Over the years, I have casually observed that parents and providers who are asked how often the baby should eat often recite a time increment, with seemingly no recognition that

timing is only an estimate, whereas feeding cues are a definitive way of determining when infants need to eat. Another problem is that sometimes staff tell parents that the time does not matter, but later ask "How many minutes did he nurse on each side?" This mixed message is not conducive to cue-based feedings.

In summary, restricting breastfeeding frequency or duration has no apparent benefit but many adverse effects. Cue-based feedings—feeding whenever the infant shows signs of hunger and continuing until he shows signs of satiation—has multiple advantages for both the mother and the infant.

STEP 9: Give No Artificial Teats or Pacifiers (Also Called Dummies or Soothers) to Breastfeeding Infants

Pacifiers and Artificial Nipples

The use of pacifiers and artificial nipples recently has become highly controversial. Although the "Ten Steps to Successful Breastfeeding" prohibits the use of pacifiers and artificial nipples for breast-fed infants, health care providers and consumers, until the last year or two, have been plagued with little research to substantiate WHO's recommendation against the use of these devices.

To understand the issues, it is important to first differentiate between the pacifier and the artificial nipple. Artificial nipples—sometimes called *artificial teats*—are placed atop bottles of fluid and the infant initiates nutritive sucking to get the palatable fluid into his oral cavity.

As described in Chapter 3, imprinting on artificial objects can occur; whether sucking the artificial nipple causes so-called nipple confusion is uncertain. However, many reports from mothers and health professionals, both in the published literature[176,177] and clinical practice, suggest that it is difficult for some infants to attach to the mother's nipple after they have learned to suck the artificial nipple. Although no cause-and-effect studies have been conducted to confirm this phenomenon, it has been clearly established that the mechanism used to suck an artificial nipple is different from that used to suck a human nipple.[178-181] Further discussion of artificial nipples, including the different types of artificial nipples and their effects, is found in Chapter 16. Here the discussion is confined to pacifiers.

Pacifiers—sometimes called *dummies, soothers,* or *comforters*—have an interesting history, as described by Kramer and colleagues.[199] Quoting others, they explain that small clay pacifiers have been found in graves dating back to about 1000 BC,[182] but in the early 1900s, the pacifier was referred to as a product of "perverted American ingenuity,"[183] an "instrument of torture,"[184] and a "curse of babyhood."[185] In stark contrast, however, in contemporary American society, the pacifier has become a routinely purchased and used apparatus. Multiple brands and styles of pacifiers are available,[186] and more than half of parents offer pacifiers.[187-190] About 94% of parents who use pacifiers introduce them before 2 weeks of age.[191]

Parents, or even health care providers, often rationalize the use of pacifiers and express a belief that the pacifier is a harmless, or perhaps even a necessary, device. There is some evidence that level of infant tension may be a reason for offering the pacifier in the first place.[192] They often express—correctly so—that infants have a high sucking need, but they express little or no acknowledgment that suckling the breast meets that need. In one study, *all* parents offered a pacifier to settle a fussy infant.[193] Although ample evidence shows that pacifiers calm the infant who is undergoing invasive procedures (e.g., heelsticks,[194-196] circumcision,[197] or venipuncture[198]), no evidence indicates that general "fussiness" is alleviated by the pacifier.[199] It is likely that pacifier use is more rooted in culture and that it meets the parents' need, not necessarily the infant's.

It is sometimes difficult to interpret the results of studies because parents who use pacifiers have both sociodemographic characteristics and parenting behaviors that are different from those of nonusers. For example, parents who are younger and have less education are more likely to offer a pacifier[200]; these characteristics are also associated with early weaning. Similarly, those who offer pacifiers are less consistent in encouraging their toddlers to brush their teeth.[201,202] This suggests that parents who offer pacifiers may have less motivation to be consistent in health promotion behaviors such as breastfeeding.

Effects of Pacifiers on Breastfeeding

Pacifiers appear to have a negative effect on latch-on problems. Righard observed that pacifier use was common among infants who had incorrect latch-on[203] and that these latch-on problems were more prevalent among infants who had had regular pacifier use than infants in a control group who had not.[204] Righard and Alade showed that mothers of infants who use a pacifier for more than 2 hours per day experience more breastfeeding problems,[96] and this has been corroborated by others.[205,206] Furthermore, Centuori and colleagues observed that pacifier use during the hospitalization is significantly related to nipple soreness during that time ($p = .02$).[207] At 12 weeks, mothers who offer a pacifier are more likely to describe breastfeeding as "inconvenient" and to report an insufficient milk supply compared with those who do not.[189]

Pacifier use has been associated with decreased frequency of feedings[189,206] and as a way to terminate the feeding.[206,208] Decreased frequency of breastfeeding, of course, can interfere with milk supply and increases the probability of conception.[209]

Several studies have been conducted to determine the effects of pacifiers on breastfeeding and early weaning. Studies in Sweden,[96,208,210] England,[211] New Zealand,[212,213] Brazil,[205,206,214] Finland,[215] Italy,[127,207] and the United States[189] have shown that pacifier use is associated with breastfeeding attrition. However, these descriptive studies do not substantiate a cause-and-effect relationship; there is only an association. Furthermore, in some of the studies, the actual amount of pacifier use was measured ("in the mouth time"), whereas in other studies it was not; there is a positive correlation between increased use and early breastfeeding termination. However, it appears that pacifier use is unrelated to weaning before 3 months, but not thereafter.[189]

One quasi-experimental study carried out in Canada reported an association between pacifier use and early weaning.[199] When one is interpreting results of this study, however, it is important to note that although subjects were randomized and assigned to either an experimental or control group, the groups were not "pacifier" versus "non-pacifier." Rather, the intervention consisted of instructing parents in the control group about avoidance of pacifier use and alternative consoling techniques, whereas parents in the control group were simply given instructions about consoling techniques. Parents in the experimental group

were less likely to use a pacifier, as described earlier. When the randomization was ignored, however (i.e., the investigators looked at both the control and the experimental groups), pacifier use and early termination of breastfeeding were strongly correlated. This is consistent with the earlier studies described here. A summary of studies related to the effects of pacifiers on early termination of breastfeeding is found in Table 8-1.

The study conducted by Victora and colleagues[206] and described further in the Research

RESEARCH HIGHLIGHT

Do Pacifiers Affect Breastfeeding?

Citation: Victora CG, Behague DP, Barros FC et al. Pacifier use and short breastfeeding duration: cause, consequence, or coincidence? *Pediatrics* 1997; 99:445-453.

FOCUS

This prospective study used a combination epidemiologic and ethnographic approach. The epidemiologic aim was to (1) describe pacifier use and breastfeeding patterns, (2) investigate the association between pacifier use and subsequent breastfeeding, (3) check reverse causality; (4) understand the mechanisms mediating the association, (5) rule out a large number of possible confounding variables, and (6) identify factors that may modify the relation of pacifiers to breastfeeding. The ethnographic study aimed to explore (1) how much and why mothers value pacifier use, (2) how mothers stimulated pacifier use, (3) how readily the infants actually take the pacifiers, and (4) the presence of self-selection.

RESULTS

Almost half of the mothers took the pacifiers to the hospital, and about 85% of mothers were using pacifiers 1 month after birth. Some who did not use pacifiers while they were breastfeeding used them after weaning, suggesting reverse causality. Bottles were a possible confounding factor because more than 84% of 1-month-old infants used bottles. There was a strong relationship between pacifier use at 1 month

and breastfeeding discontinuation; greater use of the pacifier (more hours per day) varied directly with discontinuation of breastfeeding. Furthermore, mothers saw the pacifier as a "luxury," and many strongly stimulated the infant to accept the pacifier, even after he refused it. Mothers who used the pacifier with greater intensity (more hours per day and more stimulation to get the infant to accept it) had breastfeeding behaviors that restricted infant-led feeding.

STRENGTHS, LIMITATIONS OF THE STUDY

A large sample size (605 subjects) and the careful attention to confounding variables were clear strengths of this study. The study was conducted in Brazil, and few of the infants were exclusively breastfed, both of which limit the generalizability of the findings to other populations.

CLINICAL APPLICATION

Like earlier studies, this study shows an association between pacifier use and early discontinuation of breastfeeding. However, this is the first study to suggest that pacifiers may not be the culprit in early discontinuation of breastfeeding. Rather, the observation that the woman values the pacifier and uses it as one way to restrict infant-led breastfeeding interaction underscores the need to increase consumer education and change the cultural paradigm. Professionals need to help mothers develop realistic expectations about newborns' need for frequent feedings and comfort.

Table **8-1** EFFECTS OF PACIFIERS ON EARLY TERMINATION OF BREASTFEEDING

Author	Country	N	Time of Measurement	Design	Outcome	Comments
Aarts, 1999[210]	Sweden	506	Every 14 days	Descriptive, longitudinal, prospective	Pacifier use associated with fewer feedings in a 24-hr period, early discontinuation of total breast-feeding, and earlier discontinuation of exclusive breastfeeding when compared with no pacifier use.	These associations were not found for thumb-suckers.
Barros et al., 1995[205]	Brazil	605	1, 4, 6 mo	Descriptive, longitudinal, prospective	Significantly greater risk for discontinuing breast-feeding before 1 mo.	All infants were of rooming-in; effects of pacifier remained even after adjusting for confounding factors.
Hornell et al., 1999[208]	Sweden	506	Every 14 days	Descriptive, longitudinal, prospective	Significantly greater risk for discontinuing breastfeeding before 6 mo when a pacifier was used ($p < .03$). Pacifier use was correlated to feeding frequency.	Multiparae only.
Howard et al., 1999[248]	U.S.	265	2, 6, 12, 24 wk and thereafter every 90 days until weaning occurred	Descriptive, longitudinal, prospective	Introduction of a pacifier before 6 wk was significantly associated with earlier discontinuation of full breastfeeding.	Pacifier use was correlated with breastfeeding frequency.
Kramer et al., 2001[199]	Canada	258	4, 6, 9 wk	Controlled and descriptive, double-blind	Daily use or any use of pacifier decreased significantly when parents were taught other methods for comforting infant. Pacifier use did not improve fussy behavior. When random allocation was ignored, daily pacifier use was strongly associated with discontinuation of breastfeeding before 3 mo.	Authors conclude that "pacifier use is a marker of breastfeeding difficulties or reduced motivation to breastfeed, rather than a true cause of early weaning."

Continued

Table **8-1** EFFECTS OF PACIFIERS ON EARLY TERMINATION OF BREASTFEEDING—CONT'D

Author	Country	N	Time of Measurement	Design	Outcome	Comments
Righard & Alade, 1992[96]	Sweden	82	4-6 days, 4 mo	Descriptive, longitudinal, prospective	Exclusively breastfeeding mothers were more likely to wean before 4 mo if they had used a pacifier for more than 2 hr a day than if they had not used the pacifier.	The intervention was to help correct faulty positioning, not to withhold a pacifier.
Righard & Alade, 1997[191]	Sweden	82	4-5 days, 4 mo	Descriptive, longitudinal, prospective	Exclusively breastfeeding mothers were more likely to have weaned by 4 mo if they used a pacifier than if they had not (p < .03). Pacifier users also had incorrect sucking technique.	Difficult to determine whether weaning was associated with pacifier because the poor latch could impede milk transfer and therefore breastfeeding continuation.
Riva et al., 1999[127]	Italy	1601	1, 3, 6, 12 mo	Descriptive, longitudinal, prospective	Whether fully or partially breastfeeding, mothers were more likely to wean if they introduced a pacifier within 1 mo of birth (p < .1).	Breastfeeding defined according to WHO. No attempt was made to quantify the extent of pacifier use.
Schubiger et al., 1997[122]	Switzerland	602	Day 5, then 2 mo, 4 mo, 6 mo	Quasi-experimental, longitudinal, prospective	With random assignment to control or experimental group, there was no significant difference in continuation of breastfeeding whether using or not using a pacifier.	Only study to restrict both pacifiers and supplementation in the experimental group. In the experimental group, 46% violated the study protocol (i.e., offered supplements and pacifiers to infants).

Victora et al., 1993[249]	Brazil	354	Data reported in 1 mo intervals from 1 to 18 mo	Descriptive, longitudinal	By 1 month of age, 67% of breastfed infants were using a pacifier on a daily basis, and 94% were supplemented with other fluids. By 1 month of age, only 249 were still being breastfed. Those who used the pacifier any amount of time were 2.7 times more likely to be weaned before 6 mo than those who did not use it at all (p < .001). Amount of use was directly related to weaning trend.	Even when adjusted for age and supplementation, trend persisted. Unclear when data was obtained (prospective or retrospective maternal recall).
Victora et al., 1997[206]	Brazil	450	1, 3, 6 mo	Descriptive, longitudinal, prospective	Mothers offered strong stimulation for infants to take the pacifier. Those who sucked pacifier regularly were 4 times more likely to be weaned by 6 months than nonusers.	This was the only study that looked at both epidemiologic and ethnographic factors.
Vogel et al., 2001[213]	New Zealand	350	1, 2, 3, 6, 9, 12 mo	Descriptive, prospective, longitudinal	Daily pacifier users were at greater risk for early weaning, but "less-than-daily use" was not associated with time of weaning. Primiparae were more likely to use a pacifier than multiparae. Confidence was also related to pacifier use.	Mothers were asked prenatally about their intentions to use the pacifier postnatally.

Highlight, addressed not only the question of breastfeeding continuation but also the characteristics of the mothers who depend on the pacifier to comfort and quiet their children. This study is most enlightening because it gives the reader an opportunity to understand the interrelationship between parenting behaviors and breastfeeding outcomes. That is, mothers who offer pacifiers tend to have a more restricted style of breastfeeding, and this behavior, not the pacifier, may explain the early termination of breastfeeding (Fig. 8-4). Because of this ethnographic component, it is difficult to determine whether pacifiers per se are the culprit in early breastfeeding attrition.

Other Effects of Pacifiers

Pacifiers have had negative effects on situations other than breastfeeding. Infections, dental problems, neurobehavioral difficulties, and other problems are also associated with pacifier use.

Infections

Infections are more prevalent among infants who use a pacifier. Most notably, otitis media is common among pacifier users.[200,216] More specifically, episodes of acute otitis media are 50%[217] to 100%[218] greater among pacifier users. In a meta-analysis of 22 studies, pacifier use was identified as a risk factor for otitis media in six different countries.[219] Furthermore, the routine use of pacifiers has been positively associated with higher rates of oral *Candida* infections.[220,221]

Dental Problems

Pacifier use, which typically begins in infancy, has been associated with dental problems when preschoolers continue to suck a pacifier.[188,215,216,222] Although these studies address older children, there is an important implication for the newborn period, namely, the introduction of a pacifier. The mouthing of pacifiers is significantly more likely to continue at 19 to 36 months, compared with nonpacifier mouthing, which lasts 0 to 18 months.[223]

Neurobehavioral and Neurocognitive Problems

Pacifier use has been associated with several neurobehavioral and neurocognitive problems. The effects on intelligence, sleep, and the risk of sudden

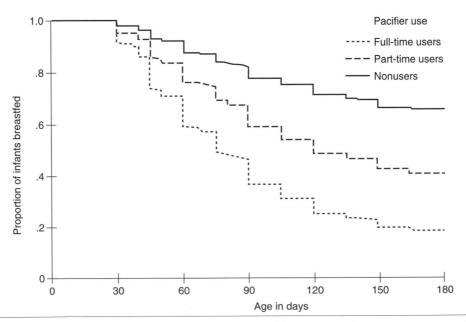

FIGURE 8-4 Proportion of infants who were breastfed up to 6 months of age according to frequency of pacifier use at 1 month. *(From Victora CG, Behague DP, Barros FC et al. Pediatrics 1997;99:445-453.)*

infant death syndrome (SIDS) and attachment behaviors are especially notable.

Pacifier use independently predicts intelligence quotients (IQs), which are lower among children who have used a pacifier in infancy.[224] Although Barros and colleagues[214] also found that pacifier use during infancy was the most important predictor of later intelligence, the relationship between IQ and pacifier use disappeared when they adjusted for breastfeeding duration. This suggests that pacifier use decreases the amount of human milk that is consumed by the infant, and the lack of human milk—not necessarily the pacifier per se—predicts lower intelligence.

It appears that children do not modulate their own sleep behavior when they use a pacifier[225] and auditory thresholds are different when they use a pacifier.[226] Similarly, pacifier sucking has no significant effects on electroencephalographic (EEG) activity, which relates to sleep-wake cycles.[227] This may have some implications for SIDS, although what, if any, relationship exists, is unclear. The relationship of the pacifier to SIDS is unclear.[228]

Lehman and colleagues conducted an especially interesting longitudinal study to evaluate healthy mother-infant attachment. Unlike children with soft-object attachments, who were rated as securely attached to their mothers at 12 months and 30 months, those who had attached to the pacifier were less often rated as securely attached to their mothers.[229]

Interpretation of these studies should reflect an understanding that confounding factors in the subjects (e.g., socioeconomic factors) make it difficult to come to any clear conclusions. A cause-and-effect relationship between pacifiers and untoward outcomes has not been established; only associations have been made at this point.

Barriers to and Strategies for Reducing or Eliminating Pacifiers

Perhaps the biggest barrier to reducing or eliminating pacifier use in the hospital or shortly thereafter at home is that parents and health care providers believe that they are helpful, or at least harmless for healthy term newborns. Reducing or eliminating pacifier use in hospitals involves a two-pronged approach, modifying the beliefs of staff and parents.

Staff members who believe pacifiers are harmless or desirable may not be willing to read and interpret the results of research studies. But those who are merely uninformed or believe that pacifiers are harmless are often jolted out of complacency when they are informed of the many disadvantages of the pacifier. A bullet-point list, placed in a strategic place on the unit and enumerating the problems associated with pacifiers, can be very thought provoking and helpful in changing practice. Furthermore, there should be some discussion in the hospital about informed consent for using pacifiers, and a form for that purpose, perhaps modeled after an existing one,[230] should be designed. It cannot be said with certainty that pacifiers are "bad," but there is ample evidence that they carry potential harm. There is little or no research showing any potential *benefit* to pacifier use for healthy term infants who are not experiencing any painful stimuli.

A more recent barrier to elimination of hospital use of pacifiers is that pacifiers are now required to meet standards for pain management in infants who are undergoing invasive procedures or painful stimuli, such as circumcision. Clearly, the pacifier has been shown to be more effective in pain management than sweet solutions.[198] The thorny and practical question, however, is how to have these pacifiers on the clinical units without having them indiscriminately distributed, and thus interfering with breastfeeding. The most logical approach is to write a policy or protocol that addresses the broader issue of pain management. In this way, there is a medical indication for the use of a pacifier.

Parents have some similar but different barriers that relate to pacifiers. They often report the fear that if children do not have a pacifier, they will suck their thumbs or digits. The parent rationalizes that the pacifier can be discontinued if it is thrown away, but the thumbs or other digits are always available to the child. This rationale, however, is faulty. It appears that children mouth pacifiers significantly longer than thumbs or digits, regardless of age.[223,231] Furthermore, even though pacifiers "prevent" sucking of digits,[231] this is not necessarily desirable. Digit sucking helps the infant console himself and self-modulate his sleep-states, whereas pacifier use does not.[225]

Educating parents can help overcome their barrier to eliminating pacifiers.[232] Mothers who receive education about pacifiers use them less frequently and breastfeed their infants more frequently.[233] Kramer's recent and controlled study showed that when parents learned of the detrimental effects of pacifiers and alternative ways of consoling their infants, pacifier use decreased.[199] Furthermore, with so much evidence about negative effects associated with pacifiers, it may be unconscionable to offer pacifiers to infants without obtaining informed consent from their parents.

Parents who use pacifiers generally restrict breastfeeding, as previously described. Help them explore their feelings about how, when, and why they restrict breastfeeding, including "holding off" a feeding. Keep a clear emphasis on ways to let the infant control the feeding frequency, pace, and termination rather than having the parent control these factors by using the pacifier or some other method. Parents who are merely uninformed but open to new information may be surprised to know that pacifier use does not result in less fussiness,[199] and they may be grateful for alternative comfort techniques.

Finally, boost mothers' confidence. Victora and colleagues,[206] in their carefully designed study, showed that mothers who had more self-confidence were less likely to wean if they used the pacifier. This is a recurring theme throughout the breastfeeding literature; maternal self-confidence varies directly with both the initiation and continuation of breastfeeding.

In summary, pacifiers provide no benefit for the infant, unless they are medically indicated. Negative effects on breastfeeding technique and the continuation of breastfeeding, as well as other negative effects, are associated with pacifier use. Overcoming the barriers to pacifiers, through a two-pronged educational program that aims to change both the knowledge and the attitudes of parents and providers, can be effective.

STEP 10: Foster the Establishment of Breastfeeding Support Groups and Refer Mothers to Them on Discharge from the Hospital or Clinic

POSTPARTUM SUPPORT

WHO says that mothers "should also be able to describe [how to find] a breastfeeding support group (if adequate support is not available in their own families) or to report that the hospital will provide follow-up support on breastfeeding if needed. The nursing [supervisor] should be aware of any breastfeeding support groups and . . . describe a way mothers are referred to them. Alternatively, she or he should be able to describe a system of follow-up support for all breastfeeding mothers after they are discharged (early postnatal or lactation clinic checkup, home visit, telephone call)."[41]

WHO has purposely omitted a clear definition of "support groups" because it is likely that social norms throughout the world vary so substantially that a prescribed form or format for one particular group would not be useful. In general, however, U.S. support groups cluster largely around (1) those that emanate from the health care system and consist of in-person or telephone contact by licensed professionals; (2) mother-to-mother support groups, usually without direct professional supervision; and (3) peer counselors who provide support for individual mothers, often in conjunction with professional supervision.[20] Variations of all these support options exist.

Effects of Support Programs

Support programs offered by professionals who practice in health care systems are generally effective in breastfeeding continuation. Most quasi-experimental studies addressing professional support in relation to breastfeeding outcomes have been conducted abroad.[97,234-238] A few have been conducted in the United States and generally offer either in-person instruction and support, telephone follow-up, or both. Hall looked at the effects of giving a postpartum slide presentation to married primiparae; this program did not significantly increase breastfeeding at 6 weeks.[239] Frank and colleagues showed that postpartum counseling (in-hospital visits, eight phone calls and 24-hour telephone paging service) delayed the introduction of solid foods, but the effect on continuation of breastfeeding at 4 months was nonsignificant compared with cohorts who had only "routine" hospital care.[139] Saunders and Carroll showed that mothers who experienced a combination of supportive interventions (an in-hospital visit, phone call at 4 to 5 days postpartum, and one support class at 2 weeks postpartum) were more likely to continue breastfeeding at 16 weeks when compared with mothers who received only routine care.[240] One study among low-income mothers showed no difference in the time of weaning between groups that received routine or intensive postpartum support.[241]

Support programs that use individual peer-counselors (rather than group support meetings) were at first studied outside of the United States.[56,58,242] Fig. 8-5 shows the effectiveness of a home-based counseling program among Mexican mothers. Mounting evidence in the United States has suggested that peer counselor interactions improve breastfeeding initiation or continuation rates. It is difficult to ascertain exactly what is effective because the studies are often dissimilar. In some studies, trained peer counselors implement a fairly structured program, whereas in others, untrained peer counselors simply "encourage" breastfeeding. The contact varies substantially; in some cases, peer counselors make one or many

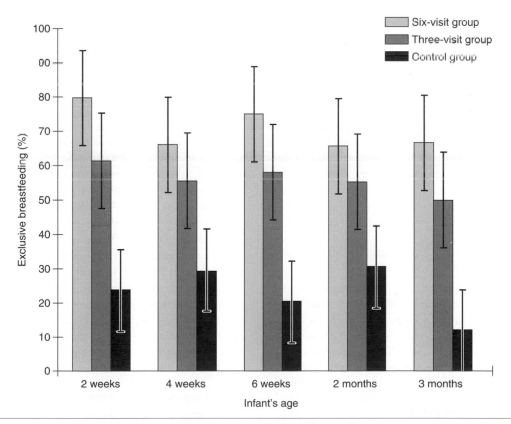

FIGURE **8-5** Proportion of mothers who exclusively breastfed their infants by infant age and study group. *(From Morrow AL, Guerrero ML, Shults J et al.* Lancet *1999;353:1226-1231.)*

in-home visits, whereas in others, they may provide anywhere from one telephone call to unlimited phone availability.

An impressive prospective study was recently conducted in Canada. A total of 256 primiparae were randomly assigned to either conventional care (clinic, telephone, and community health nurse follow-up) or to the experimental group (unlimited telephone contact with a trained peer counselor). Mothers who had peer counselors were significantly more likely to be exclusively breastfeeding at 3 months compared with those who had access to only the conventional care ($p < .01$). To date, this is arguably the most carefully designed and well-controlled study that supports the efficacy of trained peer counselors.[243]

Mother-to-mother support through group meetings has formally existed since the 1950s when La Leche League was founded. Group meetings of La Leche League members continue today, as do meetings of mothers in numerous hospitals, churches, and other places, but the efficacy of support through the group meeting has not been established. In 1976 one cross-sectional study described how women who participated in La Leche League meetings in the United States were more likely to delay the introduction of solids until after 4 to 6 months postpartum.[244] Mothers who attend mother-to-mother support groups attribute breastfeeding continuation to the support they receive from the group,[245] especially in gaining skills to cope with criticism for long-term breastfeeding.[246]

Barriers to and Strategies to Promote Community Support

Little, if any, information is available in the published literature to substantiate the barriers to community breastfeeding support, far less the strategies to overcome such barriers. Barriers to and strategies for community support can be described in terms of actions for health care services, peer-counselor programs, and mother-to-mother support groups.

Health Care Services

Health care services have relatively slow to develop community-based support mechanisms. Although the Women, Infants, and Children

(WIC) programs have begun doing this, many mothers do not qualify for and therefore do not participate in WIC. Hospitals, where more than 95% of women deliver their babies, would be the logical hub for postpartum support follow-up groups, but such programs, if they exist, are often limited to a brief telephone contact with little or no structure in terms of problem solving. Unfortunately, administrators who make financial decisions are often unaware of either the need for postpartum support or its efficacy (as previously described) among their particular population.

Those aiming to convince hospital administrators to implement a postpartum support program should begin by documenting the breastfeeding attrition rate and recording the problems identified in the postpartum period. This can be done through a formal survey, a less formal recording, or even a QI project.

I developed a way to track the topics for telephone calls fielded by our hospital staff. I did it by reviewing literally hundreds of records until I could discern a pattern of common concerns and questions. I finally identified six main categories, with the final category being "other," which contained a place for a write-in description. At the end of each quarter, I was able to show my boss the number of calls about each topic (e.g., "sore nipples"), the number of total calls, and the follow-up result. With such information firmly in hand, the viability of the program was more likely than if I had no data about the nature, frequency, and outcomes of the calls. Telephone contact, without in-person assistance, has limited value. However, it is a start, and being able to show the needs and the efficacy of the support is likely to pave the way for a more elaborate program. Administrators are more willing—or at least less resistant—to fund programs for which there is clear documentation of the needs and outcomes of the program.

Peer-Counselor Programs

In my experience, one of the big problems with "peer support" is finding true peers who are willing to commit to a period of time to help a mother choose or initiate breastfeeding. Often, the "peers" who are willing to help are the mature, married, educated, socially advantaged women. They are likely to be influential among mothers who are similar to themselves, but they are unlikely to have much influence with the adolescent, unmarried, or socially disadvantaged women who have little confidence and need the greatest amount of support. The key is to identify those women who typify your client population and who have had a rewarding breastfeeding experience and recruit them early on as peer counselors.

Peer counseling programs should be designed with a structure that is compatible with the resources of the sponsoring hospital or other agency. Resources—human, material, and financial—need to be evaluated before beginning the program so that the services offered can realistically continue for an indefinite amount of time.

Support programs, whether they are professionally driven, peer driven, or professionally driven and peer supported, should have some clear objectives and strategies before they are developed (Box 8-6).

Box 8-6 KEY ELEMENTS TO CONSIDER IN BUILDING SUPPORT PROGRAMS

- What is the greatest need among antepartum and postpartum women in your population? In my hospital, I was able to identify that the greatest number of reported postpartum problems were related to perceived insufficient milk supply. This, then, became one of the driving forces in structuring the program.
- What is the main aim of the program? Is it to provide encouragement and support or to solve emergent or ongoing health problems? (Problem-oriented programs should be professionally driven, even though they may be peer supported.)
- Who is the target audience? What are the demographics or characteristics of the target audience? Will the target audience be antenatal or postnatal mothers, or both?
- What will be the primary means of contact? Telephone? (If so, does the mother call the peer and/or professional, or does the professional and/or peer initiate the call, or either?) Are there set times for the calls, or are they ad hoc? Home visits? If so, are there limits to the number of visits that can realistically be provided? What about electronic means of communication? (This a vast, untapped resource!)
- What are the resources for the program, in terms of human, material, and financial resources? What groups are available in the community to provide additional resources or augment efforts? For example, would the local spa be willing to donate a full-

body massage to women who act as peer counselors? Would the local beauty salon be willing to offer a coupon for one free haircut to women who breastfeed for at least 2 months? (These are great strategies for businesses to increase their visibility and/or clientele, and they are often willing to use these strategies.) How can media coverage be used to gather momentum for the program and get the attention of others in the community who may be willing to provide resources?
- How can the program become a collaborative project in the community? A hospital or other agency generally needs to take the lead, but programs are more likely to be successful if they have a collaborative component.
- How will the program be evaluated? Program evaluation is often overlooked. As a result, these are the first programs to be cut when the budget gets tight because the efficacy of the program has not been shown. The program should be evaluated in terms of clinical outcomes (usually breastfeeding initiation and/or continuation, although it could be morbidity, rehospitalization, or any number of other indicators), client satisfaction, staff satisfaction, and financial viability.[49]
- How will the success of the program be publicized? Presuming that the program evaluation shows its efficacy, good publicity is likely to increase the visibility and therefore the participation—and often the financial viability—of the program.

Mother-to-Mother Support Groups

Mother-to-mother support groups are probably underused in the United States. Unfortunately, one of the barriers that I have noted over many years of clinical practice is that sometimes mother-to-mother groups are perceived as fanatical. This image is a huge barrier that the groups themselves must work to overcome. I cannot solve that problem, so I try to stay alert to groups that are less radical in their approach and steer mothers to groups that show more respect for a continuum of choices rather than a set "standard" for all to meet.

A big problem with organized mother-to-mother support groups is that they are virtually nonexistent in very rural areas. I have never been completely successful in solving that problem, but I have discovered a few strategies that provide a starting point from which to work. First, help a frustrated mother establish phone contact with a mother in a neighboring community or e-mail contact with a mother who is willing to successfully resolve her questions and concerns. If she has a gratifying experience, she might later be persuaded to start a support group in her community because she realizes the extent of the need. Multiple groups now exist in Internet chat rooms, or e-mail lists can be used as a remote means of having mother-to-mother support.

I also believe that churches are a vast untapped resource for establishing mother-to-mother support groups for breastfeeding. In the parish where I am registered, along with a neighboring parish, a scheduled monthly meeting is designed to provide a forum for discussing parenting issues; the meetings consist of a speaker and a fun event (e.g., viewing a videotape or having a picnic). This forum can serve as a way to target mothers who need an offshoot group that focuses on breastfeeding. Nurses and other health care providers can plant the seed of interest by offering to be the guest speaker (and presenting a breastfeeding topic) at one of the monthly meetings.

In summary, programs that offer postpartum support to mothers have been shown to increase the continuation of breastfeeding. These programs may be based in the health care system, or they may be mother-to-mother support groups or lay counselors. Research has not shown precisely how to establish these groups, but some questions for getting started are provided.

CONCLUSION

The Ten Steps to Successful Breastfeeding, established by WHO in 1989, are an evidence-based approach for achieving better clinical outcomes. Because UNICEF, the World Health Organization, the AAP, the U.S. government and others recognize the Ten Steps as a critical component of maternity care, it seems surprising that all facilities that offer maternity services have not embraced this model of evidence-based care for mother and newborns.

Those who formulate a long-term plan that embodies teamwork and skill can implement multiple strategies to overcome individual, interpersonal, and system-level barriers to the Ten Steps. While I was preparing this edition, I had the privilege of presenting the BFHI award to Kaiser Permanente Hospital in Hayward, California. Staff there did not seem exhausted from their efforts to achieve the award. Rather, they seemed exhilarated. In joining their celebration, I perceived that the cooperation and camaraderie among staff members, although sparked by a desire to achieve the award, would continue to be fueled by their overwhelming sense of accomplishment and that the benefits of the *process,* as well as the program, would endure indefinitely.

REFERENCES

1. WHO and UNICEF. *Protecting, promoting, and supporting breast-feeding: the special role of maternity services.* Geneva, Switzerland: World Health Organization; 1989.
2. Winikoff B, Laukaran VH, Myers D et al. Dynamics of infant feeding: mothers, professionals, and the institutional context in a large urban hospital. *Pediatrics* 1986;77:357-365.
3. Ellis DJ. The impact of agency policies and protocols on breastfeeding. *NAACOGS Clin Iss Perinat Womens Health Nurs* 1992;3:553-559.
4. Syler GP, Sarvela P, Welshimer K et al. A descriptive study of breastfeeding practices and policies in Missouri hospitals. *J Hum Lact* 1997;13:103-107.
5. Kovach AC. Hospital breastfeeding policies in the Philadelphia area: a comparison with the ten steps to successful breastfeeding. *Birth* 1997;24:41-48.

6. Stokamer CL. Breastfeeding promotion efforts: why some do not work. *Int J Gynaecol Obstet* 1990;31(Suppl 1): 61-65.

7. Reiff MI, Essock-Vitale SM. Hospital influences on early infant-feeding practices. *Pediatrics* 1985;76:872-879.

8. Garforth S, Garcia J. Breast feeding policies in practice—'no wonder they get confused'. *Midwifery* 1989;5:75-83.

9. Cunningham WE, Segree W. Breast feeding promotion in an urban and a rural Jamaican hospital. *Soc Sci Med* 1990;30:341-348.

10. Levitt CA, Kaczorowski J, Hanvey L et al. Breast-feeding policies and practices in Canadian hospitals providing maternity care. *CMAJ* 1996;155:181-188.

11. Pichaipat V, Thanomsingh P, Pudhapongsiriporn S et al. An intervention model for breast feeding in Maharat Nakhon Ratchasima Hospital. *Southeast-Asian J Trop Med Public Health* 1992;23:439-443.

12. McDivitt JA, Zimicki S, Hornik R et al. The impact of the Healthcom mass media campaign on timely initiation of breastfeeding in Jordan. *Stud Fam Plann* 1993;24:295-309.

13. Bradley JE, Meme J. Breastfeeding promotion in Kenya: changes in health worker knowledge, attitudes and practices, 1982-89. *J Trop Pediatr* 1992;38:228-234.

14. Valdes V, Perez A, Labbok M et al. The impact of a hospital and clinic-based breastfeeding promotion programme in a middle class urban environment. *J Trop Pediatr* 1993;39:142-151.

15. Popkin BM, Canahuati J, Bailey PE et al. An evaluation of a national breast-feeding promotion programme in Honduras. *J Biosoc Sci* 1991;23:5-21.

16. Winikoff B, Myers D, Laukaran VH et al. Overcoming obstacles to breast-feeding in a large municipal hospital: applications of lessons learned. *Pediatrics* 1987;80:423-433.

17. Shariff F, Levitt C, Kaczorowski J et al. Workshop to implement the baby-friendly office initiative. Effect on community physicians' offices. *Can Fam Physician* 2000; 46:1090-1097.

18. Kramer MS, Chalmers B, Hodnett ED et al. Promotion of Breastfeeding Intervention Trial (PROBIT): a randomized trial in the Republic of Belarus. *JAMA* 2001;285:413-420.

19. Marker CS. *Setting standards for professional nursing.* St. Louis: Mosby; 1988.

20. World Health Organization. *Evidence for the ten steps to successful breastfeeding.* Geneva: World Health Organization; 1998.

21. World Health Organization. *International code of marketing of breast-milk substitutes.* Geneva: World Health Organization; 1981.

22. Wright A, Rice S, Wells S. Changing hospital practices to increase the duration of breastfeeding. *Pediatrics* 1996;97:669-675.

23. Biancuzzo M. Staff nurse preceptors: a program they "own." *Clin Nurse Spec* 1994;8:97-102.

24. Powers NG, Naylor AJ, Wester RA. Hospital policies: crucial to breastfeeding success. *Semin Perinatol* 1994;18:517-524.

25. Spisak S, Gross SS. *Second follow-up report: the Surgeon General's workshop on breastfeeding and human lactation.* Washington DC: National Center for Education in Maternal and Child Health; 1991.

26. Anderson E, Geden E. Nurses' knowledge of breastfeeding. *J Obstet Gynecol Neonatal Nurs* 1991;20:58-64.

27. Hayes B. Inconsistencies among nurses in breastfeeding knowledge and counseling. *J Obstet Gynecol Neonatal Nurs* 1981;10:430-433.

28. Crowder DS. Maternity nurses' knowledge of factors promoting successful breastfeeding. A survey at two hospitals. *J Obstet Gynecol Neonatal Nurs* 1981;10:28-30.

29. Lewinski CA. Nurses' knowledge of breastfeeding in a clinical setting. *J Hum Lact* 1992;8:143-148.

30. Barnett E, Sienkiewicz M, Roholt S. Beliefs about breastfeeding: a statewide survey of health professionals. *Birth* 1995;22:15-20.

31. Bagwell JE, Kendrick OW, Stitt KR et al. Knowledge and attitudes toward breast-feeding: differences among dietitians, nurses, and physicians working with WIC clients. *J Am Diet Assoc* 1993;93:801-804.

32. Sarett HP, Bain KR, O'Leary JC. Decisions on breast-feeding or formula feeding and trends in infant-feeding practices. *Am J Dis Child* 1983;137:719-725.

33. Beshgetoor D, Larson SN, LaMaster K. Attitudes toward breast-feeding among WIC employees in San Diego County. *J Am Diet Assoc* 1999;99:86-88.

34. Howard CR, Schaffer SJ, Lawrence RA. Attitudes, practices, and recommendations by obstetricians about infant feeding. *Birth* 1997;24:240-246.

35. Freed GL, Clark SJ, Sorenson J et al. National assessment of physicians' breast-feeding knowledge, attitudes, training, and experience. *JAMA* 1995;273:472-476.

36. Guise JM, Freed G. Resident physicians' knowledge of breastfeeding and infant growth. *Birth* 2000;27:49-53.

37. Schanler RJ, O'Connor KG, Lawrence RA. Pediatricians' practices and attitudes regarding breastfeeding promotion. *Pediatrics* 1999;103:E35.

38. Schwartz K. Breast-feeding education among family physicians. *J Fam Pract* 1995;40:297-298.

39. Burglehaus MJ, Smith LA, Sheps SB et al. Physicians and breastfeeding: beliefs, knowledge, self-efficacy and counseling practices. *Can J Public Health* 1997;88:383-387.

40. Naylor AJ, Creer AE, Woodward-Lopez G et al. Lactation management education for physicians. *Semin Perinatol* 1994;18:525-531.

41. WHO/UNICEF. The global criteria for the WHO/UNICEF baby friendly hospital initiative. In WHO/UNICEF. *Baby friendly hospital initiative part II: hospital level implementation.* Geneva: WHO/UNICEF; 1992.

42. Iker CE, Mogan J. Supplementation of breastfed infants: does continuing education for nurses make a difference? *J Hum Lact* 1992;8:131-135.

43. Becker GE. Breastfeeding knowledge of hospital staff in rural maternity units in Ireland. *J Hum Lact* 1992;8:137-142.

44. Westphal MF, Taddei JA, Venancio SI et al. Breast-feeding training for health professionals and resultant institutional changes. *Bull World Health Organ* 1995;73:461-468.

45. Taddei JA, Westphal MF, Venancio S et al. Breastfeeding training for health professionals and resultant changes in breastfeeding duration. *Sao Paulo Med J* 2000; 118:185-191.

46. Rea MF, Venancio SI, Martines JC et al. Counselling on breastfeeding: assessing knowledge and skills. *Bull World Health Organ* 1999;77:492-498.

47. Sloper K, McKean L, Baum JD. Factors influencing breast feeding. *Arch Dis Child* 1975;50:165-170.

48. Valdes V, Pugin E, Labbok MH et al. The effects on professional practices of a three-day course on breastfeeding. *J Hum Lact* 1995;11:185-190.

49. Biancuzzo M. Developing a poster about a clinical innovation. Part I: Ideas and abstract. *Clin Nurse Spec* 1994;8:153-155, 172.

50. Biancuzzo M. Developing a poster about a clinical innovation. Part II: Creating the poster. *Clin Nurse Spec* 1994;8:203-207.

51. Biancuzzo M. Developing a poster about a clinical innovation. Part III: Presentation and evaluation. *Clin Nurse Spec* 1994;8:262-264.

52. Kaplowitz DD, Olson CM. The effect of an education program on the decision to breastfeed. *J Nutr Educ* 1983;15:61-65.

53. Wiles LS. The effect of prenatal breastfeeding education on breastfeeding success and maternal perception of the infant. *J Obstet Gynecol Neonatal Nurs* 1984;13:253-257.

54. Kistin N, Benton D, Rao S et al. Breast-feeding rates among black urban low-income women: effect of prenatal education. *Pediatrics* 1990;86:741-746.

55. Pugin E, Valdes V, Labbok MH et al. Does prenatal breastfeeding skills group education increase the effectiveness of a comprehensive breastfeeding promotion program? *J Hum Lact* 1996;12:15-19.

56. Burkhalter BR, Marin PS. A demonstration of increased exclusive breastfeeding in Chile. *Int J Gynaecol Obstet* 1991;34:353-359.

57. Davies-Adetugbo AA. Sociocultural factors and the promotion of exclusive breastfeeding in rural Yoruba communities of Osun State, Nigeria. *Soc Sci Med* 1997;45:113-125.

58. Morrow M. Breastfeeding in Vietnam: poverty, tradition, and economic transition. *J Hum Lact* 1996;12:97-103.

59. Long DG, Funk-Archuleta MA, Geiger CJ et al. Peer counselor program increases breastfeeding rates in Utah Native American WIC population. *J Hum Lact* 1995;11:279-284.

60. Valdes V, Pugin E, Schooley J et al. Clinical support can make the difference in exclusive breastfeeding success among working women. *J Trop Pediatr* 2000;46:149-154.

61. O'Campo P, Faden RR, Gielen AC et al. Prenatal factors associated with breastfeeding duration: recommendations for prenatal interventions. *Birth* 1992;19:195-201.

62. Britton JR, Britton HL, Gronwaldt V. Early perinatal hospital discharge and parenting during infancy. *Pediatrics* 1999;104:1070-1076.

63. Winterburn S, Fraser R. Does the duration of postnatal stay influence breast-feeding rates at one month in women giving birth for the first time? A randomized control trial. *J Adv Nurs* 2000;32:1152-1157.

64. Winikoff B, Baer EC. The obstetrician's opportunity: translating "breast is best" from theory to practice. *Am J Obstet Gynecol* 1980;138:105-117.

65. Widstrom AM, Wahlberg V, Matthiesen AS et al. Short-term effects of early suckling and touch of the nipple on maternal behaviour. *Early Hum Dev* 1990;21:153-163.

66. Klaus MH, Kennell JH. *Parent-infant bonding.* 2nd ed. St. Louis: Mosby; 1982.

67. Taylor PM, Maloni JA, Brown DR. Early suckling and prolonged breast-feeding. *Am J Dis Child* 1986;140:151-154.

68. Righard L, Alade MO. Effect of delivery room routines on success of first breast-feed. *Lancet* 1990;336:1105-1107.

69. Gonzales RB. A large scale rooming-in program in a developing country: the Dr. Jose Fabella Memorial Hospital experience. *Int J Gynaecol Obstet* 1990:31(Suppl 1):31-34.

70. U.S. Committee for UNICEF and Wellstart International. *Guidelines and evaluation criteria for hospital/birthing center level implementation.* New York: UNICEF; 1996.

71. Salariya EM, Easton PM, Cater JI. Duration of breastfeeding after early initiation and frequent feeding. *Lancet* 1978;2:1141-1143.

72. Lindenberg CS, Cabrera Artola R et al. The effect of early post-partum mother-infant contact and breast-feeding promotion on the incidence and continuation of breastfeeding. *Int J Nurs Stud* 1990;27:179-186.

73. Taylor PM, Maloni JA, Taylor FH et al. Extra early mother-infant contact and duration of breast-feeding. *Acta Paediatr Scand Suppl* 1985;316:15-22.

74. Sosa R, Kennell JH, Klaus M et al. The effect of early mother-infant contact on breast feeding, infection and growth. *Ciba Foundation Symposium* 1976;45:179-193.

75. DeChateau P, Wiberg B. Long-term effect on mother-infant behaviour of extra contact during the first hour post partum. I. First observations at 36 hours. *Acta Paediatr Scand* 1977;66:137-143.

76. Ali Z, Lowry M. Early maternal-child contact: effects on later behaviour. *Dev Med Child Neurol* 1981;23:337-345.

77. Perez-Escamilla R, Pollitt E, Lonnerdal B et al. Infant feeding policies in maternity wards and their effect on breastfeeding success: an analytical overview. *Am J Public Health* 1994;84:89-97.

78. Kurinij N, Shiono PH. Early formula supplementation of breast-feeding. *Pediatrics* 1991;88:745-750.

79. DiGirolamo AM, Grummer-Strawn LM, Fein S. Maternity care practices: implications for breastfeeding. *Birth* 2001;28:94-100.

80. Chua S, Arulkumaran S, Lim I et al. Influence of breast-feeding and nipple stimulation on postpartum uterine activity. *Br J Obstet Gynaecol* 1994;101:804-805.

81. Christensson K, Siles C, Moreno L et al. Temperature, metabolic adaptation and crying in healthy full-term new-

borns cared for skin-to-skin or in a cot. *Acta Paediatr* 1992; 81:488-493.

82. Christensson K, Cabrera T, Christensson E et al. Separation distress call in the human neonate in the absence of maternal body contact. *Acta Paediatr* 1995;84:468-473.

83. Varendi H, Christensson K, Porter RH et al. Soothing effect of amniotic fluid smell in newborn infants. *Early Hum Dev* 1998;51:47-55.

84. Humenick SS. The clinical significance of breastmilk maturation rates. *Birth* 1987;14:174-181.

85. Newton M, Newton N. Postpartum engorgement of the breast. *Am J Obstet Gynecol* 1951;61:664-667.

86. Daly SE, Hartmann PE. Infant demand and milk supply. Part 1: Infant demand and milk production in lactating women. *J Hum Lact* 1995;11:21-26.

87. Daly SE, Hartmann PE. Infant demand and milk supply. Part 2: The short term control of milk synthesis in lactating women. *J Hum Lact* 1995;11:27-37.

88. Klaus MH, Kennell JH, Klaus PH. *Bonding: building the foundations of secure attachment and independence.* Boston: Addison-Wesley; 1995.

89. Kennell JH, Klaus MH. Bonding: recent observations that alter perinatal care. *Pediatr Rev* 1998;19:4-12.

90. Lawrence RA, Lawrence RM. *Breastfeeding: a guide for the medical profession.* 5th ed. St. Louis: Mosby; 1999.

91. Neville MC, Morton J, Umemura S. Lactogenesis. The transition from pregnancy to lactation. *Pediatr Clin North Am* 2001;48:35-52.

92. DeChateau P, Holmberg H, Jakobsson K et al. A study of factors promoting and inhibiting lactation. *Dev Med Child Neurol* 1977;19:575-584.

93. American Academy of Pediatrics Committee on Fetus and Newborn. Routine evaluation of blood pressure, hematocrit, and glucose in newborns. *Pediatrics* 1993;92:474-476.

94. Widstrom AM. Gastric suction in healthy newborn infants: effects on circulation and developing feeding behavior. *Acta Paediatr Scand* 1987;76:566-572.

95. Perez-Escamilla R, Maulen Radovan I, Dewey KG. The association between cesarean delivery and breast-feeding outcomes among Mexican women. *Am J Public Health* 1996;86:832-836.

96. Righard L, Alade MO. Sucking technique and its effect on success of breastfeeding. *Birth* 1992;19:185-189.

97. Jones DA, West RR. Effect of a lactation nurse on the success of breast-feeding: a randomised controlled trial. *J Epidemiol Community Health* 1986;40:45-49.

98. Perez-Escamilla R, Segura-Millan S, Pollitt E et al. Effect of the maternity ward system on the lactation success of low-income urban Mexican women. *Early Human Development* 1992;31:25-40.

99. Hofmeyr GJ, Nikodem VC, Wolman WL et al. Companionship to modify the clinical birth environment: effects on progress and perceptions of labour, and breast-feeding. *Br J Obstet Gynaecol* 1991;98:756-764.

100. Schy DS, Maglaya CF, Mendelson SG et al. The effects of in-hospital lactation education on breastfeeding practice. *J Hum Lact* 1996;12:117-122.

101. Labbok M, Krasovec K. Toward consistency in breastfeeding definitions. *Stud Fam Plann* 1990;21:226-230.

102. Gunnlaugsson G, Einarsdottir J. Colostrum and ideas about bad milk: a case study from Guinea-Bissau. *Soc Sci Med* 1993;36:283-288.

103. Zimmerman DR, Bernstein WR. Standing feeding orders in the well-baby nursery: "Water, water everywhere . . .". *J Hum Lact* 1996;12:189-192.

104. Perez-Escamilla R, Segura Millan S, Canahuati J et al. Prelacteal feeds are negatively associated with breast-feeding outcomes in Honduras. *J Nutr* 1996;126:2765-2773.

105. Host A. Importance of the first meal on the development of cow's milk allergy and intolerance. *Allergy Proc* 1991;12:227-232.

106. Goldberg NM, Adams E. Supplementary water for breast-fed babies in a hot and dry climate—not really a necessity. *Arch Dis Child* 1983;58:73-74.

107. Ashraf RN, Jalil F, Aperia A et al. Additional water is not needed for healthy breast-fed babies in a hot climate. *Acta Paediatr* 1993;82:1007-1011.

108. Sachdev HP, Krishna J, Puri RK et al. Water supplementation in exclusively breastfed infants during summer in the tropics. *Lancet* 1991;337:929-933.

109. Verronen P, Visakorpi JK, Lammi A et al. Promotion of breast feeding: effect on neonates of change of feeding routine at a maternity unit. *Acta Paediatr Scand* 1980;69:279-282.

110. DeCarvalho M, Hall M, Harvey D. Effects of water supplementation on physiological jaundice in breast-fed babies. *Arch Dis Child* 1981;56:568-569.

111. Nylander G, Lindemann R, Helsing E et al. Unsupplemented breastfeeding in the maternity ward. Positive long-term effects. *Acta Obstet Gynecol Scand* 1991;70:205-209.

112. Martin-Calama J, Bunuel J, Valero MT et al. The effect of feeding glucose water to breastfeeding newborns on weight, body temperature, blood glucose, and breastfeeding duration. *J Hum Lact* 1997;13:209-213.

113. World Health Organization (WHO). *Hypoglycaemia of the newborn.* Geneva: World Health Organization; 1997.

114. Ojofeitimi EO, Olaogun AA, Osokoya AA et al. Infant feeding practices in a deprived environment: a concern for early introduction of water and glucose D water to neonates. *Nutr Health* 1999;13:11-21.

115. Almroth S, Mohale M, Latham MC. Unnecessary water supplementation for babies: grandmothers blame clinics. *Acta Paediatr* 2000;89:1408-1413.

116. Scariati PD, Grummer-Strawn LM, Fein SB. Water supplementation of infants in the first month of life. *Arch Pediatr Adolesc Med* 1997;151:830-832.

117. American Academy of Pediatrics and The American College of Obstetricians and Gynecologists. *Guidelines for perinatal care.* 3rd ed. Elk Grove Village, IL: American Academy of Pediatrics; 1992.

118. Committee on Nutrition American Academy of Pediatrics. *Pediatric nutrition handbook.* 3rd ed. Elk Grove Village IL: American Academy of Pediatrics; 1993.

119. Shrago L. Glucose water supplementation of the breastfed infant during the first three days of life. *J Hum Lact* 1987;3:82-86.

120. American Academy of Pediatrics Work Group on Breastfeeding. Breastfeeding and the use of human milk. *Pediatrics* 1997;100:1035-1039.

121. Drewett RF, Woolridge MW, Jackson DA et al. Relationships between nursing patterns, supplementary food intake and breast-milk intake in a rural Thai population. *Early Hum Dev* 1989;20:13-23.

122. Schubiger G, Schwarz U, Tonz O. UNICEF/WHO Baby-Friendly Hospital Initiative: does the use of bottles and pacifiers in the neonatal nursery prevent successful breast-feeding? Neonatal Study Group. *Eur J Pediatr* 1997;156:874-877.

123. Gray-Donald K, Kramer MS, Munday S et al. Effect of formula supplementation in the hospital on the duration of breast-feeding: a controlled clinical trial. *Pediatrics* 1985;75:514-518.

124. Carbonell X, Botet F, Figueras J et al. The incidence of breastfeeding in our environment. *J Perinat Med* 1998;26:320-324.

125. Feinstein JM, Berkelhamer JE, Gruszka ME et al. Factors related to early termination of breast-feeding in an urban population. *Pediatrics* 1986;78:210-215.

126. Blomquist HK, Jonsbo F, Serenius F et al. Supplementary feeding in the maternity ward shortens the duration of breast feeding. *Acta Paediatr* 1994;83:1122-1126.

127. Riva E, Banderali G, Agostoni C et al. Factors associated with initiation and duration of breastfeeding in Italy. *Acta Paediatr* 1999;88:411-415.

128. Greer FR, Apple RD. Physicians, formula companies, and advertising. A historical perspective. *Am J Dis Child* 1991;145:282-286.

129. Hayden GF, Nowacek GA, Koch W et al. Providing free samples of baby items to newly delivered parents. An unintentional endorsement? *Clin Pediatr Phila* 1987;26:111-115.

130. Howard FM, Howard CR, Weitzman M. The physician as advertiser: the unintentional discouragement of breast-feeding. *Obstet Gynecol* 1993;81:1048-1051.

131. Skipper A, Bohac C, Gregoire MB. Knowing brand name affects patient preferences for enteral supplements. *J Am Diet Assoc* 1999;99:91-92.

132. Gius MP. Using panel data to determine the effect of advertising on brand-level distilled spirits sales. *J Stud Alcohol* 1996;57:73-76.

133. Howard CR, Howard FM, Weitzman ML. Infant formula distribution and advertising in pregnancy: a hospital survey. *Birth* 1994;21:14-19.

134. Howard C, Howard F, Lawrence R et al. Office prenatal formula advertising and its effect on breast-feeding patterns. *Obstet Gynecol* 2000;95:296-303.

135. Evans CJ, Lyons NB, Killien MG. The effect of infant formula samples on breastfeeding practice. *J Obstet Gynecol Neonatal Nurs* 1986;15:401-405.

136. Dungy CI, Losch ME, Russell D et al. Hospital infant formula discharge packages. Do they affect the duration of breast-feeding? *Arch Pediatr Adolesc Med* 1997;151:724-729.

137. Bliss MC, Wilkie J, Acredolo C et al. The effect of discharge pack formula and breast pumps on breastfeeding duration and choice of infant feeding method. *Birth* 1997;24:90-97.

138. Dungy CI, Christensen-Szalanski J, Losch M et al. Effect of discharge samples on duration of breast-feeding. *Pediatrics* 1992;90:233-237.

139. Frank DA, Wirtz SJ, Sorenson JR et al. Commercial discharge packs and breast-feeding counseling: effects on infant-feeding practices in a randomized trial. *Pediatrics* 1987;80:845-854.

140. Bergevin Y, Dougherty C, Kramer MS. Do infant formula samples shorten the duration of breast-feeding? *Lancet* 1983;1:1148-1151.

141. Guthrie GM, Guthrie HA, Fernandez TL et al. Infant formula samples and breast feeding among Philippine urban poor. *Soc Sci Med* 1985;20:713-717.

142. Clarke LL, Deutsch MJ. Becoming baby-friendly. One hospital's journey to total quality care. *AWHONN Lifelines* 1997;1:30-37.

143. Merewood A, Philipp BL. Becoming baby-friendly: overcoming the issue of accepting free formula. *J Hum Lact* 2000;16:279-282.

144. Merewood A, Philipp BL. Implementing change: becoming baby-friendly in an inner city hospital. *Birth* 2001;28:36-40.

145. Jackson EB, Olmsted RW, Foord A et al. A hospital rooming-in unit for four newborn infants and their mothers: descriptive account of background, development and procedures with a few preliminary observations. *Pediatrics* 1948;1:28-43.

146. Kennell JH, Klaus MH. Early mother-infant contact. Effects on the mother and the infant. *Bull Menninger Clin* 1979;43:69-78.

147. Buxton KE, Gielen AC, Faden RR et al. Women intending to breastfeed: predictors of early infant feeding experiences. *Am J Prev Med* 1991;7:101-106.

148. Procianoy RS, Fernandes Filho PH et al. The influence of rooming-in on breastfeeding. *J Trop Pediatr* 1983;29:112-114.

149. Elander G, Lindberg T. Hospital routines in infants with hyperbilirubinemia influence the duration of breast feeding. *Acta Paediatr Scand* 1986;75:708-712.

150. Syafruddin M, Djauhariah AM, Dasril D. A study comparing rooming-in with separate nursing. *Paediatr Indones* 1988;28:116-123.

151. Yamauchi Y, Yamanouchi I. The relationship between rooming-in/not rooming-in and breast-feeding variables. *Acta Paediatr Scand* 1990;79:1017-1022.

152. Waldenstrom U, Swenson A. Rooming-in at night in the postpartum ward. *Midwifery* 1991;7:82-89.

153. Keefe MR. Comparison of neonatal nighttime sleep-wake patterns in nursery versus rooming-in environments. *Nurs Res* 1987;36:140-144.

154. Keefe MR. The impact of infant rooming-in on maternal sleep at night. *J Obstet Gynecol Neonatal Nurs* 1988;17:122-126.

155. Buranasin B. The effects of rooming-in on the success of breastfeeding and the decline in abandonment of children. *Asia Pac J Public Health* 1991;5:217-220.

156. Lvoff NM, Lvoff V, Klaus MH. Effect of the Baby-Friendly Initiative on infant abandonment in a Russian hospital. *Arch Pediatr Adolesc Med* 2000;154:474-477.

157. Norr KF, Roberts JE, Freese U. Early postpartum rooming-in and maternal attachment behaviors in a group of medically indigent primiparas. *J Nurse Midwifery* 1989;34:85-91.

158. Prodromidis M, Field T, Arendt R et al. Mothers touching newborns: a comparison of rooming-in versus minimal contact. *Birth* 1995;22:196 200.

159. Dharamraj C, Sia CG, Kierney CM et al. Observations on maternal preference for rooming-in facilities. *Pediatrics* 1981;67:638-640.

160. Cadwell K. Using the quality improvement process to affect breastfeeding protocols in United States hospitals. *J Hum Lact* 1997;13:5-9.

161. Hull V, Thapa S, Pratomo H. Breast-feeding in the modern health sector in Indonesia: the mother's perspective. *Soc Sci Med* 1990;30.625-633.

162. Suradi R. Rooming-in for babies born by caesarean section in Dr. Cipto Mangunkusumo General Hospital Jakarta. *Paediatr Indones* 1988;28:124-132.

163. Anderson GC. Risk in mother-infant separation postbirth. *Image J Nurs Sch* 1989;21:196-199.

164. Howie PW, Houston MJ, Cook A et al. How long should a breast feed last? *Early Hum Dev* 1981;5:71-77.

165. Diaz S, Herreros C, Aravena R et al. Breast-feeding duration and growth of fully breast-fed infants in a poor urban Chilean population. *Am J Clin Nutr* 1995;62:371-376.

166. DeCarvalho M, Robertson S, Merkatz R et al. Milk intake and frequency of feeding in breast fed infants. *Early Hum Dev* 1982;7:155-163.

167. Illingworth RS, Leeds MD, Stone DGH. Self-demand feeding in a maternity unit. *Lancet* 1952;1:683-687.

168. Yamauchi Y, Yamanouchi I. Breast-feeding frequency during the first 24 hours after birth in full-term neonates. *Pediatrics* 1990;86:171-175.

169. DeCarvalho M, Robertson S, Friedman A et al. Effect of frequent breast-feeding on early milk production and infant weight gain. *Pediatrics* 1983;72:307-311.

170. Daly SE, Kent JC, Owens RA et al. Frequency and degree of milk removal and the short-term control of human milk synthesis. *Exp Physiol* 1996;81:861-875.

171. DeCarvalho M, Klaus MH, Merkatz RB. Frequency of breast-feeding and serum bilirubin concentration. *Am J Dis Child* 1982;136:737-738.

172. DeCarvalho M, Robertson S, Klaus MH. Does the duration and frequency of early breastfeeding affect nipple pain? *Birth* 1984;11:81-84.

173. Slaven S, Harvey D. Unlimited suckling time improves breast feeding. *Lancet* 1981;1:392-393.

174. Renfrew MJ, Lang S, Martin L et al. Feeding schedules in hospitals for newborn infants. *Cochrane Database Syst Rev* 2000:CD000090.

175. Martines JC, Ashworth A, Kirkwood B. Breast-feeding among the urban poor in southern Brazil: reasons for termination in the first 6 months of life. *Bull World Health Organ* 1989;67:151-161.

176. Musoke RN. Breastfeeding promotion: feeding the low birth weight infant. *Int J Gynaecol Obstet* 1990:31 Suppl 1:57-59.

177. Mohrbacher N, Stock J. *The breastfeeding answer book.* 2nd ed. Schaumburg IL: La Leche League International; 1996.

178. Ardran GM, Kemp FH, Lind J. A cineradiographic study of bottle feeding. *Br J Radiol* 1956;31:11-22.

179. Ardran GM, Kemp FH, Lind J. A cineradiographic study of breast feeding. *Br J Radiol* 1958;31:156-162.

180. Weber F, Woolridge MW, Baum JD. An ultrasonographic study of the organisation of sucking and swallowing by newborn infants. *Dev Med Child Neurol* 1986;28:19-24.

181. Nowak AJ, Smith WL, Erenberg A. Imaging evaluation of artificial nipples during bottle feeding. *Arch Pediatr Adolesc Med* 1994;148:40-42.

182. Gorelick L. On the use of pacifiers in preventing malocclusion. *N Y State Dent Journal* 1955;21:3-10.

183. Pedley TF. The rubber teat and deformities of the jaws. *Dent Rec* 1907;27:176-177.

184. Pritchard E. "Comforter" otitis media. *Lancet* 1911;2:851.

185. King FT. *Feeding and care of baby.* London: McMillan; 1923.

186. Turgeon-O'Brien H, Lachapelle D, Gagnon PF et al. Nutritive and nonnutritive sucking habits: a review. *ASDC J Dent Child* 1996;63:321-327.

187. Cullen A, Kiberd B, McDonnell M et al. Sudden infant death syndrome—are parents getting the message? *Ir J Med Sci* 2000;169:40-43.

188. Larsson E. Sucking, chewing, and feeding habits and the development of crossbite: a longitudinal study of girls from birth to 3 years of age. *Angle Orthod* 2001;71:116-119.

189. Howard CR, Howard FM, Lanphear B et al. The effects of early pacifier use on breastfeeding duration. *Pediatrics* 1999;103:E33.

190. Kelmanson IA. Use of a pacifier and behavioural features in 2-4-month-old infants. *Acta Paediatr* 1999;88:1258-1261.

191. Righard L, Alade MO. Breastfeeding and the use of pacifiers. *Birth* 1997;24:116-120.

192. Lundqvist C, Hafstrom M. Non-nutritive sucking in full-term and preterm infants studied at term conceptional age. *Acta Paediatr* 1999;88:1287-1289.

193. Vogel A, Mitchell EA. Attitudes to the use of dummies in New Zealand; a qualitative study. *N Z Med J* 1997;110:395-397.

194. Campos RG. Soothing pain-elicited distress in infants with swaddling and pacifiers. *Child Dev* 1989;60:781-792.

195. Corbo MG, Mansi G, Stagni A et al. Nonnutritive sucking during heelstick procedures decreases behavioral distress in the newborn infant. *Biol Neonate* 2000;77:162-167.

196. Field T, Goldson E. Pacifying effects of nonnutritive sucking on term and preterm neonates during heelstick procedures. *Pediatrics* 1984;74:1012-1015.

197. Gunnar MR, Fisch RO, Malone S. The effects of a pacifying stimulus on behavioral and adrenocortical responses to circumcision in the newborn. *J Am Acad Child Psychiatry* 1984;23:34-38.

198. Carbajal R, Chauvet X, Couderc S et al. Randomised trial of analgesic effects of sucrose, glucose, and pacifiers in term neonates. *BMJ* 1999;319:1393-1397.

199. Kramer MS, Barr RG, Dagenais S et al. Pacifier use, early weaning, and cry/fuss behavior: a randomized controlled trial. *JAMA* 2001;286:322-326.

200. North Stone K, Fleming P, Golding J. Socio-demographic associations with digit and pacifier sucking at 15 months of age and possible associations with infant infection. The ALSPAC Study Team. Avon Longitudinal Study of Pregnancy and Childhood. *Early Hum Dev* 2000;60:137-148.

201. Paunio P, Rautava P, Sillanpaa M. The Finnish Family Competence Study: the effects of living conditions on sucking habits in 3-year-old Finnish children and the association between these habits and dental occlusion. *Acta Odontol Scand* 1993;51:23-29.

202. Gizani S, Vinckier F, Declerck D. Caries pattern and oral health habits in 2- to 6-year-old children exhibiting differing levels of caries. *Clin Oral Investig* 1999;3:35-40.

203. Righard L. Are breastfeeding problems related to incorrect breastfeeding technique and the use of pacifiers and bottles? *Birth* 1998;25:40-44.

204. Righard L. Early enhancement of successful breastfeeding. *World Health Forum* 1996;17:92-97.

205. Barros FC, Victora CG, Semer TC et al. Use of pacifiers is associated with decreased breast-feeding duration. *Pediatrics* 1995;95:497-499.

206. Victora CG, Behague DP, Barros FC et al. Pacifier use and short breastfeeding duration: cause, consequence, or coincidence? *Pediatrics* 1997;99:445-453.

207. Centuori S, Burmaz T, Ronfani L et al. Nipple care, sore nipples, and breastfeeding: a randomized trial. *J Hum Lact* 1999;15:125-130.

208. Hornell A, Aarts C, Kylberg E et al. Breastfeeding patterns in exclusively breastfed infants: a longitudinal prospective study in Uppsala, Sweden. *Acta Paediatr* 1999;88:203-211.

209. Huffman SL. Maternal and child nutritional status: its association with the risk of pregnancy. *Soc Sci Med* 1983;17:1529-1540.

210. Aarts C, Hornell A, Kylberg E et al. Breastfeeding patterns in relation to thumb sucking and pacifier use. *Pediatrics* 1999;104:e50.

211. Clements MS, Mitchell EA, Wright SP et al. Influences on breastfeeding in southeast England. *Acta Paediatr* 1997;86:51-56.

212. Ford RP, Mitchell EA, Scragg R et al. Factors adversely associated with breast feeding in New Zealand. *J Paediatr Child Health* 1994;30:483-489.

213. Vogel AM, Hutchison BL, Mitchell EA. The impact of pacifier use on breastfeeding: a prospective cohort study. *J Paediatr Child Health* 2001;37:58-63.

214. Barros FC, Victora CG, Morris SS et al. Breast feeding, pacifier use and infant development at 12 months of age: a birth cohort study in Brazil. *Paediatr Perinat Epidemiol* 1997;11:441-450.

215. Karjalainen S, Ronning O, Lapinleimu H et al. Association between early weaning, non-nutritive sucking habits and occlusal anomalies in 3-year-old Finnish children. *Int J Paediatr Dent* 1999;9:169-173.

216. Watase S, Mourino AP, Tipton GA. An analysis of malocclusion in children with otitis media. *Pediatr Dent* 1998;20:327-330.

217. Niemela M, Pihakari O, Pokka T et al. Pacifier as a risk factor for acute otitis media: a randomized, controlled trial of parental counseling. *Pediatrics* 2000;106:483-488.

218. Jackson JM, Mourino AP. Pacifier use and otitis media in infants twelve months of age or younger. *Pediatr Dent* 1999;21:255-260.

219. Uhari M, Mantysaari K, Niemela M. A meta-analytic review of the risk factors for acute otitis media. *Clin Infect Dis* 1996;22:1079-1083.

220. Darwazeh AM, al Bashir A. Oral candidal flora in healthy infants. *J Oral Pathol Med* 1995;24:361-364.

221. Mattos-Graner RO, de Moraes AB, Rontani RM et al. Relation of oral yeast infection in Brazilian infants and use of a pacifier. *ASDC J Dent Child* 2001;68:33-36.

222. Ogaard B, Larsson E, Lindsten R. The effect of sucking habits, cohort, sex, intercanine arch widths, and breast or bottle feeding on posterior crossbite in Norwegian and Swedish 3-year-old children. *Am J Orthod Dentofacial Orthop* 1994;106:161-166.

223. Juberg DR, Alfano K, Coughlin RJ et al. An observational study of object mouthing behavior by young children. *Pediatrics* 2001;107:135-142.

224. Gale CR, Martyn CN. Breastfeeding, dummy use, and adult intelligence. *Lancet* 1996;347:1072-1075.

225. Pollard K, Fleming P, Young J et al. Night-time non-nutritive sucking in infants aged 1 to 5 months: relationship with infant state, breastfeeding, and bed-sharing versus room-sharing. *Early Hum Dev* 1999;56:185-204.

226. Franco P, Scaillet S, Wermenbol V et al. The influence of a pacifier on infants' arousals from sleep. *J Pediatr* 2000;136:775-779.

227. Lehtonen J, Kononen M, Purhonen M et al. The effect of nursing on the brain activity of the newborn. *J Pediatr* 1998;132:646-651.

228. Fleming PJ, Blair PS, Pollard K et al. Pacifier use and sudden infant death syndrome: results from the CESDI/SUDI case control study. CESDI SUDI Research Team. *Arch Dis Child* 1999;81:112-116.

229. Lehman EB, Denham SA, Moser MH et al. Soft object and pacifier attachments in young children: the role of security of attachment to the mother. *J Child Psychol Psychiatry* 1992;33:1205-1215.

230. Bull P. Consent to supplement newborn infants. *J Hum Lact* 1986;2:27-28.

231. Vadiakas G, Oulis C, Berdouses E. Profile of non-nutritive sucking habits in relation to nursing behavior in preschool children. *J Clin Pediatr Dent* 1998;22:133-136.

232. Perez A. The effect of breastfeeding promotion on the infertile postpartum period. *Int J Gynaecol Obstet* 1990;31(Suppl 1):29-30.

233. Benitez I, de la Cruz J, Suplido A et al. Extending lactational amenorrhoea in Manila: a successful breast-feeding education programme. *J Biosoc Sci* 1992;24:211-231.

234. Houston MJ, Howie PW, Cook A et al. Do breast feeding mothers get the home support they need? *Health Bull Edinb* 1981;39:166-172.

235. Saner G, Dagoglu T, Uzkan I et al. Promotion of breast feeding in the postpartum mother. *Turk J Pediatr* 1985;27:63-68.

236. Neyzi O, Gulecyuz M, Dincer Z et al. An educational intervention on promotion of breast feeding complemented by continuing support. *Paediatr Perinat Epidemiol* 1991;5:299-303.

237. Neyzi O, Olgun P, Kutluay T et al. An educational intervention on promotion of breast feeding. *Paediatr Perinat Epidemiol* 1991;5:286-298.

238. Haider R, Islam A, Hamadani J et al. Breast-feeding counselling in a diarrhoeal disease hospital. *Bull World Health Organ* 1996;74:173-179.

239. Hall JM. Influencing breastfeeding success. *J Obstet Gynecol Neonatal Nurs* 1978;7:28-32.

240. Saunders SE, Carroll J. Post-partum breast feeding support: impact on duration. *J Am Diet Assoc* 1988;88:213-215.

241. Grossman LK, Harter C, Sachs L et al. The effect of post-partum lactation counseling on the duration of breast-feeding in low-income women. *Am J Dis Child* 1990;144:471-474.

242. Davies Adetugbo AA. Promotion of breast feeding in the community: impact of health education programme in rural communities in Nigeria. *J Diarrhoeal Dis Res* 1996;14:5-11.

243. Dennis CL, Hodnett E, Gallop R et al. The effect of peer support on breast-feeding duration among primiparous women: a randomized controlled trial. *CMAJ* 2002;166:21-28.

244. Meara H. A key to successful breast-feeding in a non-supportive culture. *J Nurse Midwifery* 1976;21:20-26.

245. Ryan K, Beresford RA. The power of support groups: influence on infant feeding trends in New Zealand. *J Hum Lact* 1997;13:183-190.

246. Kendall Tackett KA, Sugarman M. The social consequences of long-term breastfeeding. *J Hum Lact* 1995;11:179-183.

247. Lawrence RA. Breastfeeding in Belarus. *JAMA* 2001;285:463-464.

248. Howard CR, Howard FM, Lanphear B et al. The effects of early pacifier use on breastfeeding duration. *Pediatrics* 1999;103:E33.

Managing Newborns with Common Breastfeeding Challenges

BASIC NEEDS FOR WELL INFANTS

Feeding is one of multiple tasks that must be established and integrated for the infant's successful adaptation to extrauterine life. The newborn must accomplish biologic tasks—establishing and maintaining respiration, circulatory changes, and thermoregulation—in addition to ingesting, retaining, and digesting nutrients. Furthermore, the newborn must accomplish behavioral tasks—establishing a regulated behavioral tempo, processing, storing and organizing multiple stimuli, and establishing a relationship with caregivers and the environment.[1]

Biologic Tasks

Throughout life, organisms must maintain homeostasis. The fetus, however, uses different mechanisms than the newborn to maintain homeostasis. The transition to extrauterine life has some points that are pertinent to feeding in general and breastfeeding in particular.

Gastrointestinal and Metabolic Needs and Function

Before birth, the fetus obtained all of its nutrients through the placenta. After birth, however, the nutrients from human milk must first pass through the digestive tract before they can be used for metabolism. The normal functioning of the digestive tract and the newborn's metabolic needs and function are briefly reviewed here to provide a basis for clinical management.

Metabolism and Hormonal Regulation. Metabolism is the use of the nutrients from food after it has been digested, absorbed, and circulated to the cells.[2] Metabolism—the use of nutrients—

can be either catabolic (decomposition, or breakdown) or anabolic (synthesis, or building of molecules). The basal metabolic rate is the rate of nutrient use under basal conditions, that is, being awake but resting and being in a postabsorptive state (not digesting food) and a thermoneutral environment.

During metabolism, energy is expended. *Energy* is "the capacity to do work or to produce a change in matter. Applied to nutrition, energy deals mostly with the chemical energy obtained from foods."[3] One kilocalorie of energy is the amount of energy required to raise the temperature of 1 kg of water from 14.5° to 15.5° C (i.e., 1° C). The term *kilocalorie* is usually used to describe energy needs with respect to nutrition. The commonly used *calorie* (e.g., 1 oz of artificial milk has 20 calories) refers to the scientifically correct term, *kilocalorie* (abbreviated kcal).

Energy is required for the basic needs of metabolism, including respiration, circulation, maintenance of electrochemical gradient across cell membranes, and maintenance of body temperature.[3] Infants use nutrients to maintain this basic metabolic rate, but they also use nutrients for growth and activity. During the first 4 months after birth, about 50% to 60% of kilocalories are used to maintain the infant's basic metabolic rate, 25% to 40% are for growth, and 10% to 15% are for activity.

Metabolism—the use of digested nutrients—has two central concepts that are critical to breastfeeding management: (1) how metabolism is regulated and (2) how metabolism is related to the newborn's energy requirements and the macronutrients that human milk provides.

Regulation of Metabolism. Metabolism must be regulated in some way. The neurologic and endocrine systems are regulatory in nature, but both are immature at birth. Reflexes, part of the neurologic system, are primitive, but they are sufficiently developed to sustain extrauterine life. The endocrine system has hormones that regulate the two processes of metabolism: catabolic and anabolic.

Hormones, although present and functioning, may sometimes be produced in limited quantities or may be unable to fully meet the dynamic changes associated with the transition to extrauterine life. Hormones related to food and fluid regulation predispose the newborn to some risks. For example, antidiuretic hormone (ADH), which inhibits diuresis, is produced in limited quantities, resulting in many voidings per day and hence a higher susceptibility to dehydration. Glucagon and insulin are the hormones most closely associated with glucose regulation.

Energy Requirements. Well infants require 90 to 120 kcal/kg/24 hr.[3] About 40 to 60 of those kilocalories are needed to maintain basic metabolic functions. It is important to remember, however, that basal metabolic requirements are measured at room temperature when the subject has an empty stomach and is physically and emotionally quiet. Therefore, when food is ingested and assimilated, metabolic needs increase. The well infant also has activity and growth needs, so sufficient kilocalories should be ingested to support these needs.

Macronutrients in Human Milk. Macronutrients vary in human milk, as described in Chapter 4. The macronutrients—carbohydrates, proteins, and fats—can be either broken down or synthesized through metabolic processes, as shown in Table 9-1. Proteins are synthesized from other substances, whereas carbohydrates and fats are broken down.

Carbohydrates. Carbohydrates (sugars) supply energy; they spare the metabolism of protein and fat. Glucose, a monosaccharide (simple sugar), is the form of carbohydrate used by cells for energy. This simple sugar is derived from the digestion and metabolism of disaccharides and more complex carbohydrates such as starch and glycogen. Each gram of carbohydrate has 4 kcal. About 38% of the calories in human milk are supplied by the disaccharide *lactose*.

Carbohydrate metabolism is both catabolic and anabolic. Through catabolism, more complex carbohydrates are broken down into simple sugars; through anabolism, simple sugars are synthesized into glycogen. The catabolic process breaks down human milk lactose into glucose and galactose so that it can be used in cells. The anabolic process synthesizes glycogen, stored in the liver, beginning at around 9 weeks of gestation. Glycogen stores are used for such events as hypoxia during labor, the work of breathing, or cold stress. Newborns use stores from gestation because they have a limited ability to produce glucose from glycogen; hence, their blood sugar levels can drop rapidly.

Blood glucose levels are regulated by hormonal and neural influences. The sugar-regulating hormones include insulin (secreted by β-cells of the pancreas), glucagon (secreted by α-cells of the pancreas), epinephrine, adrenocorticotropic hormone (ACTH), growth hormone, thyroid-stimulating hormone, and thyroid hormone. Ideally, the newborn should have blood sugar levels above 60 mg/dl, but a blood sugar level above 40 mg/dl is acceptable.

Proteins. In contrast to carbohydrates and fats, whose primary function is to provide energy, proteins are primarily concerned with building tissue (anabolism). Each gram of protein has 4 kcal. Although the amount varies with the stage of lactation, about 7% of the calories in human milk are supplied by protein (whereas 9% to 11% are supplied by protein in artificial milk).[3] Metabolizing protein increases the basal metabolic requirement for kilocalories by as much as 30%, whereas the metabolism of carbohydrate and fat increases it by only 4% and 6%, respectively.[4] Simply stated, it takes more energy to metabolize protein than to metabolize carbohydrate or fat. Human milk is significantly lower in protein than cow's milk, home-prepared evaporated milk formulas, or commercially prepared artificial milks; therefore it minimizes the increase in the infant's basal metabolic requirement.

Table **9-1** DEFINITIONS

Term	Definition	Key Point
Glucagon	A hormone, produced by α-cells in the islets of Langerhans, that stimulates the conversion of glycogen to glucose in the liver	Hormone
Glucose	Monosaccharide; major source of energy occurring in human and animal body fluids	Simple sugar
Glycogen	A polysaccharide that is the major carbohydrate stored in animal cells; it is formed from glucose and stored chiefly in the liver and, to a lesser extent, in muscle cells	Complex sugar
Glycogenolysis	The breakdown of glycogen to glucose	Breakdown of complex sugar to simple sugar
Glycogenesis	The synthesis of glycogen from glucose	Formation of complex sugar from simple sugar
Glycolysis	A series of catalyzed reactions, occurring within cells, by which glucose and other sugars are broken down to yield lactic acid or pyruvic acid, releasing energy in the form of adenosine triphosphate; may be aerobic (accomplished with oxygen) or anaerobic (accomplished without oxygen)	Breakdown of simple and complex sugars
Glyconeogenesis	The formation of glycogen from fatty acids and proteins rather than carbohydrates	Formation of complex sugar from noncarbohydrates
Ketogenic response	The mobilization of fat stores to produce glycerol, free fatty acids, and ketone bodies which are then used as energy sources instead of glucose and glycogen	A glucose sparing response

Source: *Mosby's medical, nursing, and allied health dictionary.* 6th ed. St. Louis: Mosby, 2002.

Fats. Like carbohydrates, fats are used for energy. Fats and fatty acids are essential for infants; cholesterol is especially important because it contributes to brain development, and myelinization of the nervous system is not complete until age 2. Essential fatty acids, which cannot be synthesized, must be consumed; these are present in human milk, as described in Chapter 4. Human milk has about 9 kcal per gram of fat. In the breastfed infant, about 55% of the calories consumed are from fat, whereas only about 48% of the calories in artificial milk are from fat.

Lipid metabolism can be either catabolic or anabolic (lipogenesis). Most lipids, including triglycerides, cholesterol, phospholipids, and prostaglandins, can be synthesized through lipogenesis. Some, however, are essential fatty acids, which are used for growth and tissue maintenance (rather than energy only). Fat in human milk is easier for infants to digest than the fat in cow's milk because of the position of the fatty acids on the glycerol molecule and because of natural lipase activity.

Gastrointestinal Function. The gastrointestinal tract makes essential nutrients available to all cells throughout the body. This is accomplished by ingestion (taking in), digestion (breaking down), motility (movement—peristalsis and segmentation of undigested nutrients), secretion of digestive juices, absorption (movement of digested nutrients), and elimination.

Ingestion. Ingestion—the transfer of milk—is discussed in Chapter 7. Through ingestion of human milk, the infant takes in six main nutrients: carbohydrates, proteins, fat, vitamins, minerals, and water. Human milk provides energy: a total of about 67 kcal/100 ml (20 kcal/oz).[5] Very little energy (calories) comes from protein; the greatest amount is provided by fat, as shown in Fig. 9-1.

Digestion. Digestion, or the breakdown of food, is accomplished by either mechanical or chemical means. It occurs in the mouth, stomach, and intestines. Mechanical digestion involves mastication (chewing—for solid foods only), deglutition (swallowing), peristalsis (the undulating movement), and segmentation (mixing move-

ment). The newborn digests human milk primarily through swallowing and an undulating movement that begins in the tongue and continues throughout the gastrointestinal tract. Chemical digestion promotes the breakdown of carbohydrate, fat, and protein to absorbable units through hydrolysis. Chemical digestion relies on digestive enzymes.

Secretion. The presence of secreted enzymes promotes the chemical digestion of food. Digestive enzymes are secreted into the lumen of the gastrointestinal tract. Important enzymes for human digestion include salivary amylase, lingual lipase, gastric lipase, peptidases, and pancreatic amylase. However, pancreatic amylase, lipase, and saliva are scarce at birth. In human milk the presence of mammary amylase (highest in colostrum) compensates for the decreased pancreatic amylase. Bile salts in human milk are critical for the emulsification and absorption of fats.

Motility. The undulating movements of the gastrointestinal tract start with the tongue and continue throughout. Colostrum is important because it acts as a laxative on the gut, thereby facilitating the excretion of unneeded substances, most notably bilirubin, as described later in this chapter.

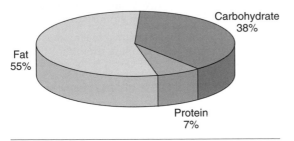

FIGURE **9-1** Energy content of human milk. High fat is needed for brain development. Lactose, the carbohydrate in human milk, is easily broken down into simple sugars for energy. Low protein requires little energy to metabolize.

𝒪CLINICAL SCENARIO

Kilocalorie Requirements

A mother says that her newborn weighs 7½ pounds and feeds 10 times in a 24-hour period. She would like to know how many ounces he would need to consume at each feeding to get the minimum amount of calories for his current weight.
1. What is the answer to her question?
2. She doubts that she has that much milk. How could you help her visualize what a small amount this is?

Answer

As specified earlier, the well newborn needs 90 to 120 kcal (or, as the mother would say, "calories") per kilogram per 24 hours. First, there are about 2.2 lb/kg, so the newborn weighs 3.41 kg. Human milk varies, but for the sake of simplicity,

figure that there are 20 kcal per ounce of milk (and there are exactly 20 kcal per ounce of standard artificial milk). Using the formula of 90 to 120 kcal per kilogram of body weight per 24 hours, this newborn would require about 307 to 409 calories per 24 hours. This would be supplied in 15.4 to 20.5 ounces of milk per day. If the newborn feeds 10 times per day, he would need to consume 1.5 to 2.1 ounces each time.

Mothers often fear that they do not have enough milk. It would be helpful to fill a medicine cup with 23 ml and tell the newborn's mother that is all she would need to have in each breast for each feeding. Another way to visualize this is by using the teaspoon. One and a half ounces is approximately equivalent to 9 teaspoons, or 4½ teaspoons per breast.

Absorption. As the digested nutrients move through the gastrointestinal tract, they cross the intestinal wall into the internal environment through the process of absorption. The newborn is unable to absorb some ingested nutrients. For example, infants can take in great quantities of iron in iron-fortified artificial milk, but they absorb them rather inefficiently. Substances that are indigestible and not needed are not absorbed into the internal environment but instead are eliminated.

Elimination. Newborns have three distinct types of stools, as described in Table 9-2. The first stool is called *meconium*. The next stool is a transitional stool, and the last is a milk stool. Infants who are exclusively breastfed will have softer stools because of the whey/casein ratio in human milk. The stools of artificially fed infants are more rubbery because of the more rubbery curd produced by the comparatively greater amounts of casein in artificial milk.

Cardiopulmonary Function

For the fetus the placenta provides both nutrients and oxygen. In contrast, the newborn has two separate systems: one for nutrients and one for oxygen. After birth the transition from fetal to postnatal circulation involves the immediate functional closure of the foramen ovale, followed by the ductus arteriosus around the fourth day after birth, and later the ductus venosus. If the ducts fail to close, various types of congenital cardiac defects result. Cardiac defects increase the metabolic rate and therefore the amount of energy needed to maintain basal metabolic rate, activity, and growth.

The newborn obtains oxygen through the lungs—breathing. Usually, infants with a respiratory

Table 9-2 STOOL PATTERNS OF NEWBORNS

Stool Pattern	Appears	Composed of	Clinical Description	Teaching Implications
Meconium	Within first 24 hours	• Amniotic fluid and related constituents • Sluffed-off mucosal cells • Possibly blood; from maternal vaginal vault or from minor bleeding of alimentary tract	Black or dark green, very sticky	Stools should *not* continue to be dark brown/black for more than 3-5 days
Transitional stools	By 2-3 days after initiation of feeding	• Meconium • Milk curds	Greenish brown to yellowish brown, pasty, less sticky than meconium	Should not continue more than 4-7 days
Milk stools	By 4-7 days after initiation of feeding	Milk curds; higher in whey than in curd content; hence, human-milk stools are less rubbery than those excreted by artificially fed infants	Stools from breastfed infants are yellow (look like cottage cheese and mustard mixed together) with a nonoffensive odor Stools from artificially fed infants are pale yellow to light brown, with more rubbery consistency, and a more offensive odor	During the newborn period, it is common for stooling to occur with nearly every feeding; thin milk stools do not mean the baby has diarrhea; later in infancy, thin stools may indicate there has been more consumption of hindmilk than foremilk

rate exceeding 60 breaths per minute have difficulty coordinating breathing and suckling and are considered tachypneic; most hospital protocols do not allow these infants to take oral feedings. Newborns older than 32 to 34 weeks of gestation can and do coordinate sucking, swallowing, and breathing and therefore ingest nutrients and fluid and then digest and eliminate food.

Thermoregulation

To prepare for the transition to extrauterine life, "brown fat" is deposited in the fetus around the twenty-eighth week of gestation. This specialized fat is highly vascular and is specifically designed for heat production. Deposits of this brown fat are located in the axilla, the area of the scapula, and the neck muscles, as well as around the kidneys and adrenals. Before birth, the fetus's temperature is dependent on the mother's temperature. Usually, the fetus's temperature is approximately 0.5° C (0.9° F) higher than that of the mother—around 37.6° to 37.8° C (99.7° to 100.0° F).[6] Immediately upon birth, the newborn is thrust into a significantly colder environment. Typically, delivery rooms are cool, and the newborn arrives covered with amniotic fluid, which makes him colder because of evaporative heat loss. The newborn's thermoregulatory system is not as well developed as that of adults. Therefore hypothermia, as discussed later in this chapter, often develops.

Fluid Balance

For newborns, small fluctuations have a great effect on fluid balance. To avoid or minimize problems, clinicians involved in breastfeeding management need to understand water requirements and observe water losses.

Normal infants require about 80 to 100 ml of water per kilogram of body weight per 24 hours.[4] Human milk consists of about 87% water. Several studies, beginning more than two decades ago and confirmed recently,[7] have shown that exclusively breastfed healthy infants less than 4 months old do not require extra water even if they are in a hot, dry climate (as explained in Chapter 8).

Water loss is the total of insensible water loss and renal water loss. It is more difficult to deter-

mine insensible losses (e.g., losses that occur through the normal functions of breathing), but it is fairly simple to observe urine output. If the newborn is less than 48 hours old, total urinary output should be 250 to 400 ml/day; after 48 hours of age, output of less than 15 to 60 ml/kg/day is considered oliguria.[6]

Newborns have some special characteristics related to fluid balance. Under normal circumstances, infants are born with extra fluids "on board," and some fluid loss (and therefore weight loss) occurs during the first few days after birth. Sometimes, however, these extra fluids are diminished or depleted because the mother has been dehydrated during the childbearing experience—a long labor, multiple episodes of vomiting, or large blood losses all contribute to maternal dehydration. Therefore, before judgments are made about the infant's fluid needs or losses, the intrapartum history should be considered.

Behavioral Tasks
Sleep-Wake Continuum

Infants are not simply asleep or awake. Rather, the sleep-wake continuum, shown in Fig. 9-2, ranges from deep sleep or lethargy to extreme irritability or crying.[8] How or whether an infant controls or modifies his response varies according to which particular sleep or awake state he is experiencing. The facial "brightness" is usually the most distinguishing factor that alerts the caregiver to the newborn's state, as shown in Fig. 9-2.[9] Clues as to which state the newborn is in include body activity, eye movements, facial movements, breathing pattern, and level of response as summarized in Table 9-3.

Sensory Needs, Stimuli, and Relationship with Caregivers

The five senses are developed to varying degrees in the newborn. At birth, visual acuity is limited. The newborn can best see objects that are about 8 to 12 inches away—about the distance of the mother's face from the infant while at the breast. Hearing acuity for a newborn is similar to that for an adult. Newborns are readily consoled by familiar sounds, such as the mother's heartbeat, that are audible during breastfeeding. Smell is well developed and more

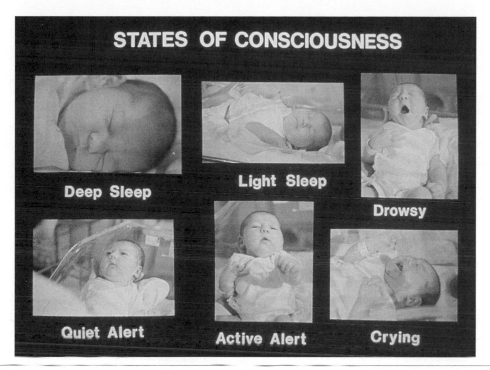

FIGURE **9-2** Summary of sleep-wake states of newborn. States of consciousness: deep sleep, light sleep, drowsy, quiet-alert, active-alert, crying. *(From* Early parent-infant relationships *[video]. White Plains, NY: March of Dimes Birth Defects Foundation; 1991.)*

functional than in adults; newborns can smell their mother's milk, and, if left to their own instincts, will find the breast to get the milk.[10] The sense of taste is fully functioning at birth, with newborns able to distinguish between sweet, sour, bitter, and tasteless solutions. The sweetness of the mother's milk usually elicits an eager suck because of the pleasant taste the newborn experiences. Touch is especially important for the newborn. He perceives tactile sensation in any part of the body, but the perioral area is the most sensitive.

ASSESSING RISKS FOR WELL INFANTS

Most newborns accomplish the biologic or behavioral tasks easily and quickly. Some, however, have slight deviations or delays that affect breastfeeding.

Lethargy or Sleepiness

Often, the newborn who is lethargic or sleepy does not feed well. Lethargy occurs with certain situ-

ations, for example, with hyperbilirubinemia. In many cases, however, the lethargy is part of the normal physiologic state that the infant experiences. Breastfeeding can be best accomplished when the infant is in the optimal state of alertness.

Effect on Breastfeeding

Breastfeeding should commence when the term infant is in the quiet-alert state. Infants who are in deep sleep or light sleep will not breastfeed. Infants who are drowsy may begin to breastfeed but may return to sleep states. These infants may benefit from alerting techniques, as shown in Box 9-1. The infant who is in the active-alert state is distracted by his own hunger; these infants may need to be consoled before they can successfully breastfeed, as shown in Box 9-2. It is extremely difficult to coax the crying newborn to breastfeed. He is often so frustrated that he is disinterested in any further stimuli. Furthermore, lengthy periods of crying will cause him to take in air, and hence he may have

Table 9-3 INFANT STATE CHART (SLEEP AND AWAKE STATES)

STATE is a group of characteristics that regularly occur together: body activity, eye movements, facial movements, breathing pattern, and level of response to external stimuli (e.g., handling) and internal stimuli (e.g., hunger)

	Characteristics of State					
	Body Activity	Eye Movements	Facial Movements	Breathing Pattern	Level of Response	Implications for Caregiving
Sleep States						
Deep sleep	Nearly still, except for occasional startle or twitch	None	Without facial movements, except for occasional sucking at regular intervals	Smooth and regular	Threshold to stimuli is very high, so that only very intense or disturbing stimuli will arouse infants	Caregivers trying to feed infants in deep sleep will probably find the experience frustrating. Infants will be unresponsive, even if caregivers use disturbing stimuli (flicking feet) to arouse infants. Infants may only arouse briefly and then become unresponsive as they return to deep sleep. If caregivers wait until infants move to a higher, more responsive state, feeding or caregiving will be much more pleasant.
Light sleep	Some body movements	Rapid eye movements (REM); fluttering of eyes beneath closed eyelids	May smile and make brief fussy or crying sounds	Irregular	More responsive to internal and external stimuli; when these stimuli occur, infants may remain in light sleep, return to deep sleep, or to deep sleep, or to drowsy	Light sleep makes up the highest proportion of newborn sleep and usually precedes wakening. Due to brief fussy or crying sounds made during this state, caregivers who are not aware that these sounds occur normally may think it is time for feeding and may try to feed infants before they are ready to eat.
Awake States						
Drowsy	Activity level variable, with	Eyes open and close	May have some facial	Irregular	Infants react to sensory stimuli although	From the drowsy state, infants may return to sleep or awaken

State	Body activity	Eyes	Face	Breathing	Responsiveness	Implications for caregiving
	mild startles interspersed from time to time; movements usually smooth	occasionally, are heavy lidded with dull, glazed appearance	movements, often there are none, and the face appears still		responses are delayed; state change after stimulation often noted	further. In order to awaken, caregivers can provide something for infants to see, hear, or suck because this may arouse them to a quiet alert state, a more responsive state. Infants left alone without stimuli may return to a sleep state.
Quiet alert	Minimal	Brightening and widening of eyes	Faces have bright, shining, sparkling looks	Regular	Infants attend most to environment, focusing attention on any stimuli that are present	Infants in quiet alert state provide much pleasure and positive feedback for caregivers. Providing something for infants to see, hear, or suck will often maintain this state. In the first few hours after birth, most newborns commonly experience a period of intense alertness before going into a long sleeping period.
Active alert	Much body activity; may have periods of fussiness	Eyes open with less brightening	Much facial movement; faces not as bright as quiet alert state	Irregular	Increasingly sensitive to disturbing stimuli (hunger, fatigue, noise, excessive handling)	Caregivers may intervene at this stage to console and to bring infants to a lower state.
Crying	Increased motor activity, with color changes	Eyes may be tightly closed or open	Grimaces	More irregular	Extremely responsive to unpleasant external or internal stimuli	Crying is the infant's communication signal. It is a response to unpleasant stimuli from the environment or from within infants (fatigue, hunger, discomfort). Crying tells us the infant's limits have been reached. Sometimes infants can console themselves and return to lower states. At other times they need help from caregivers.

Adapted from Brazelton TB, Nugent JK. *Neonatal behavioral assessment scale.* 3rd ed. London: MacKeith Press; 1995.

<u>Box</u> **9-1**   ALERTING INFANTS

GENERAL PRINCIPLES OF ALERTING INFANTS

- Infants tend to be alert immediately after birth and then move into a deep sleep. This is followed by highly individualized sleep-wake patterns.
- Infants tend to sleep much of the first 2 weeks (especially the first 2 to 3 days).
- An infant in deep sleep does not breastfeed well. Maternal analgesia, anesthesia, sedatives, and magnesium sulfate, as well as infant jaundice, may augment sleepiness.
- Noxious stimuli should not be used to alert infants. Noxious stimuli include pinching, thumping the feet, and so on. Infants should associate feedings with pleasure, not discomfort. Frantically crying infants do not breastfeed effectively.

TECHNIQUES FOR ALERTING INFANTS

- Unswaddle, undress to diaper
- Change diaper
- Talk to the infant
- Gently stimulate extremities by stroking, massaging
- Apply a cool cloth to face
- Hold the infant upright
- Use motion; simulate motion within the uterus by gently bouncing the infant (never shake the infant)
- Turn the infant from side to side
- Elicit "doll's eye reflex" but avoid jackknifing

Modified from Bocar D. *Breastfeeding educator program resource notebook.* Oklahoma City: Lactation Consultant Services; 1997.

the feeling of a full stomach. (Burping may be necessary *before* feeding.) Just as an adult is not very good at performing his or her daily job when tired or frustrated, so too an infant is considerably less effective when he has been asked to do his "job" under less than optimal circumstances. These suboptimal circumstances can be avoided with good clinical management.

Clinical Management Strategies

One simple guideline should govern clinical management: A sleepy baby will not eat, and a hungry baby will not sleep! The feeding experience is enhanced when the mother responds to early hunger cues (see Box 7-1), and the infant is in the quiet-alert state; this is most likely to happen when the care provider, parents, and environment foster easy access to the breast, as shown in Box 9-3.

Newborns spend most of the first 24 hours sleeping. Waking them will not necessarily result in a good feeding during this first day. The World Health Organization (WHO) states, "Interval between feeds varies considerably particularly in the first few days of life. There is no evidence that long interfeed intervals adversely affect health of newborns who are kept warm and who are breastfed when they show signs of hunger."[11] Infants who have risk factors for hypo-

glycemia should be awakened every 3 hours using the alerting techniques shown in Box 9-1.

Food-Fluid-Warmth Relationship

Thermoregulation is critical for newborns. Similarly, nutrients and fluids are essential for survival. Because the thermoregulatory mechanism and the ingestion, digestion, and utilization of nutrients and fluids are interrelated, their relationship is influenced by breastfeeding, which supplies calories, fluids, and skin-to-skin warmth. Therefore any alteration in breastfeeding can positively or negatively affect the infant's serum glucose level or temperature. Conversely, any alteration in the infant's serum glucose level or temperature can affect breastfeeding behavior. The following sections aim to explain the physiologic basis for the food-fluid-warmth relationship.

Hypoglycemia

Glucose needs and regulation start long before birth. During pregnancy, glucose is delivered to the fetus via the placenta. Typically, fetal glucose levels are about 70% to 80% of the maternal serum levels. (Hence, the importance of regulation for diabetic mothers.) For example, if the gravida's serum

Box 9-2 Consoling Infants

GENERAL PRINCIPLES OF CONSOLING

- *Frantically crying* infants need consoling before they go to the breast.
- *Fussy* infants can be consoled at the breast.
- If an infant has his tongue elevated against the hard palate, consoling techniques should be used before offering the breast.
- Respond quickly to signs of discontent; infant calms more rapidly and learns trust.
- Infants may need interactions and/or stimulation (stimulation may distract from discomfort).
- Always rule out hunger; if an infant responds to rooting reflex, offer the breast; use consoling techniques to calm the infant before breastfeeding, but not as a substitution for a feeding.
- No technique works every time; try different techniques at different times, or combine techniques.

TECHNIQUES FOR CONSOLING INFANTS
Provide Kinesthetic Stimulation

- Keep the infant in warm, humid environment
- Physical security: swaddling, flexion with head support, "nesting" with soft, supportive linens creates physical security
- Holding
- Gentle motion in all three planes: side to side, up and down, front to back (amount of motion similar to intrauterine motion)
- Carry, rock, swing, gently bounce (never shake infants!)
- Skin-to-skin contact
- Tactile stimulation
- Massaging/stroking: massaging or stroking in the direction of hair growth is consoling; massaging or stroking against hair growth is stimulating

Provide Auditory Stimulation

- Parent's voice (infants are more responsive to familiar parental voices)
- Talking (infants are more responsive to high-pitched voice tones)
- Soft, rhythmic sounds at about 60 to 100 beats per minute; singing, humming, nursery rhymes, metronome
- White noise (monotone constant sound that reduces stimulation from other sounds (e.g., sound of clothes dryer, vacuum cleaner, TV "off" channel)

Provide Visual Stimulation

- Human face with eye contact
- Mirrors, lights, ceiling fans, mobiles
- Pictures with black-and-white geometric figures
- Primary colors (especially red and yellow)

Provide Gustatory and Olfactory Stimulation

- Expressing colostrum
- Placing colostrum or mother's milk on lips
- Offering clean parental finger to suck (health care providers should use glove)
- If parent is unavailable, caregiver may wear parent's unwashed clothing

Combine Consoling Techniques

- Placing the infant in an infant seat on top of an operating clothes dryer within parental view; moist, warm area with rhythmic motion and sounds
- Taking the infant for a car ride in infant seat (physical security, gentle motion, white sound)

Modified from Bocar DL. *Breastfeeding educator program resource notebook*. Oklahoma City: Lactation Consultant Services; 1997.

glucose is 70 to 80 mg/dl as it should be, the fetal level will be around 49 to 64 mg/dl. The glucose supports not only fetal metabolism but also growth and development. After about 24 weeks of gestation, glycogen is stored in the liver and the muscles, and it increases in quantity as term gestation approaches.

Glucose supply from the placenta is abruptly terminated once the umbilical cord is severed. Birth is a critical turning point because newborns "must transform themselves from a state of net glucose intake and glycogen synthesis to one of glucose production and regulation."[12] After birth, the infant must obtain energy from both exogenous

Box 9-3   PRIORITIES FOR CARE: ACCESS TO THE BREAST

- Encourage mothers and newborns to share a room.
- Watch for signs of alertness, as shown in Fig. 9-2.
- Teach parents to watch for *early* hunger cues (see Box 7-1).
- Encourage mothers to breastfeed at night.
- Be an advocate for decreasing other interactions and treatments that occur in hospitals and interfere with the breastfeeding experience (visitors, discharge photos, routine hearing tests).
- Discourage time-limited feedings.
- Emphasize the importance of adequate help at home so that the mother can focus on the newborn's needs.

Box 9-4   CLINICAL SIGNS ASSOCIATED WITH HYPOGLYCEMIA*

- Changes in levels of consciousness
  - Irritability
  - Lethargy
  - Stupor
- Apnea, cyanotic spells
- Coma
- Feeding poorly, after feeding well
- Hypothermia
- Hypotonia, limpness
- Tremor
- Seizures

From Cornblath M, Hawdon JM, Williams AF. *Pediatrics* 2000;105:1141-1145.
*Clinical signs should be alleviated with concomitant correction of plasma glucose levels.

and endogenous sources. Locating and finding his mother's breast, he can successfully obtain the exogenous source of energy. The endogenous source, however, is glucose that is available from a balance of gluconeogenesis, glycogenolysis, and ketogenesis; tissue glucose oxidation occurs in target organs.[12] The most common target organ is the brain. The newborn mounts adaptive responses, including mobilization of glucose and fatty acids from glycogen and triglyceride depots.[13] Even when glucose levels drop after prolonged intervals (more than 8 hours) between breastfeedings, it appears that newborns have a marked ketogenic response (see definition in Table 9-1) that spares glucose utilization in the brain.[13] Through this ketogenic response, fat stores are used as alternative energy sources (alternatives to glucose) until the onset of lactogenesis stage II, after glycogen in the liver and muscle have been depleted. This response is limited in preterm infants, who have immature livers and decreased availability of the enzymes involved in fat breakdown.

Fortunately, newborns also have glycogen stores, but these stores are used up within about 2 to 3 hours after birth. Although the stores of glycogen do exist, glycogenolysis appears to be depressed in newborns, resulting in decreased serum blood glucose. After the glycogen stores are used, the newborn uses fat for metabolism. Hence,

the adaptation to extrauterine life results in fluctuations in newborn glucose supply and utilization while regulatory mechanisms are still immature. The fluctuation in newborn glucose supply and utilization is normal; the newborn is mounting an adaptive response to the external environment. Stressors in the external environment, most notably hypothermia, increase energy needs that sometimes exceed the newborn's ability to provide the necessary energy substrate.

Clinical signs and symptoms of hypoglycemia are listed in Box 9-4.[14] The exact incidence of newborn hypoglycemia is unknown, but it appears to be somewhere around 14%[15] to 15%.[16] When it occurs, it is often associated with disease.[15]

Multiple definitions have been formed over the past several decades, but because experts have disagreed on the definition of euglycemia for newborns, it has been difficult to define hypoglycemia. Perhaps the most useful definition is that offered by Cornblath who says, "[Hypoglycemia is] the concentration of glucose in the blood or plasma at which the individual demonstrates a unique response to the abnormal milieu caused by the inadequate delivery of glucose to a target organ, for example, the brain."[14] Hypoglycemia is a common metabolic problem,[16] but its signs and symptoms can easily be mistaken for other clinical phenomenon. Therefore the presence of specific signs and symptoms is helpful but not sufficient for diagnosing hypoglycemia in the newborn.

Similarly, most experts, including Cornblath, are reluctant to define hypoglycemia by using only one number (i.e., the mg/dl) because the "number" at which newborns experience difficulty varies with several factors, including feeding method (human or artificial milk).[17]

Risk Factors. Some newborns are at especially high risk for hypoglycemia, as shown in Box 9-5. There is some suggestion that infants whose mothers have had dextrose infusions intrapartally are more at risk for hypoglycemia, but this has not been confirmed.[18]

Glucose Monitoring and Interpretation. Glucose monitoring for the newborn requires a clear protocol about who, when, and how often to monitor, as well as by what method. Unless there are risk factors for hypoglycemia, it is unnecessary to routinely test for hypoglycemia.[11,19] Screening of infants of diabetic mothers should occur within 30 minutes of birth and no later than 2 hours for newborns with other risk factors.[20] Thereafter, blood glucose levels can be measured at 1 hour before and 3 hours after feedings, until stable.

Box **9-5**   RISK FACTORS OF HYPOGLYCEMIA

A. Associated with changes in maternal metabolism
   1. Intrapartum administration of glucose
   2. Drug treatment
      a. Terbutaline, ritodrine, propranolol
      b. Oral hypoglycemic agents
B. Associated with neonatal problems
   1. Idiopathic condition or failure to adapt
   2. Perinatal hypoxia-ischemia
   3. Infection
   4. Hypothermia
   5. Hyperviscosity
   6. Erythroblastosis fetalis, fetal hydrops
   7. Other (iatrogenic causes, congenital cardiac malformations)
C. Intrauterine growth restriction
D. Hyperinsulinism
E. Endocrine disorders
F. Inborn errors of metabolism

From Cornblath M, Hawdon JM, Williams AF. *Pediatrics* 2000;105:1141-1145.

Most brands of reagent strips are not accurate for newborns.[14,21] Reagent strips are affected by the newborn's hematocrit level. Because they were designed to be used with adults, the strips yield inaccurate results when used with newborns, who have higher hematocrits. The reagent strips can be considered only a screening device, but if used properly, they are useful for this purpose.

If a reagent strip is not used, interpretation of results should be done with a clear understanding of whether the laboratory used whole blood or serum when performing the test. Glucose levels are higher in whole blood than in serum, so interpreting laboratory data depends on the technique used. Serum glucose levels may differ between breastfed and artificially fed newborns.[22]

Effect on Breastfeeding and Clinical Management Strategies. Exclusive breastfeeding should suffice for healthy, term, appropriate-for-gestational-age (AGA) newborns who exhibit no symptoms.[11] In one study no cases of hypoglycemia were reported among 203 unsupplemented breastfed infants.[23] Hoseth concludes that "Very few healthy, breastfed, term infants of appropriate size for gestational age have low blood glucose levels."[24] Most times, the symptoms of hypoglycemia occur fairly soon after birth. Those who experience transient symptoms, however, should be treated according to protocol based on national and international recommendations. Furthermore, a follow-up plan should be in place; although hypoglycemia after hospital discharge is unlikely, it is possible. One report described three breastfed infants who experienced transient hypoglycemia after early discharge.[25]

A healthy term infant who is mildly hypoglycemic is usually willing to suckle. Suckling while skin-to-skin with his mother and with his back covered usually improves the infant's glucose levels. Moderate hypoglycemia can cause lethargy, so some nursery protocols call for giving the infant some artificial milk (assuming expressed human milk is unavailable) until he perks up enough to suckle. If the infant is markedly hypoglycemic, however, he will require more aggressive interventions; nursery protocols can be modeled after the Academy of Breastfeeding Medicine's hypoglycemia protocol.[20] Furthermore, the infant who is hypoglycemic is at risk for hypothermia. WHO summarized recommendations for newborns with hypoglycemia.[11] The following points are especially pertinent:

- Hypoglycemia is most likely to occur in the first 24 hours of life.
- Newborns who have risk factors for hypoglycemia, including those who are preterm or neurologically impaired, should be awakened every 3 hours.
- WHO states, "Healthy newborns show signs of readiness to feed when they are hungry, but the interval between feeds varies considerably, particularly in the first few days of life. There is no evidence that long interfeed intervals adversely affect healthy newborns who are kept warm and who are breastfed when they show signs of hunger. An infant who shows no signs of hunger or is unwilling to feed should be examined to exclude underlying illness"[11] (p. 1).

Transient hypoglycemia is the reflection of a normal adaptive response. Hypoglycemia that persists (meaning the symptoms do not resolve) is abnormal; it is not the result of underfeeding, and it requires prompt medical follow-up. Identification of infants at risk for hypoglycemia usually makes prevention possible. If a medical diagnosis of hypoglycemia is confirmed, supplementation is indicated. However, an attempt to preserve the breastfeeding relationship should be made.

Hypothermia

Hypothermia commonly occurs in newborns. An understanding of the newborn's thermoregulatory mechanisms helps the nurse avoid the potential consequences of heat loss and recognize its effect on breastfeeding.

Thermoregulatory Mechanisms. The newborn tries to maintain homeostasis with a temperature of about 36.5° to 37.5° C (97.7° to 99.5° F), but he may easily lose heat and need to produce heat. One concept is central to the understanding of heat production: Heat is produced through the metabolism of foods. It follows, then, that if one does not have enough food for metabo-

lism, a decreased body temperature results. The thermoregulatory mechanism strives to maintain homeostasis in the presence of heat production and heat loss.

Infants can produce a little heat simply by increasing activity. The main way of producing heat in the neonate, however, is through nonshivering thermogenesis through the metabolism of brown adipose tissue. Contrary to the adult, in whom nonshivering thermogenesis is controlled by epinephrine, nonshivering thermogenesis in the neonate is controlled through norepinephrine. When norepinephrine is released, it increases the body's metabolic rate and stimulates brown fat to release glycerol and fatty acids that act as fuel. In essence, the newborn burns fat to keep warm. This mechanism indeed keeps the infant warm, but once supplies of brown fat are exhausted, they are not replenished. Hypothermia becomes a real threat.

Newborns are especially at risk for heat loss because of their larger body surface area in relation to their body mass, the close proximity of their blood vessels to the skin, and their immature thermoregulatory mechanisms. Because heat is produced through only one means—the metabolism of nutrients—the infant who is hypothermic will soon become hypoglycemic. Hypothermia triggers increased metabolism—the infant will be burning calories just to keep warm—resulting in hypoglycemia. Hypothermia or hypoglycemia can be life threatening to a newborn.

Heat loss occurs because of stresses on metabolism (i.e., the infant has an increased basal metabolic rate for whatever reason) or through the environment. Common examples of metabolic stressors include prematurity, cardiac defects, acidosis, and infection. After birth, the infant is exposed to various environmental stressors. Infants lose heat through four processes in the environment: evaporation, radiation, conduction, and convection. Heat loss can result in hypothermia, as described previously. The skin is the primary site of sensory receptors that alert the body to environmental temperature changes. These receptors relay the information to the hypothalamus in the brain. The hypothalamus is the control center for thermoregulation; it coordinates both heat production and heat loss, but its function is immature in the newborn. Usually, this "thermostat" works reasonably well to keep the infant within the normal range (from 36.5° to 37.5° C). However, it can be impaired by oxygen deprivation, alterations in central nervous system functioning (e.g., birth trauma), or maternal drug consumption.

Consequences of Heat Loss. Newborns who experience heat loss can quickly become hypothermic. Infants lose heat by one of four mechanisms: conduction, radiation, convection, or evaporation. Aside from losing heat, however, infants can become hypothermic if they are hypoglycemic. For this reason, it is imperative to recognize that these conditions are likely to coexist, and an effective breastfeeding session is likely to prevent or minimize either condition. Table 9-4 summarizes physiologic problems associated with hypothermia and hyperthermia.

Effect on Breastfeeding and Clinical Management Strategies. Infants who are on the low side of normal temperature should be offered the breast to obtain additional energy (calories) and skin-to-skin warmth. Hypothermia in the presence of a warm environment and adequate breastfeeding requires medical follow-up; such a situation may indicate that the infant has a higher metabolic need, as is seen with cardiac defects, sepsis, and other problems.

Hyperthermia

Hyperthermia is somewhat uncommon in newborns and often is the result of overdressing the infant. If it is accompanied by the signs and symptoms listed in Table 9-4, it may be a sign of inadequate fluid intake, or it at least requires further follow-up.

Inadequate Fluids

Generally speaking, infants who are taking in adequate amounts of human milk are consuming adequate amounts of fluids. Infants can and do get dehydrated, however. There are three types of dehydration: isotonic (also called *isonatremic*), hypotonic (hyponatremic), and hypertonic (hypernatremic). Isotonic dehydration is usually associated with the use of artificial milk. Hyponatremic dehy-

dration has been associated with premature infants who have had fortified milk.[26] The important thing is not the label but rather the early recognition that there is a problem.

Cases of hypernatremic dehydration[27,28] have been associated with breastfeeding, but a series of clinical management errors, including poor breastfeeding management, a delay in seeking help for worrisome factors, and not being seen by a physician, were all apparent in those cases that resulted in serious morbidity. In other cases, existing factors such as infant craniofacial defects and lactation failure following postpartum hemorrhage should have been noted and followed up on before serious consequences ensued.[29] Scare stories in the popular press describe desperate scenarios in which newborns have been severely dehydrated,[30] and in the professional literature, lack of adequate breastfeeding has been identified as a possible sole cause of dehydration.[31]

Hypernatremic dehydration may be subtle in breastfed newborns. In one report of five newborns, none had overt physical signs but had lost more than 10% of their body weight. Their parents reported only decreased output and sleepiness or irritability. At the time of hospital admission, some still did not have the "typical" signs of dehydration.[32] All five, however, were born to mothers who had no experience or little experience ("unsuccessful with previous baby") breastfeeding.[32] It is therefore important to emphasize to parents that if breastfeeding is going well, dehydration is unlikely to occur, but worrisome signs need to be reported promptly.

Clinical Signs of Dehydration. Typically, professional education emphasizes a sunken fontanel as a sign of dehydration in the newborn. However, this is a very late sign. Like other problems that can be detected, dehydration is easier to manage in the early phases. Several earlier signs of dehydration are clues that, if left uncorrected, indicate a dangerous situation. Table 9-5 shows that most clinical signs of isonatremic dehydration appear "normal" during the early phases of dehydration; signs and symptoms of hypernatremic dehydration are less obvious, which means the clinical assessment usually underestimates the magnitude of hydration.[33] Note that one of the earliest signs of dehydration is pallor, which warrants follow-up.

Table **9-4**   COMPARISON OF HYPOTHERMIA AND HYPERTHERMIA

	Hypothermia	Hyperthermia
Definition	**Temperature <36.5° C (97.7° F)**	**Temperature >37.5° C (99.5° F)**
Possible causes	*Physiologic problems* • *Hypoglycemia* • *Prematurity* • *Sepsis* • *Hypoxia* • *SGA or IUGR* *Conduction:* infant has been on a cold surface *Radiation:* isolette or room too cold *Convection:* drafts in room, portholes of isolette open *Evaporation:* giving a bath or not drying thoroughly after bath, wet diapers, clothes, blankets; not drying the newborn immediately after birth	*Physiologic problems* • *Tachypnea* • *Septicemia* • *Dehydration* *Conduction:* infant has been on a warm surface or wrapped in warm blankets *Radiation:* warmer or isolette temperature is too high
Physical signs	• Mottling • Cold extremities • Lethargy • Poor feeding • Low serum blood glucose levels	• Tachypnea • Red skin (plethoric) • Low serum blood glucose • Occasionally, infant will have sweat on forehead
Corrective strategies	Dependent on cause, but some general suggestions include the following: • Hypoglycemia: feed infant and listen for swallowing; check blood glucose 1 hour later, then after feeding, every 3 hours until stable • Hypoxia: work with physician to identify and ameliorate cause • Conduction losses: pad cold surfaces with blankets • Radiation losses: keep room warmer, use a second blanket • Convection losses: decrease drafts, or move infant away from drafts • Evaporation losses: dry immediately after birth; keep under warmer for bath; cover dry head with cap; keep in dry clothes and diapers; use upside-down T-shirt as "pajama" bottoms. • Refer to primary health care provider if hypothermia persists	Hyperthermia happens infrequently in newborns; corrective strategies depend on cause, but some general suggestions include the following: • Check setting if infant is in warmer or isolette; it is especially easy for isolettes to overheat • Check pulse and respirations; this infant may be ill • Undress infant; wipe with cool cloth if indicated • Refer to primary health care provider ifabove actions do not correct the hyperthermia

IUGR, Intrauterine growth restriction; *SGA,* small for gestational age.

Table 9-5 SIGNS AND SYMPTOMS RELATED TO DEGREE OF DEHYDRATION*

Parameter	Mild	Moderate	Severe
Weight loss	3%-5%	10%	15%
Skin color	Pale	Gray	Mottled
Skin turgor	May be elastic	Decreased elasticity	Tenting
Mucous membranes	Slightly dry	Dry	Dry, parched, collapse of sublingual veins
Eyes	Probably normal	Decreased tears	Sunken; absence of tears, soft globes
Central nervous system	Alert but calm	Somewhat decreased	Distal pulse not palpable
Pulse			
Quality	Strong	Somewhat increased	Markedly tachycardic
Rate	Probably normal	Somewhat increased (orthostatic changes)	Markedly tachycardic
Capillary refill	Norm (<2 sec)	2-4 sec Orthostatic decrease	>4 sec Decreased while supine
Blood pressure	No change Probably	Elevated specific	Less than 0.5 ml/kg/hr
Urine	normal or slightly decreased volume	gravity, decreased volume	over past 12-24 hr; may be anuric
Clinical implications	Assess closely; implement preventative measures Notify primary health care provider and record observations	Initiate interventions as ordered; goal is to avoid severe problem Continue to assess; record observations Help mother and family understand effect on feeding	Continue to implement medical interventions as ordered Help mother to continue breastfeeding efforts, even if separated from infant (see Chapter 15)

Modified from Hoekelman RA, Adam HM, Nelson NM et al. *Primary pediatric care.* 4th ed. St. Louis: Mosby; 2001.
*The table is best used to judge severity in infants with isonatremic dehydration; those with hypernatremic dehydration have the same signs, but they are more subtle and therefore are more likely to be underestimated.

Infants who are jaundiced are often dehydrated,[34] so parents of jaundiced infants should be instructed on how to detect signs of dehydration. Increased body temperature within the first week of life, presumably related to decreased body water, is a sign of dehydration.[32]

Effect on Breastfeeding and Clinical Management Strategies. Dehydration is a medical diagnosis that should be managed by the pediatrician or primary care provider. It is certainly possible that good breastfeeding management can alleviate the problem, but supplementation may be indicated in some situations. Supplementation can upset the supply-and-demand phenomenon, so the benefit of supplementing must always outweigh any possible risks.

Hyperbilirubinemia and Jaundice

Early studies showing a direct relationship between breastfeeding and elevated bilirubin levels were interpreted to mean that breastfed infants were more at risk for jaundice than artificially fed cohorts.[35-39] These studies, however, were conducted when breastfed newborns routinely had restricted feedings, and there is an inverse relationship between frequency of feeding during the first few days and incidence of jaundice[40,41] (Fig. 9-3).

Definitions and Descriptions

Understanding the relevant terms helps clarify common misconceptions about jaundice and the breastfed newborn. *Bilirubin* is the orange-yellow pigment of bile. Resulting from the breakdown of red blood cells, it is therefore an end product of

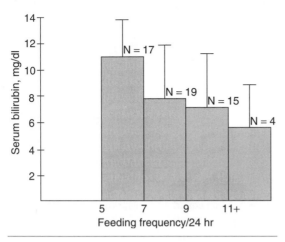

FIGURE **9-3** Relationship of mean frequency of feedings during first 3 days of life and serum bilirubin concentrations (*r* = .361, *p* < .01). Vertical bars represent standard deviations. *(From DeCarvalho M, Klaus MH, Merkatz RB. Am J Dis Child 1982;136:737-738.)*

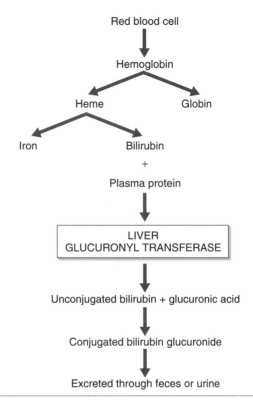

FIGURE **9-4** Formation of bilirubin from red blood cells. Bilirubin is excreted primarily through the feces; it can be reabsorbed if feces remain in the colon too long. *(From Wong D. Whaley & Wong's nursing care of infants and children. 6th ed. St. Louis: Mosby, 1999.)*

digestion and is simply excreted. *Jaundice* is a symptom of increased levels of bilirubin, which are caused by problems with production, transport, metabolism, and excretion.

Bilirubin. Bilirubin is present in the developing fetus from the first trimester, with most of it formed by the breakdown of hemoglobin. Hemoglobin catabolizes into the heme and the globin (protein) components; the heme component is then converted into biliverdin, which is later reduced to bilirubin by enzymes.

Production. The major sites of bilirubin production are the spleen and the liver, but all body tissues can form bilirubin from hemoglobin. Fig. 9-4 summarizes the processes. The amount of bilirubin produced varies inversely with gestational age; the lower the gestational age, the more bilirubin is produced. Furthermore, the amount of bilirubin that is considered "normal" varies according to how many days old the infant is. Although there are two forms of bilirubin, direct and indirect, serum levels are frequently calculated as "total" (TSB) when one is speaking of the normal range for serum levels in the newborn.

Transport. Table 9-6 describes pertinent differences between direct and indirect bilirubin.

Bilirubin produced outside the liver is transported to the liver via the plasma; there it undergoes conjugation to direct bilirubin, which is more soluble. Indirect bilirubin is transported via the plasma and is bound to albumin.

Metabolism. In the small intestine, conjugated (i.e., water-soluble) bilirubin undergoes further catabolism in the intestinal tract to form urobilinogen and stercobilinogen. This accounts for the yellow-orange color that contributes to the color of feces.

Excretion. Indirect bilirubin is not readily excreted in the urine because it is fat soluble. Direct bilirubin is a major component of bile and feces, and it is excreted through the intestines. Because bilirubin is excreted primarily in the feces, giving

Table **9-6**   Comparison of Direct and Indirect Bilirubin

	Direct Bilirubin	Indirect Bilirubin
Terms	"Bilirubin diglucoromide"	"Bilirubin"
Status	Conjugated	Unconjugated
Soluble	Soluble in aqueous solution	Insoluble in aqueous solution
Deviations	May be increased in the following conditions: • Biliary atresia • Biliary hypoplasia • Hepatitis • Cystic fibrosis • Trisomy 18 • Dubin-Johnson syndrome • Choledochal cysts • Galactosemia • α_1-Antitrypsin deficiency	**Increased Production of Bilirubin** Extravascular hemolysis • Bruising • Petechiae • Enclosed hemorrhage (intracranial bleed) Intravascular hemolysis • Polycythemia • Rh incompatibility • ABO incompatibility • Intrinsic red cell abnormalities • Hemolysis from drug toxicity **Transport Deficiencies** • Acidosis • Prematurity • Hypoglycemia • Hypothermia **Increased Conjugation in the Liver** • Prematurity • Hypoxia **Decreased Intestinal Excretion** • Antibiotic therapy • Intestinal obstruction **Metabolic Problems** • Infants of diabetic mothers • Hypothyroidism • Amino acid deficiency diseases

breastfed newborns water will not prevent or minimize jaundice; one cannot "flush" the bilirubin out through the urinary tract. In breastfed infants, greater stool output has been associated with greater excretion of bilirubin in the feces and lower serum bilirubin concentrations.[42]

Hyperbilirubinemia. Elevated levels of bilirubin result in an observable symptom called *jaundice.* Jaundice is the yellowish color that is observable when the infant's skin is blanched. Usually, jaundice is visible when bilirubin levels are above 5 mg/dl. A slightly elevated bilirubin level results in jaundice in the upper part of the body; higher levels affect the upper and lower body. In other words, the lower on the body that the jaundice can be observed, the higher the bilirubin level is. Elevated levels are treated medically with blood transfusions (for pathologic jaundice) and/or phototherapy.

Newborns, with their higher-than-adult hematocrit levels and immature livers, normally have increased levels of bilirubin. The decision to initiate medical treatment for increased bilirubin levels is dependent on the bilirubin level in relation to the infant's age.

Four types of jaundice exist: physiologic jaundice, pathologic jaundice, breastfeeding jaundice, and breast-milk jaundice. Table 9-7 compares three types of jaundice. Clinical management, including breastfeeding management, differs depending on the type of jaundice and the infant's age in days.

Physiologic Jaundice. Physiologic jaundice, sometimes called *idiopathic jaundice,* appears after the infant is 24 hours old and indicates a sluggish

Table 9-7 COMPARISON OF TYPES OF JAUNDICE*

	Physiologic Jaundice (Idiopathic Jaundice)	Pathologic Jaundice	Breast-Milk Jaundice
Onset	About 48 hr after birth	<24 hr after birth	About 7 days
Peak	72 hr in term infant	24 hr in term infant	2 wk
Duration	Variable; recedes after 72 hr	Variable; rapid rise in bilirubin that recedes with treatment	Variable; 2-16 wk
Cause	Alteration primarily in bilirubin excretion	As a result of pathologic condition, alteration in bilirubin 1. Production 2. Transport 3. Conjugation 4. Excretion	Substance in some mothers' milk that exhibits certain enzyme activity in baby's liver, resulting in a slower breakdown and secretion of bilirubin
	These alterations are due to physiologic conditions and require monitoring and possible intervention	These alterations are due to pathologic conditions and require additional medical evaluation and treatment	
Risk factors	Prematurity, delayed passage of stool	Hemolytic disease of newborn, some maternal diseases or drug ingestion, other	Mothers who have had previous baby with breast-milk jaundice
Treatment	Day-dependent	Phototherapy Blood transfusion	Phototherapy if bilirubin level is excessive

Modified from Biancuzzo M. *Breastfeeding the healthy newborn: a nursing perspective*. White Plains, NY: March of Dimes Foundation; 1994.
*Breast*feeding* jaundice is described and discussed in the accompanying text. Breastfeeding jaundice is caused by poor intake and is best managed by the techniques described in Chapter 7.

bilirubin excretion. It has two phases: Phase 1 (first 5 days) is characterized by a relatively rapid rise in serum unconjugated bilirubin, peaking at about 5 mg/dl on day 3, with a sharp decline about day 5. Phase 2 begins around the fifth day; at that time, serum unconjugated bilirubin concentration slowly declines until it reaches an adult level at around 11 to 14 days of life.[43]

Pathologic Jaundice. Pathologic jaundice appears before the newborn is 24 hours old and usually indicates increased serum bilirubin synthesis or decreased clearance. Pathologic jaundice in the newborn often results from a blood disorder, such as Rh or ABO incompatibility, or from a pathologic condition of the hepatic system. Newborns affected with pathologic jaundice require intervention as directed by their primary health care provider.

Breastfeeding Jaundice. Breastfeeding jaundice should be distinguished from breast-milk jaundice. Breastfeeding jaundice is related to the lack of feeding, not the consumption of human milk. Gartner and Herschel describe breastfeeding jaundice as the equivalent of adult "starvation jaundice."[44] With an onset of earlier than 5 days, the mechanism of this type of jaundice is poorly understood, and the resulting increase in bilirubin is simply caused by an inadequate milk intake. This type of jaundice is not compared with other types of jaundice on the accompanying tables because its causes and cures are usually fairly simple. Early and frequent feedings with audible swallowing are the key to prevention and treatment of breastfeeding jaundice. A delayed passage of meconium also is likely to increase the rise of serum bilirubin levels because bilirubin that remains in the colon is reabsorbed.

Breast-Milk Jaundice. Breast-milk jaundice is a condition related to the presence of an unidentified substance in human milk, not lack of feeding.

β-Glucuronidase was thought to be a main causative factor, but this remains unproven.[45] The exact component or combination of components responsible for the existence of this condition remains unknown,[46] but the effect is the enhanced absorption of unconjugated bilirubin. With an onset after 5 to 7 days, peak bilirubin concentrations occur between the fifth and fifteenth day,[43] and jaundice continues as long as until the twenty-eighth day.[47]

Effect on Breastfeeding and Clinical Management Strategies

Misconceptions about how to manage the breast-fed infant who has been diagnosed with jaundice are common. Priorities for breastfed infants are listed in Box 9-6. Some mothers may recall that their last jaundiced infant was forbidden to breastfeed or that they were encouraged to give the infant water between feedings. Both of these strategies are outdated and are not based on research results or physiologic principles. It has long been established that there is no difference in peak serum bilirubin levels between those who

have been supplemented with water and those who have not,[48] as shown in the Research Highlight box.

Mothers with jaundiced infants may have questions about "pumping and dumping" their milk; Table 9-8 answers some of these and other related questions with respect to which type of jaundice the infant is experiencing. Appendix B lists patient education materials on the topic of jaundice.

Assessment and management of jaundice before hospital discharge is critical because a large portion of newborns are readmitted to the hospital for jaundice.[34,49] Although prematurity and short stay are risk factors for readmission of jaundiced newborns,[50] longer stays may not be an effective strategy.[51] Rather, identifying newborns who are at risk and initiating early and aggressive follow-up in the outpatient setting are perhaps more realistic approaches.

Breastfed infants who are at high risk for jaundice include those who have lost significant amounts of weight[52] and/or those who have been supplemented.[53] Asian[54] and American Indian[55] newborns tend to have higher levels of serum

Box 9-6   Priorities for Care: The Jaundiced Newborn

- Discourage the use of water supplementation. The practice of giving supplementary water continues, despite the landmark study nearly two decades ago showing that water supplements did not lower the serum bilirubin level.[48] Furthermore, the American Academy of Pediatrics states that "supplementing with water or dextrose water does not lower the bilirubin level in jaundiced, healthy, breast-feeding infants."[67]
- Advocate for continuation of breastfeeding. The American Academy of Pediatrics clearly states, "The AAP discourages the interruption of breastfeeding in healthy term newborns and encourages continued and frequent breastfeeding (at least eight to ten times every 24 hours)."[67]
- Explain the importance of frequent feedings. Infants who breastfeed more than eight times per 24 hours have significantly lower bilirubin levels than those whose feedings are limited.

- Promote early feedings at the breast. Colostrum has a laxative effect on the gut, which helps bilirubin to be excreted.
- Monitor intake and output. Note the time of the first stool. Continue to note the quantity and quality of voidings and stools and weight loss. Call the pediatrician or primary care provider about data that appear worrisome.
- Lead efforts to minimize maternal-infant separation when the hyperbilirubinemia is treated with phototherapy. Advocate for the newer fiberoptic treatment because it is more conducive to keeping the mother and infant together. Separation in and of itself can breed problems with breastfeeding, so keeping the dyad together is optimal.
- Teach the parents how to blanch for jaundice. In addition, provide a card describing worrisome signs, and a clear idea of when to call the primary health care provider.

RESEARCH HIGHLIGHT

Water Does not Prevent Jaundice

Citation: DeCarvalho M, Hall M, Harvey D. Effects of water supplementation on physiological jaundice in breast-fed babies. *Arch Dis Child* 1981;56:568-569.

FOCUS

This prospective study of 175 healthy term newborns was designed to determine the effects of water supplementation on bilirubin levels. Fifty-five newborns were given no water; 120 were given water ad libitum at the end of each breastfeeding.

RESULTS

There was no significant difference between the two groups when peak serum bilirubin levels and incidence of phototherapy were compared. Bilirubin peaked at 4 days in both the control and the study groups.

STRENGTHS, LIMITATIONS OF THE STUDY

Only infants who had no risk factors for jaundice were included in this study conducted in London. All newborns began breastfeeding within the first 3 hours of life and continued to breastfeed on demand, although the number of feedings per day was not specified.

CLINICAL APPLICATION

The practice of giving water to newborns was begun without any scientific evidence to support the claim that it prevents or minimizes jaundice, yet it still exists in some hospitals. The results of this study should be considered when updating jaundice protocols in hospitals. Giving water probably interferes with the mechanisms that *do* minimize or prevent jaundice. For example, when the infant consumes water, he is likely to breastfeed fewer times in a day, and a later study by the same author[40] shows that frequent feedings are beneficial in minimizing bilirubin levels. Furthermore, the same author[42] shows that lower serum bilirubin levels are associated with greater stool output—which is enhanced by colostrum, not water—and lowered bilirubin levels.

---

bilirubin compared with whites or African-Americans. Boys and those with cephalohematomas or bruising are also at risk.[52] Predischarge measurement of total serum bilirubin would help target newborns who are at risk.[56] An increase in staff nurse support of protocols that are conducive to unrestricted breastfeeding, of course, would help in prevention.[57] A recent study has shown that infants who are fed a casein-hydrolysate formula, rather than human milk or a standard formula, had lower bilirubin levels.[58]

WELL INFANTS WHO NEED EXTRA HELP

Normal, healthy term newborns and their mothers can usually succeed at breastfeeding with little assistance. Some situations, however, may require a little extra help. Mothers who breastfeed multiple-birth infants and those who tandem breastfeed are common examples.

Multiple Gestation

The percentage of multiple births is the highest reported in at least 50 years.[59] Of those infants born in 1996, 2.7% were multiple births, the most frequent type of which is twins. Often, mothers of multiple infants erroneously assume that breastfeeding is not a realistic possibility. The many benefits of breastfeeding that are conferred to singletons are multiplied with twins or higher order multiples, however, so mothers should be counseled about breastfeeding as soon as they realize they are carrying multiple fetuses.

Breastfeeding two offspring can seem daunting. The true challenge, however, is usually not breastfeeding per se, or even feeding. The transition to parenthood and/or basic caregiving for a singleton within a growing family is often overwhelming, so the mother and her partner are understandably more overwhelmed by meeting the many needs of multiple infants. Furthermore, multiple

Table 9-8 COMPARISON OF BREASTFEEDING MANAGEMENT STRATEGIES FOR DIFFERENT TYPES OF JAUNDICE

	Physiologic Jaundice	Pathologic Jaundice	Breast-Milk Jaundice
Onset (clue)	About 48 hr after birth	Anytime after birth	About 7 days
Initiation of breastfeeding	Early initiation decreases threat	Early initiation desirable	Unrelated to condition
Weaning	Not necessary	Not necessary	Not necessary
Interruption of breastfeeding	Not necessary	Not necessary	Rarely, if ever, necessary to interrupt breastfeeding for diagnosis[68]
Supplementation			
• Indication	If baby is too lethargic to suckle	If baby is too lethargic to suckle	Likely to be ordered if bilirubin levels are excessively high
	Dependent on hydration status and/or phototherapy	Dependent on hydration status and/or phototherapy	May need formula to dilute effect on bilirubin
• With water?	No	No	No
• With artificial milk?	Acceptable if supplementation is indicated and human milk is unavailable	Acceptable if supplementation is indicated and human milk is unavailable	Yes, every other feeding
• With expressed mother's own milk	If supplementation is indicated, this is best option	If supplementation is indicated, this is best option	Not appropriate
• With banked donor milk	Yes, if mother has insufficient volume	Yes, if mother has insufficient volume	Yes, if available
Expressing breast milk			
Frequency	Express milk after any skipped or partial feedings	Express milk after any skipped or partial feedings	Express milk after any skipped or partial feedings
Save and feed	Yes	Yes	No—may be unusable after 1 month of age
Discard	No	No	Yes
Helpful devices			
Wallaby phototherapy unit	Safe and effective; improves mother's access to newborn	Safe and effective; improves mother's access to infant	No data to determine effectiveness with this group; good for home care
Nursing supplementers (see Chapter 16)	Probably not indicated if infant can suckle	May be helpful for baby who is lethargic or who has weak suck	May be helpful for supplementation

Modified from Biancuzzo M. *Breastfeeding the healthy newborn: a nursing perspective.* White Plains, NY: March of Dimes Foundation; 1994.

gestation may result in preterm birth; hence, the mother may arrive home with one but not all infants.

It is critical for the mother to produce an adequate volume of milk to meet the needs of her infants. This can be accomplished through frequent feedings. There is a direct relationship between frequency of breastfeeding sessions and milk production for singletons, as well as for twins and triplets.[60] Quadruplets have successfully breastfed and have made mean weight gains of 30 to 54 g per day.[61]

With adequate stimulation, a mother of twins will produce more than 800 ml of milk per day.[60] If artificial milk is introduced, suckling is decreased and milk synthesis is decreased as well. This is usually accompanied by the cascade of deleterious effects that occur with milk stasis. Exclusively breastfeeding twins for several months is a realistic option. Success has been associated with more frequent episodes of pumping during the first few days (for infants who are unable to suckle) and increased support from the nursing staff.[62]

Some women are reluctant to breastfeed multiples because they have heard that doing so will make their nipples twice as sore as breastfeeding a singleton. This may be true, but only if the soreness is the result of poor latch-on or incorrect use of a pump—it should not be the result of multiple infants suckling at the breast. Some breast and nipple problems, however, do seem to be more prevalent in mothers of multiples. Mastitis, for example, is commonly seen in these situations. It is likely that mastitis occurs because of increased milk synthesis and incomplete removal of milk at each feeding (see Chapter 12). Thrush that occurs in one infant requires immediate treatment not only of that infant but of the others as well. There is no reason, however, to "assign" a breast to a particular infant when there is an outbreak of thrush.

The infants may suckle simultaneously or separately. There are advantages and disadvantages to both strategies. Simultaneous feedings save time, however, so mothers should be persuaded to at least learn this option. There are no rules for how to accomplish breastfeeding multiples, however. Several positions for simultaneous feedings offer specific advantages, as shown in Table 9-9, and include[63] (1) the double football (or double clutch hold); (2) the cradle-football (or parallel hold); and (3) the double cradle (crisscross or V-hold), as shown in Figs. 9-5 to 9-7.

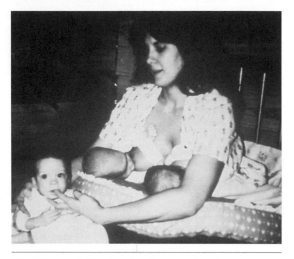

FIGURE **9-5** Double football hold. *(Courtesy Jane Bradshaw, Forest, VA.)*

Feeding one twin and then the other is referred to as *alternate feeding*. In alternate feeding the hungrier infant demands to be fed and therefore sets the pace as the mother then wakens the second infant. Some mothers have successfully breastfed for several months using alternate feedings and enjoy the one-on-one contact. This approach is quite acceptable, and breastfeeding may continue nicely despite the extra time required.

Sometimes the mother assigns one breast to one infant and one to the other, but this is not recommended. A more abundant supply may be created on one side if one infant suckles more vigorously and removes more milk there.

Whether the infants are ill or well, the mother should be discouraged from breastfeeding one and artificially feeding another. She may experience differences in bonding/attachment, and all infants benefit from and deserve human milk.

Priorities for teaching mothers of multiples are listed in Box 9-7. Professional literature about breastfeeding multiples is somewhat limited. However, Gromada[64] describes in detail the importance of prenatal preparation (including the decision to breastfeed, social support assessment, and the development of goals and plans specific to multiples), circumstances surrounding the initiation of lactation for multiples, interventions to

Table **9-9** BREASTFEEDING MULTIPLES: COMPARING STRATEGIES

Positioning for More Than One Infant	Advantages	Limitations
Alternate The mother feeds first one infant and then the other	• May be easier for mother to manage in the beginning • Gives "private time" with each infant	• More time consuming • Difficulty letting down when other baby is waiting to eat and crying • More difficult to meet needs of both babies at once; may require another person to feed the other baby who is hungry but not at the breast
Simultaneous Feeding Two infants are fed at the same time; these include the following: • Double football (double clutch)	• More time efficient • Easier to meet the needs of both babies at once • Allows mother better head control of smaller, fussier infants because her hands are more free • Hands more free to position both infants because pillows function as a sort of extra "hand" • Usually able to support each breast for latch-on and/or throughout the feeding	• Requires more coordination to latch-on and reposition infants • Requires a couch or large chair for support on both sides
• Cradle/football (parallel hold)	• Can alternate positioning; thus each infant exercises both eyes for eye contact	• Hands not free to reposition infants • Difficult for mother to support her breasts prior to latch-on
• Double cradle (crisscross or V-hold) both infants in cradle position	• Allows for eye contact between mother and both infants	• Difficult to use until after infants have gained more head control

promote maintenance of lactation, and alternative plans for carrying out the feedings. This article, although somewhat dated, is still well worth reading. Twins and higher-order multiples are at risk for inadequate intakes, so frequent weight checks, preferably in the convenience of the parent's home, should be scheduled.[65] Cobedding—a strategy that I began suggesting to parents more than 20 years ago—has recently been shown to be beneficial for feeding and sleep-wake states.[66] Suggestions for educational materials for parents of multiples are listed in Appendix B.

Tandem Breastfeeding

Tandem breastfeeding means that the mother is breastfeeding two siblings of different ages at the same time (Fig. 9-8). Usually, the mother becomes pregnant while breastfeeding a toddler or preschooler and then wishes to breastfeed the newborn upon his arrival. The mother may feel uneasy about lactating while she is pregnant and may require reassurance and approval. Some women experience contractions when they are breastfeeding, however. Therefore if mothers are at high risk for preterm labor, the potential threat to the

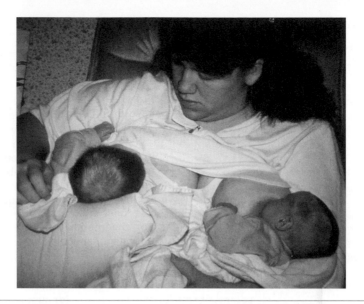

FIGURE **9-6** Cradle/football (or parallel) hold. *(Courtesy Jane Bradshaw, Forest, VA.)*

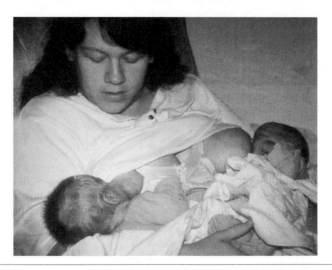

FIGURE **9-7** Double cradle hold (also called crisscross or V-hold). *(Courtesy Jane Bradshaw, Forest, VA.)*

fetus—an early birth resulting from contractions—may outweigh the potential benefits the older child receives from breastfeeding. Mothers are likely to experience increased nipple soreness because of the hormonal changes of pregnancy, and positioning the older child at the breast with the enlarging abdomen may be awkward.

Colostrum is produced as the pregnancy advances to term, but the colostrum tastes saltier than the milk the older child is accustomed to. The older child may have loose stools because of the colostrum's laxative effect. Sometimes the older child weans himself at this point. If he does not, however, tandem breastfeeding can continue as

Box 9-7 Priorities for Care: Breastfeeding Education for Mothers of Multiples

- Applaud mother's breastfeeding efforts and help her to find lifestyle adjustments that facilitate breastfeeding.
- Teach the mother about adequate rest and nutrition and about positions for simultaneous breastfeeding.
- Verify proper latch-on to avoid sore nipples and other problems that become magnified with multiple infants.
- Access material and human resources: find support services in the community and provide

helpful literature before hospital discharge. Help mother to ask for practical help from family and friends.
- Emphasize that adequate stimulation is critical to adequate milk supply and that adequate consumption of hindmilk by all infants is critical; pump if indicated. Provide list of reassuring signs.
- Refer to support services. See Appendix A for contact information for support groups for parents of multiples.

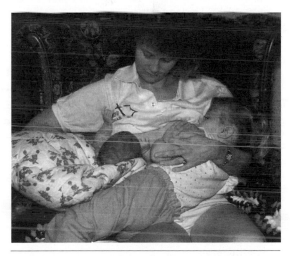

FIGURE 9-8 Tandem nursing. An infant and his older sibling are suckling at the same time. *(Copyright Debi Bocar, Lactation Consultant Services, Oklahoma City, OK.)*

long as the mother wishes. After delivery, these mothers will experience some degree of postpartum engorgement, although less than that experienced by mothers who are not tandem breastfeeding. The most important priority is the mother's nutritional status; sufficient stores of nutrients—most notably calcium—are needed, and the mother's own body becomes deficient in response to the extra demands to make milk. (See Clinical Scenario box in Chapter 2.)

No rules govern the pattern of breastfeeding: Frequency, duration, and whether the siblings suckle simultaneously or separately are all determined by what works best for the mother and her family. Some recommendations to aid in successful tandem breastfeeding are described in Box 9-8. Some consumer education materials are listed in Appendix B.

Tandem breastfeeding is for some people but not for others. Some men and women may consider this practice natural and acceptable; others are repulsed by it. The mother deserves support for her decision and should not be discouraged because of cultural biases of health care providers. If the mother approaches the idea of tandem breastfeeding enthusiastically but later decides that it is not for her, she may need help to gently wean the older child.

SUMMARY

The transition to extrauterine life requires several adaptations for the newborn. The newborn's metabolism is immature, and he may need changes in the environment or food to meet his biologic needs and achieve homeostasis. Human milk provides nutrients, including energy, to help the newborn establish and maintain circulatory, respiratory, thermoregulatory, and gastrointestinal function. Behavioral tasks such as sleep-wake cycles and sensory needs are an integral factor in the breastfeeding experience. Newborns are especially at risk for hypoglycemia, hypothermia, and

Box 9-8   Priorities for Care: Tandem Breastfeeding

- The newborn has priority at the breast. The older sibling can increase intake of solid foods during the first 3 to 5 days after birth so that the newborn receives adequate colostrum. The mother may fear that the older child will consume the younger child's portion, but this is unlikely given that human milk is synthesized according to supply and demand.
- Reassure the mother that any change in behavior from the older child—being repulsed by the engorgement or being thrilled with the bountiful supply—is okay. Things will return to "normal" in a few days.
- Suggest many different ways to position two siblings at the breast if the mother wishes to breastfeed simultaneously, as described in Figs. 9-5 to 9-8.
- Reassure the mother that it is not necessary to discontinue breastfeeding or limit feedings to one breast if one child becomes ill. After the onset of symptoms, the siblings have already been sharing the breast for several days.
- Help the mother identify ways to get some time to herself because she may be feeling that her body is no longer her own. Even a short walk alone can be helpful.
- Identify calcium-rich foods and encourage the mother to consume these foods in substantial quantities.

hyperbilirubinemia. These conditions can be minimized or overcome by good breastfeeding management. Newborns who are generally healthy but have some special situation (e.g., those whose mother is breastfeeding a twin or an older sibling) can breastfeed successfully if their mothers adapt good breastfeeding principles to the special situation.

REFERENCES

1. Lowdermilk DL, Perry SE, Bobak IM. *Maternity & women's health care.* 7th ed. St. Louis: Mosby; 2000.
2. Thibodeau GA, Patton KT. *Anatomy & physiology.* 4th ed. St. Louis: Mosby; 1999.
3. Committee on Nutrition American Academy of Pediatrics. *Pediatric nutrition handbook.* 4th ed. Elk Grove Village, IL: American Academy of Pediatrics; 1998.
4. Behrman RE, Kliegman RM, Arvin AM, editors. *Nelson textbook of pediatrics.* 16th ed. Philadelphia: WB Saunders; 2000.
5. Vorherr H. Human lactation and breast feeding. In Larson BL, editor. *Lactation.* New York: Academic Press; 1978.
6. Blackburn S, Loper DL. *Maternal, fetal, and neonatal physiology: a clinical perspective.* Philadelphia: WB Saunders; 1992.
7. Cohen RJ, Brown KH, Rivera LL et al. Exclusively breastfed, low birthweight term infants do not need supplemental water. *Acta Paediatr* 2000;89:550-552.
8. Brazelton TB. *Neonatal behavioral assessment scale.* Philadelphia: Lippincott; 1984.
9. Barnard K. *Early parent-infant relationships.* White Plains, NY: March of Dimes Foundation; 1978.
10. Varendi H, Porter RH. Breast odour as the only maternal stimulus elicits crawling towards the odour source. *Acta Paediatr* 2001;90:372-375.
11. World Health Organization (WHO). *Hypoglycaemia of the newborn.* Geneva: World Health Organization; 1997.
12. Eidelman AI. Hypoglycemia and the breastfed neonate. *Pediatr Clin North Am* 2001;48:377-387.
13. Hawdon JM, Ward Platt MP, Aynsley-Green A. Patterns of metabolic adaptation for preterm and term infants in the first neonatal week. *Arch Dis Child* 1992;67:357-365.
14. Cornblath M., Hawdon JM, Williams AF. Controversies regarding definition of neonatal hypoglycemia: suggested operational thresholds. *Pediatrics* 2000;105:1141-1145.
15. Pildes R, Forbes AE, O'Connor SM et al. The incidence of neonatal hypoglycemia: a completed survey. *J Pediatr* 1967;70:76-80.
16. Cornblath M. Neonatal hypoglycemia 30 years later: does it injure the brain? Historical summary and present challenges. *Acta Paediatr Jpn* 1997;39(Suppl 1):S7-S11.
17. Kalhan S, Peter-Wohl S. Hypoglycemia: what is it for the neonate? *Am J Perinatol* 2000;17:11-18.
18. Srinivasan G, Pildes RS, Cattamanchi G et al. Plasma glucose values in normal neonates: a new look. *J Pediatr* 1986;109:114-117.
19. American Academy of Pediatrics Committee on Fetus and Newborn. Routine evaluation of blood pressure, hematocrit, and glucose in newborns. *Pediatrics* 1993;92:474-476.
20. Academy of Breastfeeding Medicine. Guidelines for glucose monitoring and treatment of hypoglycemia in term breastfed neonates. *ABM News and Views* 1999;5. Available at http://www.bfmed.org/protos.html.
21. Cornblath M, Schwartz R, Aynsley-Green A et al. Hypoglycemia in infancy: the need for a rational definition. A Ciba Foundation discussion meeting. *Pediatrics* 1990;85:834-837.

22. Heck LJ, Erenberg A. Serum glucose levels in term neonates during the first 48 hours of life. *J Pediatr* 1987;110:119-122.

23. Nylander G, Lindemann R, Helsing E et al. Unsupplemented breastfeeding in the maternity ward. Positive long-term effects. *Acta Obstet Gynecol Scand* 1991;70:205-209.

24. Hoseth E, Joergensen A, Ebbesen F et al. Blood glucose levels in a population of healthy, breast fed, term infants of appropriate size for gestational age. *Arch Dis Child Fetal Neonatal Ed* 2000;83:F117-F119.

25. Moore AM, Perlman M. Symptomatic hypoglycemia in otherwise healthy, breastfed term newborns. *Pediatrics* 1999;103:837-839.

26. Kloiber LL, Winn NJ, Shaffer SG et al. Late hyponatremia in very-low-birth-weight infants: incidence and associated risk factors. *J Am Diet Assoc* 1996;96:880-884.

27. Thullen JD. Management of hypernatremic dehydration due to insufficient lactation. *Clin Pediatr Phila* 1988;27:370-372.

28. Cooper WO, Atherton HD, Kahana M et al. Increased incidence of severe breastfeeding malnutrition and hypernatremia in a metropolitan area. *Pediatrics* 1995;96:957-960.

29. Livingstone VH, Willis CE, Abdel-Wareth LO et al. Neonatal hypernatremic dehydration associated with breast-feeding malnutrition: a retrospective survey. *CMAJ* 2000;162:647-652.

30. Helliker K. Dying for milk. Some mothers, trying in vain to breast-feed, starve their infants. *The Wall Street Journal* 1994;(July 22)1, 4.

31. Oddie S, Richmond S, Coulthard M. Hypernatraemic dehydration and breast feeding: a population study. *Arch Dis Child* 2001;85:318-320.

32. Ng PC, Chan HB, Fok TF et al. Early onset of hypernatraemic dehydration and fever in exclusively breast-fed infants. *J Paediatr Child Health* 1999;35:585-587.

33. Hoekelman RA, Adam HM, Nelson NM et al. *Primary pediatric care.* 4th ed. St. Louis: Mosby; 2001.

34. Liu S, Wen SW, McMillan D et al. Increased neonatal readmission rate associated with decreased length of hospital stay at birth in Canada. *Can J Public Health* 2000;91:46-50.

35. Butler DA, MacMillan JP. Relationship of breast feeding and weight loss to jaundice in the newborn period: review of the literature and results of a study. *Cleve Clin Q* 1983;50:263-268.

36. Johnson CA, Lieberman B, Hassanein RE. The relationship of breast feeding to third-day bilirubin levels. *J Fam Pract* 1985;20:147-152.

37. Kivlahan C, James EJ. The natural history of neonatal jaundice. *Pediatrics* 1984;74:364-370.

38. Maisels MJ, Gifford K. Normal serum bilirubin levels in the newborn and the effect of breast-feeding. *Pediatrics* 1986;78:837-843.

39. Schneider AP II. Breast milk jaundice in the newborn. A real entity. *JAMA* 1986;255:3270-3274.

40. DeCarvalho M, Klaus MH, Merkatz RB. Frequency of breast-feeding and serum bilirubin concentration. *Am J Dis Child* 1982;136:737-738.

41. Yamauchi Y, Yamanouchi I. Breast-feeding frequency during the first 24 hours after birth in full-term neonates. *Pediatrics* 1990;86:171-175.

42. DeCarvalho M, Robertson S, Klaus M. Fecal bilirubin excretion and serum bilirubin concentrations in breast-fed and bottle-fed infants. *J Pediatr* 1985;107:786-790.

43. Gartner LM, Lee KS. Jaundice in the breastfed infant. *Clin Perinatol* 1999;26:431-445.

44. Gartner LM, Herschel M. Jaundice and breastfeeding. *Pediatr Clin North Am* 2001;48:389-399.

45. Yigit S, Ciliv G, Aygun C et al. Breast milk beta-glucuronidase levels in hyperbilirubinemia. *Turk J Pediatr* 2001;43:118-120.

46. Maruo Y, Nishizawa K, Sato H et al. Prolonged unconjugated hyperbilirubinemia associated with breast milk and mutations of the bilirubin uridine diphosphate-glucuronosyltransferase gene. *Pediatrics* 2000;106:E59.

47. Crofts DJ, Michel VJ, Rigby AS et al. Assessment of stool colour in community management of prolonged jaundice in infancy. *Acta Paediatr* 1999;88:969-974.

48. DeCarvalho M, Hall M, Harvey D. Effects of water supplementation on physiological jaundice in breast-fed babies. *Arch Dis Child* 1981;56:568-569.

49. Brown AK, Damus K, Kim MH et al. Factors relating to readmission of term and near-term neonates in the first two weeks of life. Early Discharge Survey Group of the Health Professional Advisory Board of the Greater New York Chapter of the March of Dimes. *J Perinat Med* 1999;27:263-275.

50. Hall RT, Simon S, Smith MT. Readmission of breastfed infants in the first 2 weeks of life. *J Perinatol* 2000;20:432-437.

51. Grupp-Phelan J, Taylor JA, Liu LL et al. Early newborn hospital discharge and readmission for mild and severe jaundice. *Arch Pediatr Adolesc Med* 1999;153:1283-1288.

52. Centers for Disease Control and Prevention. Kernicterus in full-term infants—United States, 1994-1998. *JAMA* 2001;286:299-300.

53. Bertini G, Dani C, Tronchin M et al. Is breastfeeding really favoring early neonatal jaundice? *Pediatrics* 2001;107:E41.

54. Itoh S, Kondo M, Kusaka T et al. Differences in transcutaneous bilirubin readings in Japanese term infants according to feeding method. *Pediatr Int* 2001;43:12-15.

55. Saland J, McNamara H, Cohen MI. Navajo jaundice: a variant of neonatal hyperbilirubinemia associated with breast feeding. *J Pediatr* 1974;85:271-275.

56. Bhutani VK, Johnson L, Sivieri EM. Predictive ability of a predischarge hour-specific serum bilirubin for subsequent significant hyperbilirubinemia in healthy term and near-term newborns. *Pediatrics* 1999;103:6-14.

57. Janken JK, Blythe G, Campbell PT et al. Changing nursing practice through research utilization: consistent support for breastfeeding mothers. *Appl Nurs Res* 1999;12:22-29.

58. Gourley GR, Kreamer B, Cohnen M et al. Neonatal jaundice and diet. *Arch Pediatr Adolesc Med* 1999;153:184-188.

59. March of Dimes: *National perinatal statistics: live births.* White Plains, NY:March of Dimes. Available at http://www.modimes.org/HealthLibrary2/InfantHealthSta tistics/stats.htm#PrematurityandLowBirthweight.

60. Saint L, Maggiore P, Hartmann PE. Yield and nutrient content of milk in eight women breast-feeding twins and one woman breast-feeding triplets. *Br J Nutr* 1986;56:49-58.

61. Mead LJ, Chuffo R, Lawlor Klean P et al. Breastfeeding success with preterm quadruplets. *J Obstet Gynecol Neonatal Nurs* 1992;21:221-227.

62. Hattori R, Hattori H. Breastfeeding twins: guidelines for success. *Birth* 1999;26:37-42.

63. Sollid DT, Evans BT, McClowry SG et al. Breastfeeding multiples. *J Perinat Neonatal Nurs* 1989;3:46-65.

64. Gromada KK. Breastfeeding more than one: multiples and tandem breastfeeding. *NAACOGS Clin Iss Perinat Womens Health Nurs* 1992;3:656-666.

65. Gromada KK, Spangler AK. Breastfeeding twins and higher-order multiples. *J Obstet Gynecol Neonatal Nurs* 1998;27:441-449.

66. Nyqvist KH, Lutes LM. Co-bedding twins: a developmentally supportive care strategy. *J Obstet Gynecol Neonatal Nurs* 1998;27:450-456.

67. American Academy of Pediatrics. Provisional Committee for Quality Improvement and Subcommittee on Hyperbilirubinemia. Practice parameter: management of hyperbilirubinemia in the healthy term newborn. *Pediatrics* 1994;94:558-565.

68. Gartner LM. Neonatal jaundice. *Pediatr Rev* 1994;15:422-432.

Strategies for Breastfeeding the Preterm Newborn

Preterm birth can affect newborn behavior in general and breastfeeding specifically. Infants who are born before term have physiologic alterations that cause them to have greater needs than infants who have the benefit of remaining in utero for the full gestation. These alterations, although not necessarily pathologic, can alter feeding management. The infant's increased nutritional needs, along with his limited capabilities to suckle, require some special feeding strategies.

Some infants are born so much before term that they are unable to accomplish direct breastfeeding (suckling at their mothers' breasts) and therefore experience indirect breastfeeding (human milk given via some other means). Ultimately, however, the goal is to achieve full, direct breastfeeding. The purpose of this chapter is to help nurses use strategies that facilitate direct breastfeeding (suckling) for preterm infants, even when indirect or supplemented feedings may be simultaneously required.

When feeding decisions are made, issues of gestational age should not be confused with issues of weight. Infants can be classified according to gestation (preterm, term, postterm),[1] weight only (low birth weight [LBW], very low birth weight [VLBW], or extremely low birth weight [ELBW]), and gestation in relation to age[2] (weight appropriate for gestational age, small for gestational age, or large for gestational age). These classifications are explained in Box 10-1. Infants of the same gestational age can have weights that are very different from one another, and they look very different from one another (Fig. 10-1).

Having acknowledged these clear classification differences, however, in this chapter, the word *preterm* is used when referring to infants born before 35 weeks of gestation because breastfeeding management for them differs substantially from that required for term infants. Generally, feeding management for infants who are technically preterm but born nearer to term is about the same as feeding management for infants who are full term.

The infant who is born many weeks before term may begin his life with all of his body systems underdeveloped to meet even basic survival needs. (The severity of the problem is directly proportional to the degree of prematurity.) Preterm infants have several immature bodily functions, as described in Table 10-1. All of these difficulties will become apparent as the infant attempts oral feedings, whether those feedings are through an artificial nipple or at the mother's breast. A developmental care approach,[3-5] including kangaroo care described in Chapter 14, should be instituted for optimal breastfeeding experiences. For the most part, however, suckling directly at the breast (direct breastfeeding) is generally more beneficial for the preterm infant.

Preterm infants often have other factors that influence breastfeeding. For example, multiple gestation is commonly associated with preterm birth. Preterm infants born from multiple gestation can usually initiate and continue breastfeeding with relatively little assistance. Direct breastfeeding can be achieved with few modifications even in twins born at 35 weeks of gestation.[6] However, infants with defects are often born before term, and these infants experience many difficulties with breastfeeding as a result of their immaturity and their underlying pathologic condition. Sometimes, a preterm birth is preceded by months of maternal illness and/or hospitalization. Although this is

Box **10-1** COMPARISON OF WEIGHT AND GESTATION STATUS

Gestational age is merely the number of weeks that have elapsed between the onset of the last menstrual period (not the presumed time of conception) and the delivery date. (The phrase *postmenstrual age [PMA]* is functionally equivalent to *gestational age,* because both reflect dates that are based on the onset of the last menstrual period.) Following the onset of the last menstrual period, and regardless of their weight, infants born

- before 37 completed weeks of gestation (259 days) are considered preterm.[1]
- from 37 completed weeks plus one day (260 days) through 42 completed weeks of gestation (294 days) are considered to be at term.
- after 42 completed weeks of gestation (295 days) and later, following the onset of the last menstrual period, are considered postterm.

Weight: Regardless of their gestation, infants who weigh less than 2500 g but more than 1500 g at birth are low birth weight (LBW). Infants who weigh less than 1500 g but more than 1000 g at birth are considered very low birth weight (VLBW). Infants who weigh less than 1000 g at birth are extremely low birth weight (ELBW).

Infants' weight and age are combined to form yet another classification.[2] Infants who are

- appropriate for gestational age (AGA) have weights that fall between the 10th and 90th percentiles in comparison with other infants of the same gestational age. (The specific gestational age does not matter.)
- small for gestational age (SGA) are those whose weights fall below the 10th percentile in relation to weights of other infants of the same gestational age. (N.B.: Infants who are SGA are not necessarily preterm.)
- large for gestational age (LGA) have weights that fall above the 90th percentile in relation to other infants of the same gestational age at the same number of weeks of gestation (i.e., their weight is considered in relation to infants born at the same number of weeks of gestation).

Three infants of the same gestational age but different weights are shown in Fig. 10-1.

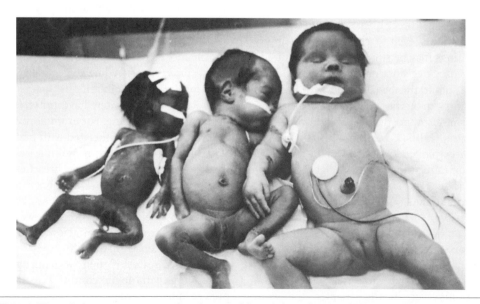

FIGURE **10-1** Three infants, same gestational age, with weights of 600, 1400, and 2750 g, respectively, from left to right. *(From Korones SB.* High-risk newborn infants. *4th ed. St. Louis: Mosby, 1986.)*

Table **10-1** POSSIBLE PROBLEMS AND BREASTFEEDING MANAGEMENT FOR PRETERM NEWBORNS

Immaturity of Several Systems	Clinical Problem	Goals and Clinical Strategies	Rationale
Cardiopulmonary	Increased need for oxygen	Conserve oxygen: • Keep baby warm—skin-to-skin contact is effective • Breastfeed; this requires less oxygen than bottle feeding • Respirations >60-70; do not feed infant (or per nursery protocol)	Hypothermia burns calories; when calories are spent, oxygen is consumed
	Unalert (sleepy) infant attempting to feed	Minimize factors that contribute to sleepy infant at breast: • Plan to breastfeed at baby's peak alert times • Use alerting techniques described in Chapter 9 • Unwrap baby if temperature is stable • Evaluate amount of supplementation infant has had	Stimulation may help infant to suckle successfully
	Infant tires easily when fed	Optimize chances for milk transfer at breast: • Use warm cloth or other techniques to elicit milk-ejection reflex • Offer frequent feedings (i.e., every 2-3 hr) • Watch for signs of overstimulation	Best efforts are usually at beginning of feeding
Neuromuscular/ neuroendocrine (suck/swallow problems)	Poor coordination of suck-swallow reflex	If infant can coordinate suck/swallow, offer the breast	It is no more difficult to suck/swallow at breast than it is at bottle
	Absent or weak suck	Preterm infant may "practice" sucking between feedings Dancer hand is an option but not imperative Consider using a nursing supplementer (see Chapter 16)	

Continued

Table **10-1**   Possible Problems and Breastfeeding Management for Preterm Newborns—cont'd

Immaturity of Several Systems	Clinical Problem	Goals and Clinical Strategies	Rationale
	Difficulty latching on	Make sure baby opens wide; tickle lower lip Decrease overful nipple if mother is engorged	
	Nipple confusion	Ideally, offer only the breast; this is not always possible Alternatives include gavage, medicine cup, syringe	
Gastrointestinal/ nutritional	Increased incidence, longer duration of jaundice	Increase feedings of colostrum	Bilirubin is excreted primarily through the gut, and colostrum acts as a laxative on the gut
	Need for calories, fluids, nutrients to support growth	Increase calories, fluids, and nutrients Use combination plan: offer direct feeding and express milk for indirect feeding	Milk fortifier provides nutrients and calories (see Chapter 15) Direct breastfeeding alone may be inadequate for newborn needs and/or maternal stimulation

Box **10-2** GOALS AND PRIORITIES FOR CARE: THE PRETERM INFANT

ANTEPARTUM PERIOD

- Assist the mother to recognize that breast-feeding is not only possible but optimal for a preterm infant.
- Acknowledge that direct breastfeeding—feeding the newborn directly at the breast—may not be possible at first. If it is not, indirect breastfeeding—expressing milk and giving it through a supplemental device—is an interim strategy.
- Facilitate contact with a local support group, especially one that includes mothers who have successfully breastfed preterm infants. La Leche League can help. Tertiary care centers that handle many preterm births may have established their own support group.
- Collaborate with other members of the health care team, including the registered dietitian, breastfeeding specialist, neonatologist, pediatrician, and others to identify strategies and options for supplemental feeding. These should be thought of as options, not necessarily as closed cases.
- Mobilize equipment; be sure that a suitable pump—preferably with a double accessory kit as described in Chapter 14—will be available in the hospital and after discharge.
- Ensure that educational media will be available and accessible at the hospital when the infant is delivered.

IMMEDIATE POSTPARTUM PERIOD

- Initiate or reinforce actions listed for the antepartum period.
- Assist the infant who can coordinate suck/swallow/breathe to achieve good positioning and latch-on.
- Provide mother with a list of worrisome signs and a list of phone numbers to call for help.
- Give suggestions to improve milk supply (see Chapters 7 and 14).
- Provide a list of pump rental depots and ask the neonatologist to prescribe a pump. Having a prescription may enable the mother to obtain reimbursement from her health insurance company.

CONTINUATION OF BREASTFEEDING

- Bolster the mother's confidence in her ability to provide for her infant.
- Reinforce to the mother her infant's capabilities; suggest strategies that will help him overcome his limitations with suckling.
- Reassure mother that infant is "getting enough."
- Help the mother to understand why the neonatologist has ordered a quota of milliliters of milk that her infant must consume at each feeding; help her understand that supplementation with fortifier or artificial milk may be necessary to meet this quota.
- Discuss devices, other than bottles, that can be used to supplement the preterm infant (see Chapter 16).
- Determine whether the infant has adequate weight gain by using test-weighing; collaborate with the entire health care team if he does not.
- Be sure that the infant can successfully ingest and retain enough human milk to make adequate weight and length gains. According to the AAP, the VLBW or ELBW infant who is consuming preterm human milk should have about 180 to 200 ml/kg per day during the first 2 to 3 weeks.[24] After about the first 3 to 4 weeks, the protein content of preterm milk drops and is inadequate to meet nutritional needs, and although the mother's milk is still appropriate, a strategy for providing adequate protein must be implemented.
- Ensure that the infant gets the hindmilk because the high fat content of hindmilk is essential for energy needs and brain growth.
- Determine whether the mother is developing an adequate supply of milk; initiate interventions if she is not (see Chapters 7 and 14). Kangaroo care can be especially helpful in developing an adequate milk supply for preterm infants.[100]
- Advocate for the use of banked donor milk if the mother's milk supply is insufficient to meet the infant's need.
- Anticipate discharge if the infant makes *consistent* weight gains, and if his weight approaches at least 2 kg and if other clinical factors are stable.

unfortunate, it does allow some advanced planning to help the mother and family meet the goals and priorities for feeding of preterm infants (Box 10-2). If a premature birth cannot be anticipated in the prenatal period, however, the postpartum mother may need help with her decision to initiate and continue breastfeeding.

MATERNAL LACTATION FOR THE PRETERM INFANT

Although it seems obvious, it bears emphasizing that direct breastfeeding will never occur unless the mother decides to lactate for her infant. Generally, mothers of preterm infants or infants who require special care are less likely to initiate breastfeeding than mothers of term infants.[7-9] This may be either related to or exacerbated by the commonly observed situation in which nurses and other health care providers erroneously assume that breastfeeding is too stressful for the infant or that providing milk is too stressful for the otherwise stressed mother. In a supportive environment, however, mothers who did not plan to breastfeed their term infant are often willing and even eager to breastfeed their preterm infant (personal observation). Mothers often say, "I just wish I could do something to help him," which gives members of the health care team an opportunity to say, "Actually, there is something that you can do for him that none of us can do for him."

Effect of the Health Care System

Anecdotal reports and various abstracts have suggested that health care professionals may be in a pivotal position with respect to the feeding decision for the very preterm infant, but published studies on the topic are sparse. In one study, however, mothers of preterm infants said that encouraging words from health care providers were powerful motivators that "outweighed the efforts" of long-term milk expression during the infants' hospitalization.[10]

Educational and supportive programs for preterm mothers have reportedly increased the incidence and duration of breastfeeding in the United States, but these nonexperimental studies have provided no data on the incidence or duration before implementation of the program.[11,12]

A recent experimental study showed that such a program did not increase duration among mothers of VLBW infants in Canada.[13] Presumably, this might be explained by the high level of motivation among mothers of these infants. A controlled study in Germany recently showed that multiple pregnancy and gestational age of greater than 29 weeks were associated with prolonged feeding of mother's milk, as were maternal age (older than 35) and spontaneous pregnancy.[14]

Anticipatory Guidance

The nurse must provide some anticipatory guidance for the mother who has chosen to breastfeed her preterm infant. First, a certain amount of anxiety about the infant's clinical condition and the consequent unplanned separation can be especially distressing and must be addressed. Mothers should be reassured, however, that this separation will not preclude successful breastfeeding.[15] (Chapter 14 discusses support for the mother who has an unplanned separation from her infant.)

The mother may have difficulty with accomplishing milk transfer when the infant is suckling, and she can benefit from the strategies discussed later in this chapter. If the infant cannot suckle, milk expression will be necessary for a while. Milk volume is a critical issue for the mother of a preterm infant, however, and deserves special mention.

Milk volume is minimal immediately after birth, and the mother who is expressing milk for her preterm infant may be especially discouraged that she has expressed only a few drops of colostrum into the collection container. She may be comforted by knowing that preterm newborns have a very small stomach capacity. Chapter 14 gives specific suggestions for helping mothers deal with this situation, including storing the milk in very small containers so that it does not appear "lost" in a large-volume container.

After the first few days, mothers of preterm infants tend to have a supply of milk that exceeds what their infants will suckle because preterm newborns have a lower suction pressure and inconsistent sucking patterns.[16-20] The same is true if they have initiated milk expression for the infant who cannot suckle.

The volume of milk produced varies directly with the frequency and degree of breast emptying, as explained in Chapter 7. Strategies for achieving adequate breast emptying when the infant is not suckling are described in Chapter 14. The aim of these strategies is to help the mother produce about 750 ml of milk per day by about the end of the second week postpartum.[21] The infant may not need that much; it is likely that he will need only about 500 to 600 ml per day, or perhaps less. A target exceeding what the infant will need in one day is recommended, however, because mothers need a bit of a "stash" of milk for days when milk supply dwindles, as occurs after a prolonged time of expressing in the absence of a suckling infant.

Maternal milk volume does dwindle in the absence of a suckling infant. In one study, mothers were unable to maintain lactation for 40 days.[22] This happens because the mechanical stimulation, although efficient, is not as efficient as the vigorously suckling infant. It also happens because mothers typically maintain the same pumping regimen, whereas if they were suckling a term infant, they would receive stimulation and breast emptying in response to the infant's appetite and growth needs. Expressing about 5 minutes after the last drops of milk have been obtained is a good way to simulate this.

Production of less than 350 ml per day is worrisome. At this point, strategies to increase milk volume should be initiated. Stress is likely to interfere with both milk production and milk let-down,[23] and certainly, mothers of preterm infants are likely to feel stressed or report feeling stressed (personal observation).

BASIC FEEDING DECISIONS

Three feeding decisions need to be made. Decisions about the choice of milk, the route of administration, and the feeding schedule are pertinent for the preterm infant.

Choice of Milk: Understanding Infants' Needs and Capabilities

Preterm infants may be fed mothers' own milk, fresh or frozen; mothers' milk, modified; banked donor milk; or artificial milk (see Chapter 15).

Decision makers should choose milk for a preterm infant with a clear understanding of his needs.

Choice Based on Overall Needs

Like term infants, preterm infants need to meet their basic needs for metabolic function and growth. The needs to consume energy, to build more tissue, and to regulate bodily functions are extraordinary in very preterm infants.

Need for Increased Energy. Preterm infants require more energy (from carbohydrates, proteins, and fats) because of their high metabolic rates. Data on the exact needs of those who are 34 to 36 weeks of gestation are sparse; the needs of those who are younger have been more well defined.

LBW and VLBW infants need at least 100 to 120 kcal/kg/day to support metabolic function and normal growth and development.[24] To achieve this, the infant must take in around 140 to 200 ml/kg/day of milk. (Milk differs in caloric values.*) Infants with problems such as bronchopulmonary dysplasia or other serious problems need a minimum of 120 to 150 kcal/kg/day. Preterm infants may have difficulty taking in and retaining these amounts of kilocalories. First, the preterm newborn's stomach capacity is fairly small. He also tires easily and therefore often consumes little volume in feeding. Those who are suckling their mother's breasts often tire before they get the energy-rich hindmilk, and hence they make poor weight gains. Finally, some preterm infants, because of their clinical condition, are fluid restricted. Most energy comes from fat and carbohydrate sources. The stable, growing preterm infant needs about 10 to 14 g/kg/day of carbohydrate and about 5 to 7 g/kg/day of fat.[24]

Need to Build More Tissue. Preterm infants need to build more tissue because the greatest amount of tissue accretion occurs during the third trimester of gestation. Building tissue requires greater amounts of protein. The preterm infant needs to achieve a weight gain of approximately

---

*At 1 week, *preterm* human milk provides about 670 kcal/L, and at 4 weeks, about 700 kcal/L. Caloric value of preterm formulas are listed on the labels.

15 g/kg/day. To achieve that growth, he will need to consume 3.0 to 3.8 g/kg/day of protein.[24]

Need to Regulate Bodily Function. Like term infants, preterm infants need vitamins and minerals to regulate body processes. Mineral requirements of the VLBW infant are higher than those for larger preterm infants; sodium and potassium requirements are estimated to be 2.0 to 3.0 mEq/kg/day higher, and even greater for ELBW infants.[24] Magnesium, calcium, and phosphorus are needed in greater amounts as well.

Preterm infants need increased amounts of calcium and phosphorus for bone mineralization and metabolism. Calcium is needed for bone mineralization because the greatest amount of bone mineralization happens during the last trimester of gestation—a time that is shortened for the infant who is born significantly before term—and during early infancy. Preterm infants need about 100 to 192 mg of calcium per 100 kcal.[24] Phosphorus is needed, among other reasons, because it enhances the absorption of calcium and decreases urinary calcium and magnesium excretion. Preterm infants need about 50 to 117 mg of phosphorus per 100 kcal.[24] When there is an extreme deficit of phosphorus, calcium absorption is impaired. Optimal mineral requirements for the ELBW infant have not been well established.[25]

Preterm infants are born with lower body stores of vitamins; they also have poor enteric absorption of vitamins.[26] Recently, controversy over vitamin E has evoked much discussion in the literature. It has been concluded that vitamin E supplementation is not routinely necessary for healthy premature infants gestational age 30 weeks ± 1.7 weeks or older.[27] A thorough discussion of vitamin needs for LBW and VLBW preterm infants is described in detail by Yu.[26]

Choices of Milk: Examining Advantages and Disadvantages

Ideally, the choice of milk is selected based on the advantages and risks of human and artificial milk. In most cases the advantages of human milk for the preterm infant exceed the advantages of artificial milk and the few risks that are associated with human milk.

Human Milk. The American Academy of Pediatrics (AAP) has given a strong statement that human milk is best for all infants, including preterm and LBW infants.[28,29] Since the publication of their paper, experts assert that human milk may also be best for VLBW infants.[30] The AAP cites evidence that breastfeeding and human milk provide unparalleled advantages in term of nutrition and antiinfective, immune, and bonding factors. This is true for term infants, but it may be especially true for the preterm infant who has the aforementioned extraordinary needs.

Nutrition. The mother's own milk (MOM) is best for preterm infants because mothers of these infants have what is commonly called *preterm milk.* Preterm milk differs in composition from term milk. The first study, conducted by Atkinson and colleagues in 1978, showed that there is an association between the degree of prematurity and the concentration of protein and lipids found in preterm milk.[31] Summarizing more than 25 studies that have been conducted since, Atkinson asserts that these data have been confirmed by other researchers.[32] Differences between term milk and preterm milk, as shown in Table 10-2, are the values analyzed 22 to 30 days after birth of the preterm infant; milk during the earlier postpartum period has even higher concentrations for most nutrients, with the exception of fat, lactose, and energy.[32]

In general, the concentration of nutrients in preterm milk during the first 28 days or so closely aligns with the needs of preterm infants 1500 to 1800 g. That is, preterm milk contains more of the nutrients that preterm infants have a greater need for. Human milk offers many nutritional advantages for helping the infant meet his needs for increased energy, tissue building, and regulation of bodily function.

Meeting Energy Needs. Preterm milk does not provide significantly more calories than term milk.[33] Therefore VLBW or ELBW infants need extra nutrients (and therefore extra kilocalories) that can be provided by adding fortifiers to human milk. Other ways to meet this requirement for VLBW or ELBW infants is to use 150 ml/kg/day of specially designed (24-kcal/oz) artificial milk (see Chapter 15).

Table **10-2**   SOME NUTRITIONAL DIFFERENCES IN THE HUMAN MILK FROM MOTHERS OF PRETERM VERSUS THOSE OF TERM INFANTS*

Days after Delivery	3 Days	7 Days	28 Days	Term Milk
Proteins, g	3.2	2.4	1.8	1.3
Fats, g	1.6	3.8	7.0	4.2
Carbohydrates, g	6.0	6.1	7.0	4.2
Calcium, mg	21.0	25.0	22.0	35.0
Phosphorus, mg	9.5	14.0	14.0	15.0
Energy, kcal	51.0	68.0	71.0	71.0

From Aguayo J. *Early Hum Dev* 2001;65(Suppl):S19-S29.
*Nutrients per 100 ml.

Fat is the most variable component of human milk. This is an especially important factor when evaluating whether the preterm infant is getting adequate calories. Milk fat tends to differ according to all of the factors enumerated in Chapter 4. For the preterm infant, factors include the method by which the mother expressed milk, the use of tubes for feeding (fat can stick to the tube), and separation of fat that occurs when milk has been standing. Because fat varies from woman to woman, day to day, and even from hour to hour, it is useful to determine the milk's creamatocrit, as described later in this chapter.

Meeting Needs for Building Body Tissue. Preterm milk is dramatically higher in protein than term milk. Nitrogen, a building block of protein, is high in preterm milk and may help support the higher anticipated rates of growth. Human milk is beneficial for growth and development, particularly with respect to development of the brain and retina.

Fats and fatty acids are important in tissue building also. Preterm infants especially need cholesterol, which is a necessary component for brain development. Human milk appears to be the ideal food for neurodevelopmental needs.[34] Cholesterol is present only in human milk but absent from artificial milk. Lucas and colleagues' 1992 study caused quite a stir in the professional and the consumer literature; it showed that 7½- to 8-year-olds who were born preterm and fed mother's milk had higher intelligence quotients (IQs) than their artificially fed cohorts.[35] This study was particularly significant because it showed the value of human

milk only—not the process of breastfeeding (i.e., the infants were fed by tube). Retinal function also is improved when preterm infants are fed human milk, with its long-chain fatty acids, as opposed to artificial milk with corn oil–based fatty acids.[36]

Human milk is especially beneficial because of the very-long-chain fatty acids docosahexaenoic acid (DHA; a derivative of linolenic acid) and arachidonic acid (AA; a derivative of linoleic acid), as described in Chapter 4. "AA and DHA acids are major components of cell membranes and are of special importance to the brain and blood vessels" (p. 275S), and the worst case scenario of lack of DHA and AA could be cell death in the brain.[37] ELBW infants, who have subsequent IQs as much as 13 points lower than term infants, can enjoy the cognitive benefits that human milk's DHA confers, even though evidence among this population is currently somewhat sparse.[38] New formulas containing DHA and AA are described in Chapter 15.

Meeting Needs for the Regulation of Bodily Functions. Some vitamins and minerals that help regulate body processes are more abundant in preterm milk than in term milk. Unfortunately, the amounts of calcium and phosphorus are about the same in preterm and term milk, so the amount is inadequate to completely meet the needs of many preterm infants.

Preterm infants have immature kidney functioning and are therefore less able to tolerate high renal solute loads. Human milk has a lower potential renal solute load than artificial milk, as shown in Fig. 10-2. This lower renal solute load occurs because levels of protein, sodium, phosphorous,

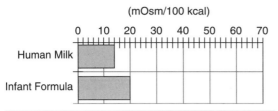

(mOsm/100 kcal)

FIGURE **10-2** Potential renal solute load for human milk and formula. Note that "Infant Formula" is representative of the major commercial infant formulas. *(Data from Committee on Nutrition, American Academy of Pediatrics. Pediatric nutrition handbook. 4th ed. Elk Grove Village, IL: American Academy of Pediatrics; 1998.)*

and potassium are lower in human milk than in artificial milk. The relatively low levels of these constituents require less water for excretion; hence, lower levels of water are lost when the infant consumes human milk. This water conservation results in a more stable body temperature because water is a factor in thermoregulation.

Antinfective and Host Defense Properties. The preterm infant's life is threatened by actual or potential infections; he is vulnerable not only because of preterm status but also because of invasive technology and exposure to staff who have cared for other potentially infected infants.

✐CLINICAL SCENARIO

Breastfeeding Infants Born Preterm

Baby Megan and Baby Gretchen were born at 35 weeks of gestation. Baby Megan weighed 2245 g at birth, and Baby Gretchen weighed 2740 g at birth. These fraternal twins went to the NICU for sepsis workups and were then admitted to the regular nursery at age 2 days. The infants are now about 72 hours old, floppy, and vigorously sucking 60 ml of artificial milk from a bottle at one feeding.

In checking the graph, you see that 10% of infants born at 35 weeks of gestation weigh less than 1750 g. Also, 10% of infants born at 35 weeks weigh more than 3000 g.

How would you classify Baby Megan?

❑ Term
❑ Preterm
❑ Low birth weight
❑ Very low birth weight

❑ Average for gestational age
❑ Small for gestational age
❑ Large for gestational age

The mother is about 72 hours postpartum and has seen the twins only briefly for one time. She was admitted to the high-risk postpartum floor and is making a steady recovery. She has a history of infertility × 19 years and desperately wants to breastfeed these infants. What *immediate* priorities do you see?

1.
2.
3.

What problems could you anticipate for these twin girls, and what strategies would you use to overcome the difficulties?

Possible Problems	Strategies

Review your list of immediate priorities. Now, what do you see as critical priorities for discharge?

1.
2.
3.

What other issues might you want to address?
Readers are encouraged to discuss this scenario among their colleagues because often there is no one right answer.

Preterm infants, who are especially vulnerable to respiratory and gastrointestinal infection, particularly benefit from the infection protection properties of human milk, most notably secretory IgA, but also lysozyme, lactoferrin, and other protective components (see Chapter 4).

The incidence of various infections is lower when preterm infants are fed their mother's milk during the day (and artificial milk at night) compared with infants who have only formula.[39] The reduction of sepsis among VLBW infants who are fed human milk is dramatic.[40] Furthermore, protection from infection endures whether the infant ingests fresh mother's milk or pasteurized donor milk.[41]

The higher protein content of preterm milk (in comparison with term milk) helps explain why its antiinfective properties such as immunoglobulins (which are protein components) are greater. For example, sIgA, the antiinfective that provides so much protection against respiratory and gastrointestinal infection, is nearly doubled in preterm colostrum (about 310 mg/g of protein) compared with term colostrum (about 168 mg/g of protein). Furthermore, phagocytic cells—cells that engulf pathogenic organisms—are enhanced by colostrum. Preterm colostrum contains higher numbers of phagocytic cells than term colostrum.[42]

Oligosaccharides are important in host defense. These carbohydrate polymers may be digested and have structures that mimic specific bacterial antigen receptors, thereby preventing bacteria from attaching to the mucosa in the host. This protection by human milk oligosaccharides may facilitate the digestion of lactose and therefore is especially beneficial to the preterm infant.[43]

Because they have immature digestive tracts, preterm infants have more difficulty digesting—breaking down—nutrients they have ingested. Human milk, with its lower casein/whey ratio, is ideal for preterm infants because it is more easily digested and absorbed than artificial milk. Infants who are born preterm are particularly at risk for developing necrotizing enterocolitis (NEC), an acute inflammatory disease that occurs in the intestines; necrosis of intestinal tissue may follow. This condition can be life threat-ening. Infants who are exclusively artificially fed are 6 to 10 times more likely to develop NEC than those who are exclusively fed human milk; those who had mixed feedings (human milk and artificial milk) were 3 times more likely to be affected than those who were exclusively fed human milk.[44] In one study of 12 preterm infants with gastroschisis repairs, none of the infants who were exclusively fed human milk developed NEC, as opposed to 30% of those who were exclusively fed formula.[45]

The bifidus factor, available in human milk, results in gram-positive beneficial (normal) intestinal flora, rather than the gram-negative pathogenic bacteria found in the gut. Furthermore, constipation or "hard stools" or infrequent stools are a common problem for preterm infants. Those who are fed artificial milk are more likely to have stools with a higher solid content than infants who are fed human milk.[46]

Bonding and Maternal Benefits. The effects of bonding appear to be magnified in the preterm situation. It appears that breastfeeding and lactation actually have positive effects on mothers, as evidenced by studies that have shown that breastfeeding and lactation help mothers cope with the situation.[10] If a mother is unwilling to breastfeed, other options need to be explored.

The superiority of bonding through breastfeeding has never been disputed, nor is it likely to be. Breastfeeding offers the pleasurable sensory stimuli, but the extent to which this is mimicked in bottle-feeding is extremely little indeed.

The nutritional and protective benefits of human milk are clear, but the human milk alone is inadequate for those who are VLBW or ELBW. In these cases, additional nutrients must be added through human milk fortifier.

There are a few potential disadvantages of human milk. Given alone, human milk is inadequate to meet the nutritional needs of the VLBW or ELBW infant. Although the protective components of human milk reduce the infant's risk of infection, pathogens can and are transmitted through human milk and can have serious consequences. For example, the risk of transmission of cytomegalovirus seems to loom especially high for the preterm newborn.[47,48] Other bacteria in the mother's milk—coagulase-negative staphylococci, α-hemolytic streptococci, and diphtheroids—are sometimes present, but whether they represent a clinical hazard is uncertain.[49] Overall, the consensus among experts is that human milk, when fortified for infants who weigh less than 1500 g, if given at volumes of at least 180 ml/kg/day, is ideal.[41] In a few cases, artificial milk may be appropriate for preterm infants.

Artificial Milk. Perhaps the one most clear-cut reason for using artificial milk is that the mother has decided not to lactate for the infant. Other times, artificial milk is used as a supplement for infants who are primarily breastfed but have circumstances that dictate this "supplementation."

Supplementation, too, is a tricky term. Very preterm infants who cannot obtain all of their nourishment by suckling the breast (direct breastfeeding) are often given supplements of their mother's milk (indirect breastfeeding) or even artificial milk. Supplementation can also mean adding to their diet extra energy and nutrients, as are found in human milk fortifier or artificial milk designed for premature infants. Unlike term infants, who, as a group, have clearly understood nutritional and developmental needs and for whom there is a clear definition of supplementation, preterm infants require thoughtful management to compensate for a variety of circumstances that occur with each individual.

Route of Administration

Some decision must be made about how to administer the nutrition that has been chosen for the infant. The most basic decision is whether the feeding will be enteral (through the gastrointestinal tract, including, but not limited to, oral feedings) as opposed to parenteral (intravenously). If the infant has been born significantly before term or if he has had significant pathology, parenteral feedings generally continue until the attending physician determines that the infant can tolerate enteral feedings. Early enteral feedings tend to increase intestinal lactase activity in preterm infants, which is a marker of intestinal maturity.

For the ELBW infant, "trickle feedings" (TF) or "gastric priming" is often implemented. TF is "the administration of nutritionally inconsequential quantities of [oral] feed while the main route for nutrition is parenteral"[50] (p. 228). The rationale for TF is that "small volumes of milk promote maturation of gut function while avoiding the possible disadvantages or difficulties of full-volume enteral feeding"[50] (p. 228). This early gut priming appears to be beneficial.[51]

In the past, arbitrary criteria were used to determine when direct breastfeeding could be initiated. Infants who were an arbitrarily determined number of weeks' corrected age or who weighed an arbitrarily determined number of grams were allowed to breastfeed. Similarly, many infants were required to demonstrate that they could feed with an artificial nipple before they were allowed to suckle directly at the breast. All of these rules were based on the idea that suckling the breast was more difficult than suckling the bottle. Finally, nursery protocols are using evidence to make these determinations.

Preterm newborns can better maintain their transcutaneous oxygen pressure and body temperature while breastfeeding than while bottle-feeding,[52,53] as described in the Research Highlight box. Because the preterm infant is likely to have weak or absent cough or gag reflexes, aspiration is possible, but it is less likely with breastfeeding than with bottle-feeding. Furthermore, if the infant does aspirate, human milk is less irritating to the bronchial tree than artificial milk. Generally, however, infants with respiratory rates of over 60 to 70 are allowed nothing by mouth, and enteral or parenteral feeding must be implemented. Improved oxygenation has been repeatedly shown to occur when preterm infants suckle the breast rather than suck a rubber nipple (Fig. 10-3).[52-55]

Feeding Frequency

Although demand feedings are optimal for term infants, "demand" or cue-based feedings are usually not appropriate for very preterm infants. Preterm infants have immature neuroregulatory mechanisms that make their sleep cycles and states different from those of term infants; therefore relying solely on state behavior and feeding cues may not ensure adequate intake for these infants.

RESEARCH HIGHLIGHT

Breastfeeding Is Easier Than Bottle-Feeding

Citation: Meier P. Bottle- and breast-feeding: effects on transcutaneous oxygen pressure and temperature in preterm infants. *Nurs Res* 1988;37:36-41.

FOCUS

Five preterm infants who weighed less than 1500 g at the initial oral feeding were continuously monitored during 71 feeding episodes (32 bottle-feeding and 39 breastfeeding episodes). Each infant served as his own control; that is, the same infants were studied while breastfeeding and bottle-feeding at different times. The investigator measured body temperature and qualitative and quantitative differences in transcutaneous oxygen pressure (tcPo$_2$).

RESULTS

The tissue oxygenation of the infant's skin (tcPo$_2$) differed markedly from breastfeedings to bottle-feedings during the episode, immediately postfeed, and 10 minutes postfeed. Typically, bottle-fed infants had a decline in tissue oxygenation during the period of intake, a return to near-baseline levels as sucking ceased, a plateau at or near baseline when the infant rested and burped, and a gradual decline in tissue oxygenation from the end of the feeding until about 10 minutes after the feeding was completed. The lowest oxygenation was always recorded while the infant was sucking the bottle nipple. In breastfed infants fluctuations in tissue oxygenation from baseline were minimal, as opposed to the large declines from baseline that occurred during bottle-feeding. Breastfeedings generally lasted longer than bottle-feedings; the author suggests that infants may be unable to tolerate longer bottle-feedings because fatigue results from ventilatory disruption. Temperature increases were significant during breastfeeding but not during bottle-feeding (see Fig. 10-3).

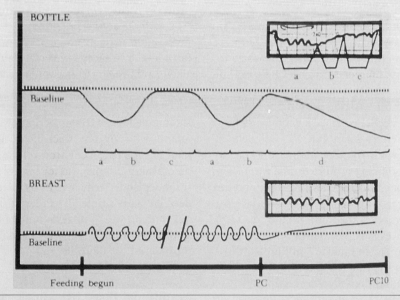

FIGURE **10-3** Schematic of typical tcPo$_2$ patterns during bottle-feeding and breastfeeding. Note in bottle-feeding (BoF) *(a)* decline, *(b)* recovery, *(c)* plateau, and *(d)* decline between end of feeding (PC) and 10 minutes postfeeding (PC10). Both schematics have been magnified somewhat for clarity. Also note interruption in the breastfeeding (BrF) line to show that BrFs were generally longer than BoFs. Inserts are from actual tcPo$_2$ recordings. *(From Meier P. Nurs Res 1988;37:36-41.)*

Continued

RESEARCH HIGHLIGHT—CONT'D

CLINICAL APPLICATION

This well-controlled study, although performed on only a few infants, looked at many feeding episodes. The dramatic difference in oxygenation while breastfeeding as opposed to bottle-feeding gives strong direction for hospital protocols. Infants should not be required to tolerate bottle-feeding before attempting breastfeeding. Caregivers and parents should recognize that breastfeeding is less disruptive to respiratory efforts and temperature is enhanced when the preterm infant is put to breast. The results from this study were similar to results in a 1997 study by Blaymore Bier and colleagues.[101]

Sleep-Wake States

Term and near-term infants are generally fed when they exhibit early feeding cues, which occur when they are in the quiet alert state. This may or may not be appropriate for infants who are very preterm, however.

First, infants who are very preterm simply sleep more than other infants,[56] both immediately after birth and throughout the neonatal period.[57] On day 1, preterm infants sleep an average of 17.57 hours, compared with term infants who sleep 14.78 hours. The number of total hours of sleeping decreases over 28 days: Preterm infants sleep an average of 17.15 hours per day, and term infants sleep an average of 11.94 hours on the twenty-eighth day after birth.

Preterm infants do exhibit different behaviors when they are in different sleep-wake states, but the challenge for feeding is to recognize when the states occur. Summarizing landmark studies, Medoff-Cooper explains that "Generally, behavioral states in preterm infants are less well defined and lack clarity while the transitions from state to state are longer, making it more difficult to recognize the beginning of one behavioral state and the ending of another"[58] (p. 65).

The sleep-wake states observable in term infants are not exactly the same as sleep-wake states found in preterm infants,[59] nor are the associated behaviors the same. Preterm infant behaviors are described in the following sections.[60]

Quiet Waking. The infant's eyes are open or opening and closing slowly. Motor activity is typically low and respiration is fairly even, but the infant may be active for brief periods when clearly alert or drowsy.

Active Waking. The infant's eyes are usually open, dull, and unfocused. The infant may be fussing or crying. Motor activity varies but is typically high. During periods of high-level activity or crying, the eyes may close.

Sleep-Wake Transition. The infant shows behaviors of both wakefulness and sleep. There is generalized motor activity, and although the eyes are typically closed, they may open and close rapidly. Brief fussy vocalizations may occur.

Active Sleep. The infant's eyes are closed. Respiration is uneven and primarily costal in nature. Sporadic motor movements occur, but muscle tone is low between these movements. Rapid eye movement (REM) occurs intermittently in this state.

Quiet Sleep. The infant's eyes are closed. Respiration is relatively regular and abdominal. A tonic level of motor tone is maintained, and motor activity is limited to occasional startles, sighs, or other brief discharges.

The type of sleep that occurs also may affect feeding behavior. Over a period of at least 1 week, infants who are less than 35 weeks of gestation (and not in critical condition) have more frequent quiet waking, active waking, and sleep-wake transition episodes; the length of sleep states does decrease across time.[60,61] Preterm infants who are less than 30 weeks of gestation are less efficient at feeding when they spend greater amounts of time throughout the day in sleep states or drowsy states as opposed to alert states.[62]

Traditional Fixed Schedules

Fixed schedules are usually every 3 hours for a minimum of eight feedings per day. If the infant is very preterm or has special needs, he may be fed as often as every 2 hours, for a total of 12 feedings per day. This may be appropriate while the infant is being fed human (or artificial) milk through a bottle or a nasogastric tube. At some point, however, the goal is to help him achieve a demand feeding pattern much like that of term infants.

Modified-Demand Feedings

Infants who are preterm, LBW, or VLBW are sometimes allowed to be on a modified-demand schedule. That is, the caregiver offers feedings as frequently as the infant exhibits hunger cues, but no less frequently than some predetermined interval. Infants who are on the modified-demand schedules are evaluated for adequate volume intake and overall growth.

Preterm infants may exhibit hunger cues that are very subtle or so inconsistent that feeding only on cue results in an insufficient quantity of milk intake.[19,20] Therefore some "modified-demand" feedings are often appropriate for very preterm infants, rather than true cue-based feedings.

There is currently no clear definition for modified demand feedings for preterm infants. One report describes a model that encourages initiation of suckling when hunger cues are present and the infant is consuming a prescribed volume or "quota" of milk over a brief, predetermined interval (e.g., having the infant take in 45 ml or more over 4 hours).[63] In this model the mother uses test weights before and after feedings; if the infant does not consume his quota of milk at the breast over the specified interval, extra milk may be given as a supplement at the end of the time interval. As the infant consumes more milk, the time interval is lengthened. This is continued until there is no need for the supplemental milk (usually mother's milk). Hence, this model focuses on volume of milk that is consumed during a period of about 4 hours, as verified with test-weighing before and after feedings.

Another model of modified-demand feedings for preterm infants emphasizes offering the breast when very early feeding cues are present, having the mother wake the infant and offer the breast at that time, and completing a minimum number of feedings during a 24-hour period.[64] If the infant is taking only very small volumes of fluid, the physician prescribes a fixed volume (8 times a day for those who weigh around 1600 g or more; 12 times

for those who are smaller) and the infant is awakened at set intervals. When the infant takes about half of the prescribed volume—perhaps 20 ml of a 45 ml quota—the mother is encouraged to disregard the time and offer the breast as soon as she notes signs of her infant's wakefulness. The total volume needed over 24 hours is calculated, and the total of actual intake over the 24-hour period is assessed. The mother continues to suckle the infant whenever he appears to go from a sleep to an alert state and shows interest in feeding. Many mothers have spontaneously commented that this shift in timing is what really makes a difference to overall intake. Over a period of days, the number of feedings is reviewed. If adequate weight gains are occurring, the mother continues to offer the same number and frequency of feedings, even if the infant "forgets" to wake up and needs the mother's encouragement to achieve a sufficient number of feedings. This continues until the infant has a more mature sleep-wake pattern. Hence, this model focuses on infant behavior and the number and frequency of feedings in relation to weight gains over 24 hours (or preferably, 48 or 72 hours).

There are no published studies showing outcomes of demand or modified demand feeding regimens for preterm breastfed infants, but several have been conducted among preterm bottle-fed infants. The earliest was conducted a half-century ago[65] and is supported by more recent studies.[66-69] Some of these studies have included a few breastfed infants, but none articulate the results in terms of outcomes for the breastfed infants. However, modified demand feedings have been implemented for breastfed infants.

NUTRITIVE FEEDING BEHAVIORS OF PRETERM INFANTS

Reflexes associated with feeding appear at different points in fetal development. Sucking and swallowing occur early in gestation,[70-72] as shown in Table 10-3, but the coordination of sucking, swallowing, and breathing occurs much later. Table 10-3 describes feeding behaviors in general terms, but there are distinct differences among individuals.[73] Nonnutritive behaviors have been described in

Table **10-3** NORMAL SEQUENCE OF FETAL ORAL MOTOR DEVELOPMENT

Gestational Age	Oral-Facial Reflex
9 wk	Purposeful oral-buccal movement starts
10-14 wk	Swallow develops; by the twelfth week fluid can be swallowed by most fetuses
18-24 wk	Suckling begins to appear
24-27 wk	Gag reflex appears and becomes stronger until 40 wk; strength diminishes to that of an adult by about 6 mo of age
by 25 wk	Phasic bite reflex and transverse tongue reflex appear
32 wk	Rooting reflex appears and becomes stronger until 40 wk; this reflex disappears by 3 mo of age

From Dowling D, Danner SC, Coffey P. *Breastfeeding the infant with special needs.* White Plains, NY: March of Dimes Foundation; 1997.

some detail,[74] but nutritive behaviors have not been as well described.

Like term infants, preterm infants exhibit nutritive sucking behaviors that can be observed and quantified—number of sucks, number of sucking bursts (episodes of several consecutive sucks), swallows, and pauses between the suck/swallow reflex. Several tools have been developed to observe the efficiency of breastfeeding for term infants, but only one has been developed for preterm infants. The Preterm Infant Breastfeeding Behavior Scale (PIBBS), developed by Nyqvist and colleagues,[75] as shown in Table 10-4, allows the observer to score the infant's rooting, areolar grasp, latch-on, suckling, longest suckling burst, and swallowing.

Unlike term infants, whose feeding behaviors are, by definition, "mature," preterm infants have feeding behaviors that mature over time. In bottle-fed infants, these behaviors, described as *progressive* as the infant gains more experience in suckling, have been delineated as immature, transitional, or mature. Initially, preterm infants have an immature suck-swallow pattern that consists of frequent mouthing and short sucking bursts; swallows and long pauses[56] occur between the sucking bursts.[76] After they have more experience, an increased number of sucks and sucking bursts occur. Then they exhibit a pattern wherein bursts of 5 to 10 sucks occur along with occasional bursts of greater than 10 sucks per sucking burst.[77,78] Finally, a pattern that more closely resembles that of term infants is exhibited: a more rhythmic suck-swallow pattern, with up to 30 consecutive sucks per burst and frequent swallows, with a sequential coordination of suck-swallow-breath.[79,80] Maturation of

oral motor skills occurs over time.[81] Also, it appears that maternal awareness and assistance can help develop infant feeding skills.[82]

Detailed studies describing the development of nutritive behavior have been conducted in Sweden by Nyqvist and her colleagues.[83] They described breastfeeding behavior in terms of gestational age (GA) and postmenstrual age (PMA). (*GA* refers to the number of weeks in utero since the last menstrual period; *PMA* refers to the number of weeks since the mother's last menses and is often used to describe extrauterine maturational level. PMA is equivalent to corrected age.) They showed that infants can initiate breastfeeding as early as 27.9 weeks PMA, although some delayed until 35.9 weeks PMA. Regardless of their GA, infants responded by rooting and inefficient suckling on the first contact with the mother's breast. Efficient rooting, areolar grasp, and latch-on were observed at 28 weeks PMA. Repeated bursts of 30 or more sucks were observed at 32 weeks PMA. Nutritive suckling, defined as intake of at least 5 ml as verified by test-weighing before and after the feeding, occurred as early as 30 weeks PMA. Of the 71 singletons in the study, 57 (80%) were able to achieve full, direct breastfeeding at a mean of 36 weeks PMA (range of 33.4 to 40.0 weeks PMA). The large range of variability in the time required for individuals to exhibit certain feeding behaviors on the PIBBS or to achieve full breastfeeding leads to the question of what factor or factors are associated with such achievements.

Surprisingly, breastfeeding behavior and establishment of full breastfeeding were not entirely explained by gestational age. Rather, a short gestation was associated with a high PIBBS score during

Table 10-4   PRETERM INFANT BREASTFEEDING BEHAVIOR SCALE (PIBBS)

Scale Items	Maturational Steps	Score
Rooting	Did not root	0
	Showed some rooting behavior	1
	Showed obvious rooting behavior	2
Areolar grasp (how much of the breast was inside the baby's mouth)	None, the mouth only touched the nipple	0
	Part of the nipple	1
	The whole nipple, not the areola	2
	The nipple and some of the areola	3
Latched on and fixed to the breast	Did not latch on at all so the mother felt it	0
	Latched on for ≤5 min	1
	Latched on for 6-10 min	2
	Latched on for ≥11-15 min	3
Sucking	No sucking or licking	0
	Licking and tasting, but no sucking	1
	Single sucks, occasional short sucking bursts (2-9 sucks)	2
	Repeated short sucking bursts, occasional long bursts (≥10 sucks)	3
	Repeated (≥2) long sucking bursts	4
Longest sucking burst	1-5 consecutive sucks	1
	6-10 consecutive sucks	2
	11-15 consecutive sucks	3
	16-20 consecutive sucks	4
	21-25 consecutive sucks	5
	≥26 30 consecutive sucks	6
Swallowing	Swallowing was not noticed	0
	Occasional swallowing was noticed	1
	Repeated swallowing was noticed	2

From Nyquist KH et al. *Early Hum Dev* 1999;55:252.

weeks 32 to 37 PMA; it appears that latch-on and suckling and swallowing are probably more influenced by the early exposure to the breast than to the infant's gestational age.[84] This provides evidence that breastfeeding should be initiated as soon as the infant can be transferred from the warmer and maintain cardiorespiratory stability.

A most interesting case study[85] shows how one infant, born at 27 weeks and 4 days and weighing 1177 g, was first given the opportunity to suckle when she was 11 days old (i.e., exactly 29 weeks PMA). The mother was shown how to observe for subtle cues that her infant was displaying (including approach/avoidance behaviors), and the infant was able to take in 11 ml of her mother's milk.

Intake, a prominent worry among mothers of preterm infants described later in the chapter,

should be observed and the results communicated to mothers. Beginning at 30 weeks PMA, infants can take at least 5 ml while suckling at the breast, and at 32 weeks PMA, they can take about 80% of the prescribed volume of milk. Full, direct breastfeeding can be accomplished as early as 33 weeks PMA.[86]

In a separate but related study, Nyqvist and colleagues described the sucking and sucking bursts among 26 preterm infants.[87] The infants were from 32.1 to 37.1 weeks PMA and were clinically stable, with no history of significant disease. The investigators looked at the number of sucks per sucking burst, the length of sucking bursts, the intensity of sucks, and the duration of the sucks. Infants had a mean number of 8 sucks per burst (range of 2 to 33 sucks per burst), with the longest sucking bursts having a median of 28 sucks (with a range of 5 to 96 sucks). Duration of sucking was from 0.6 to

1.1 seconds. Interestingly, this study showed that clinical observation (the nurse counting and timing) was not significantly different from the results reported with electromyography.

STRATEGIES TO PROMOTE DIRECT BREASTFEEDING

Direct breastfeeding may not be immediately possible for the infant who is VLBW or ELBW. The goal, however, is to achieve direct breastfeeding for these infants by the time they reach 38 weeks' corrected age or sooner. When newborns are finally free from monitoring and other devices, they need tactile, kinesthetic, and auditory stimulation.[88] Breastfeeding meets all of these needs, usually simultaneously. The first breastfeeding sessions may consist of little more than rooting and nuzzling the mother's breast. The aim, however, is to gradually increase the amount of milk consumed directly at the breast so that, eventually, the entire feeding is accomplished through direct breastfeeding. (Indirect breastfeeding—providing human milk through some indirect means—may supplement the direct breastfeeding for a while.) To achieve full, direct breastfeeding, a few strategies need to be used. Recognizing and responding to the infant's behaviors and capabilities are strategies that facilitate this goal.

Recognizing Infant State and Readiness to Suckle

Central nervous system functions that regulate behavioral states are not mature until the infant reaches full term. Consequently, preterm infants do not have clearly defined sleep-wake states or hunger-satiety behaviors like term infants. Infants who are only a few weeks preterm may exhibit subtle or inconsistent cues of wakefulness or hunger when they awaken, whereas those born several weeks before term often "forget" to wake up unless they are stimulated to do so. In either case, mothers need to be taught to observe for the very early signs of hunger, including those listed in Chapter 7, but also some that are less well recognized, such as when the infant is slightly squirming or raising his

eyebrows. When these signs occur, mothers need to gently employ the alerting techniques[89] described in Box 7-1 and offer the breast.

Achieving Optimal Milk Transfer and Intake

Suckling directly at the breast—direct breastfeeding—is certainly the goal to be achieved. To achieve optimal milk transfer and intake, however, infants need to obtain an adequate seal, adequate negative pressure, and an adequate suckling mechanism, as described in Chapter 11. Preterm infants often have difficulty achieving this because their neuromuscular function is underdeveloped. However, most of these problems can be overcome or minimized by using special positioning techniques.

Special Positioning Techniques

Any position can certainly be used for the preterm infant. However, because the preterm infant is often hypotonic and because muscles that extend his neck are more well developed than those that flex his neck, it is often best to use a position that allows the mother to better support the infant's head. The so-called cross-cradle hold or transitional hold, shown in Fig. 10-4, is often very helpful with these infants, as is the football hold. Both of these positions enable the mother to support the infant's head with her hand, and her wrist can then be used to direct a slight gentle pressure of the infant's body toward her breast. These positions can help compensate for the infant's hypotonia and provide a little more stability to prevent loss of a good seal on the nipple/areola. A pillow or two helps the infant avoid "reaching" for the breast. This minimizes muscle exertion and helps the neck to be flexed, rather than extended, which is imperative for achieving a good seal.

Special Latch-On Techniques

Negative pressure is often inadequate when preterm infants suckle, and therefore the nipple/areola complex is not held in place. Inadequate negative pressure can sometimes be overcome by grasping the infant's cheeks, as shown

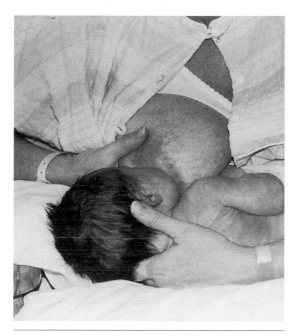

FIGURE **10-4** Transitional hold, sometimes also called the cross-cradle hold. *(Copyright Kay Hoovor.)*

in Fig. 11-15. The Dancer hand, so named for nurse midwife Sarah Coulter Danner and the late Dr. Edward Cerutti, is accomplished by having the mother form a "cup" with her hand; she then holds the breast with the lower fingers and the infant's cheeks with her thumb and forefinger, as shown in Fig. 11-15. This hold is helpful for the newborn who needs a little extra help getting an adequate seal around the breast. This may include preterm infants, or infants with craniofacial defects, as described in Chapter 11. Sometimes, the infant needs chin support only, as shown in Fig. 11-14; this is a variation of the Dancer hand.

Although chin support has not been studied among preterm breastfed infants, it has been helpful for bottle-fed preterm infants.[90] There are no published reports of positioning at the breast that enhance latch-on for preterm infants. However, clinical experience has shown that some strategies appear to be effective.

Especially large breasts or long nipples—a significant problem for term infants—are particularly problematic for preterm infants who have a very small mouth. To minimize problems with the long nipples, help the infant to open wide. This is best accomplished by brushing his lips with the mother's nipple when he is on the verge of the quiet alert state but still a little sleepy.

Nipple shields (see Fig. 12-2) have been reported to significantly increase the amount of milk that a preterm infant can transfer to himself.[18] A closer look at the study methodology, however, casts doubt on this correlation. First, infants included in the study were those who were having difficulty latching on, and no other attempts to correct latch-on were reported. Second, the subjects—really part of a larger study—received the intervention when the nurse "felt they would increase the volume of milk consumed," which introduced the potential for experimental bias. There was no control group. The 34 infants served as their own controls, but only two measurements were reported: milk intake during one feeding with the shield and milk intake during the next feeding without the shield. (N.B.: the comparison was shield/no-shield, but never no-shield/shield.) When the ultrathin silicone nipple shield was used, overall mean milk transfer was significantly greater (18.4 ml versus 3.9 ml; $p <$ .0001). The explanation for the greater milk intake was that "negative pressure appears to be generated in the small chamber between the tip of the maternal nipple and the interior of the shield"[18] (p. 111). This explanation is inadequate, however, because negative pressure was never measured and principles of physics do not support such an explanation. The more likely explanation is that the shield, which has some texture in comparison to the bare skin, offers some resistance to slippage, so it is likely that the infant was able to attain a better seal and thereby show a better intake.

Developing a Plan to Achieve Full, Direct Breastfeeding

A plan to achieve full, direct breastfeeding involves not only the special positioning and latch-on techniques previously mentioned but also a methodic plan to move towards full, direct breastfeeding. Such a plan is described in Chapter 14. An integral part of that plan is kangaroo care, which is beneficial not only as a means to facilitate direct breastfeeding but also for a variety of physiologic and psychologic reasons, as described in Chapter 14. Hypothermia, for which the preterm infant is particularly at risk, is less likely if kangaroo care is implemented. The preterm infant who is exposed to many nosocomial pathogens in the critical care environment has the benefit of his mother's specific antibodies when he is held skin-to-skin.

Verifying Milk Transfer and Adequate Intake

Milk transfer must be verified. For infants who suck a bottle, determining milk intake is a fairly simple matter; the amount of milk that is left in the container after a feeding is simply subtracted from the amount that was originally poured into the container. For infants who suckle their mother's breasts, however, there is no "window" to see how

RESEARCH HIGHLIGHT

Kangaroo Care Improves Outcomes, Including Continuation of Breastfeeding

Citation: Charpak N, Ruiz-Pelaez JG, Figueroa de CZ et al. A randomized, controlled trial of kangaroo mother care: results of follow-up at 1 year of corrected age. *Pediatrics* 2001;108:1072-1079.

FOCUS

In Botagá, Colombia, Charpak and colleagues conducted a randomized clinical trial of kangaroo mother care (KMC) and traditional care for infants who weighed less than 2000 g at birth. After infants who were ineligible for the study because of severe clinical conditions (e.g., encephalopathy, bronchopulmonary dysplasia) were excluded, 777 were randomized to receive KMC or traditional care. Upon discharge, infants in the KMC group were held in an upright position attached for 24 hours a day to their mother's (or another caregiver's) chest until they no longer accepted the kangaroo position. Follow-up visits were done at 1, 3, 6, 9, and 12 months of corrected age.

RESULTS

Growth index of head circumference was significantly greater in the KMC group, but developmental indices were similar to the infants in the traditional group. Infants who weighed less than 1500 g at birth and were given KMC were discharged earlier than those who were given traditional care. Although the incidence of infection was about the same, the severity

was less among KMC infants. Cumulative mortality was always lower in the KMC group, and the measurements of mortality at 3 and 9 months almost reached statistical significance. Continuation of any breastfeeding was more likely among participants in the KMC group at 3 months, but continuation of exclusive breastfeeding was about the same between the groups throughout the study period.

STRENGTHS, WEAKNESSES OF THE STUDY

Randomization and a large study population were major strengths of this study. Also, investigators made a clear distinction between exclusive and partial breastfeeding so that readers could draw appropriate conclusions.

CLINICAL APPLICATIONS

Consistent with other studies, the results of this study show the efficacy of KMC for low-birth-weight infants, who pose a significant public health problem throughout the world. Whether in low-income countries where technology is often unavailable or in high-income countries where technology is depended upon, KMC can be used as a therapeutic intervention for low-birth-weight infants. Technology, while appropriate in some circumstances, is not always superior to simple interventions, such as KMC, in facilitating better clinical outcomes.

much was in the breast before the feeding, and hence there needs to be some way to accurately determine the volume of milk that the infant consumed. In addition, some infants are not sucking or suckling; there needs to be some way to evaluate milk intake for them, too.

Schanler and colleagues[21] delineate five methods to evaluate milk intake: (1) observing the infant's suck and swallow, (2) observing maternal perceptions of the milk-ejection reflex, (3) determining the degree of change in breast fullness, (4) pulling back on an indwelling orogastric tube to measure gastric milk volume, and (5) test-weighing. They point out that the first three methods are somewhat subjective and that the faster motility rates that occur with human milk feedings[91] may result in underestimation of intake. They propose that test-weighing is most accurate. With use of the electronic scales, test-weighing allows accurate determination of the infant's intake, understanding that 1 g of weight gain is approximately equal to 1 ml of intake.

Test-Weighing

Test-weighing—weighing the infant before and after the feeding—was not helpful a few decades ago when nurseries had only a balance scale on which to weigh the infants. Now, however, with electronic scales, often accurate to within 2 g, test-weights can be carried out with meaningful results. Estimations by experienced clinicians and mothers are inaccurate when compared to the test-weighings.[19,20]

Clinicians who fear that it may cause mothers undue anxiety have sometimes objected to test-weighing. In clinical practice, certainly, it is not uncommon to notice that mothers give messages that indicate that their "performance" is being evaluated, but so far, the evidence to support or refute these clinical observations is unclear. Studies conducted among women who have been discharged from the hospital have shown that some women felt reassured by the test-weights.[17] Whether these results can be extrapolated to mothers of hospitalized infants, however, has not been proven; these women have infants who are much more vulnerable, and it may be that test-weighings do add to their anxiety. In any event,

test-weighing should certainly not be done routinely, and a clear indication for the need for test-weighing should be established.

Appropriate Weight Gains

Appropriate weight gains for preterm infants have not yet been documented in research studies.[92] However, in general, the AAP has recommended that the rate of intrauterine growth is a desirable goal for the preterm infant.[93] Ongoing evaluation of infant weight after hospital discharge is essential, however, along with other nutritional parameters. Table 10-5 shows values that are helpful for assessment of growth and nutritional status. Weight gain, of course, is related to overall energy and nutrient intake.

Energy and Nutrient Intake

It is imperative for infants to take in enough food energy to maintain metabolism and grow, as described earlier. Preterm infants who are suckling their mothers' breasts are particularly vulnerable to not consuming enough calories, because often, they are too tired to get the energy-rich hindmilk that they would obtain at the end of the feeding. A few strategies can be used to overcome this. First, if infants are getting any of their mother's milk via indirect feedings, the milk can be tested for creamatocrit. *Creamatocrit*, a term originally coined by

Table **10-5** ASSESSMENT OF GROWTH AND NUTRITIONAL STATUS*

Characteristic	Values Indicating Deficiency
Growth	
Weight	< 25 g/day
Length	< 1 cm/wk
Head circumference	< 0.5 cm/wk
Biochemical measurements	
Phosphorus	< 4.5 mg/dl
Alkaline phosphatase	> 450 IU/L
Urea nitrogen	< 5 mg/dl
Transthyretin (prealbumin)	< 10 mg/dl
Retinol binding protein	< 2.5 mg/dl

From Hall RT. *Pediatr Clin North Am* 2001;48:455.
*Four to six weeks posthospital discharge in preterm infants ≤34 weeks of gestation or ≤1800 g birth weight.

Lucas,[94] is the percentage of fat that is in the milk. Originally, this was determined only by health care providers, but more recently, mothers themselves have been able to accurately determine the cream-atocrit of their milk.[95] Some infants have clear intake deficits in the first few weeks.[96]

Alternatively, infants can be allowed to suckle at the breast until they tire, and then they can be given the hindmilk by gavage. If infants are making poor weight gains, the physician may prescribe the hindmilk only[97] (accomplished by having the mother express the foremilk into one container, and then expressing the hindmilk into a separate container).

DISCHARGE PLANNING

The adage that discharge planning should begin at the time of admission is often ignored when it comes to feeding issues. In some cases, discharge is planned to occur within a few hours or already in progress and someone finally realizes that the infant has yet to be suckled at his mother's breast (personal observation). The shear mechanics of getting the infant to suckle so that the expert observer can be certain that milk transfer is actually occurring is often impossible. (For example, the mother has arranged for transportation home, and her "ride" as arrived.) The ethics of this situation, however, are disturbing. In some cases, infants are knowingly sent home with the primary means of nutrition being accomplished by gavage, and yet there is no evidence to support the efficacy of this practice. Raddish and Merritt[98] suggest that discharge of preterm infants should be evidence-based using clearly established criteria. They also point out that several questions related

---

Box 10-3 Discharge Planning Priorities for the Low-Birth-Weight Infant: Feeding Issues

- Be certain that someone who can accurately evaluate breastfeeding has observed at least one (preferably more) successful feeding directly at the breast before discharge.
- Give parents a clear message about feedings at home in terms of what, how, how often, and how much to offer.
- Give parents clear, written directions about signs of adequate intake and output, and what to do if either is inadequate.
- Set a plan in motion for infants who are discharged when they are not yet exclusively breastfeeding. These infants and their mothers need follow-up to facilitate direct, exclusive breastfeeding.
- When possible, arrange follow-up with a pediatrician, clinic, or community health nurse that facilitates convenient follow-up and weight checks that will be done on the same scale in the place where the next weight check is most likely to take place, which includes the home.
- Recognize that the infant and his parents may live many miles from the tertiary care facility where he has been hospitalized. Hence, parents cannot quickly or conveniently return for advice, follow-up, or replacements.

- Make sure that milk fortifier or special formula (e.g., Neosure) is available locally for infants for whom it has been prescribed. Often, this is not in stock, so before discharge, make sure it has been ordered through a pharmacy near the family's home. If possible, provide the family with a few "doses" that they can take with them when the infant is discharged.
- If it is prescribed, teach the parent how to mix the formula. (The special formulas are usually not available to consumers in the ready-to-feed bottles.)
- Help parents anticipate and solve possible problems with equipment that may be required for feeding after discharge. For example, if the infant is discharged with an indwelling nasogastric tube, teach the parents how to reinsert the tube if it becomes dislodged and how to check for proper placement. Similarly, if an infant is using the Haberman feeder (see Chapter 16), warn parents that if no milk comes out of the bottle, it is probably because the filter is worn out or dislodged.
- Be certain that the mother can identify at least three people who will be available and supportive of her efforts to breastfeed.

to feeding issues are unanswered, including the following:

- How is nutrition best provided while transitioning to home?
- In infants whose mothers desire exclusive breastfeeding, should gavage feeds be used to supplement to avoid bottle-feedings?
- How long should human milk be fortified and when should supplemented artificial milks be used and for what period of time postdischarge should these more expensive special-discharge artificial milks be used?
- What other supplements, such as inositol, vitamins, or antioxidants, should be provided to achieve optimal growth and development?

These and other questions remain. However, it is advisable to establish clear priorities for discharging the infant that reflect the AAP's statement on discharge for the high-risk neonate[99] (Box 10-3). Discharge planning should include a plan for full breastfeeding. Such a plan is described in Chapter 14.

After hospital discharge, mothers of term infants often wonder if they "have enough" milk, but mothers of preterm infants worry about whether the infant is "getting enough" milk.[17] These are two separate and distinguishable concepts, and discharge planning should reflect a plan to deal with the latter for mothers of preterm infants.

SUMMARY

Suckling directly at the breast may be difficult or even impossible for infants who are born several weeks before term. Basic feeding decisions, including what the infant should be fed as well as how and how often to feed, should be made with the underlying conviction that breastfeeding and human milk are optimal for preterm infants. Nutritive feeding behaviors of preterm infants can be somewhat different from those exhibited by term infants, and an understanding of these behaviors—by both the caregivers and the parents—helps optimize the suckling experience when it does occur. Strategies for promoting direct suckling of the breasts should be based on the existing body of research and should reflect an understanding of both the infant's capabilities and limitations.

REFERENCES

1. American Academy of Pediatrics and the American College of Obstetrics and Gynecology. *Guidelines for perinatal care.* 4th ed. Elk Grove Village, IL: American Academy of Pediatrics; 1997.
2. Battaglia FC, Lubchenco LO. A practical classification of newborn infants by weight and gestational age. *J Pediatr* 1967;71:159-163.
3. Als H, Lawhon G, Duffy FH et al. Individualized developmental care for the very low-birth-weight preterm infant. Medical and neurofunctional effects. *JAMA* 1994;272:853-858.
4. Als H. Developmental care in the newborn intensive care unit. *Curr Opin Pediatr* 1998;10:138-142.
5. Mouradian LE, Als H, Coster WJ. Neurobehavioral functioning of healthy preterm infants of varying gestational ages. *J Dev Behav Pediatr* 2000;21:408-416.
6. Biancuzzo M. Breastfeeding preterm twins: a case report. *Birth* 1994;21:96-100.
7. Lefebvre F, Ducharme M. Incidence and duration of lactation and lactational performance among mothers of low-birth-weight and term infants. *Can Med Assoc J* 1989;140:1159-1164.
8. Ellerbee SM, Atterbury J, West J. Infant feeding patterns at a tertiary-care hospital. *J Perinat Neonat Nurs* 1993;6:45-55.
9. Ryan AS. The resurgence of breastfeeding in the United States. *Pediatrics* 1997;99:E12.
10. Kavanaugh K, Meier P, Zimmermann B et al. The rewards outweigh the efforts: breastfeeding outcomes for mothers of preterm infants. *J Hum Lact* 1997;13:15-21.
11. Bell EH, Geyer J, Jones L. A structured intervention improves breastfeeding success for ill or preterm infants. *MCN Am J Matern Child Nurs* 1995;20:309-314.
12. Meier PP, Engstrom JL, Mangurten HH et al. Breastfeeding support services in the neonatal intensive-care unit. *J Obstet Gynecol Neonatal Nurs* 1993;22:338-347.
13. Pinelli J, Atkinson SA, Saigal S. Randomized trial of breastfeeding support in very low-birth-weight infants. *Arch Pediatr Adolesc Med* 2001;155:548-553.
14. Killersreiter B, Grimmer I, Buhrer C et al. Early cessation of breast milk feeding in very low birthweight infants. *Early Hum Dev* 2001;60:193-205.
15. Nyqvist KH, Ewald U. Successful breast feeding in spite of early mother-baby separation for neonatal care. *Midwifery* 1997;13:24-31.
16. Hill PD, Ledbetter RJ, Kavanaugh KL. Breastfeeding patterns of low-birth-weight infants after hospital discharge. *J Obstet Gynecol Neonatal Nurs* 1997;26:189-197.
17. Kavanaugh K, Mead L, Meier P et al. Getting enough: mothers' concerns about breastfeeding a preterm infant after discharge. *J Obstet Gynecol Neonatal Nurs* 1995;24:23-32.
18. Meier PP, Brown LP, Hurst NM et al. Nipple shields for preterm infants: effect on milk transfer and duration of breastfeeding. *J Hum Lact* 2000;16:106-114.

19. Meier PP, Engstrom JL, Fleming BA et al. Estimating milk intake of hospitalized preterm infants who breastfeed. *J Hum Lact* 1996;12:21-26.

20. Meier PP, Engstrom JL, Crichton CL et al. A new scale for in-home test-weighing for mothers of preterm and high risk infants. *J Hum Lact* 1994;10:163-168.

21. Schanler RJ, Hurst NM, Lau C. The use of human milk and breastfeeding in premature infants. *Clin Perinatol* 1999;26:379-398.

22. Lucas A, Fewtrell MS, Morley R, et al. Randomized outcome trial of human milk fortification and developmental outcome in preterm infants. *Am J Clin Nutr* 1996;64:142-151.

23. Lau C. Effects of stress on lactation. *Pediatr Clin North Am* 2001;48:221-234.

24. Committee on Nutrition, American Academy of Pediatrics. *Pediatric nutrition handbook.* 4th ed. Elk Grove Village, IL: American Academy of Pediatrics; 1998.

25. Rigo J, De Curtis M, Pieltain C et al. Bone mineral metabolism in the micropremie. *Clin Perinatol* 2000;27:147-170.

26. Yu VY. Enteral feeding in the preterm infant. *Early Hum Dev* 1999;56:89-115.

27. Kaempf DE, Linderkamp O. Do healthy premature infants fed breast milk need vitamin E supplementation: alpha- and gamma-tocopherol levels in blood components and buccal mucosal cells. *Pediatr Res* 1998;44:54-59.

28. American Academy of Pediatrics. Work group on breastfeeding. Breastfeeding and the use of human milk. *Pediatrics* 1997;100:1035-1039.

29. American College of Obstetricians and Gynecologists. *ACOG Educational Bulletin #258. Breastfeeding: Maternal and infant aspects.* Washington, DC: ACOG; 2000.

30. Lawrence RA. Breastfeeding support benefits very low-birth-weight infants. *Arch Pediatr Adolesc Med* 2001;155:543-544.

31. Atkinson SA, Bryan MH, Anderson GH. Human milk: difference in nitrogen concentration in milk from mothers of term and premature infants. *J Pediatr* 1978;93:67-69.

32. Atkinson SA. Human milk feeding of the micropremie. *Clin Perinatol* 2000;27:235-247.

33. Anderson DM, Williams FH, Merkatz RB et al. Length of gestation and nutritional composition of human milk. *Am J Clin Nutr* 1983;37:810-814.

34. Uauy R, De Andraca I. Human milk and breast feeding for optimal mental development. *J Nutr* 1995;125:2278S-2280S.

35. Lucas A, Morley R, Cole TJ et al. Breast milk and subsequent intelligence quotient in children born preterm. *Lancet* 1992;339:261-264.

36. Hoffman J. Congenital heart disease: incidence and inheritance. *Pediatr Clin North Am* 1990;37:25-43.

37. Crawford M. Placental delivery of arachidonic and docosahexaenoic acids: implications for the lipid nutrition of preterm infants. *Am J Clin Nutr* 2000;71:275S-284S.

38. Reynolds A. Breastfeeding and brain development. *Pediatr Clin North Am* 2001;48:159-171.

39. Narayanan I, Prakash K, Bala S et al. Partial supplementation with expressed breast-milk for prevention of

40. Hylander MA, Strobino DM, Dhanireddy R. Human milk feedings and infection among very low birth weight infants. *Pediatrics* 1998;102:E38.

41. Schanler RJ. Suitability of human milk for the low-birth-weight infant. *Clin Perinatol* 1995;22:207-222.

42. Straussberg R, Sirota L, Hart J et al. Phagocytosis-promoting factor in human colostrum. *Biol Neonate* 1995;68:15-18.

43. Schanler RJ. The role of human milk fortification for premature infants. *Clin Perinatol* 1998;25:645-657, ix.

44. Lucas A, Cole TJ. Breast milk and neonatal necrotising enterocolitis. *Lancet* 1990;336:1519-1523.

45. Jayanthi S, Seymour P, Puntis JW et al. Necrotizing enterocolitis after gastroschisis repair: a preventable complication? *J Pediatr Surg* 1998;33:705-707.

46. Quinlan PT, Lockton S, Irwin J et al. The relationship between stool hardness and stool composition in breast- and formula-fed infants. *J Pediatr Gastroenterol Nutr* 1995;20:81-90.

47. Vochem M, Hamprecht K, Jahn G et al. Transmission of cytomegalovirus to preterm infants through breast milk. *Pediatr Infect Dis J* 1998;17:53-58.

48. Hamprecht K, Maschmann J, Vochem M et al. Epidemiology of transmission of cytomegalovirus from mother to preterm infant by breastfeeding. *Lancet* 2001;357:513-518.

49. Hodge D, Puntis JW. The use of expressed breast milk for the premature newborn. *Clin Nutr* 2000;19:75-77.

50. Newell SJ. Enteral feeding of the micropremie. *Clin Perinatol* 2000;27:221-234.

51. Schanler RJ, Shulman RJ, Lau C et al. Feeding strategies for premature infants: randomized trial of gastrointestinal priming and tube-feeding method. *Pediatrics* 1999;103:434-439.

52. Meier P. Bottle- and breast-feeding: effects on transcutaneous oxygen pressure and temperature in preterm infants. *Nurs Res* 1988;37:36-41.

53. Meier P, Anderson GC. Responses of small preterm infants to bottle- and breast-feeding. *Am J Matern Child Nurs* 1987;12:97-105.

54. Chen CH, Wang TM, Chang HM et al. The effect of breast- and bottle-feeding on oxygen saturation and body temperature in preterm infants. *J Hum Lact* 2000;16:21-27.

55. Dowling DA. Physiological responses of preterm infants to breast-feeding and bottle-feeding with the orthodontic nipple. *Nurs Res* 1999;48:78-85.

56. Hack M, Muszynski SY, Miranda SB. State of awakeness during visual fixation in preterm infants. *Pediatrics* 1981;68:87-92.

57. Ardura J, Andres J, Aldana J et al. Development of sleep-wakefulness rhythm in premature babies. *Acta Paediatr* 1995;84:484-489.

58. Medoff-Cooper B, McGrath JM, Bilker W. Nutritive sucking and neurobehavioral development in preterm infants

infection in low-birth-weight infants. *Lancet* 1980;2:561-563.

from 34 weeks PCA to term. *MCN Am J Matern Child Nurs* 2000;25:64-70.

59. Lundqvist-Persson C. Correlation between level of self-regulation in the newborn infant and developmental status at two years of age. *Acta Paediatr* 2001;90:345-350.

60. Holditch-Davis D, Edwards LJ. Temporal organization of sleep-wake states in preterm infants. *Dev Psychobiol* 1998;33:257-269.

61. Davis DH, Thoman EB. Behavioral states of premature infants: implications for neural and behavioral development. *Dev Psychobiol* 1987;20:25-38.

62. Daniels H, Devlieger H, Casaer P et al. Feeding, behavioural state and cardiorespiratory control. *Acta Paediatr Scand* 1988;77:369-373.

63. Meier PP. Breastfeeding in the special care nursery. Prematures and infants with medical problems. *Pediatr Clin North Am* 2001;48:425-442.

64. Nyqvist KH. Personal communication. 2001.

65. Horton FH, Lubchenco LO, Gordon HH. Self-regulatory feeding in a premature nursery. *Yale J Biol Med* 1952;24:263-272.

66. Collinge JM, Bradley K, Perks C et al. Demand vs. scheduled feeding for premature infants. *J Obstet Gynecol Neonatal Nurs* 1982;11:362-367.

67. Saunders RB, Friedman CB, Stramoski PR. Feeding preterm infants. Schedule or demand? *J Obstet Gynecol Neonatal Nurs* 1991;20:212-218.

68. Pridham KF, Kosorok MR, Greer F et al. Comparison of caloric intake and weight outcomes of an ad lib feeding regimen for preterm infants in two nurseries. *J Adv Nurs* 2001;35:751-759.

69. McCain GC, Gartside PS, Greenberg JM et al. A feeding protocol for healthy preterm infants that shortens time to oral feeding. *J Pediatr* 2001;139:374-379.

70. de Vries JI, Visser GH, Prechtl HF. The emergence of fetal behaviour. I. Qualitative aspects. *Early Hum Dev* 1982;7:301-322.

71. de Vries JI, Visser GH, Prechtl HF. The emergence of fetal behaviour. II. Quantitative aspects. *Early Hum Dev* 1985;12:99-120.

72. Roodenburg PJ, Wladimiroff JW, van Es A et al. Classification and quantitative aspects of fetal movements during the second half of normal pregnancy. *Early Hum Dev* 1991;25:19-35.

73. de Vries JI, Visser GH, Prechtl HF. The emergence of fetal behaviour. III. Individual differences and consistencies. *Early Hum Dev* 1988;16:85-103.

74. Lundqvist C, Hafstrom M. Non-nutritive sucking in full-term and preterm infants studied at term conceptional age. *Acta Paediatr* 1999;88:1287-1289.

75. Nyqvist KH, Rubertsson C, Ewald U et al. Development of the preterm infant breastfeeding behavior scale (PIBBS): a study of nurse-mother agreement. *J Hum Lact* 1996;12:207-219.

76. Gryboski JD. Suck and swallow in the premature infant. *Pediatrics* 1969;43:96-102.

77. Hack M, Estabrook MM, Robertson SS. Development of sucking rhythm in preterm infants. *Early Hum Dev* 1985;11:133-140.

78. Palmer MM. Identification and management of the transitional suck pattern in premature infants. *J Perinat Neonat Nurs* 1993;7:66-75.

79. Bu'Lock F, Woolridge MW, Baum JD. Development of coordination of sucking, swallowing and breathing: ultrasound study of term and preterm infants. *Dev Med Child Neurol* 1990;32:669-678.

80. Medoff-Cooper B, Weininger S, Zukowsky K. Neonatal sucking and clinical assessment tool: preliminary findings. *Nurs Res* 1989;38:162-165.

81. Lau C, Kusnierczyk I. Quantitative evaluation of infant's nonnutritive and nutritive sucking. *Dysphagia* 2001;16:58-67.

82. Lau C, Schanler RJ. Oral motor function in the neonate. *Clin Perinatol* 1996;23:161-178.

83. Nyqvist KH, Sjoden PO, Ewald U. The development of preterm infants' breastfeeding behavior. *Early Hum Dev* 1999;55:247-264.

84. Hedberg Nyqvist K, Ewald U. Infant and maternal factors in the development of breastfeeding behaviour and breastfeeding outcome in preterm infants. *Acta Paediatr* 1999;88:1194-1203.

85. Nyqvist KH, Ewald U, Sjoden PO. Supporting a preterm infant's behaviour during breastfeeding: a case report. *J Hum Lact* 1996;12:221-228.

86. Nyqvist KH. The development of preterm infants' milk intake during breastfeeding. Influence of gestational age. *J Neonatal Nurs* 2001;7:48-52.

87. Nyqvist KH, Farnstrand C, Eeg-Olofsson KE et al. Early oral behaviour in preterm infants during breastfeeding: an electromyographic study. *Acta Paediatr* 2001;90:658-663.

88. Klaus MH, Kennell JH. *Parent-infant bonding.* 2nd ed. St. Louis: Mosby; 1982.

89. McCain GC. Facilitating inactive awake states in preterm infants: a study of three interventions. *Nurs Res* 1992;41:157-160.

90. Hill AS, Kurkowski TB, Garcia J. Oral support measures used in feeding the preterm infant. *Nurs Res* 2000;49:2-10.

91. Cavell B. Gastric emptying in infants fed human milk or infant formula. *Acta Paediatr Scand* 1981;70:639-641.

92. Hall RT. Nutritional follow-up of the breastfeeding premature infant after hospital discharge. *Pediatr Clin North Am* 2001;48:453-460.

93. American Academy of Pediatrics Committee on Nutrition. Nutritional needs of low-birth-weight infants. *Pediatrics* 1985;75:976-986.

94. Lucas A, Gibbs JA, Lyster RL et al. Creamatocrit: simple clinical technique for estimating fat concentration and energy value of human milk. *Br Med J* 1978;1:1018-1020.

95. Griffin TL, Meier PP, Bradford LP et al. Mothers' performing creamatocrit measures in the NICU: accuracy, reactions, and cost. *J Obstet Gynecol Neonatal Nurs* 2000;29:249-257.

96. Embleton NE, Pang N, Cooke RJ. Postnatal malnutrition and growth retardation: an inevitable consequence of current recommendations in preterm infants? *Pediatrics* 2001;107:270-273.

97. Valentine CJ, Hurst NM, Schanler RJ. Hindmilk improves weight gain in low-birth-weight infants fed human milk. *J Pediatr Gastroenterol Nutr* 1994;18:474-477.

98. Raddish M, Merritt TA. Early discharge of premature infants. A critical analysis. *Clin Perinatol* 1998;25:499-520.

99. American Academy of Pediatrics. Committee on Fetus and Newborn. Hospital discharge of the high-risk neonate—proposed guidelines. *Pediatrics* 1998;102:411-417.

100. Charpak N, Ruiz-Pelaez JG, Figueroa de CZ et al. A randomized, controlled trial of kangaroo mother care: results of follow-up at 1 year of corrected age. *Pediatrics* 2001;108:1072-1079.

101. Blaymore Bier JA, Ferguson AE, Morales Y et al. Breastfeeding infants who were extremely low birth weight. *Pediatrics* 1997;100:E3.

Strategies for Breastfeeding the Compromised Newborn

Breastfeeding occurs within the context of the many biologic and behavioral tasks the infant must accomplish. When an infant is compromised in some way, breastfeeding, which is both a biologic and a behavioral task, is affected. The purpose of this chapter is to help the nurse manage breast-feeding within the broader context of the health-illness continuum. Pathophysiology is discussed in relation to breastfeeding (the activity) and human milk (the source of nutrition). It would not be practical to list every disease entity here, but one specific prototype is given to each class of problems to demonstrate how the infant's capabilities and limitations define his specific needs and management strategies.

ALTERATIONS IN NUTRIENT NEEDS AND SUPPLY

Nutrients—sources of energy, vitamins, and minerals—are essential for survival. Usually, the supply of nutrients that the infant ingests, digests, and absorbs is more or less equivalent to his needs. Difficulties arise when the infant's *need* for nutrients is about normal, but his net ingestion, digestion, and absorption of nutrients are insufficient. Other times, the infant has a high need (e.g., he has a higher metabolic rate), but the supply of nutrients (milk) is sufficient for an infant with normal needs.

The normal, healthy term infant requires about 90 to 120 kcal/kg/day for basal needs, growth, and activity. Energy requirements are greater, however, when infants have an increased metabolic rate. The term *metabolic rate* means "the amount of energy released in the body in a given time by catabolism. It represents energy expended for accomplishing various kinds of work. In short, metabolic rate actually means catabolic rate, or rate of energy release."[1] When certain conditions are present (infection, cardiac dysfunction, prematurity, surgery), the metabolic rate is accelerated; more energy is released to meet the increased need for nutrients to the cells. To meet these demands, these infants also need an increase in intake. Furthermore, energy—kilocalories—alone will not suffice. Compromised infants may need an increase in other nutrients, such as vitamins and minerals.

Infections

Infants who have infections require a greater amount of energy because their metabolic rate is increased.[2] Preterm infants are 10 times more likely to experience infection, and boys are more vulnerable than girls. The clinical signs and symptoms of sepsis are listed in Box 11-1; these are subtle and often overlooked. "Poor feeding" and "disinterested" behavior should not be mistaken for breastfeeding problems. These manifestations, especially when they occur in the presence of other signs of sepsis or in a newborn at risk for infection, should be reported to the primary caregiver.

Often, infants have been exposed to infections in utero, as is the case with amnionitis, endometritis, or a urinary tract infection. If so, these infants can experience respiratory distress and apnea, and hence feeding is hampered. Whether the infection was transmitted from the mother in utero or was acquired by the infant postnatally, good lines of communication among the physician, the mother, and the nursing staff will enhance breastfeeding efforts. In most cases, transmission of the infection

BOX 11-1   SIGNS OF NEONATAL SEPSIS

Signs may be subtle and nonspecific. They include the following:

- Respiratory distress
- High-pitched cry
- Lethargy
- Temperature instability (hypothermia or hyperthermia)
- Hypotonia
- Vomiting
- Jaundice
- Diarrhea
- Abdominal distention
- Poor feeding
- Apnea
- Cyanotic spells
- Seizures
- Poor perfusion
- Petechiae
- Purpura

Source: Seidel HM, Rosenstein BJ, Pathak A. *Primary care of the newborn.* 2nd ed. St. Louis: Mosby; 1997.

is not exacerbated by breastfeeding (see Chapter 13).

Alterations in Gastrointestinal Function

Alterations in gastrointestinal function cause obstruction and result in differing symptoms. (Lawrence and Lawrence discuss various disorders along with their clinical manifestations and treatment, so details of each disorder are not described here.[3]) Alterations in gastrointestinal function often result in separation from the mother, at least temporarily. Chapter 14 suggests strategies to deal with separation issues.

Some common gastrointestinal disorders affect the breastfeeding couplet, either because the diagnosis has not yet been made or because the clinical interpretations of the problem differ according to whether the infant is breastfed or bottle-fed. Problems that may not be immediately diagnosed include tracheoesophageal fistula (TE fistula) and tracheoesophageal atresia (TE atresia). Data about problems such as diarrhea and regurgitation are interpreted differently, depending on the method of feeding.

Gastroesophageal Reflux

Regurgitation occurs in about half of all infants who are 1 to 3 months old, peaks at about 4 months, and subsides by 7 months.[4] Regurgitation and gastroesophageal reflux (GER), although common in the artificially fed newborn, are possible but unlikely for the breastfed newborn. Therefore the breastfed newborn who exhibits GER requires medical evaluation. If GER does occur in breastfed infants, episodes are of significantly shorter duration than those observed in formula-fed infants.[5] Sandifer's syndrome is a rare manifestation of GER; affected children exhibit the reflux along with abnormal movements of the head, neck, and upper part of the trunk. In 65 children described in the literature, only 2 were breastfed.[6] Therefore it is unlikely that breastfed newborns who exhibit these signs have a "breastfeeding problem," and they should receive prompt medical follow-up.

Interventions for GER are initiated less frequently than parental reports of GER.[4] Current "therapy" should begin with reassurance of the parents and maternal dietary modifications.[7] If GER is left uncorrected, however, it can result in lower overall energy intakes.[8] GER is sometimes alleviated by holding the infant in an upright position.

In the breastfed infant a variation of reflux can be caused by oversupply of maternal milk. Although it is somewhat uncommon, high volumes of foremilk consumption (in relation to hindmilk) can be the cause of failure to thrive (FTT). This situation, reported by Woolridge,[9] was successfully managed by interventions that increased the transfer of hindmilk and gradually reduced the production of foremilk. (The more likely scenario, however, is that oversupply results in colic.)

Colic, Colitis, and Milk-Protein Allergy

The etiology of colic is poorly understood, but it is apparently related to a combination of biologic and psychosocial factors that lead to a fussy period each day. Typically, the fussy period—with loud crying and drawing of the legs up to the abdomen—occurs in the evening and lasts for a few hours. In addition to the behavioral symptoms, numerous other symptoms are present, including GER and persistent constipation.[10]

Unfortunately, when infants exhibit signs of colic, mothers often become fretful about breastfeeding and switch to artificial feeding. The American Academy of Pediatrics advises that infants often do not improve with the artificial feeding.[11] This switch would prove beneficial only if the infant were allergic to his mother's milk, which although possible, is highly unlikely.

Colic can occur in conjunction with maternal oversupply of milk. Typically, the infant will have made good weight gains but is fussy and irritable with watery or foamy stools that are indicative of lactose overload. Sometimes, the infant is allergic to cow-milk protein, as described in the following section.

Although it is not uncommon for breastfed infants to exhibit "colicky" behaviors, there are very few published reports of exclusively breastfed infants having proctocolitis (not to be confused with enterocolitis).[12-16] Most infants began showing symptoms around 4 weeks of age and had blood in their stools. (Since the 1940s, rectal bleeding has been associated with cow's milk ingestion.) The mean onset of colitis and rectal bleeding is 5 weeks, with a range of 1 to 8 weeks.[16]

Cow's milk protein has been implicated as a possible reason for proctocolitis and colic symptoms. Certainly, this is fathomable in infants who are consuming cow's milk–based formulas. One clinical expert, however, reports being suspicious more than 20 years ago that perhaps colic in breastfed infants is caused by the bovine protein present in milk secreted by mothers who consume dairy products.[17] More recently, it has been shown that proteins ingested by the mother are secreted in her milk.[18-20] Double-blind crossover studies have shown that bovine whey proteins could elicit symptoms of colic in breastfed and formula-fed infants.[21-23]

Some clinicians have found that eliminating the offending protein from the maternal diet is an effective way to resolve the colitis and/or colic.[12,15,17,24] In studies of 85 breastfed infants with colic, 56% of the infants had a resolution of colic symptoms after cow's milk had been strictly eliminated from the maternal diets.[25,26] If the offending protein is eliminated—either with formula substitution or dairy elimination in the maternal diet—clinical resolution of the bleeding occurs within 72 to 96 hours.[27] One study recommends about 4 days of a casein-hydrolysate formula-feeding for the infant while the mother abstains from dairy products, in preparation for reestablishing breastfeeding on the fifth day. Often, however, mothers do not seek or are not given help, colic runs its course, and breastfeeding continues.

Vomiting and Diarrhea

Vomiting, especially projectile vomiting, is not normal in the breastfed infant and requires immediate medical follow-up because it is common in disorders of the central nervous system.[28]

It is unusual for a breastfed newborn to have diarrhea. Normal stools are typically very soft. Excessively thin stools may indicate an inadequate consumption of the hindmilk. If diarrhea is observed in the infant, prompt referral for medical diagnosis and treatment is needed.

Tracheoesophageal Fistula and Tracheal Atresia

TE fistulas and tracheal atresias are rare congenital defects of the gastrointestinal tract that occur around the fourth week of gestation. During fetal development, the foregut usually lengthens and separates longitudinally, and each longitudinal portion separates to form two channels, the esophagus and the trachea. In normal development (1) both proximal and distal segments of the esophagus *connect* to the stomach, and (2) the esophagus completely *separates* from the trachea or bronchus.

When these two channels do not separate properly, a *fistula* and/or *atresia* results. A TE fistula is an abnormal opening between the trachea and the esophagus—the trachea fails to separate from the esophagus. An atresia is an abnormal occlusion, or discontinuous character of a channel. There are five types of atresia and fistula, as shown in Fig. 11-1. The most common situation is that in which the proximal segment of the esophagus dead-ends (an atresia) and an abnormal opening

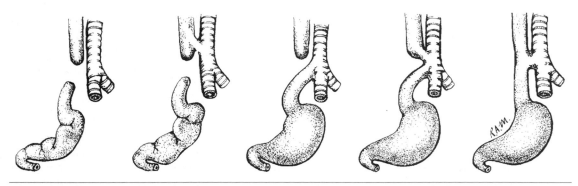

FIGURE 11-1. Five most common types of esophageal atresia and tracheoesophageal fistula. *(From Wong D:* Whaley & Wong's nursing care of infants and children. *6th ed. St. Louis: Mosby; 1999.)*

(fistula) exists between the distal segment of the esophagus and the trachea (or primary bronchus). Clinical symptoms include the following:

- Frothy saliva in the mouth and nose
- Drooling, often accompanied by choking and coughing
- Swallowing milk normally, followed by sudden coughing and gagging, with fluid returning through the nose and mouth
- Becoming cyanotic and apneic as the overflow of milk or saliva is aspirated into the trachea or bronchus, when there is a proximal esophageal pouch (most cases)[29]

Any infant who has a known or suspected TE fistula should not be put to the breast. TE fistulas are known if they are seen on ultrasound and are suspected if the mother has polyhydramnios. If the mother has polyhydramnios, a feeding tube should be passed to confirm esophageal patency before the newborn suckles. The objective is to have the infant undergo surgery as soon as possible, so feeding is contraindicated to prevent aspiration of milk, which is likely if uncorrected.

Slow Weight Gain

Slow weight gain has not been well-understood in the breastfed infant. First, some nurses and primary care providers have assumed that exclusively breastfed infants will follow the traditional National Center for Health Statistics (NCHS) reference growth curves, but studies show that they do not.[31-34] These and more recent studies[35] have shown that breastfed infants tend to be larger initially, particularly in the first 28 days.[32] Adopted in 1978 by the World Health Organization, traditional growth references were based on the NCHS data that rely on longitudinal growth studies conducted by the Fels Research Institute from 1929 to 1975. (Even when used for formula-fed children, these charts are more of a *reference* for comparison than a *standard* that the infant must achieve.[36]) Furthermore, because breastfed infants self-regulate their intake, they ingest less than bottle-fed cohorts, and they tend to have a lower metabolic rate than formula-fed infants, so no apparent adverse effects are associated with the lower intake and slower weight gain.[37] Criticized by internationally recognized experts,[38,39] the traditional growth charts have recently been replaced (see http://www.cdc.gov/growthcharts). (Oddly, however, the charts still do not address the normal growth patterns for breastfed newborns, that is, during the first 28 days.)

Adding to the mystique surrounding slow weight gain is that multiple authorities and clinicians conceptualize the problem differently. Powers[40] summarizes several conceptual schema, including those based on *rate* of weight gain,[3] chronology[41] (change in growth over time), energy balance (intake, losses, metabolic demands),[3] behavioral (content versus fretful),[42] possible etiology,[3,43] compartmental[3] (maternal milk production, infant milk intake, dyad milk transfer), occurrence (common versus rare),[40] and appearance[40] (apparently healthy versus known illness). One of the most useful frameworks, however, is that described by Lawrence and Lawrence[3] and shown in Fig. 11-2.

Some experts[3] distinguish between infants who are simply slow to gain (i.e., those who are generally healthy) and infants who have FTT. The FTT terminology can add to the confusion, however, because it has been defined generically as follows: (1) "The rate of gain in weight is less than the -2SD value during an interval of 2 months or longer for infants less than 6 months of age or during an interval of 3 months or longer for infants over 6 months of age," and (2) "the weight for length is less than the 5th percentile."[44] This definition, however, is not entirely applicable to the breastfed infant. Lawrence and Lawrence more clearly define

FTT in breastfed infants in terms of their ability to regain and maintain their birth weight and then exhibit growth.[3]

Some infants are "slow to gain." Unlike FTT infants who show worrisome signs, infants who are slow to gain generally show signs of wellness along with slow but steady progress, as shown in Table 11-1. They do gain weight, but their rate of weight gain is considerably slower than expected.

The label, however, is less important than recognizing that a problem exists, finding a root cause for the problem, and initiating corrective strategies. Sometimes, however, the nurse or other care provider does not have a clear understanding of growth in the breastfed infant, and the situation is exacerbated because the provider gives (1) no advice (or unqualified) advice to supplement; (2)

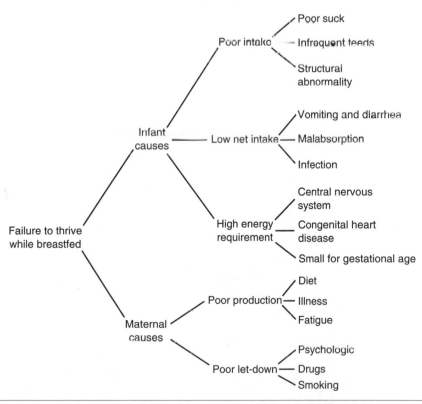

FIGURE **11-2** Diagnostic flowchart for failure to thrive. *(From Lawrence RA, Lawrence RM: Breastfeeding: a guide for the medical profession. 5th ed. St. Louis: Mosby; 1999.)*

Table 11-1 PARAMETERS FOR EVALUATION OF BREASTFED INFANTS

Infant Who Is Slow to Gain Weight	Infant with Failure to Thrive
Alert, healthy appearance	Apathetic or crying
Good muscle tone	Poor tone
Good skin turgor	Poor turgor
At least 6 wet diapers/day	Few wet diapers
Pale, dilute urine	"Strong" urine
Stools frequent, seedy (or if infrequent, large and soft)	Stools infrequent, scanty
Eight or more nursings/day, lasting 15-20 min	Fewer than 8 feedings, often brief
Well-established let-down reflex	No signs of functioning let-down reflex
Weight gain consistent but slow	Weight erratic—may lose

From Lawrence RA, Lawrence RM. *Breastfeeding: a guide for the medical profession.* 5th ed. St. Louis: Mosby; 1999.

inaccurate, useless, or inconsistent advice; (3) telephone-only advice; or (4) delayed advice. No advice is given when the parent does not initiate contact or the provider does not identify a problem. Problems also occur when the provider gives inaccurate or useless advice or when advice differs from one or more providers. For example, telling the mother to feed more frequently is useless if the breast is not being emptied and if milk transfer is not occurring, as described in Chapter 7. Telephone-only advice, although probably adequate in many cases, limits the provider to determining the follow-up, based on the history alone (as reported by the mother or, often, someone else) rather than direct observation and physical assessment. Delayed advice often results when the nurse or other provider is in the "wait and watch" mode or the "avoid supplementation at all costs" mode, and the infant becomes clinically unstable when an earlier follow-up might have prevented further problems.

Assessment. Although growth problems can occur at any time, the discussion here is focused largely on problems that occur during the neonatal period because that is the scope of this book. It is not uncommon to see growth problems in the first 3 months, however. Growth problems that occur thereafter are less common and likely to be the result of disease, if all was going well previously.

Early identification of growth problems is dependent on early, ongoing, and complete assessment. Some infants are particularly at risk for slow growth, including those who are born around 35 to 38 weeks (and are therefore treated as "term" infants), those who are preterm, and those who experience compromised status as described throughout this chapter. (Infants with structural or neurologic problems are especially at risk.) Although it is wise to schedule a follow-up visit for all newborns a few days after hospital discharge, it is imperative to do so for those who are at risk for weight-gain problems.[45]

History-Taking. A good interview and history begin when the mother walks in the door (or, perhaps, when you walk in her door at home). Questions that the provider might not have thought to ask or misleading responses to the interviewer's questions can be correctly interpreted when the skilled clinician astutely observes nonverbal behavior and the environment. For example, when one is making a home visit, walking into a room that is blue with smoke may contradict the mother who reports that she smokes two or three cigarettes per day. Or, the infant who comes into the office with a pacifier in his mouth signals the need for more vigorous inquiries about the number of feedings per day and the intervals between feedings.

Infant History. History of the infant is important. The perinatal history, including the mode of birth, Apgar scores, and similar data, can be helpful in identifying causative problems of slow weight gain. A history of sleep and output patterns is also useful.

History of feeding is especially important. Some data about frequency and duration can be obtained through the interview. (Because mothers may want to respond with the "right answer," however, direct observation of a feeding is invaluable.) Restricted feedings, long intervals, sleeping through the night, offering of water, and use of nipple shields can all be corrected by some simple interventions, as listed in Table 11-2. Frantz[46] suggests this simple mismanagement contributes substantially to weight-gain problems for the newborn.

Maternal History. A maternal history, including current and past obstetric history, medical and surgical history, family history, and psychosocial history (see Chapter 6), helps identify problems with maternal milk production, ejection, and transfer. Asking about family history of atopy can be especially important because infants who are allergic to milk proteins ingested by the mother may, as a result, have weight-gain problems. Frantz, Fleiss, and Lawrence[47] have developed an excellent history form that captures pertinent points of the mother's social and health habits, infant's behaviors, birth history, and family history. This comprehensive but easy-to-use form is shown in Fig. 11-3.

Physical Examination. A complete physical assessment of the mother and the infant is indicated when infants have slow growth. The physical assessment includes a direct observation of the breastfeeding dyad.

Maternal Physical Examination. Examination of the mother's breasts is an important component of the assessment process when the infant has slow weight gain. All of the points mentioned in Chapter 6 should be included, with special attention to breast changes (day-to-day changes that occur with lactogenesis, as well as changes in fullness of the breast before and after a feeding). Reports of sore breasts require further follow-up because mothers with sore breasts sometimes give fewer feedings or abbreviated feedings. Sore nipples have been associated with slow weight gain.[48]

Low milk supply is a likely cause of slow weight gain.[40] Factors that interfere with milk production, ejection, and transfer should be identified and modified if possible. However, lactation is not regulated by the mammary gland alone, and a complete physical examination, including examination of the thyroid, may be indicated. (Sometimes, one of the first signs of hypothyroidism is a low milk supply.)

Direct observation of the feeding provides important clues about whether the weight-gain problem is related to breastfeeding management or if instead a more serious pathologic problem is present. Absence of a good latch-on is worrisome. Similarly, subtle signs may indicate trouble. The infant who is always slightly hypothermic, for example, requires further investigation, as does the infant who seems overly fatigued while feeding. Reassuring signs should be present. Audible swallowing is a very reassuring sign that milk transfer is occurring, but if the infant has a high metabolic need, the quantity he is ingesting may sometimes be insufficient to meet that need. *Lack of audible swallowing, however, is always a worrisome sign.* Although the seriousness of FTT should not be underestimated, many problems are simple and can be easily corrected.

Infant Physical Assessment. Typically, physical assessment of the infant begins with measuring the infant's weight, length, and head circumference.[49] Weight gain is only one consideration of growth and should be considered along with other physical assessment data and measurements, including length, head circumference, and skinfold thickness. Although it is only one factor for consideration, weight loss is often the trigger for action. Unfortunately, the action is sometimes based on data that are obtained incorrectly or recorded inaccurately. Therefore a few common-sense rules bear repeating when weight discrepancies are noted:

- Weigh the infant on an electronic scale that is accurate to within 2 g. Weights obtained by using the balance scales are not completely accurate.
- Be sure that the electronic scale is in proper working order.
- Weigh using the same scale, and with approximately the same amount of clothing, each time weight is assessed. (Nude weights are generally done during at least the first month of life.)

Table **11-2** SIMPLE MISMANAGEMENT OF BREASTFEEDING A NEWBORN

Assessment	Intervention	Rationale
Mother removes infant before he is finished or adheres to a preset time guideline	Encourage mother to let infant self-limit feedings by monitoring swallows; teach swallow sounds	Breastfed newborns take 10- to 60-minute feedings, mean of 31 min; length of feeding is equal to quantity of nutritive suckle
	Explain about overdressing; may need to unwrap and wake infant to finish feeding	Overheated infants decrease suckling; swaddled newborns assume sleep state
	Switch to second breast when swallows slow or stop, and back to first breast again *if* infant is interested	Offering both breasts stimulates better milk volume; pauses may not mean newborn is finished; feeding refusal when switched may mean newborn is finished
Consistently long intervals between feedings (4 hr or more for newborn)	Feed more *often;* do not adhere to formula-fed 4-hr schedule	Breastfed newborns usually feed every 2-3 hr; some infants cluster feed after a long sleep period
	Discourage pacifier during first weeks	Desire to suckle is a survival mechanism but may indicate real need to feed; more suckling equals more milk volume
	Wake sleepy infants, feed *at least* 8 times every 24 hr	Drugs during labor, maternal postpartum drugs, or hyperbilirubinemia may cause infant to sleep *too* much
Trying to get infant to "sleep through the night" before 8-12 wk	Dispel myths that parents should promote long infant sleep periods by letting infant cry or using pacifier	Newborns need to feed throughout a 24-hour period; most do not sleep for a 6-hr stretch until 8-12 wk of age
	Tell mother "power" feedings are at night the first 3 weeks; she should rest during the day	Prolactin levels are high when mother sleeps; newborns feed best at night during the first 3 weeks
Mother offering more water than breast milk, thinking she is supposed to or because of fear of jaundice	Discontinue water for more frequent breast-milk feedings	No extra water is needed because of the lower solute load of breast milk, if the infant is feeding frequently
		Water not proven to lower bilirubin levels faster than milk feedings; bilirubin also excreted in stool with milk feedings
Mother using nipple shield	Discontinue shield Use feeding tube device if infant will not breastfeed well	Shield reduces available milk by 22%-66%

From Frantz KB. *NAACOGS Clin Issu Perinat Womens Health Nurs* 1992;3:647-655. Copyright Kittie Frantz.

No. _____
Date _____

Slow Gaining Special History

Mother

Name _____

A. Diet
    1. Do you eat regular meals? _____ How do you rate the kind of food you eat?
       excellent ❏ good ❏ poor ❏
    2. Do you take vitamins? _____ If so, what? _____
       _____
    3. Do you take brewer's yeast? _____
    4. Are you worried about your weight? _____

B. Health
    1. Are you in good health? _____ If not, describe problems _____
       _____
    2. Are you taking any medications? _____ Birth control pills? _____
       Prescriptions? _____ Nonprescription medicines? _____
    3. Have you had any thyroid problems at any time in your life? _____
       Are thyroid medications being taken now? _____ What kind? _____
       _____
       Dosage _____ Last time you had your blood tested for thyroid _____
    4. Do you have any blood pressure problems? _____

C. Habits
    1. Do you smoke? _____ Which brand? _____
       How many per day? _____
    2. Do you drink coffee? _____ How many cups per day? _____
       Do you drink caffeinated sodas? _____ How many caffeinated sodas per day? _____
    3. Do you drink alcohol? _____ How much per day? _____
       week? _____ month? _____

D. Nursing
    1. When the infant nurses, do you feel tingling ❏ burning ❏ filling feeling ❏
       leaking on other side ❏ nothing ❏
       other _____
    2. Do you have a quiet environment for nursing? _____ If not, why? (describe)
       (Example, loud music, freeway noise, dogs barking) _____
       _____
    3. Do you own a rocking chair? _____

E. Social environment
    1. Do you have a busy life-style? _____ If so, why? (name activities) _____
       _____
       _____
    2. Marriage relationship is good ❏ average ❏ poor ❏
    3. Do you have other children? _____ Ages _____
       Breastfed? _____ How long? _____
    4. Do you have any source of anxiety or tension? _____ If so, describe _____

FIGURE **11-3** Slow-gaining special history. *(From Lawrence RA, Lawrence RM:* Breastfeeding: a guide for the medical profession. *4th ed. St. Louis: Mosby; 1994.)* *Continued*

- Verify that the last weight was recorded correctly. A simple but frequent error occurs when converting metric to U.S. measurements, and vice versa.
- If a significant and otherwise unexplained discrepancy occurs, reweigh the infant. If the discrepancy still exists after double-checking, follow up with appropriate data gathering and physical assessment.

Infant

Name _____ Date of birth _____

1. How often is infant fed? _____
2. Breast milk only? _____ Other? _____
   Does he feed at each breast at each feeding? _____ How long on each breast? _____
3. How long does infant take to finish a feeding? _____ Does infant pause often during feeding? _____
4. Who initiates end of feeding? you ❑   infant ❑
5. How do you rate his sucking? poor ❑   weak ❑   average ❑   strong ❑
6. Is he burping easily? _____ What technique is used? _____
   When is he burped? _____
7. Is a pacifier used? _____ What kind? _____
   How much usage? _____
8. Number of wet diapers per day _____ Are ultra-absorbent diapers used? _____
9. Number of stools per day _____ consistency _____ color _____
10. Infant is active ❑   average ❑   placid ❑
11. Night sleep pattern: time put to bed _____ Is this on a regular basis? _____
    List awake times _____
12. Is infant healthy? _____ Any problems since birth? _____ If so, what? _____
    _____
    _____
    Jaundice? _____ How high was the bilirubin level? _____
    Had any medications? _____ If so, what? _____
13. Ever had a urinalysis? _____ When? _____
    Any other test (especially those for slow weight gain)? _____ If so, what? _____
    _____
    Where? _____

Birth history

1. Type of delivery: vaginal ❑   CS ❑   If CS, scheduled ❑   or emergency ❑?
2. Labor: yes ❑   no ❑   Length of time _____
3. Were medications given during labor or delivery? _____ If so, what? _____
   _____
4. Was it a difficult birth? _____ If so, describe problem _____
   _____
5. First time infant put to breast was _____ hr after birth. Did infant take it easily? _____
6. Where was the birth? Home birth ❑   Hospital with rooming-in ❑
   Hospital with infant only in the nursery ❑   Were you separated from infant for any length of time?_____
   If so, why? _____
   _____
7. Any medications taken during pregnancy? _____ If so, what? _____
   _____
8. Any medications taken after birth? _____ If so, what? _____
   _____

Family history

1. Have previous infants or relatives with failure to thrive? yes ❑   no ❑
2. Have history of metabolic or malabsorption disease? yes ❑   no ❑
3. Infant has cystic fibrosis? yes ❑   no ❑
4. Infant has milk allergy? yes ❑   no ❑
5. Other _____

FIGURE **11-3,** cont'd

A complete physical assessment is still needed, however; looking at growth parameters, although necessary, is not sufficient. Other assessment data may help determine whether the observed problems are the result of breastfeeding management or if they are symptoms of disease. Priorities for physical assessment include the following:

- *Vital signs:* Vital signs are indeed *vital;* if the infant's vital signs are outside of normal parameters, further follow-up is imperative. For example, hypothermia may indicate an inadequate caloric intake, hyperthermia may suggest dehydration, tachycardia may indicate a high metabolic rate, and tachypnea may be a clear sign that the infant cannot successfully eat and breathe at the same time.

- *Infant behavior:* Infants who are hyperalert or lethargic, those who are irritable or excessively sleepy, or those who are sleepy after 3 to 5 minutes of suckling may not be getting enough milk. Similarly, those who are ravenously hungry or those who are indifferent to food ("good babies") are likely to have insufficient intakes.

- *Signs of dehydration* (described in Chapter 9) result from insufficient fluid. Sunken fontanels are one of the last signs of dehydration.

- *Pathologic conditions* put the infant at risk for weight-gain problems. Also, oral-motor examination should be performed. Clefts have been known to go undetected for some time, however, so a repeat digital examination of the oral cavity is indicated if any of the following are observed: poor infant weight gain, absence of or limited audible swallowing, or persistently sore maternal nipples.

FTT may be a symptom of disease rather than a breastfeeding problem. Lukefahr lists underlying illness causing FTT in breastfed infants according to age and notes that in the newborn group, 7% had an underlying pathologic condition.[41] The take-home message is simple: Not all worrisome signs and symptoms can be corrected by better breastfeeding management; rather, they should be reported and medical follow-up should be initiated. Red flags, including those listed in Box 11-2, require clear problem identification and, if needed, referral. It is absolutely imperative to complete a thorough history and physical assessment of the mother and the infant before choosing clinical management strategies.

Box 11-2 Red Flags for Continued Growth Problems

"Red flags" that warrant follow-up include, but are not limited to, when the newborn:

- Does not have adequate intake and output (see Chapter 7)
- Has clinical signs of dehydration, regardless of age
- Has clinical signs of disease, regardless of age
- Loses ≥10% of birth weight
- Weighs less than his birth weight after 2 weeks of age
- Is preterm and has not gained in length, weight, and head circumference at approximately the same rate as he would be experiencing if he were still in utero
- Is compromised and is not ingesting, digesting, and retaining enough calories to support activity and growth (beyond basal needs)

CLINICAL SCENARIO

The Breastfed Infant Who Fails to Thrive

The pediatrician, Dr. R., calls and asks you to do a home visit for a newborn whom she has diagnosed as having failure to thrive. The newborn has no known defects, anomalies, or unusual circumstances. You arrive at an upper-middle-class home and meet a married couple in their early forties and their 3-week-old baby, Joshua. Mrs. A., a short woman, appears to be recovering from her cesarean delivery, but you notice that she has flat nipples and large breasts. She holds Joshua in a cradle position, and he arches his back, screams, and will not take the breast.

What are your first assessments for the mother-baby dyad?

What is your first intervention? Assuming that you have corrected the basic technique, what else may help?

Readers are encouraged to discuss this scenario among their colleagues because often there is no one right answer.

Clinical Management Strategies. The primary goals in cases of slow weight gain are to identify the underlying reason for the problem and to initiate corrective strategies. Breastfeeding problems require better breastfeeding management; pathologic situations require medical management. In either case, corrective strategies should be based on exact causes.

If the primary care provider determines that no pathologic condition is present, establish goals and priorities for the breastfed infant with weight-gain problems as shown in Box 11-3. Identify the two or three most pressing problems that interfere with transfer of adequate amounts of milk; correct these problems. Continue to gather data and monitor progress, and report any changes—those that are reassuring and those that are worrisome—to the primary health care provider. The overarching strategy is to provide increased food energy available to the infant (including increased maternal milk production) and increased breast emptying.

Increasing Milk Production. Use any or all of the strategies listed in Chapter 7 for the slow-gaining situation. Galactagogues should especially be considered if simpler methods are not effective. Switch-nursing, sometimes recommended, is effective *only* if the mother is taught to switch sides immediately after she feels a let-down. (The extra stimulation is good, but switch-nursing 5 minutes after let-down is counterproductive because then the infant suckles only the foremilk.)

Consider the advantages of offering the hindmilk only. The hindmilk has more than twice as many calories as foremilk, and this will aid in weight gain. This is an especially useful strategy for the infant who suckles fairly well at the beginning of the feeding but then tires easily and rarely or never gets the hindmilk. Mothers can obtain the hindmilk by expressing the foremilk into one container, and later, expressing the hindmilk into another.

Box 11-3   GOALS AND PRIORITIES FOR CARE: WEIGHT-GAIN PROBLEMS

Correct simple mismanagement: See discussion in the text. Poor latch-on or restricted feedings are common causes of weight loss in the newborn.

Ensure complete evaluation: In some cases, failure to thrive may be a symptom of a pathologic condition rather than a breastfeeding problem.

Increase milk production: The simplest intervention here is to express milk after every feeding in which the infant was unsuccessful in "emptying" the breast.

Supplement as prescribed: Exclusive breastfeeding may not be the treatment of choice for an infant who has been diagnosed with failure to thrive. This may indeed be a time when supplementing is the safest approach. Supplementation, however, does not need to occur via bottle. Several alternative feeding methods may be used (see Chapter 16).

Promote maternal food, fluid, and rest: Although milk production is not dependent on the quantity or quality of food and fluids consumed, hormonal changes that occur when the mother is having a nourishing snack before or during breastfeeding do seem to improve milk production. A woman who is well rested can more readily have a milk-ejection reflex than one who is chronically fatigued.

Facilitate interdisciplinary collaboration: Often, this is a multifactorial clinical situation that requires everyone's expertise. It is imperative, however, that everyone give the mother the same message and that the members of the health care team do not have turf battles. Clear communication, negotiation, and respect for everyone's input—especially the mother's— are essential. Scaring the mother by suggesting that she is "starving" her infant is counterproductive, but a high degree of complacency is undesirable, too.

Offer appropriate guidelines: Create a simple 3 × 5 card that lists reassuring signs on one side and worrisome signs on the other. This card should be fairly brief and should use simple words. The card should also contain the names and phone numbers of three support people (list these on the reassuring side) and the names and phone numbers of three places to call in case of an emergency.

Suggest a nursing supplementer if the infant is given human milk, donor milk, or artificial milk in addition to direct breastfeeding, because it provides extra food energy for the infant and increased stimulation for the mother.

Plan to work collaboratively with the primary health care provider, whose philosophy about supplementation may differ from your own. Avoid a turf battle; otherwise, the mother may get mixed messages about who is "right" or "wrong" about clinical management. This is no time to insist on exclusive breastfeeding. Rather, acknowledge that supplementation may be essential for sustaining life. Donor milk is the better alternative, but if it is unavailable, the benefits of artificial milk may outweigh any potential risks. Misgivings about the use of bottles and "nipple confusion" are understandable; this is a point for negotiation. Most primary health care providers prescribe only the supplementation, not the method by which it should be delivered. Help the parents weigh the advantages of several alternative feeding methods and identify one that will work (see Chapter 16). The point here is to expedite feeding—to provide adequate calories, nutrients, and fluids—not to have a philosophic discussion about the use of bottles.

Provide sensitive teaching and counseling for parents of infants with poor or slow weight gain. Discuss many assessment findings with the mother, not just weight gain or loss, or she may interpret weight-gain problems as her fault. It is extremely difficult for women to hear that their infants are not gaining weight satisfactorily; they often interpret this situation as a sign of their own inadequacy in providing nutrition for the infant. Mothers may be tempted to discontinue breastfeeding and to give a bottle instead. Handle this issue carefully. On one hand, certain circumstances may dictate that the infant receive at least some artificial milk, so if artificial milk is medically indicated, avoid giving the impression that it is "bad." On the other hand, if the mother's anxieties and frustrations have driven the decision to discontinue breastfeeding, help her overcome these negative feelings. In all cases, give practical advice for achieving milk transfer, reassure her that she is doing the right thing, and give truthful information about her infant's status. Reinforce the importance of having the infant, not the mother, control the frequency and duration of feeding.

Supplementation. Supplementation with formula meets the goal of providing increased food energy for the infant. However, it defeats the goal of getting more breast stimulation and emptying. Supplementation with the mother's own milk, therefore, would be ideal.

Powers defines supplementation for the slow-growing infant as intake other than that which the infant obtains directly at the breast.[50] If the infant is clinically stable and exhibiting hunger cues, supplementation may be unnecessary if the underlying problem can be quickly identified and a corrective strategy immediately implemented to reverse the weight lose trend. For example, this might be appropriate when a 4-day-old newborn weighs 10% less than birth weight, has had two wet diapers and no stools in the past 2 days, and dry lips but a moist tongue. The mother has small lesions on her breast and milk supply has not yet become copious. Presuming that the mother is receiving adequate instruction on breastfeeding and lactation, feeding the expressed milk is an acceptable strategy if an in-person reassessment of the infant status and maternal lactogenesis can occur within the next 24 hours.

Supplementation with expressed mother's milk or donor milk (or formula) is indicated if the clinical condition of the infant is worrisome. Supplementing the infant during the feeding (with a nursing supplementer) or after the feeding with a cup, dropper, or other device are options (see Chapters 15 and 16). In the absence of an acute problem that requires more aggressive therapy, oral feedings can be continued and the frequency of breast stimulation and emptying increased. Initially, the infant may be prescribed 50 ml/kg per day, divided into six to eight feedings, in addition to what he suckles at the breast.[50] (The amount is gradually increased according to the infant's appetite.) For example, this might be appropriate in a 19-day-old infant who is still 7% below birth weight and reportedly has 4 to 6 wet diapers, one brown bowel movement per day, suckles about 6 times a day, and sleeps through the night.

Evaluation. Never assume that strategies for improving the infant's weight gain are successful. Evaluate and reevaluate whether milk transfer is actually occurring. If it is not, the short-term goal is to "empty" the mother's breast, and the longer-term goal is to achieve effective latch-on. In the meantime, supplementation may be appropriate. Weight checks should continue on a regular basis until the problems are satisfactorily resolved. This may be every 2 days or every 7 days, depending on the severity of the problem.[40]

Test-weighing before and after feeding can certainly be done, but there are some drawbacks to doing this. First, test-weighing can make the mother feel performance-driven, which is counterproductive if she is already stressed and having difficulty experiencing a let-down. Second, the amount of milk ingested shows only what was consumed at that feeding, and because infants typically take fairly different amounts of milk from one feeding to another, this information is not reflective of a 24-hour intake pattern. In addition, test-weighing is accurate only with an electronic scale.

Other evaluations may be needed, such as general laboratory tests for the mother and/or infant, and can be used to rule out disease. Thyroid function or other endocrine tests may be ordered for the mother. Measuring maternal serum prolactin levels is rarely helpful.[40]

Cardiac Defects

The cardiovascular system has a twofold purpose: (1) to deliver oxygen and nutrients to meet the metabolic needs of every cell in the body and (2) to remove waste products such as carbon dioxide. Infants with cardiac defects have increased metabolic needs and therefore require more calories.

Infants with cardiac defects are likely to experience problems that will influence feeding practices, including low tolerance for activity and energy expenditure. Problems and goals vary slightly from one cardiac defect to another, but general goals and priorities for care are those listed in Table 11-3. Ventricular septal defects are discussed in the fol-

lowing section as a prototype to demonstrate care for the cardiac infant.

Ventricular Septal Defects

Incidence and Implications. Ventricular septal defect (VSD) is the most common congenital cardiac defect, occurring in about 25% of all cardiac defect cases. VSDs are congenital problems that result when the septum (wall) between the left and right ventricle of the heart fails to close completely at 4 to 8 weeks of gestation, creating an opening, or *communication,* between the ventricles through which blood can flow. This, of course, results in altered circulation. With a VSD, whether or not shunting occurs depends on several factors, but the size of the defect is the most important.

A small communication (less than 0.5 cm) is called *restrictive;* that is, the blood is largely restricted to one ventricle or the other and does not offer resistance to flow, and the pressures in the two ventricles may differ. Right ventricular pressure is normal, and left pressure is increased. Therefore the higher left-sided pressure may shunt blood from left to right (left-to-right shunting), but the volume of shunted blood may be minimal because the communication is so small. Small defects usually do not have clinical signs and symptoms that are immediately evident, and they are likely to be identified when the examiner auscultates the newborn's heart on routine examination. These defects often close spontaneously, and surgery is not recommended under most circumstances.

Some communications may be so large (greater than 1.0 cm) that the septum is completely absent and the infant has only one common ventricle. These larger defects are called *nonrestrictive;* that is, there is no resistance to blood flow. Here the severity and the direction of the shunting vary. These large defects result in feeding difficulties and dyspnea. The infant is usually not cyanotic—this is an acyanotic defect—but duskiness is likely to be seen, particularly when the infant feeds. A septal defect most commonly involves the membrane part of the septum, but it can involve the muscle part of the septum. In either case the size of the defect can be relatively small or large, and the size of the

Table 11-3   Possible Problems and Breastfeeding Management for Newborns with Alterations in Cardiac Function

Problem	Clinical Strategy	Rationale
Activity intolerance	Short, frequent feeds Stop feeding if signs of fatigue develop: • Cyanosis • Tachypnea • Dyspnea • Oxygen saturation below 87% • Infant takes himself off the breast but looks exhausted rather than peaceful (a well newborn who is satiated would take himself off the breast, but he looks peaceful, not exhausted) If infant exhibits the above signs for three consecutive feedings, stop feeding and call physician or primary care provider Consider using a nursing supplementer, which may conserve energy Keep drafts off the infant; place blanket over infant's back, and use skin-to-skin contact with mother	To minimize fatigue and decrease cardiac demands Infant has better chance of getting greater intake with less energy exerted Cold stress increases oxygen consumption
Tachypnea and/or dyspnea	Infant may be NPO if respiratory rate is greater than 70 (or per hospital policy); initiate gavage feeding Encourage use of human milk	To minimize risk of aspiration, as coordination of suck/swallow/breathe is more difficult Greater volume of artificial milk is needed to gain the same amount of nutrients because nutrients are better absorbed from human milk
Fluid volume excess (if congestive heart failure develops)	Monitor intake and output; consider test-weighing Explain rationale for use of powder fortifier, if ordered	Powdered milk fortifier minimizes fluid volume given
Possible hypothermia	Keep infant warm Encourage breastfeeding	Conserves oxygen and nutrients breast Milk is at body temperature, and lactating is warm

Continued

Table 11-3   POSSIBLE PROBLEMS AND BREASTFEEDING MANAGEMENT FOR NEWBORNS WITH ALTERATIONS IN CARDIAC FUNCTION—CONT'D

Problem	Clinical Strategy	Rationale
Risk for slow growth or failure to thrive	Be sure infant gets the hindmilk! "Emptying" one breast completely to get the hindmilk is better than going to both breasts, but not getting hindmilk	Rich in fat and calories
	Listen for audible swallowing	To verify milk transfer
	Monitor weight	To ensure that infant is getting enough calories, especially if the infant is fluid restricted
	Explain rationale for artificial supplementation to mother if it is ordered	Infant may not be able to get all needed nutrition from the breast
Risk for hypoxia	Encourage feeding at the breast if mother is available	Po$_2$ of oxygen is less labile when feeding at the breast, rather than using a rubber nipple
	Respond and offer other breast promptly when infant is hungry	Crying increases oxygen consumption
	Encourage intake of human milk	Iron is better absorbed from human milk than from artificial milk; Fe is necessary for O$_2$
Risk for respiratory infection	Encourage intake of human milk	Presence of immunoglobulins mobilizes infant's natural defenses and minimizes threat of infection
Risk for separation from mother	Suggest creating a supply of frozen mother's milk if infant is scheduled for surgery	To facilitate use of human milk and preserve breastfeeding relationship

defect is most influential in determining whether there is a left-to-right shunt.

Infants with cardiac defects can and should breastfeed; those with cyanotic defects will have more difficulties than those with acyanotic defects, but bottle-feeding those infants will be problematic also. Unfortunately, however, mothers of infants with cardiac defects are more likely to bottle-feed than to breastfeed.[51]

Human milk, although ideal for all infants, is especially beneficial for the infant with cardiac defects. These infants are especially vulnerable to infections, and the immunoglobulins found in human milk help protect them. Although infants with cardiac defects have an increased metabolism and often tire easily, they are not overstressed by breastfeeding. Suckling the breast is more physiologic for the newborn than feeding from the bottle. In one study in which infants served as their own controls, oxygen saturation measurements were significantly higher during breastfeeding than bottle-feeding, and none of the infants desaturated (SaO_2 less than 90%) during breastfeeding, whereas four did so during bottle-feedings.[52] Similarly, studies of preterm infants have examined the effects of breastfeeding and bottle-feeding on oxygenation in newborns.[53-55] The transcutaneous oxygen pressure ($tcPO_2$) levels decreased while bottle-feeding, but $tcPO_2$ levels returned to baseline or nearly to baseline while breastfeeding. These data form a basis for the recommendation that breastfeeding appears to pose relatively few difficulties in maintaining oxygenation, as opposed to bottle-feeding, and obliterates the myth that breastfeeding is more "work" than bottle-feeding.

Prenatal Assessment and Counseling. Thanks to advances in fetal imaging and ultrasound, including echocardiography, fairly accurate prenatal diagnosis of cardiac defects is now possible. Parents who are anticipating an infant with VSD should be told that breastfeeding is possible for their child and that suckling the breast and consuming human milk are particularly beneficial for the infant with a cardiac defect. Prenatal information should include information about anticipated feeding difficulties that the infant may experience.

Postpartum Period

Assessments. Sometimes, the VSD is not so obvious and may not be detected until the routine physical examination, or difficulties in feeding may hasten the physical examination because infants generally do become dyspneic while feeding. Newborns who have not been diagnosed with a cardiac defect may exhibit mild symptoms or difficulties; they may breastfeed immediately after birth, and these symptoms are unlikely to interfere with continued efforts to breastfeed. Newborns with more dramatic symptoms need a complete medical evaluation before further feeding—by breast or bottle—occurs. Symptoms can be subtle or severe, and the severe symptoms may indicate a life-threatening problem.

VSDs can occur as isolated defects or associated with other congenital cardiac defects. A VSD might go undetected for the first 3 or 4 days after birth, and then the infant starts to exhibit symptoms when he is home. Because feeding is the time when the infant increases his activity and hence his oxygen consumption, parents may wonder about the behavior the infant is manifesting.

Infants who have VSD occasionally experience endocarditis. Infants who have large defects may experience multiple episodes of respiratory infection and congestive heart failure. They may also experience pulmonary hypertension, which is a result of high pulmonary blood flow. Their risk for pulmonary vascular disease is prevented when surgery is performed within the first year.[56] These infants are especially at risk for FTT.

The degree of difficulty with feeding and whether or not surgery is performed vary with the type and severity of the defect. Small defects do not require surgery, and generally feeding progresses without problems. The infant may, however, show signs of difficulty. Large defects require medical management and/or surgery. The aim of medical management is to control episodes of congestive heart failure, and the goal of surgery is to prevent pulmonary vascular disease. The goal of therapeutic management is maintenance of normal growth.

Clinical Management Strategies. Mothers have reported several difficulties associated with breastfeeding an infant with a cardiac defect, including their own fatigue and anxiety, separation from their infants, and a lack of support from health care providers.[57] The infant, of course, exhibits signs of fatigue, and the mother will sometimes try to stimulate the infant to continue eating. However, feeding should be carried out with the recognition that it requires expenditure of energy for the infant. The infant should not be hurried or prodded; jiggling or prodding any infant who eats slowly is often counterproductive. The mother should be advised to terminate the feeding when the infant shows signs of being too tired to continue. These signs might include dyspnea, marked tachypnea, and/or cyanosis; in addition, when the infant stops, he looks exhausted (in contrast to the well infant, who spontaneously comes off the breast but looks peaceful).

Conclusions about Breastfeeding Management. Infants with cardiac impairment can breastfeed. The stress these infants experience relates to the expenditure of energy during the feeding. Breastfeeding, however, should be thought of as an intervention for these infants because it conserves oxygen and provides needed amounts of nutrients and antiinfective properties. With good observation skills and some very simple interventions to enhance the experience, breastfeeding can often continue with few, if any, problems.

ALTERATIONS IN NEUROLOGIC FUNCTION

Term infants often experience fluctuations in neurophysiologic responses during the transition from intrauterine to extrauterine life. After an uneventful birth, relatively common alterations, such as hypothermia and hypoglycemia (as described in Chapter 9), are merely a result of the normal newborn's adaptation to extrauterine life and have little effect on breastfeeding.

Newborns may also have transient alterations in neurologic status related to unfavorable perinatal events. Hypoxic-ischemic brain injury, resulting in birth asphyxia and later some residual hypoxia, is the most common cause of neurologic impairment in newborns. Infants who have experienced decreased oxygenation during labor, poor Apgar scores, respiratory difficulties caused by respira-

tory distress syndrome or recurrent apnea, or any type of cardiac insufficiency (defects, persistent pulmonary hypertension, respiratory failure secondary to sepsis) are at risk for neurologic impairment. (Preterm infants may experience several of these problems.) These factors may preclude or hamper initial breastfeeding sessions, and the severity and duration of the clinical manifestation is directly related to the severity and duration of the oxygenation deprivation.

Some newborns have pathologic conditions such as Down syndrome or other pathologic conditions that result in long-term alterations in neurologic function. Serious neurologic impairments require some special management in terms of the nutrition required and the feeding technique. Breastfeeding is usually possible for infants with these and similar difficulties and is best managed with a clear understanding of how anatomy and physiology are affected.

Structure and Function

Muscles of the head and neck are less directly involved in breastfeeding, but they do influence feeding success. In the well infant, muscles that extend the neck are usually better developed than those that bring the head forward, requiring the caregiver to support the head to keep it aligned with the rest of the newborn's body. This head lag is even more pronounced in infants with weak head and neck muscles, as is typically found in neurologically impaired infants. These weak muscles make positioning at the breast somewhat more difficult. Muscular deficits may or may not be associated with impaired reflexes.

Oral, buccal, lingual, and pharyngeal muscles are directly involved in breastfeeding, as shown in Fig. 11-4. The *masseter* and *temporalis* muscles elevate the jaw when the infant is latching on, then retract the jaw while compressing the tongue, a solid mass of skeletal muscles, against the alveolar ridge and hard palate. The *genioglossus* protrudes the tongue, and the *hypoglossus* depresses it. The glossopharyngeal muscle groups are involved in swallowing and when the infant gags. If the infant has neurologic impairments, these muscles may not be intact or they may be too weak to initiate

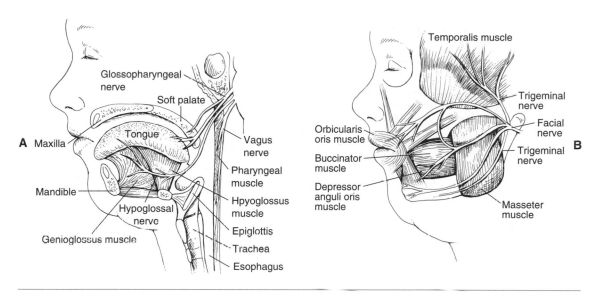

FIGURE **11-4** Muscles and nerves used in suckling and swallowing. **A,** Sagittal section. **B,** Lateral view.

and/or sustain successful suckling. Similarly, the muscle response may be delayed, or the infant may be hypersensitive to stimuli, and the muscle response may therefore occur too early.

Nerves innervate the muscles involved in breastfeeding. The *trigeminal* nerve (cranial nerve V) innervates muscles of the mandible (jaw). The *facial* nerve (cranial nerve VII) innervates muscles of the face, including the buccinator, lower lip, and chin muscles. The *glossopharyngeal* nerve (cranial nerve IX) innervates sensations of the tongue, and the *hypoglossal* nerve (cranial nerve XII) innervates tongue movements. The glossopharyngeal and the *vagus* (cranial nerve X) nerves innervate muscles of the posterior pharynx, palate, and epiglottis.

Breastfeeding is accomplished by intact structure and function of the oral cavity—the lips, cheeks, tongue, and hard and soft palates, as well as the jaw. When a *stimulus* occurs to the nerve in any one of these structures, it forms the beginning of a reflex arc. When a *nerve* impulse passes over the reflex arc, a predictable response to the stimulus, called a *reflex,* results. A reflex consists of either a muscle contraction (e.g., suckling) or glandular secretion (milk ejection is an example of a glandular reflex). Therefore, when a stimulus occurs, the

message is carried to the spinal cord and a reflex results. The reflex is accomplished by using *muscles.* For example, when the infant's cheek is touched (stimulus), he starts rooting movements (reflex) through contraction of his oral muscles.

Sucking, swallowing, gagging, and rooting are all somatic *reflexes* associated with breastfeeding. The breastfeeding infant needs not only the ability to suck and swallow—reflexes normally present very early in gestation—but also the ability to *coordinate* suck and swallow with breathing, which appears around 32 weeks of gestation. This coordination of suck and swallow is essential for milk transfer. Intact reflexes are an indication of normal neurologic functioning. Conversely, impaired reflexes are generally a result of dysfunction of the central or peripheral nervous system for a variety of reasons.

Reflexes are altered in some situations. For example, the events of labor (i.e., a particularly stressful labor that depletes the fetus's oxygen reserves) or neurologic disease can alter the infant's reflexes. (Preterm infants do not have "abnormal" reflexes, but because their nervous systems are immature, they will not exhibit reflexes equivalent to those of a term infant.) Furthermore, the

CLINICAL SCENARIO

The Infant with Neurologic and Structural Alterations

Baby Thomas was born at 40 weeks of gestation. His mother is a gravida 4, para 4, and has successfully breastfed three other infants for a substantial period of time. You are called to the pediatric floor to see Thomas when he is about 5 days old. He has been diagnosed with Pierre Robin syndrome, as shown in Fig. 11-5. He has been readmitted to the hospital for apneic episodes.

What are the three *greatest* difficulties you could anticipate for Thomas, and what recommendations could you make?

Problem	Recommendation

What are the three *greatest* difficulties you could anticipate for his mother, and what are your discharge priorities?

Problem	Recommendation

Readers are encouraged to discuss this scenario among their colleagues because often there is no one right answer.

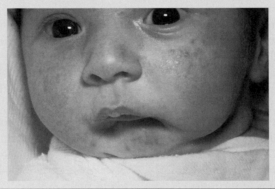

FIGURE 11-5 Infant with Pierre Robin syndrome. *(Photo taken with assistance of Ruth A. Lawrence, MD.)*

muscles of the infant's oral, buccal, lingual, and pharyngeal musculature might not be intact or might be too weak to accomplish and sustain suckling. A thorough assessment is therefore needed to optimize breastfeeding efforts.

Assessments

A few key assessments about neurologic status should be part of routine care for the infant. General assessments may affect the decision to initiate feedings or to discontinue a feeding that is in progress. More specific observations related to breastfeeding provide the basis for breastfeeding management of the infant who has alterations in neurologic functioning.

General Assessments

Sometimes infants are diagnosed at or before birth as having a neurologic deficit. Other times, however, neurologic limitations are not immediately evident. In assessing an infant it is important to first determine whether he is a candidate for oral feedings; sometimes those with severe neurologic impairment are not. Those who are candidates for oral feedings should be offered the breast, and the feeding should be monitored to see how the infant tolerates the activity.

Before and during a feeding—when the infant is interacting and using muscles and reflexes associated with feeding—are opportune times to identify signs of neurologic impairment. Altered states of consciousness, eye responses, abnormal posture and tone, abnormal reflexes, and abnormal movements, described in Table 11-4, are all clues to possible neurologic deficits.

State of consciousness is particularly important to observe; those who have an altered state of consciousness are at risk for aspiration. Eye responses are also important; for example, the preterm infant whose eyes appear glassy may be overstimulated and unable to continue the feeding. The infant's posture may also influence the feeding decision. For example, hypotonia may be difficult to distinguish from lethargy, particularly in the preterm infant. Usually, however, the lethargic infant appears disinterested in the feeding; the hypotonic infant is more likely to appear interested and willing, but unable to successfully accomplish feeding.

Infants who have any abnormal movement, including jitters or seizures, require medical follow-up. There are four types of neonatal seizures: clonic, tonic, myoclonic, and subtle. Subtle seizures may develop in either the term or preterm infant; they can be easily overlooked or mistaken for jitteriness. It is critical to distinguish jitters from seizures; infants who are jittery are likely to be hypoglycemic and should be immediately put to the breast. Infants who are having seizures may be hypoglycemic, although multiple other causes are also possible. Unlike infants with jitters, infants with suspected seizures should not receive oral feedings, pending medical confirmation, because they are at risk for aspiration. They at least require further investigation; they may also have difficulties sucking. Box 11-4 differentiates ocular movements, dominant movement, sensitivity to stimulation, and duration of jitters and seizures.[29] (Note: This box is not meant to be used for diagnosis, but rather for guidance in helping the nurse make some immediate decisions related to feeding.)

Assessments Related to Breastfeeding

Infants who are neurologically impaired may have alterations of structure, function, or both. Structural alterations may involve the face, jaw, posterior pharynx, palate, epiglottis, and tongue. Muscles of the oral, buccal, lingual, and pharyngeal musculature might not be intact, or they might be too weak to accomplish and sustain sucking. The sucking reflex will not be optimal in an infant who has dysfunction of the central or peripheral nervous system and musculature. Sometimes the muscular and reflex problems are interrelated, and sucking difficulties usually result.

Infants with neurologic impairments may have a variety of sucking disorders. These might include (1) an absent or decreased sucking reflex, (2) weakness of suckling, (3) nonrhythmic suckling, or (4) uncoordinated suck/swallow/breathe.[58] An absent

---

Box **11-4**   DISTINGUISHING BETWEEN JITTERS AND SEIZURES

	Jitters	**Seizures**
Ocular movement	Absent	Present
Dominant movement	Tremors—repetitive movement of both hands at frequency of 2 to 5 per second, lasting more than 10 minutes	Clonic jerking that cannot be stopped by flexion of the affected limb
Sensitivity to stimulation	High	Low
Persist beyond fourth day	No	Yes

Source: Wong DL. *Whaley & Wong's nursing care of infants and children.* 6th ed. St. Louis: Mosby; 1999.

Table 11-4 NEUROLOGIC STATUS AND FEEDING DECISIONS

Assessment/ Observation	Normal	Abnormal	Feeding Implications for Abnormal Reflexes
State of consciousness	Infant should respond to noxious stimuli and should become quiet after soothing or a successful feeding (see Chapter 9 for full discussion of states of consciousness)	Infant does not respond to noxious stimuli and does not become quiet after successful feeding or after attempts to soothe the infant; infants who are comatose or have alterations in their level of consciousness are very worrisome	Question whether these infants should be NPO; evaluate for other signs of neurologic impairment before initiating feeding for infants who are unresponsive or exhibit signs of alterations in consciousness
Eye responses	Around 32 weeks of gestation, infants should blink and should have extraocular movements	A fixed stare may indicate that the infant is having a seizure; "glassy" eyes while feeding may indicate that the infant is overstimulated	Term infants who stare are worrisome and require further evaluation before initiating feeding; glassy eyes, particularly in the preterm infant, suggest that the infant is tired and needs to rest
Posture and tone	Flexion of the arms, knees, and hips should be present in term infants; varying degrees of flexion will be present in preterm infants	Hypotonia or hypertonia; hypotonia is particularly relevant to the feeding experience; the infant has a "floppy" posture, making it difficult to achieve and maintain a good position at the breast	Positioning, described in the text and in boxes in this chapter, enhances feeding
Reflexes	Reflexes associated with breastfeeding (e.g., rooting, sucking, swallowing, and gagging) are indeed part of a larger assessment; observe other reflexes, including Moro, grasp, blink, tonic neck; reflexes are not fully developed in the preterm infant	Reflexes may be absent or weak, as described in the text; the infant may also have difficulty coordinating the suck and swallow reflex with breathing	Report abnormal reflex activity to the physician because the problems encountered may be beyond the scope of a "breastfeeding problem"; trying to correct a "breastfeeding problem" is futile if other reflexes are not functioning optimally
Movements	Infants should have organized movement in response to stimuli; movement should also reflect symmetry	Clonic, tonic, myoclonic, and subtle seizures	Infants who are seizing should not be fed

sucking reflex simply means that when the infant is stimulated to suck, he does not. (He may not even have a rooting reflex.) A decreased sucking reflex means that when he is presented with stimulation he responds with little sucking, or only a flutter-suck, although he may continue that sucking pattern for an extended time. That is, he cannot establish an adequate suckling mechanism. In contrast, a weak suck means that the infant can establish sucking but cannot sustain it. Nonrhythmic suckling means that the infant does not suck in a rhythm; he sucks in a disorganized way. Uncoordinated suck/swallow/breathe means that the infant may suck—and may even suck vigorously—but cannot coordinate his efforts to take in food with his efforts to take in air. These infants frequently sputter and may even become cyanotic.

Clinical Management

If sucking is absent, initiate pumping, but if the sucking reflex is present but decreased, ensure that the infant and the mother receive adequate stimulation. Use stroking and/or a cold washcloth in and around the mouth, as well as other nonnoxious interventions, to stimulate the infant. Then, try the Dancer hand, as shown in Fig. 11-6, or try pressing the chin inward slightly, as shown in Fig. 11-7. Use pillows for the hypotonic infant, and position him so that the mouth is fairly high up on the breast. In this way, an active milk-ejection reflex will not

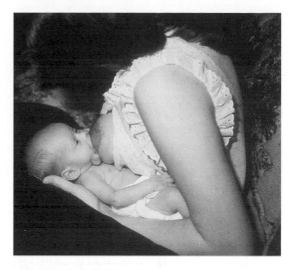

FIGURE **11-7** The infant's chin is supported by only the index finger. *(Courtesy Sarah Coulter Danner, Hot Springs, SD.)*

"choke" the infant who suckles poorly. Likewise, the mother needs adequate stimulation. Suggest a nursing supplementer (see Chapter 16) so that she receives stimulation when the infant suckles, but be prepared to express milk also.

A weak suckling reflex impedes the sucking mechanism, the negative pressure, and an adequate seal. The infant's tongue muscles are too weak to form a trough to perform the undulating motion

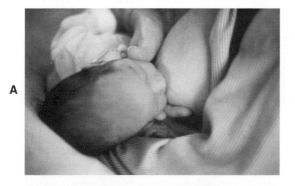 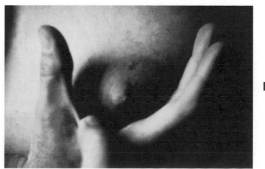

A

B

FIGURE **11-6** Dancer hand. **A,** Infant's chin rests in the V web between thumb and forefinger. **B,** The mother's finger is pointing to the place where the infant's chin should rest while breastfeeding. *(Courtesy Sarah Coulter Danner, Hot Springs, SD.)*

necessary for obtaining milk. The negative pressure, necessary for holding the nipple/areola complex in place, is inadequate, so the infant cannot achieve a good seal. Interventions that aim to overcome weak muscles and inadequate negative pressure and to organize suck patterns are most helpful for the infant who is neurologically impaired.

A nonrhythmic sucking reflex impairs primarily the sucking mechanism (i.e, the infant's ability to compress the lactiferous sinuses and achieve milk transfer). Preterm infants often have nonrhythmic sucking patterns, and a further discussion is in Chapter 10.

An uncoordinated sucking reflex reflects not only a feeding problem but also a problem breathing while eating. Sometimes, interventions that reduce the speed of maternal milk flow can help infants who exhibit an uncoordinated suckling reflex.

Interventions should be timed so that they correspond with the infant's quiet-alert state.[59] Table 11-5 describes some specific interventions that enhance suckling mechanisms for infants who have alterations in neurologic function; the categories are delineated rather arbitrarily, and each difficulty described is likely to coexist with another difficulty. For example, the previous Clinical Scenario box describes an infant with Pierre Robin syndrome; this infant exhibited neurologic difficulties as well as structural difficulties (see Fig. 11-5).

Several congenital and acquired problems are associated with neurologic impairment. Down syndrome, myelomeningocele, and hydrocephalus are but a few of the more common problems.

Down Syndrome

According to the National Down Syndrome Society, the risk of having a child with Down syndrome is about 1 in 1000 births for mothers in their twenties. The risk increases dramatically, however, if the mother is older than 35, to about 1 in every 350 births, and to about 1 in every 100 births for women who are older than 40. However, about 75% of infants born with Down syndrome are born to mothers who are younger than age 35.

Down syndrome is a congenital defect. Usually, the somatic cell nucleus contains 46 chromosomes arranged in 23 pairs; the members of each pair are virtually identical. Sometimes, however, the cell contains three, rather than two, copies of one chromosome; this is called a *trisomy*. In trisomy 21, or *Down syndrome*, as it is often called, the infant

---

ⱰCLINICAL SCENARIO

The Infant with Down Syndrome

Baby Jeffrey was born at 37 weeks of gestation. His mother (23 years old and a gravida 1, para 1) has delivered about 2 hours ago. She is quietly resting in bed, but is asking about Jeffrey. She says, "What will we do to feed him?" What are the three *greatest* difficulties you could anticipate for Jeffrey, and what recommendations could you make?

Problem	Recommendation

What are the three *greatest* difficulties you could anticipate for his mother, and what are your discharge priorities?

Problem	Recommendation

Readers are encouraged to discuss this scenario among their colleagues because often there is no one right answer.

Table 11-5 POSSIBLE PROBLEMS AND BREASTFEEDING MANAGEMENT FOR NEWBORNS WITH ALTERATIONS IN NEUROLOGIC FUNCTION

Problem	Clinical Strategies	Rationale
Impaired sucking reflexes		
Decreased sucking reflex	If sucking or rooting is *absent*, express milk Offer the breast so that it is positioned in center of mouth Press chin down as infant latches on Encourage nonnutritive sucking: • Offer textured teething toy, even for newborn • Offer breast or pacifier to suck Consider equipment (e.g., nursing supplementer; see Chapter 16)	Helps infant to *establish* and optimize (or prepare) response to reflex stimulus
Weakness of sucking	Try different positions: across lap with pillow, specially designed pillows, football hold Try Dancer hand (see Fig. 11-6) Consider infant sling Burp frequently Encourage short, frequent feeds	Helps newborns to *sustain* sucking reflex after they have established it
Nonrhythmic sucking	Hold infant across lap; use two pillows Try infant sling Burp frequently	Helps infant to maintain *rhythmic* suck
Uncoordinated suck/swallow	Position nipple so that back of neck and throat are higher than mother's nipple Have mother recline at about 30 degree angle if milk flows too fast Sit baby on extra pillows	Improves ability to exhibit long, slow, rhythmic sucks *interspersed* appropriately with breathing; milk flow is unaided by gravity when mother reclines
Low muscle tone (generalized), weak head and neck muscles	Use pillows to get infant nearer to breast instead of having infant use muscles to "reach for breast" Tap, stroke lips, cheeks, and tongue (use circular mouth exercise) Offer clean, textured teething toys dipped in breast milk Consider help of special therapist	Helps overcome or promote *muscle* tone that in turn promotes milk transfer
Hyperreflexia	Use infant sling or football hold; keep baby flexed! Tonic bite: try Dancer hand	Helps infant to flex, rather than extend, muscles
Risk for failure to thrive	Listen for audible swallowing! Emphasize importance of having infant obtain the hindmilk	Emphasizes milk transfer and promotes adequate nutrients for growth

Developed with the assistance of Sarah Coulter Danner.

has extra chromosomal material on the twenty-first chromosome. This extra genetic material alters the course of growth and development (Fig. 11-8).

Benefits of Breastfeeding an Infant with Down Syndrome

Breastfeeding is advantageous for all infants but especially for infants with Down syndrome. From

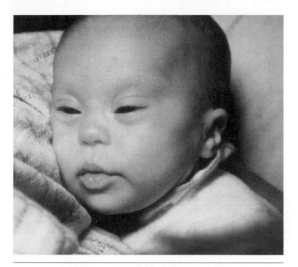

FIGURE **11-8** Infant with Down syndrome. *(Courtesy Sarah Coulter Danner, Hot Springs, SD.)*

an emotional perspective, the enhanced bonding may be particularly helpful if the mother is having difficulty accepting her newborn's condition. From a biologic perspective, breastfeeding and human milk help the infant with Down syndrome reduce the risk of morbidity associated with concomitant problems. About 30% to 40% of children with Down syndrome also have cardiac defects, predisposing them to respiratory difficulties and infection. The act of breastfeeding is beneficial to these infants because it conserves their cardiopulmonary resources and contributes to better speech development.

Prenatal Assessment and Counseling

Down syndrome can be suspected from results of prenatal blood testing (α-fetoprotein), but conclusive prenatal diagnosis is determined from the results of an amniocentesis. Women who have been told that their infants have Down syndrome may not be immediately interested in discussing feeding methods, but the topic should be addressed as soon as possible because these infants may have special feeding difficulties.

Prenatal education and counseling can be extremely helpful for the parents of a child with Down syndrome. Because it is so common

for Down syndrome to be detected prenatally and because abortion is legalized in the United States, in most cases the parents have made a conscious decision to birth and care for the infant. Therefore early discussion about effective ways to help the infant overcome his potential limitations gives a strong message of support for the parents' decision and expresses confidence in their caregiving skills. Infants with Down syndrome are more like other infants than they are different, and parents can maximize their child's potential by not placing limits on their own expectations. Early planning gives the entire health care team an opportunity to mobilize personnel and equipment that will optimize the breastfeeding experience.

Postpartum Assessment and Management

Some infants with Down syndrome are born to parents who do not have prior knowledge of the infants' condition, especially to younger mothers who have little or no prenatal care or did not opt for an amniocentesis. With or without the advanced warning, mothers may need to simultaneously grieve for the loss of a perfect child and bond with their infant.

Assessments. Assessment for breastfeeding begins with a more general assessment of the infant's ability to achieve good positioning at the breast and then with the specific neuromuscular capabilities associated with his feeding behavior. Assessment of strength and organization of suck, although helpful, is counterproductive if the examiner overstimulates the infant. (More than other newborns, infants with Down syndrome will "shut down" if they are overstimulated.) Assessment findings should be used to form a basis for clinical management.

Clinical Management Strategies. The infant with Down syndrome may have both generalized and feeding-related difficulties that will make the feeding experience frustrating whether the infant is breastfed or bottle-fed. All of the goals and priorities for the compromised infant (Box 11-5) are appropriate for the infant with Down syndrome. In addition, establish the goals and priorities found in Box 11-6.

Box 11-5   GOALS AND PRIORITIES FOR CARE: COMPROMISED INFANTS

ANTEPARTUM PERIOD

- Assist mother to recognize that breastfeeding is not only possible but optimal.
- Facilitate contact with local support groups, especially mothers who have successfully breastfed similarly affected infants (see Appendix A).
- Collaborate with other members of the health care team to identify strategies and options for supplemental feeding.
- Mobilize equipment: Be sure that a suitable pump will be available both in the hospital and after discharge.
- Ensure that educational media will be available and accessible at the hospital when the infant is delivered (see Appendix B).

IMMEDIATE POSTPARTUM PERIOD

- Initiate or reinforce actions listed for the antepartum period.
- Assist newborn to achieve good latch-on.
- Teach mother to pump or supplement, if indicated.
- Provide mother with a list of worrisome signs and a list of phone numbers to call for help.
- Give suggestions to overcome problems of engorgement in early period and diminished supply later on.
- Provide a list of pump rental depots and become the mother's advocate for getting a prescription for a pump. This prescription may enable the mother to obtain reimbursement from her health insurance company.

DISCHARGE PLANNING

- Assist the couplet to achieve excellent latch-on and audible swallowing before hospital discharge; this may not be entirely achieved because infants are being discharged early nowadays.
- Provide anticipatory guidance to help parents with the most common concerns.
- Plan for some mechanism for weighing infant to determine appropriate weight gains. How frequently the infant needs to be weighed depends largely on the infant's weight at discharge and his nutritional and general health status. Electronic scales can be rented for accurate test-weighing at home.
- Recommend appropriate resources in the community, and list phone numbers where parents can find information and support.
- If appropriate, coordinate efforts so that an electric pump can be available at home, and parents can successfully demonstrate how to use it before discharge.
- Create a list of danger signs and reassuring signs.
- Schedule follow-up visits or telephone consultation within the first week after discharge and plan for ongoing support and follow-up.

TIME PRECEDING AND FOLLOWING SURGERY IF NEEDED

- Support mother's decision to continue breastfeeding or to wean.
- Anticipate the need for milk after surgery and initiate an appropriate pumping regimen about 10 days before the surgery.
- Assist the family to ask questions pertinent to feeding after the surgery.
- Facilitate rooming-in, if feasible.

Typically, infants born with Down syndrome are hypotonic; hypotonicity hampers their ability to position themselves at the breast. The tongue is also hypotonic. If the tongue is hypotonic, the infant cannot form the trough necessary to achieve good areolar compression. This affects the infant's ability to compress the tongue against the hard palate. Furthermore, the tongue often falls to the back of the mouth, which impairs sucking motions and may result in apneic periods as well. To minimize this problem, the mother can hold the infant more upright so that gravity does not add to the problem. Frequently, the tongue protrudes, having the appearance of not quite fitting into the mouth.

Suckling at the Breast. Follow all of the directives listed in Chapter 7 to achieve good positioning and latch-on. Infants with Down

Box 11-6   GOALS AND PRIORITIES FOR CARE: DOWN SYNDROME

- Ensure adequate intake. Make sure the infant gets the hindmilk.
- Remember that growth patterns are different for infants with Down syndrome, as opposed to those for other infants, and current charts describing growth in infants with Down syndrome do not differentiate between breastfed and bottle-fed infants.[61]
- Champion breastfeeding as ideal for this infant, who is at greater risk for cardiac defects and infection.
- Promote family self-esteem and self-confidence.
- Foster family education and support through use of pamphlets, such as those listed in Appendix B, and consumer organizations

syndrome are likely to have problems—hypotonia and frequent drooling—that make it more difficult to achieve an adequate seal, adequate negative pressure, and adequate suckling mechanisms.

Possible Concurrent Problems. In about 30% to 50% of the cases, infants with Down syndrome have an accompanying congenital heart defect, which can range in severity from mild to severe (see the section on cardiac defects). This makes them more vulnerable to respiratory infections and fatigue. They are also likely to be born before term. Other concurrent problems may include hyperbilirubinemia (related to liver dysfunction), intestinal anomalies (duodenal atresia/stenosis, Hirschsprung's disease), thyroid dysfunction, and childhood leukemia. In addition, they are at high risk for otitis media and feeding difficulties.[60] Interestingly, the American Academy of Pediatrics suggests that growth should be monitored according to Cronk's growth charts for children with Down syndrome.[61] However, because we know that exclusively breastfed children who are unaffected by Down syndrome do not gain weight at the same rate as unaffected children who are formula-fed, it may be difficult to use these charts for exclusively breastfed infants affected with Down syndrome. (The charts also address infants from 1 syndrome.

month to 18 months, with no mention of neonates.)

Education, Counseling, and Support. Mothers who choose to breastfeed their infants with Down syndrome may have some difficulties that may not immediately be apparent. They may experience chronic sorrow, a continued wish for the perfect child, or guilt feelings related to the infant's condition. Increased social isolation is a continuing problem; hence, the mother may never go out of the house or seek companionship with other breastfeeding mothers. A sense of decreased family self-esteem may further affect her stress level, and marital difficulties frequently come to a head when families have a child with a serious deviation. Although there are no easy remedies to help these mothers, sensitivity, compassion, and acceptance of the infant's capabilities and limitations go a long way to support not only the breastfeeding efforts but also the family dynamics surrounding this birth. It is often helpful for parents to link with a local parent support group. The National Down Syndrome Society, listed in Appendix A, can refer parents to local groups.

Help the mother deal with issues of separation and modesty. Frequently, infants with Down syndrome go to "school" within the first few months. To maintain breastfeeding, help the mother identify ways to be present for the breastfeedings—in which case she will need to know how to breastfeed discretely—or to express and save milk to maintain supply.

Conclusions about Breastfeeding Management. Infants with Down syndrome can breastfeed. Various interventions, largely aimed at overcoming the difficulties associated with hypotonia, will improve the breastfeeding experience. Active support, instruction, and collaboration among members of the health care team are essential for breastfeeding success.

ALTERATION IN STRUCTURAL ANATOMY

Structural defects influence breastfeeding. Perhaps the most important question for infants with structural defects is, Does the infant have an adequate seal, adequate suckling mechanism, and adequate negative pressure? Whether or not the infant can breastfeed depends on the extent of the problem, but in many cases he can.[62] Infants with significant structural alterations frequently have as much or more difficulty bottle-feeding as they do breastfeeding. A broad overview of a common craniofacial defect is used here to show how to apply this idea of achieving adequate suck, seal, and negative pressure.

Cleft Lip and Palate

Incidence and Implications

Clefts occur about once in every 700 live births.[63] For most parents, the risk of having a child with a cleft is about 0.14%; this increases dramatically if they have already had a child with a cleft, if the woman or her partner has a cleft, or if their siblings or other family members are affected.

Clefting is a congenital problem. It can occur in isolation, but it is also seen in more than 150 syndromes, including Pierre Robin syndrome, Turner's syndrome, and Van der Woude's syndrome. Cleft lip, a congenital failure of fusion of the upper lip, occurs during the fifth week of gestation. The cleft may be unilateral or bilateral and may involve the alveolar ridge (gum), as shown in Fig. 11-9. When the left and the right palatal shelves fail to fuse during the seventh or eighth week of embryonic development, a cleft palate results. Cleft palates may involve the hard palate, the soft palate, or both, as shown in Fig. 11-10. Clefts of the soft palate may involve either the back of the soft palate, as shown in Fig. 11-11, or the complete soft palate, as shown in Fig. 11-12.

The degree of difficulty in feeding varies with the severity of the lesion. If the infant has only a small notch on the lip or a split uvula, feeding may not be a problem. A complete clefting of the lip, which may occur in conjunction with a cleft palate, as shown in Fig. 11-13, complicates clinical management. Clefting poses both structural and functional difficulties; the alteration in orofacial structure impacts dental, speech, and hearing function as well as feeding. With so many possible difficulties, the infant will need the many benefits of breastfeeding.

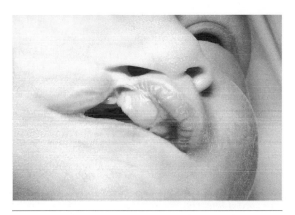

FIGURE **11-9** Cleft of lip only. *(Photo taken with assistance of Ruth A. Lawrence, MD.)*

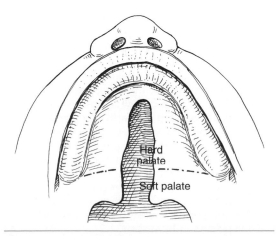

FIGURE **11-10** Cleft of soft and hard palates.

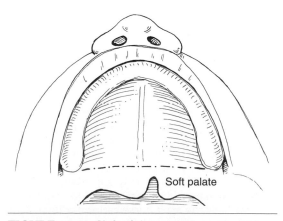

FIGURE **11-11** Cleft of the posterior soft palate.

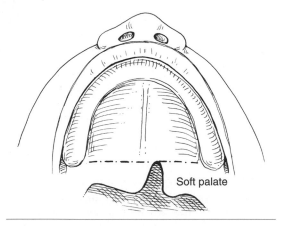

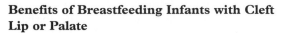

FIGURE **11-12** Cleft of the soft palate.

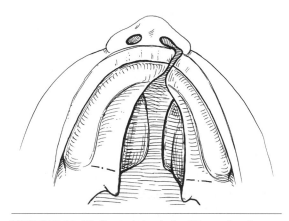

FIGURE **11-13** Complete cleft of lip and palate.

Benefits of Breastfeeding Infants with Cleft Lip or Palate

Breastfeeding is advantageous for all infants, but especially for infants with clefts. From an emotional perspective, breastfeeding is an ideal way to promote bonding for these infants whose faces are not intact. From a biologic perspective, problems associated with clefts can be overcome or minimized through human milk and the act of suckling the breast. For example, infants with cleft palates are at high risk for ear infections because the eustachian tubes easily fill with liquid when the infant swallows; breastfeeding creates less pressure in the middle ear than bottle-feeding, thereby lessening the risk of otitis media. Otitis media occurs significantly more often when the infant is fed artificial milk than when he is fed human milk, and breastfeeding duration is positively correlated with an

*C*LINICAL SCENARIO

The Infant with a Cleft Defect

You are the nurse practitioner in the nursery. Baby George has a unilateral cleft lip and appears to be breastfeeding well. However, he is losing weight. Here are his weights from the last few days:

Birth   3970 g
Day 1   3905 g
Day 2   3735 g
Day 3   3705 g
Day 4   3730 g

Would you order a supplement for this baby?

You are the lactation consultant, and the nursery staff nurses call you to see a baby with a fairly wide, unilateral cleft. You suggest that the mother try putting her thumb in the cleft, but this is not completely successful because the cleft is so wide. What else might you try?

You are the staff nurse caring for baby Kurt who has a unilateral cleft lip. His mother successfully breastfed two other children. Kurt is a vigorous nurser and has had about a 7% weight loss over the past 4 days. He is being discharged today with a bilirubin level of 12. What two priorities would you identify for Kurt's discharge planning?

You are the nurse practitioner in a busy pediatric office. Mrs. M. has been pumping for 6 months because her son was born at 32 weeks of gestation with a significant cleft of the soft and hard palate. She is tearful; her supply is dwindling, and she knows that the baby will have the cleft repaired at 8 months but is not sure she can continue pumping until then. She asks if she should quit. How would you respond, or what would you recommend?

Readers are encouraged to discuss these scenarios among their colleagues because often there is no one right answer.

occurrence of effusion.[64] The act of compressing the human nipple and areola promotes better muscle development in the face, mouth, and tongue.

Prenatal Assessment and Counseling

Prenatal assessment and counseling are pivotal for successful breastfeeding. Unless a mother has successfully breastfed before, she may lack confidence in her ability to breastfeed even under the best of circumstances. This problem escalates if clefting occurs.

If there is a family history of clefting, the pregnant woman should specifically ask the ultrasound technician to visualize the fetus's facial features. The ultrasound may not give a good indication of the width of the cleft lip, but this forewarning will mobilize the cleft team and help the family prepare for some of the infant's capabilities and limitations. If the presence of a cleft is established, a clear, consistent, collaboratively developed plan with specific strategies can overcome the anticipated feeding difficulties. Goals and priorities during the antepartum period can be found in Box 11-7.

Immediate Postpartum Period Management

The majority of mothers who intended to breastfeed opt for bottle-feeding when they discover that the infant has a cleft.[65] In some cases, exclusive breastfeeding may not be realistic, but even partial or short-term breastfeeding is laudable. Goals and priorities for the immediate postpartum period are found in Box 11-7.

Assessments. Sometimes, cleft palates are not easily identifiable. Subtle feeding cues signal a need for further physical assessment and diagnosis. For example, a clicking sound may signal the possibility of a cleft (although it is more frequently caused by poor latch-on). Other clues may be present, too. In my experience, a multipara complained of extremely sore nipples and had not experienced such intense pain when breastfeeding a normal infant. More generalized signs—dehydration,[66] chronic hypothermia, poor weight gain, lack of swallowing—require further investigation to determine the cause; sometimes clefting can be the root of these problems. Some infants who have

> ### Box 11-7 Goals and Priorities for Care: Cleft Lip
>
> **ANTEPARTUM PERIOD**
> - Assist the mother to recognize that breastfeeding is not only possible but optimal.
> - Facilitate contact with local support groups, especially mothers who have successfully breastfed cleft infants. La Leche League or About Face can help.
> - Collaborate with other members of the cleft team to identify strategies and options for supplemental feeding.
> - Mobilize equipment: Be sure that a suitable pump will be available both in the hospital and after discharge.
> - Ensure that educational media will be available and accessible at the hospital when the infant is delivered (see Appendix B).
>
> **IMMEDIATE POSTPARTUM PERIOD**
> - Initiate or reinforce actions listed for the antepartum period.
> - Assist the newborn to achieve good latch-on.
> - Teach the mother to express milk or use donor or artificial milk, if indicated.
> - Provide parents with a list of worrisome signs and a list of phone numbers to call for help.
> - Give suggestions to overcome problems of engorgement in the early postpartum period and diminished supply later on.
> - Provide a list of pump rental depots and ask the plastic surgeon, neonatologist, or other physician to write a prescription. This prescription may enable the mother to obtain reimbursement from her health insurance company.
>
> **POSTOPERATIVE PERIOD**
> - Establish or resume breastfeeding as soon as the surgeon allows.
> - Assist with latch-on and basic information if the infant has not previously suckled.
> - Reestablish a full milk supply.

experienced "feeding problems" have had undetected clefts for years.[67]

Cleft lips are quite obvious at the time of delivery. Early initiation of breastfeeding gives the infant an opportunity to experiment with latching on and suckling when the mother's breast is soft. The goal of the first feeding, however, is for warmth, bonding, and stimulation of milk supply; whether or not colostrum is obtained is less important. In subsequent feedings, however, the mother and the infant will need to learn how to successfully suckle. A good assessment improves chances for success.

The extent of the lesion generally predicts whether the newborn can accomplish the three factors necessary for successful breastfeeding.[68] First, the *seal* not only must be present but also adequate. The seal allows negative pressure and holds the nipple and areola in place, but it does not extract milk from the breast; an adequate seal can be difficult to achieve with a cleft defect. Second, the *negative pressure* must be adequate; this is accomplished in part by the motion of the tongue upon the gum and lips and areola compressing the hard palate. When both cleft lip and cleft palate are present, an adequate negative pressure will not be generated.[69] Finally, the *suckling mechanisms* must be adequate; milk flows from the nipple and swallowing occurs as a result of reflex; otherwise normal infants with a cleft can swallow normally. Problems with intraoral muscular movements are associated with bilateral cleft lips because the tongue does not stabilize the nipple. Similarly, wide cleft palates are problematic because the tongue cannot compress the nipple effectively (Table 11-6). Assessment data should be used to form clinical management strategies.

Clinical Management Strategies. The visual impact of a cleft often produces dismay and grief that require extensive support.[70] Infants with clefts of the lips and/or the alveolar ridge, however, look quite normal while breastfeeding because the breast tissue fills the cleft and camouflages it. During the first few days, parents need help to develop realistic expectations of the breastfeeding experience. They may assume that the infant's less-than-enthusiastic approach to breastfeeding is a result of the cleft defect when, in fact, many infants do not immediately latch on and suckle vigorously. Messages about the infant's limitations must be balanced with messages about his capabilities; otherwise, parents get the message that breastfeeding

will be "difficult." Switching from breast to bottle does not eliminate the difficulty. Infants with clefts continue to choke, gag, and sputter with the bottle; bottle-feeding may even exaggerate this problem.

Whether they are breastfed or bottle-fed, infants with clefts have some special difficulties. For example, they tire easily.[71] To overcome this, offer frequent feedings. Forewarn the parents that the infant may gag and have milk come back up through the nose. Reassure them that you will stay with them; it can be very frightening to see the infant struggle. Suggest holding the infant upright as much as possible to reduce this problem. These infants may take in more air than others and should be burped frequently. Have the bulb syringe handy, and teach the parents how to use it.

When the infant is suckling at the breast, be sure that the basic techniques are not overlooked so that milk transfer can be accomplished. Consider using a few specialized techniques as shown in Box 11-8, but keep in mind that frequently, you will need to use a trial-and-error process to discover which technique is needed and works best.

If an infant has a unilateral cleft, suggest that the mother point the nipple away from the cleft. (The mother will need to position the newborn so that her breast enters his mouth from the side on which the defect is located.) For example, instruct the mother whose infant has a right-sided cleft of the lip or palate to hold the infant so that his right cheek touches the breast. If this works, use the cradle hold on one side and the football hold on the other.[68]

If the infant has a bilateral defect of the palate or alveolar ridge, position him so that he squarely faces the breast. This can be accomplished by using either a sitting or straddle position (Fig. 11-14). If the lesion is large, try tipping the breast downward or angling it slightly to one side or the other.[68] Try multiple techniques and see which one works best, because what works well for one infant may not work for another infant with a technically similar but clinically unique lesion.

Evaluate and reevaluate interventions. It is all too easy to suggest intervention after intervention, only to learn much later that the infant is not gaining weight. For example, the infant often appears

Table 11-6   POSSIBLE PROBLEMS AND BREASTFEEDING MANAGEMENT FOR NEWBORNS WITH ALTERATIONS IN CRANIOFACIAL STRUCTURE OR FUNCTION

Problem	Clinical Strategies	Rationale
Risk for aspiration	Determine whether infant's respiratory status indicates or contraindicates oral feeding; withhold oral feedings if respirations are greater than 60-70, if dyspnea is present, or per hospital protocol	Increased respiratory rate makes coordination of sucking and swallowing more difficult
	Have bulb syringe handy in case infant is unable to clear his own airway; aspirate contents of mouth first, then suction nose; show parents how to use the bulb syringe	Aspirating mouth first prevents inhalation of aspirate—infant will gasp if nares are stimulated first; avoid center of mouth because this stimulates gag reflex
	Cleft palate: use upright feeding position	Milk less likely to go into cleft
Inadequate seal	Help infant to open wide (tickle bottom lip; gently press chin inward)	Essential for all infants; improves likelihood of adequate areolar grasp, and ultimately, milk transfer
	Point nipple away from cleft	Minimizes the problem
	Try using Dancer hand as shown in Fig. 11-6	Provides extra support for latch-on
	Try straddle position as shown in Fig. 11-14	Facing breast head-on makes more tissue available
	Cleft lip: place index finger on top edge of areola and middle finger on bottom; nipple will protrude as if it were full of milk	Helps areolar tissue to mold to fill the cleft
	Cleft lip: fill the cleft with mother's thumb as shown in Fig. 11-15	Minimizes amount of space that interferes with good seal
Inadequate negative pressure	Grasp both cheeks, pushing lips together	Helps create negative pressure
	Burp more frequently	Infant may swallow more air; inadequate negative pressure leads to faulty seal
Inadequate suckling	Consider pillow to help position infant	Decreases distance between infant and breast
mechanisms	Make sure neck is flexed rather than extended	Difficult to swallow with extended neck
Milk let-down too slow; baby working too hard	Hand massage first	Enhances rapid milk-ejection reflex and hastens flow of milk
Milk let-down too fast; baby gagging	Consider Australian hold, as shown in Fig. 7-13	Slows flow of milk; force of gravity pulls milk toward mother rather than toward infant

Box **11-8** Techniques for Special Feeding Challenge

- Encourage suckling when the breast is full and the nipple protrudes a bit.
- Consider using one breast at a feeding if the infant tires easily because it improves the likelihood of obtaining the hindmilk before he gets too tired.
- Try the football position or the straddle position so that the infant squarely faces the breast. Because of the size of the infant's legs, the straddle position might be less successful during the neonatal period. Using a pillow underneath the infant's buttocks may help when using the straddle position.
- Point the nipple away from the cleft.
- Place the index finger at the top edge of the areola and the middle finger on bottom to make nipple protrude.
- Hold the infant semiupright to prevent milk from coming out the nose.
- Massage or use warm compresses to improve the milk-ejection reflex. Sometimes infants find it more gratifying to get the milk with less effort.
- Tickle the lips so that the infant opens wide! When the mouth is gaping and the tongue is troughed and over the lower alveolar ridge, quickly guide the mother's arm so that she brings the infant to the breast.
- Fill the cleft lip with the mother's thumb, as shown in Fig. 11-15.
- Gently press chin inward, hook angle of the jaw as shown in Fig. 11-7, or use the Dancer hand (Fig. 11-6) to maneuver when bringing infant onto the breast to augment intraoral suction.
- Make sure neck is flexed (but not hyperflexed) rather than extended.

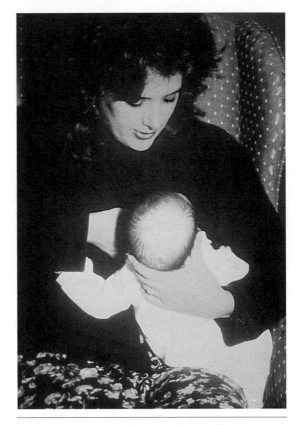

FIGURE **11-14** Modified straddle hold. *(Copyright Debi Bocar,* Lactation Consultant Services, *Oklahoma City, OK.)*

to be latched on well, but further observation reveals that air can be heard going through the cleft. This produces a soft hissing noise. Continue efforts to fill the cleft, either with a finger as shown in Fig. 11-15 or with the breast tissue. This may be a trial-and-error process at first. Audible swallowing is a very reassuring sign that optimal latch-on has been achieved. If swallowing is not audible or if air can be heard going through the cleft, the infant is not suckling effectively, even though he may appear to be making sucking motions.

Possible Concurrent Problems. If the seal, negative pressure, or suckling mechanisms are inadequate, the result will be inadequate intake. The key, therefore, is to optimize milk intake through good intervention and evaluation. Inadequate intake can and does occur to some degree, however, so be alert to common problems that may accompany cleft defects.

Jaundice is a common problem. Because the infant may have difficulty suckling well in the first few days, he may be unable to gain the laxative effects of colostrum. Sometimes an otherwise healthy infant needs to remain in the hospital for jaundice treatment after his mother has been discharged. This interruption in the normal breast-

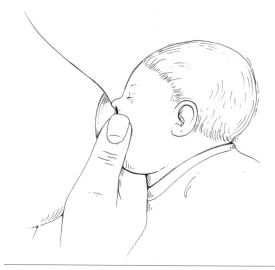

FIGURE **11-15** Mother's thumb fills the cleft.

feeding relationship can be the difference between success and failure with cleft infants. Discharge planning should include a contingency plan to treat the jaundice at home if necessary so that potential separation of the mother and infant is avoided.

Breast engorgement is a likely problem in the early days because the newborn may not be completely removing all of the milk from the breast. Any of the usual strategies for managing engorgement are appropriate. Expressing milk may be indicated as well.

A dwindling supply threatens breastfeeding if the infant is unable to suckle or becomes separated from the mother for several weeks or even months. For example, an infant with a cleft palate may be unable to suckle adequately for 8 to 10 months. Having the infant nuzzle the breast and applying warm packs applied to the breast usually enhance success, as does multiparity. The best strategy, however, is bilateral expression using an electric pump (see Chapter 14). Continuation of milk expression is often essential.[72]

FTT is a threat to any infant who cannot suckle adequately. Cleft infants are particularly at risk not only because of feeding difficulties but also because of apparently increased metabolic rates. Those with isolated clefts, however, are less likely to be at risk for FTT than those who have clefts asso-

ciated with a syndrome.[73] Giving the infant adequate time at the breast helps the infant to obtain the hindmilk that is critical for weight gain. A SOAP note from an actual patient record is found in Box 11-9.

If the infant is always hungry or hypothermic, it is likely that he is not obtaining enough milk. Supplementation is one means to achieve the goal of adequate intake,[74] but supplementing should not replace good clinical management.

Supplemental Feeding Methods. Many infants affected with cleft defects can suckle at the breast; some do as well as unaffected infants, but others need assistive devices. As early as possible, the cleft team should determine one or possibly two alternative feeding methods that can be used before and after surgery, rather than teach the parent one method and then another. A lactation supplementer can provide extra calories and promote stimulation to the breast (see Chapter 16). Each situation will require evaluation to determine what supplementation method will work best, but clear communication among the members of the cleft team and with the parents is critical to breastfeeding success. Alternative methods for giving supplemental feedings should be considered, rather than using bottles.

Various devices have been used in different facilities and in different countries. A few decades ago, the lamb's nipple and Brecht feeder, Mead-Johnson Cleft Palate Nurser, and Ross Cleft Palate Nurser were popular in the United States. In England and Australia the Rosti bottle (similar to the spoon-shaped devices distributed with liquid over-the-counter medications in the United States) has been used. Squeezable plastic bottles (usually with narrow, long crosscut nipples) have been used for cleft defects for decades and have recently been shown to be beneficial,[75] but infants appear to suckle and gain weight as well with a standard nipple that has been crosscut.[76] The Haberman feeder by Medela has an elongated nipple that can be compressed more easily than a traditional nipple, which may be helpful if the infant has difficulty getting adequate negative pressure; most mothers seem to prefer this device.[77] At the University of Rochester Medical Center, we used an Asepto-type

Box 11-9   Sample Nurse's SOAP* Note for Cleft Lip Newborn

S: "It feels much better when we do that" (when baby opens wide and is positioned tummy-to-tummy).

O: A small reddened area (a few millimeters in diameter) on right nipple. Baby does not always open wide and is not always tummy-to-tummy. Mom encouraged to elicit good open-wide before allowing latch-on and to position tummy-to-tummy. Multipara has breastfed two noncleft infants × 4-5 months each. Upon palpation, breasts do appear to be filling, congruent with mom's report of feeling full. Mom reports feeling let-down about the time that newborn has slower, rhythmic sucks. Audible swallowing. Unilateral cleft lip and cleft of alveolar ridge on right side—not a wide cleft. Shown how to tip nipple upward just until baby latches on chin first; then readjust. Also shown how to use straddle position. Dancer hand suggested as a possible option; reinforced idea of pointing nipple away from the cleft. Baby has lost 6% of birth weight and is jaundiced this morning. Sometimes takes baby off from breast and does switch-nursing; discouraged this and explained need for hindmilk. Mom and nursery staff instructed to use Asepto-type syringe or eyedropper if supplementation is ordered.

A: Infant has significant weight loss, but suckled and swallowed well at this feeding; asleep at end of feeding. Mom's milk is coming in; nipple breakdown due to baby not opening widely.

P: Reinforcement and anticipatory guidance/planning:

- Reinforce OPEN-WIDE and good positioning; make sure baby gets hindmilk.
- Give expressed pumped breast milk via Asepto syringe if supplement is ordered.
- Reassure mom that 6% weight loss is okay at this point but will need to be reevaluated in context of entire clinical picture.
- Reevaluate feeding success if mom becomes engorged.
- Begin exploring possibility of Wallaby phototherapy unit for home use if this should become necessary.
- Call me if you have questions. Thanks.

M. Biancuzzo, RN

*The SOAP format—subjective and objective data, assessment and plan—is frequently used for nurses' notes.

syringe attached to a pediatric catheter-like tube. This device works well both before and after surgery. Variations on this idea might be a regular syringe, a dental syringe, or an eyedropper. Cup feeding, described in more detail in Chapter 16, has been used successfully in supplementing infants with clefts.[78]

Education, Counseling, and Support. Intense educational support is required not only for initiating breastfeeding but also for continuing. Unfortunately, mothers report a low level of satisfaction with the education that they receive in the hospital about feeding their children with clefts.[77] Patient education materials (see Appendix B) offer little help unless they are available immediately after the infant is born. The pamphlet by Danner is outstanding; the photos are excellent and the approach is positive.

Weaning is a continuous, recurring question. The mother may want to wean before cleft lip surgery because of a "quit-while-we're ahead" attitude, out of fear that it will be impossible to reestablish breastfeeding after the surgery. A mother who wants to wean before cleft palate surgery probably has many ambivalent feelings; her infant may have never suckled at the breast and/or may do remarkably better after the palate is repaired. Breastfeeding can continue after surgery in any case, but the challenge may seem insurmountable. The mother may need help identifying her own goal, and together with the nurse she can generate strategies to best accomplish it.

Mothers can become very discouraged. Despite good clinical management and the mother's valiant efforts, I saw an infant with a cleft lip and two cleft palates who was unable to suckle effectively and required supplementation. The mother saw this as not "really" breastfeeding, and she needed support to overcome her feelings of failure. Mothers in this situation need someone to acknowledge their disappointments and redefine their contribution and motivation. It is helpful to reinforce the idea that the mother is providing the best food for the infant and to emphasize that the goal is obtaining the *milk* and suckling the breast is only one way to achieve that goal.

Assisting parents of infants affected with clefts is truly a collaborative effort that depends on the expertise of everyone on the cleft team. The Cleft Foundation (see Appendix A) can recommend a cleft team and a support group in every area of the United States.

Surgery for Cleft Lip or Palate. Most surgical repairs are done after the infant is 1 month old. Goals and priorities for the time preceding and following surgery are listed in Box 11-4. When infants require surgery, parents require both preoperative and postoperative teaching and support.

Preoperative Teaching and Support. Preoperative teaching and support should begin as soon as possible. Parents may ask how soon the cleft will be repaired. This varies dramatically from surgeon to surgeon, but the 10-10-10/10 guideline often applies. That is, some surgeons wait until the infant weighs 10 pounds and has a hemoglobin count of 10 mg/dl; cleft lips are generally repaired before 10 weeks, and cleft palates are generally repaired before 10 months. This is by no means a rule, but it serves as a general guideline. It appears that timing of the cleft lip repair does not correlate with adverse effects, and, in fact, mothers prefer the surgery during the neonatal period, rather than later.[79]

To optimize feeding efforts, parents frequently need answers to questions that have no "stock" answers because postoperative management varies considerably from surgeon to surgeon. For example, it may be difficult to predict whether an individual surgeon will use an arm restraint (these hamper feeding efforts and are being ordered less frequently because it is doubtful that they serve any useful purpose).[80] Parental concerns have been described,[81] and from these, pertinent questions have been generated in Box 11-10.

Postoperative Management. Preferences vary widely, but many surgeons will not allow the infant to suck anything—a breast, a rubber teat, or a pacifier—for approximately 10 days after a cleft repair. (Again, note the "10" guideline.) Some forbid returning to "nipple feeding" for as long as 6 weeks after a cleft lip repair.[82] The myth that delayed sucking reduces tension on the suture line

Box 11-10   GENERAL CONCERNS OF PARENTS OF INFANTS WITH CLEFT

GENERAL HOSPITAL ROUTINES
- Am I allowed to room-in with the baby?
- Are siblings allowed to visit?
- What routine procedures are performed before and after surgery?
- How long will my baby have nothing by mouth before surgery?
- How will my baby be anesthetized?
- Will I be able to visit my baby in the recovery area?

POSTSURGICAL RESTRAINTS
- Will my baby be prevented from bending his elbow?
- Will any special positioning be necessary?

LIP CARE
- Will I need to use normal saline and/or antimicrobial ointment on the suture line?
- Will a Turner's bow be used?

FEEDING
- How soon will I be able to breastfeed my baby?
- Will you write an order for my baby to be fed my milk until he can go to the breast?
- Will my baby be fed with an Asepto syringe or dropper? For how long?
- Will any obturator be used?
- How can I obtain a breast pump?

Source: Curtin G. *Perinatal Neonatal Nurs* 1990;3:80-89.

of cleft lips persists, despite research nearly two decades ago and confirmed more recently that no detrimental effects were noted when breastfeeding was initiated immediately after the surgery.[83,84] In the Third World, where breastfeeding is common, similar results have been noted and reported anecdotally to the author and in controlled studies.[85,86] The first postoperative feeding at the breast— whenever it occurs—should proceed as normally as possible. Main support measures include praise for mother's efforts, suggestions on needed adjustments, and a gentle reminder that the repair should solve, not worsen, the feeding problems created by the cleft. Often, the real problem becomes the *interruption* in breastfeeding, rather than breastfeeding per se.

Mechanical trauma to the roof of the mouth—such as trauma caused by artificial nipples—may damage cleft palate repairs. If the surgeon insists on this delay, he may be persuaded to allow a Tommy-Tippy type of cup for supplemental feedings before the end of the 10 days. If surgeons prefer to delay sucking, the infant can be fed with a tube at the side of the mouth, allowing the infant to swallow the fluid. Expressed human milk is superior to formula, so if a significant interruption in breastfeeding is anticipated, there should be a plan to help the mother express and freeze her milk before the surgery. The mother's supply may be reduced during this hiatus, but her regular supply can be reestablished fairly easily.

The palatal obturator is a prosthesis that is retained in the crevices of the mouth, providing a seal between the mouth and the nasal cavity. Few surgeons use palatal obturators these days, although they are still being made.[87] It is difficult to fit the device into the extremely small mouth of a newborn without the use of wires, which many surgeons object to. Dentists who make this prosthesis find that a proper fit is a difficult challenge even in older infants. Anecdotally, some nurses or mothers have suggested that breastfeeding is more effective with the use of the palatal obturator, but there have been no studies to confirm this possibility. Mothers also report that the obturator causes sore nipples, but again, there is no conclusive research on this issue.

Conclusions about Breastfeeding Management. Infants with cleft defects can and should breastfeed. It is best to mobilize personnel, equipment, and educational materials and active support before delivery, if possible. Special techniques and community support help overcome problems immediately after delivery and in subsequent months before and after surgery. The breastfeeding specialist has a critical role in implementing interdisciplinary care and evaluating the effectiveness of interventions.

Short or Tight Frenulum

Infants are sometimes born with a short or tight frenulum, or ankyloglossia, as shown in Fig. 11-16. As with other structural defects, the extent of the

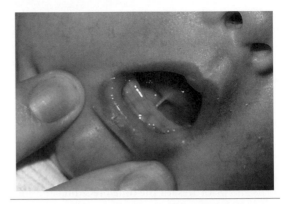

FIGURE **11-16** Newborn with ankyloglossia. *(Copyright Kay Hoover.)*

problem determines the degree of feeding difficulty encountered. Breastfeeding difficulties, including sore nipples, are more likely to occur in infants affected with ankyloglossia.[88] Although the problems are fairly easy to identify, the solutions are not.

Multiple actions related to breastfeeding these infants have been reported anecdotally, but so far no valid and reliable assessment tools have been published in the peer-reviewed literature to guide management. If the frenulum is particularly short, the pediatrician may recommend surgical repair. Protocols that outline eligibility are needed for determining which infants have surgical repair.[89]

The goal is for the infant to be able to extend his tongue enough so that he can adequately compress the lactiferous sinuses. If this is happening, further intervention is probably not necessary. Having the mother lean back and use an Australian hold is sometimes helpful because the infant's tongue is then "down" on the nipple rather than reaching upward (see Fig. 7-13).

SUMMARY

The newborn must quickly adapt to the extrauterine environment, and the processes used under most circumstances become more necessary but frequently less efficient when the infant has alterations in structural anatomy or in gastrointestinal, neurologic, or cardiorespiratory function. Infants who are born preterm may have multiple alterations, and they will require many special interventions to reach or maintain homeostasis. In many of these cases, however, special techniques can be used to help the infant suckle at the breast, which promotes optimal functioning of all systems. If the infant is unable to suckle or if breastfeeding must be interrupted for a time, the nurse needs to coordinate communication and clinical strategies to provide human milk and facilitate direct breastfeeding.

REFERENCES

1. Thibodeau GA, Patton KT. *Anatomy and physiology.* 4th ed. St. Louis: Mosby; 1999.
2. Stephensen CB. Burden of infection on growth failure. *J Nutr* 1999;129:534S-538S.
3. Lawrence RA, Lawrence RM. *Breastfeeding: a guide for the medical profession.* 5th ed. St. Louis: Mosby; 1999.
4. Nelson SP, Chen EH, Syniar GM et al. Prevalence of symptoms of gastroesophageal reflux during infancy. A pediatric practice-based survey. Pediatric Practice Research Group. *Arch Pediatr Adolesc Med* 1997;151:569-572.
5. Heacock HJ, Jeffery HE, Baker JL et al. Influence of breast versus formula milk on physiological gastroesophageal reflux in healthy, newborn infants. *J Pediatr Gastroenterol Nutr* 1992;14:41-46.
6. Corrado G, Cavaliere M, D'Eufemia P et al. Sandifer's syndrome in a breast-fed infant. *Am J Perinatol* 2000;17:147-150.
7. Vandenplas Y, Belli D, Cadranel S et al. Dietary treatment for regurgitation—recommendations from a working party. *Acta Paediatr* 1998;87:462-468.
8. Mathisen B, Worrall L, Masel J et al. Feeding problems in infants with gastro-oesophageal reflux disease: a controlled study. *J Paediatr Child Health* 1999;35:163-169.
9. Woolridge MW, Fisher C. Colic, "overfeeding," and symptoms of lactose malabsorption in the breast-fed baby: a possible artifact of feed management? *Lancet* 1988;2:382-384.
10. Moneret-Vautrin DA. Cow's milk allergy. *Allergy Immunol* 1999;31:201-210.
11. American Academy of Pediatrics Work Group on Breastfeeding. Breastfeeding and the use of human milk. *Pediatrics* 1997;100(6):1035-1039.
12. Lake AM, Whitington PF, Hamilton SR. Dietary protein-induced colitis in breast-fed infants. *J Pediatr* 1982;101:906-910.
13. Perisic VN, Filipovic D, Kokai G. Allergic colitis with rectal bleeding in an exclusively breast-fed neonate. *Acta Paediatr Scand* 1988;77:163-164.
14. Odze RD, Bines J, Leichtner AM et al. Allergic proctocolitis in infants: a prospective clinicopathologic biopsy study. *Hum Pathol* 1993;24:668-674.
15. Machida HM, Catto Smith AG, Gall DG et al. Allergic colitis in infancy: clinical and pathologic aspects. *J Pediatr Gastroenterol Nutr* 1994;19:22-26.
16. Anveden-Hertzberg L, Finkel Y, Sandstedt B et al. Proctocolitis in exclusively breast-fed infants. *Eur J Pediatr* 1996;155:464-467.
17. Lindberg T. Infantile colic and small intestinal function: a nutritional problem? *Acta Paediatr Suppl* 1999;88:58-60.
18. Cant A, Marsden RA, Kilshaw PJ. Egg and cows' milk hypersensitivity in exclusively breast fed infants with eczema, and detection of egg protein in breast milk. *BMJ (Clin Res Ed)* 1985;291:932-935.
19. Axelsson I, Jakobsson I, Lindberg T et al. Bovine beta-lactoglobulin in the human milk. A longitudinal study during the whole lactation period. *Acta Paediatr Scand* 1986;75:702-707.
20. Stuart CA, Twiselton R, Nicholas MK et al. Passage of cows' milk protein in breast milk. *Clin Allergy* 1984;14:533-535.
21. Lothe L, Lindberg T, Jakobsson I. Cow's milk formula as a cause of infantile colic: a double-blind study. *Pediatrics* 1982;70:7-10.
22. Jakobsson I, Lindberg T. Cow's milk proteins cause infantile colic in breast-fed infants: a double-blind crossover study. *Pediatrics* 1983;71:268-271.
23. Lothe L, Lindberg T. Cow's milk whey protein elicits symptoms of infantile colic in colicky formula-fed infants: a double-blind crossover study. *Pediatrics* 1989;83:262-266.
24. Hill DJ, Hudson IL, Sheffield LJ et al. A low allergen diet is a significant intervention in infantile colic: results of a community-based study. *J Allergy Clin Immunol* 1995;96:886-892.
25. Jakobsson I, Borulf S, Lindberg T et al. Partial hydrolysis of cow's milk proteins by human trypsins and elastases in vitro. *J Pediatr Gastroenterol Nutr* 1983;2:613-616.
26. Jakobsson I, Lindberg T. Cow's milk as a cause of infantile colic in breast-fed infants. *Lancet* 1978;2:437-439.
27. Lake AM. Food-induced eosinophilic proctocolitis. *J Pediatr Gastroenterol Nutr* 2000;30(Suppl):S58-S60.
28. Ravelli AM, Milla PJ. Vomiting and gastroesophageal motor activity in children with disorders of the central nervous system. *J Pediatr Gastroenterol Nutr* 1998;26:56-63.
29. Wong DL. *Whaley & Wong's nursing care of infants and children.* 6th ed. St. Louis: Mosby; 1999.
30. Lucas A, Cole TJ. Breast milk and neonatal necrotising enterocolitis. *Lancet* 1990;336:1519-1523.
31. Butte NF, Garza C, Smith EO et al. Human milk intake and growth in exclusively breast-fed infants. *J Pediatr* 1984;104:187-195.
32. Dewey KG, Heinig MJ, Nommsen LA et al. Growth of breast-fed and formula-fed infants from 0 to 18 months: the DARLING Study. *Pediatrics* 1992;89:1035-1041.
33. Dewey KG, Heinig MJ, Nommsen LA et al. Breast-fed infants are leaner than formula-fed infants at 1 y of age: the DARLING study. *Am J Clin Nutr* 1993;57:140-145.
34. Dewey KG, Peerson JM, Brown KH et al. Growth of breast-fed infants deviates from current reference data: a pooled analysis of US, Canadian, and European data sets. World Health Organization Working Group on Infant Growth. *Pediatrics* 1995;96:495-503.

35. Baxter-Jones AD, Cardy AH, Helms PJ et al. Influence of socioeconomic conditions on growth in infancy: the 1921 Aberdeen birth cohort. *Arch Dis Child* 1999;81:5-9.

36. WHO Working Group on Infant Growth. An evaluation of infant growth: the use and interpretation of anthropometry in infants. *Bull World Health Organ* 1995;73:165-174.

37. Dewey KG. Growth characteristics of breast-fed compared to formula-fed infants. *Biol Neonate* 1998;74:94-105.

38. de Onis M, Garza C, Habicht JP. Time for a new growth reference. *Pediatrics* 1997;100:E8.

39. Victora CG, Morris SS, Barros FC et al. The NCHS reference and the growth of breast- and bottle-fed infants. *J Nutr* 1998;128:1134-1138.

40. Powers NG. Slow weight gain and low milk supply in the breastfeeding dyad. *Clin Perinatol* 1999;26:399-430.

41. Lukefahr JL. Underlying illness associated with failure to thrive in breastfed infants. *Clin Pediatr (Phila)* 1990; 29:468-470.

42. Habbick BF, Gerrard JW. Failure to thrive in the contented breast-fed baby. *Can Med Assoc J* 1984;131:765-768.

43. Neville MC, Neifert MR, editors. *Lactation: physiology, nutrition and breast-feeding.* New York: Plenum Press; 1983.

44. Fomon SJ, Nelson SE. Size and growth. In Fomon SJ. *Nutrition of normal infants.* St. Louis: Mosby; 1993.

45. Neifert MR. Prevention of breastfeeding tragedies. *Pediatr Clin North Am* 2001;48:273-297.

46. Frantz KB. The slow-gaining breastfeeding infant. *NAACOGS Clin Iss Perinat Womens Health Nurs* 1992;3:647-655.

47. Frantz KB, Fleiss PM, Lawrence RA. Management of the slow-gaining breastfed baby. *Keeping Abreast* 1978;3:287.

48. Wilton JM. Sore nipples and slow weight gain related to a short frenulum. *J Hum Lact* 1990;6:122-123.

49. Yurdakok K, Ozmert E, Yalcin SS. Physical examination of breast-fed infants. *Arch Pediatr Adolesc Med* 1997;151:429-430.

50. Powers NG. How to assess slow growth in the breastfed infant. Birth to 3 months. *Pediatr Clin North Am* 2001;48:345-363.

51. Clemente C, Barnes J, Shinebourne E et al. Are infant behavioural feeding difficulties associated with congenital heart disease? *Child Care Health Dev* 2001;27:47-59.

52. Marino BL, O'Brien P, Lore H. Oxygen saturations during breast and bottle feedings in infants with congenital heart disease. *J Pediatr Nurs* 1995;10:360-364.

53. Blaymore Bier JA, Ferguson AE, Morales Y et al. Breastfeeding infants who were extremely low birth weight. *Pediatrics* 1997;100:E3.

54. Bier JB, Ferguson A, Anderson L et al. Breast-feeding of very low birth weight infants. *J Pediatr* 1993;123:773-778.

55. Meier P. Bottle- and breast-feeding: effects on transcutaneous oxygen pressure and temperature in preterm infants. *Nurs Res* 1988;37:36-41.

56. Behrman RE, Kliegman RM, Arvin AM, editors. *Nelson textbook of pediatrics.* 15th ed. Philadelphia: WB Saunders; 1996.

57. Lambert JM, Watters NE. Breastfeeding the infant/child with a cardiac defect: an informal survey. *J Hum Lact* 1998;14:151-155.

58. McBride MC, Danner SC. Sucking disorders in neurologically impaired infants: assessment and facilitation of breastfeeding. *Clin Perinatol* 1987;14:109-130.

59. Danner SC. Breastfeeding the neurologically impaired infant. *NAACOGS Clin Iss Perinat Womens Health Nurs* 1992;3:640-646.

60. American Academy of Pediatrics: Health supervision for children with Down syndrome. *Pediatrics* 2001;107:442-449.

61. Cronk C, Crocker AC, Pueschel SM et al. Growth charts for children with Down syndrome: 1 month to 18 years of age. *Pediatrics* 1988;81:102-110.

62. Biancuzzo M. Clinical focus on clefts. Yes! Infants with clefts can breastfeed. *AWHONN Lifelines* 1998;2:45-49.

63. Cleft Palate Foundation (cleftline@aol.com). Personal Communication with Amy Mackin November 28, 2001.

64. Paradise JL, Elster BA, Tan L. Evidence in infants with cleft palate that breast milk protects against otitis media. *Pediatrics* 1994;94:853-860.

65. Oliver RG, Jones G. Neonatal feeding of infants born with cleft lip and/or palate: parental perceptions of their experience in South Wales. *Cleft Palate Craniofac J* 1997;34:526-532.

66. Livingstone VH, Willis CE, Abdel-Wareth LO et al. Neonatal hypernatremic dehydration associated with breast-feeding malnutrition: a retrospective survey. *CMAJ* 2000;162:647-652.

67. Moss AL, Jones K, Pigott RW. Submucous cleft palate in the differential diagnosis of feeding difficulties. *Arch Dis Child* 1990;65:182-184.

68. Danner SC. Breastfeeding the infant with a cleft defect. *NAACOGS Clin Iss Perinat Womens Health Nurs* 1992;3:634-639.

69. Clarren SK, Anderson B, Wolf LS. Feeding infants with cleft lip, cleft palate, or cleft lip and palate. *Cleft Palate J* 1987;24:244-249.

70. Lynch MC. Congenital defects: parental issues and nursing supports. *J Perinatal Neonatal Nurs* 1989;2:53-59.

71. Styer GW, Freeh K. Feeding infants with cleft lip and/or palate. *J Obstet Gynecol Neonatal Nurs* 1981; 10:329-332.

72. Stockdale HJ. Long-term expressing of breastmilk. *Breastfeed Rev* 2000;8:19-22.

73. Avedian LV, Ruberg RI. Impaired weight gain in cleft palate infants. *Cleft Palate Journal* 1980;17:24-26.

74. Kogo M, Okada G, Ishii S et al. Breast feeding for cleft lip and palate patients, using the Hotz-type plate. *Cleft Palate Craniofac J* 1997;34:351-353.

75. Shaw WC, Bannister RP, Roberts CT. Assisted feeding is more reliable for infants with clefts—a randomized trial. *Cleft Palate Craniofac J* 1999;36:262-268.

76. Brine EA, Rickard KA, Brady MS et al. Effectiveness of two feeding methods in improving energy intake and growth of infants with cleft palate: a randomized study. *J Am Diet Assoc* 1994;94:732-738.

77. Trenouth MJ, Campbell AN. Questionnaire evaluation of feeding methods for cleft lip and palate neonates. *Int J Paediatr Dent* 1996;6:241-244.

78. Lang S, Lawrence CJ, Orme RL. Cup feeding: an alternative method of infant feeding. *Arch Dis Child* 1994;71:365-369.

79. Slade P, Emerson DJ, Freedlander E. A longitudinal comparison of the psychological impact on mothers of neonatal and 3 month repair of cleft lip. *Br J Plast Surg* 1999;52:1-5.

80. Jigjinni V, Kangesu T. Do babies require arm splints after cleft palate repair? *Br J Plast Surg* 1993;46:681-685.

81. Curtin G. The infant with a cleft lip or palate: More than a surgical problem. *J Perinatal Neonatal Nurs* 1990;3:80-89.

82. Skinner J, Arvedson JC, Jones G et al. Post-operative feeding strategies for infants with cleft lip. *Int J Pediatr Otorhinolaryngol* 1997;42:169-178.

83. Weatherley White RC, Kuehn DP, Mirrett P et al. Early repair and breast-feeding for infants with cleft lip. *Plast Reconstr Surg* 1987;79:879-887.

84. Darzi MA, Chowdri NA, Bhat AN. Breast feeding or spoon feeding after cleft lip repair: a prospective, randomised study. *Br J Plast Surg* 1996;49:24-26.

85. Fisher JC. Early repair and breastfeeding for infants with cleft lip: discussion. *Plast Reconstr Surg* 1987;79:886-887.

86. Fisher JC. Feeding children who have cleft lip or palate. *West J Med* 1991;154:207.

87. Osuji OO. Preparation of feeding obturators for infants with cleft lip and palate. *J Clin Pediatr Dent* 1995;19:211-214.

88. Messner AH, Lalakea ML, Aby J et al. Ankyloglossia: incidence and associated feeding difficulties. *Arch Otolaryngol Head Neck Surg* 2000;126:36-39.

89. Masaitis NS, Kaempf JW. Developing a frenotomy policy at one medical center: a case study approach. *J Hum Lact* 1996;12:229-232.

Strategies for Managing Breast and Nipple Problems

The mother may experience several problems during the course of lactation. Most of these problems can be prevented or alleviated by the nurse; others require the nurse's swift recognition, intervention, and perhaps referral to the primary care provider. Building on the physical assessment findings described in Chapter 6, the purpose of this chapter is to help the nurse manage common breast/nipple problems.

EARLY PROBLEMS

Breast and nipple problems can develop at any time, but generally, flat and inverted nipples, sore nipples, and engorgement are the main problems that occur during the first few days after birth.

Inverted and Pseudoinverted Nipples

Inverted nipples are those that are not everted; they do not protrude outward. Some inverted nipples are a lifelong problem, whereas others evert with gentle pressure, or even spontaneously.

Nipple Variation

Sometimes, nipples that are inverted in early pregnancy will spontaneously evert later in pregnancy. This is especially true for nulliparae.[1] Regardless of parity, nipples that were everted during the first trimester may become inverted during the third trimester. For this reason, the nipples should be assessed at least once during the first trimester (or the first visit) and during the last trimester.

Some nipples are not truly inverted; they appear inverted, but when compressed they readily evert. These are sometimes called *umbilicated nipples*.[2] In these nipples, ductal "length" is adequate, but the underlying connective tissue is deficient; hence, the nipples at rest do not protrude from the base but can be everted with the hand or by the suckling infant.

Some inverted nipples are a lifelong problem. During fetal development, the woman's nipple is formed. Usually, the lactiferous ducts open into a shallow depression called the *mammary pit*. From this pit, cells proliferate to form the nipple and the areola, and the pit elevates. When the cells proliferate but do not elevate, the nipple fibers become "tied" and the nipple is inverted; this is also called an *invaginated nipple*, as shown in Fig. 12-1. It is usually a unilateral condition. Plastic surgeons report that patients with invaginated nipples have been known to breastfeed, although the duration or success of the experience has not been described. Apparently, the degree of nipple inversion and the strength of the infant's suck determine whether breastfeeding is possible. These researchers have stated that "there is no way to predict whether a woman with invaginated nipples will be able to breastfeed or not."[2]

If the inverted nipple has been invaginated since birth, it is unlikely to be inverted at term. Surgical correction of inverted nipples is possible and was recorded as early as 1873. Recent studies have questioned how to best perform the procedure to preserve the woman's ability to breastfeed.[2] The Niplette, designed by a plastic surgeon primarily for cosmetic purposes, aims to permanently correct inverted nipples while the woman is not pregnant, or through the seventh month of pregnancy. (The Niplette therefore has limited use during pregnancy because the manufacturer's instructions prohibit use of

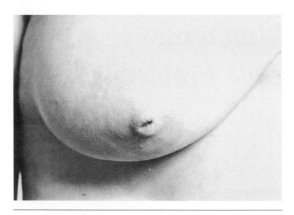

FIGURE 12-1 Simple nipple inversion with lifetime history. *(From Seidel HM et al. Mosby's guide to physical examination, 4th ed. St. Louis: Mosby; 1999.)*

the device in later pregnancy. It could be used postpartally.)

These invaginated nipples are sometimes associated with fewer ducts or abnormal ducts in the breast, and hence, there should be verification that the mother is producing enough milk. The infant should be weighed frequently during the first several days to be certain that adequate weight gain has occurred.

Treatment Strategies

Certainly, breastfeeding is not contraindicated for a woman with inverted nipples. Getting the infant to latch on to an inverted nipple, however, can be a thorny problem. Some effective and ineffective solutions are listed in Box 12-1.

Box 12-1   DO'S AND DON'TS FOR MANAGING INVERTED, PSEUDOINVERTED NIPPLES

DO'S

- Do tickle the baby's lip (with either finger or breast) until the infant opens *wide*. Look carefully; the infant can almost always open wider! This is probably the *most important* intervention for helping the infant to latch on to an inverted or pseudoinverted nipple.
- Do suggest that the infant breastfeed on the inverted side first. Infants are more hungry when they first go to the breast and may be more likely to take whatever is offered. After a few days, the nipple is frequently less inverted or less dimpled.
- Do assist the mother to roll her nipple and gently pull it out before offering the infant the breast.
- Do help the mother hold her nipple so that it protrudes. Sometimes, a scissors hold (rather than a C-hold) is all that is needed to accomplish this.
- Do try any "tricks" to entice the infant to suckle. For example, express a little colostrum onto the nipple so that the infant can taste it first.
- Do suggest wearing a breast shell between feedings.
- Do try applying the electric pump for a few seconds.

DON'TS

- Don't allow the infant to latch on in increments (i.e., have his mouth only partly open, then gradually take more of the tissue into his mouth). This will only make the mother's nipple sore.
- Don't use a syringe to "pull out" the nipple. This technique was reported anecdotally,[16] but it has no basis in scientific research. The worst case of sore nipples I have ever seen was created using this technique.
- Don't recommend Hoffman's technique. This technique, which manipulates the nipple vertically and horizontally, has never been proved (by anyone except Hoffman, several decades ago) to be effective. One study showed that it was clearly ineffective. This technique may damage nipple tissue, making the overall breast-feeding experience even more difficult.
- Don't use ice to get the nipple to protrude. Admittedly, ice will indeed cause the nipple to protrude, but it causes another problem, too. Ice interferes with the signals to the brain that create the milk-ejection reflex. If the woman is engorged, ice may be applied to relieve *breast distention after* the feeding but should never be applied to *nipples* before feeding.

Spontaneous eversion, of course, requires no treatment. If an inverted nipple persists until late in the third trimester, some interventions may be considered. The decision to use such interventions should be based on the potential risks and benefits.

Breast shells are a commonly used intervention for flat or inverted nipples. Not to be confused with nipple *shields* (shown in Fig. 12-2), breast *shells* (shown in Fig. 12-3) are designed to exert pressure on the nipple and help it protrude from the base by gentle suction. Table 12-1 shows the difference between breast shells and nipple shields.

The effectiveness of prenatal breast shells has been disputed.[3,4] Some women who wore shells prenatally were less likely to initiate breastfeeding; they complained that the shells cause discomfort, embarrassment, sweating, rash, and milk leakage.[3] For women who were highly motivated, however, these factors did not seem to be a deterrent to breastfeeding. The "negative" results are misleading because the studies looked at continuation of breastfeeding, rather than eversion of the nipple, as the outcome. Furthermore, these studies addressed *prenatal* use of the shells, and *postpartum* use has never been studied.

Until research proves that these devices do not work, they are worth trying if the previously listed inconveniences do not become deterrents for mothers. Several colleagues and I have often recommended shells and noted dramatically better clinical results. In our experience, shells do not

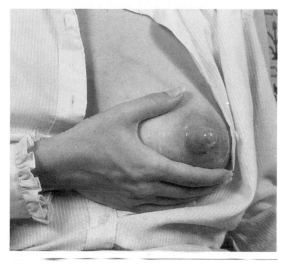

FIGURE **12-2** Nipple shields. *(Courtesy Medela, Inc., McHenry, Ill.)*

Table **12-1** Comparison of Nipple Shields and Breast Shells

	Nipple Shields	Breast Shells
Primary reason for using	Nipple is not well everted	Nipple is not well everted
Description	Shaped similar to rubber nipple	Plastic dome-shaped device
When worn	During feeding	Between feedings
Disadvantages	Abrade nipple tissue, prevent nipple from getting adequate stimulation (hence, milk supply decreases), and frequently an infant who has breastfed with a shield refuses to suckle without it; multiple studies have documented the detrimental effects of nipple shields	Usually none; can be too "tight"; this can be relieved by using a bra extender
Effectiveness	Often ineffective in solving the problem; may delay treatment of underlying problem	Can help nipples evert
Comments	Should be used only as a last-resort management strategy	Initiated prenatally if the woman has inverted or flat nipples but can be used postpartum if they were not used prenatally

Modified from Biancuzzo M. *Breastfeeding the healthy newborn*. White Plains, NY: March of Dimes Foundation; 1994.

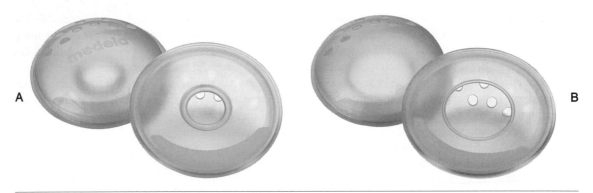

FIGURE **12-3** Breast shells. **A,** The small-hole back is used to help inverted or flat nipples to evert. **B,** The large-hole back is used if the woman is wearing the shells as a protective device for sore nipples. *(Courtesy Medela, Inc., McHenry, Ill.)*

always work, but they tend to work best when they are worn between 36 weeks of gestation and delivery, although postpartum mothers have noticed good results when these are worn between feedings. This is an area that requires further research.

Nipple shields are frequently recommended to overcome latch problems associated with inverted nipples. In nearly all cases, infants can latch on without the use of the shield. Lawrence observes that "Many lactation experts consider the use of a breast shield a sign of failure of proper lactation guidance and a preventable situation" and further asserts that "no medical problems have been identified when a shield is a good solution" (p. 262).[5] The safety and efficacy of these devices are controversial.

Some recent reports have suggested that nipple shields are safe and effective,[6-8] but results are unconvincing when methodology is scrutinized carefully. For example, one recent study[9] had a small sample size, lack of rigorous control, retrospective data, and self-selection of the subjects. Slightly less than half of the subjects were considered "successful" (breastfeeding until at least 6 weeks of age), with apparently no measure of weight gain or milk transfer and no indication if the data were statistically significant.

Other studies have demonstrated adverse effects from these devices. The older shields, which were thick and made of latex rubber ("Mexican hat" style), dramatically reduced milk supply and made the infant vulnerable to altered sucking patterns.[10] The newer type, made of thin silicone, can worsen nipple pain and damage.[11] One well-controlled study clearly showed that even the newer silicone nipple shields are associated with insufficient milk supply and all of its resultant problems, including failure to thrive.[12] There is also the possibility that some of the negative results noted in controlled studies reflect an inadequate latch-on when the shield is used. Shields have been used successfully by master clinicians, and continuation of breastfeeding and appropriate weight gains have been reported.[13]

Mothers who use shields are vulnerable to nipple skin abrasion because the shield can rub as the infant is suckling. Furthermore, it is often difficult to get the infant to accept the bare breast after he has become accustomed to using the shield. Some nurses try to wean the infant from the shield by using a scissors to cut the opening of the shield a little more each day. This can be helpful, but it is better to achieve good latch-on in the first place rather than try to "wean" the infant from the shield. (Using a makeshift nipple shield—using the latex rubber nipple from a bottle—should absolutely never be done. These seriously impede milk transfer and are likely to abrade the skin both because they were not designed to fit on humans and because they are made from latex.)

Hoffman's exercises should not be recommended. These exercises, which require the woman to stretch her nipples in both the horizontal and the vertical direction, were designed to stretch and break the fibers that "tie" the inverted nipple. In 1953 Hoffman showed good results in the two cases he described.[14] However, no research study since has shown any benefit from these exercises, and one study has shown detrimental effects.[3] Although gentle rolling and tapping are often helpful, excessive handling is not. Grasping the nipple with the thumb and forefinger, pulling the nipple out to the point of discomfort and then releasing it, has been associated with preterm uterine contractions and has not been associated with improved breastfeeding success.[15]

An anecdotal report recommended using a cut-off syringe to evert the nipples.[16] This practice is potentially harmful. I have never used this technique, but I once saw a mother who had had this technique performed by an experienced breastfeeding specialist. Hers was the worst case of damaged nipple tissue I have ever seen. The nipple had a deep ulcer, and narcotic analgesics were required to manage her pain. Furthermore, the woman's overall impression of breastfeeding was marred by this experience. It is also important to recognize that using a piece of equipment for other than its intended purpose invites litigation.

Some new devices have been manufactured that are designed to evert the inverted nipple. The Evert-It is designed to be used in the postpartum period to evert the nipple just before latch-on, as shown in Fig. 12-4. Although no scientific evidence supports this device, multiple anecdotal reports have favored it.

"Sore Nipples"

Somewhere between 11% and 96% of all breastfeeding mothers report "sore nipples."[17,18] For at least a half-century, lactating mothers have been complaining about "sore nipples."[19] The mother's complaint, however, does not make her a "complainer." When a person experiences pain, it is the body's way of alerting the brain that something is wrong; ignoring the soreness will lead to increased soreness accompanied by tissue damage. Sore nipples may include nipple pain, nipple damage, or both.[20]

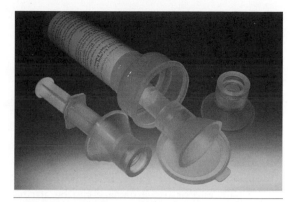

FIGURE **12-4** Evert-It. *(Courtesy Maternal Concepts, Inc. Elmwood, Wisc.)*

Nipple Pain

Sometimes, pain exists when visible damage cannot be observed. In these cases, it is important to first identify the possible source of the pain; pertinent questions such as those listed in Box 12-2 can be helpful in identifying the underlying cause. Unfortunately, many women give up breastfeeding when the source of the pain is not identified and corrected or when it is unbearable and seemingly unmanageable.

Nipple Damage

If the underlying problem is not corrected, nipple pain will eventually progress to nipple damage.

Box 12-2 QUESTIONS TO ASK ABOUT NIPPLE PAIN

- Where is the soreness?
- When did it begin?
- Is it present just at the beginning of the feeding or throughout the feeding? Or does it persist after the completion of the feeding?
- Describe the characteristics of the pain. Is it dull, shooting, or hot? (Ask for phrases to describe the pain, to elicit responses such as "like there was broken glass in my nipple" or "like it was liquid fire.")
- Describe the intensity of the pain on a scale of 1 to 10, with 1 being mild discomfort and 10 being exquisite pain.

Once the nipple skin is no longer intact, a cascade of deleterious effects follows.

Nipple damage may range from a slightly imperceptible white compression stripe to a gaping fissure. Damage to the nipple may include erythema, edema, fissures, blisters, inflamed areas, white patches, dark patches, yellow patches, peeling, pus, and ecchymosis.[21] Any lesion should be noted as completely as possible, and follow-up evaluation should be initiated.

Causes of Nipple Pain and/or Damage. Nipple pain and/or tissue damage can be attributed to one or more of four causes: (1) transient, physiologic causes; (2) incorrect attachment or removal of the infant; (3) use or misuse of equipment or commercial products; and (4) pathologic causes.[22]

Transient, Physiologic Causes. A common physiologic reason for sore nipples is the unrelieved negative pressure that occurs when there is little milk in the ducts. During the first few days, the ducts are not yet filled with a large volume of milk, and swallowing takes places infrequently, thus creating unrelieved negative pressure, which in turn may cause discomfort,[23] as shown in the Historical Highlight box on p. 344. Also, the mother is unaccustomed to having an infant suckle at the breast; peak intraoral pressures can reach as high as 135 mm Hg.[24]

Sometimes mothers of infants who are true "barracudas," as described in Chapter 7, will experience nipple soreness. This discomfort is particularly remarkable during the first few days. Assuming that the discomfort results from this suckling style, not improper positioning at the breast, a few recommendations may be helpful. First, reassure the mother that this discomfort will not last forever; it should disappear when milk supply is copious. In the meantime, suggest that she offer the least-sore breast first because the infant's suck is more vigorous on the first side. Also, suggest using different positions. Recommend that at one feeding she use the cradle position; at the next feeding, the side-lying position; at the next feeding, the football hold. Using different positions alternates where the pressure points occur and should lessen the discomfort.

Incorrect Latch-on or Removal of the Infant. There is a strong correlation between sore nipples and an incorrect infant latch-on.[23,25-27] Often, inflammation and/or abrasions and bruising of the nipple occur as a result of poor positioning. The positioning requires immediate intervention to avoid further trauma to the nipple.

If the subjective reports of pain are not accompanied by objective data that suggest the likely problems, presume that latch-on is the problem. Observe the feeding session and be especially alert to poor latch-on. Question the mother about the location of her pain. Pain that is perceived on top of the nipple is likely to be caused by poor latch-on and/or tongue thrusting. To correct the problem, observe the feeding. If the infant does not demonstrate good latch-on, initiate corrective actions. If the infant is thrusting his tongue, try inserting a gloved finger and holding the infant's tongue down for about 30 seconds before latching on. This is not always helpful, but it is worth a try. Pain that is perceived on the underside of the nipple is more likely caused by the nipple being tipped upward when the mother offers the breast. It is acceptable—perhaps even advisable—to tip the breast slightly upward so that the infant can readily latch on, chin first. However, the mother must quickly stop tipping the breast as soon as the infant has an adequate grasp of the nipple/areola or else soreness and bruising are likely to result. Use of the palmar grasp makes the mother particularly vulnerable to tipping the nipple upward during the feeding because she may exert more pressure with her thumb and displace the nipple tissue when she uses this position.

At least temporarily, engorgement results in an alteration of the contour of the nipple. The nipple/areola complex shortens in the presence of engorgement, making it more difficult for the infant to achieve good latch-on. Expressing a little milk by hand until the nipple/areola softens helps the infant achieve a proper grasp.

Blisters on the nipple are often caused when the infant's lower lip is not flanged on the breast. This should be recognized early and the infant assisted to open wide and achieve adequate latch-on. Blisters can also occur when the pump flange is not centered on the nipple.

Nipples can become sore when they are exposed to unrelieved negative pressure, such as occurs during prolonged nonnutritive suckling, a delayed let-down, or not breaking the suction before removing the infant from the breast. The nurse needs to raise the mother's awareness to these possibilities and offer corrective strategies.

Use or Misuse of Commercial Products or Equipment. Sometimes sore nipples are iatrogenic; they can occur as the result of using or misusing commercial products. For example, if the user turns the suction on too high and leaves it there, an electric breast pump will cause excessive negative pressure. (Excessive negative pressure—either high negative pressure or unrelieved negative pressure—is a common culprit for sore nipples.)

Sometimes, products meant to "help" sore nipples can actually cause the soreness. Prolonged exposure to wet nursing pads or to moisture build-up in poorly vented breast shells often results in tissue maceration and, subsequently, cracked nipples. Using plastic-lined breast pads or not replacing moist pads also creates tissue maceration. Drying the nipples by simply keeping the bra flaps down and exposing the nipples to air is perhaps the best remedy. A fairly new device, the breast leakage inhibitor system *(blis)*, is designed to help mothers avoid leakage that can result in tissue maceration and soggy underclothes.* Nipple shields can rub on the nipple skin and cause an abrasion. If the woman is allergic to creams or ointments that she applies to her nipples, she will experience the wheal and itching that typically occur with allergic reactions.

Pathologic or Anatomic Variations. If there is any alteration of the infant's orofacial structure, the mother may experience sore nipples. I am aware of one case in which the mother complained of exquisitely sore nipples. A smacking sound could be heard when the infant nursed, so everyone's first inclination was to presume that there was poor positioning. After adjusting the infant's position, however, the mother still complained of sore nipples. As it turned out, no one had given the

infant a complete digital examination of the oral cavity. When that occurred, the likely cause of the sore nipples was identified. The infant had a cleft of the soft palate. Similarly, mothers whose infants have a short frenulum are likely to complain of sore nipples.[28] However, do not assume that the cause of the mother's sore nipples is the infant's anatomy. One mother complained of very sore nipples and blamed her infant's cleft lip. When I observed the dyad breastfeeding, however, it immediately became evident that the cause of the sore nipples was a poor latch-on. When the infant opened wide and latched on, the problem of sore nipples almost immediately disappeared.

Inverted nipples may cause discomfort when the mother puts the infant to the breast. As discussed earlier, often the best treatment for inverted nipples is suckling at the breast.

The common notion that fair-skinned women are more vulnerable to nipple soreness than darker-skinned women is without substance. Although those of us in clinical practice have seen this many times and may be skeptical about the research results, to date, no controlled studies support these casual observations.[26]

Clinical Management Strategies

For more than half a century, "sore nipples" have been reported as the reason for early weaning.[18,19,29-33] However, sore nipples are not an expected consequence of breastfeeding and can usually be prevented or managed when there is a clear understanding of the root of the problem.

Over the years, several recommendations have been given for preventing and/or treating sore nipples. Some of these treatments have been shown to be ineffective; others appear to be effective. A summary of a few helpful strategies is found in Box 12-3.

Prevention Strategies. Strategies that effectively treat sore nipples do not necessarily prevent sore nipples, and vice versa. And, some strategies, presumed to be helpful, have not been proven safe or effective. These should be discontinued.

"Prevention" Strategies to Discontinue. Several decades ago, pregnant women were instructed to prepare for breastfeeding by rubbing

*The Breast Leakage Inhibitor System, *blis,* is available from Prolac, Inc., 888-410-2547 or 315-685-1955 or see http://www.blis.com.

Box 12-3   Tips for Managing Sore Nipples

- Determine the root of the problem. Otherwise, interventions may cause more harm than good.
- Instruct the mother to discontinue using practices or products that are likely to cause or exacerbate sore nipples. This includes rubbing the nipples with a towel, using soap or alcohol products, using creams or ointments that she may be allergic to, not changing wet breast pads promptly, and using nipple shields.
- Correct poor positioning. An asymmetric latch-on, incremental latch-on, "dragging" on a large breast (use rolled-up towel under the breast to alleviate drag), and sucking of

the nipple instead of the areola all contribute to sore nipples.
- Reduce pressure on the sore spot. Feed on the less-sore side first because the infant's suck is most vigorous when he starts. Alternating positions for a few days (e.g., cradle hold at this feeding, side-lying hold at next feeding, football hold at next feeding) may be helpful.
- Enhance milk-ejection reflex. Warm compresses or massaging before feeding or while the infant pauses during feeding helps an eager infant obtain milk without excessive sucks before let-down.

---

their nipples vigorously with a bath towel. This action may create rather than prevent or resolve a problem. Rubbing the nipples vigorously with a towel removes the protective epithelial cells. Furthermore, such stimulation to the breasts may stimulate uterine contractions, causing preterm labor.

Over the years, various topical creams and ointments have been recommended as a panacea for sore nipples. These include A&D ointment, bag balm, lanolin (unprocessed lanolin, made from sheep's wool), and modified lanolin (lanolin that has been processed). Some may have some therapeutic value for skin that is already broken, but none have any preventive powers.

Limitation of suckling time has been recommended for decades as a way to prevent nipple soreness, but it has never been proven effective.[34] On the other hand, "marathon" suckling in the first few days, particularly when there is little milk in the ducts, invites unrelieved negative pressure and the potential for sore nipples.

Effective Prevention Strategies. Good positioning and latch-on are likely to be the best prevention strategy for most cases of sore nipples.[27] Similarly, it is likely that avoiding a pacifier, which may interfere with suckling behavior, is a preventive strategy (see Chapter 8).

Air-drying the nipples, with the bra flaps down for several minutes, allows the nipple tissue to dry.

This reduces the possibility of having a dark environment with a sweet, moist medium for bacterial growth. The blis device also helps reduce moisture build-up. Frequent feedings, long presumed to avoid the situation of having a ravenously hungry newborn and subsequently sore nipples, has finally been shown to be effective.[35]

Treatment Strategies. Good latch-on, as described in Chapter 7, is probably the key to preventing most cases of sore nipples. If the tissue damage has already occurred, however, treatment is required.

Protective methods such as alternating positions and using shells, shields, or pads can be effective. (Shells used for protective purposes differ slightly in design from shells used to treat inverted nipples.) Dry wound healing, for example, using a hairdryer to dry the nipples, was once thought to be helpful, but this has never been proven. Although it is plausible that such a practice may prevent maceration of tissue, it is highly unlikely to have a curative effect. Starting on the less-sore side first and eliciting a milk-ejection reflex helps. Even if corrective strategies have begun, analgesics may be needed for temporary relief of the discomfort.

Moist wound healing methods are thought to be the most effective treatment for damaged nipple tissue. Modified lanolin, a popular moist wound healing method, has been shown effective in some studies[36,37] but not in others.[26,38] Warm water compresses are preferable to another commonly used intervention, tea bags.[39,40] Whether or not human milk is effective in preventing or treating traumatized nipples has yet to be completely proved. One research study showed no difference,[38] but expert clinicians are staunch defenders of this practice.[5] In some cultures human milk is used for many skin irritations. There appear to be no harmful effects, and therefore no reason to not recommend this practice, which clinical experience has shown to be beneficial.

Commercially made moist wound dressings, which have been used for chronic ulcers and surgical wounds for the last two decades or so, have recently been manufactured specifically for nipples. The first published study describing the use of the glycerine-based dressing showed no significant difference in effectiveness when compared with modified lanolin cream. The study had to be discontinued, however, because pathogens were growing on the nipples of women using the dressings. Two other unpublished studies have shown no untoward effects. One study, which compared the effectiveness of lanolin cream with the saline-based dressing, claimed that the dressing prevented nipple soreness[41] (Table 12-2). Another study, which compared the effectiveness of lanolin cream, a glycerine-based dressing, and teaching only, showed no significant difference in the dressing's ability to treat women with already damaged nipple tissue.[42] The decision to recommend or not recommend these dressings requires careful assessment and evaluation

All too often, a reasonable strategy is recommended but the problem does not resolve. Ongoing evaluation is essential, and no presumptions about problem resolution should be made. Direct observation of the nipples, questioning of the mother about her comfort, and the general status of the infant are perhaps the most important outcome criteria. If problem resolution cannot be verified, the root of the problem must continue to be pursued and corrective strategies initiated. Sore nipples are not an expected consequence of breastfeeding, but a signal for help. Breastfeeding is not meant to be painful; if it were, the species would not have survived. Causes, goals, and strategies for dealing with sore nipples are described in Table 12-3.

Engorgement

Engorgement is the distention of body tissue. The term *engorgement* means distention of mammary *tissue,* and it is a sign of milk production but is not equivalent to milk production or milk volume. Newton and Newton[43] assert that engorgement begins when milk is retained in the alveoli; the alveoli become distended and compress the surrounding ducts (Box 12-4). Engorgement involves two elements: (1) congestion and increased vascularity and (2) accumulation of milk[5] (see Historical Highlight box in Chapter 7).

Types of Engorgement

There are two types of engorgement: physiologic and pathologic. They differ primarily in degree. It is important to differentiate the two in terms of clinical recognition and management.

Physiologic Engorgement. The breasts begin to fill with milk around the second or third postpartum day, depending on how early and how frequently the infant has suckled. Some degree of engorgement is physiologic, and its absence should be considered a red flag for further follow-up. Unfortunately, the word *engorgement* has often carried a negative connotation, so the mother may need some reeducation.

Help the new mother recognize the signs and symptoms of physiologic engorgement as positive; the tissue distention heralds the "coming-in" of her milk supply. Most of all, impress upon her that when the tissue distention goes away, it does not mean that the milk goes away. She may assume that she already has an oversupply of milk and therefore may deny the infant access to the breast, thinking that more stimulation will only exacerbate the situation. Instruct her to continue breastfeeding because the degree of tissue distention is not equivalent to the degree of milk supply. To the contrary, *not* having the infant drain the breasts will only worsen the problem because milk stasis invites pathologic engorgement.

Table 12-2   Comparison of Three Types of Hydrogel Dressings

	Elasto-gel	MaterniMate	Soothie
Manufacturer	Southwest Technologies	Kendall	Puronyx
Description of dressing	Glycerin-based pad	Saline-based pad	Glycerin-based pad
Author	Brent et al.[37]	Dodd and Chalmers[41]	Cadwell[42]
Aim of study	To compare the safety and efficacy of hydrogel dressings to use of lanolin cream and shells for *treating* sore nipples	To compare the safety and efficacy of hydrogel dressings to use of lanolin cream for *preventing* sore nipples	To compare the safety and efficacy of hydrogel dressings to lanolin and shells; also, to examine the effectiveness of teaching for effective latch-on
Study design	Comparative descriptive	Comparative descriptive	Comparative descriptive
Population	Mothers referred to lactation clinic for treatment of bleeding, cracked, or crusted nipples and/or painful nipples; a total of 39% of the mothers were exclusively breastfeeding	Primiparae who had given birth within the past 24 hr and who were identified as "at risk" for sore nipples because of "frequency of feeding"	Sequential sample of Latvian women who presented to midwife with reports of nipple soreness; subjects with no known infections, abscesses, or chronic unrelated pain conditions had delivered infants with no known craniofacial anomalies; all had some nipple trauma
N	42 (21 control/21 experimental)	106 (54 control/52 experimental)	90* (15 control/15 experimental*)
Time dressing first applied	Not specified	Within 24 hr of birth	Unspecified times during the first 10 days
Time results measured	Each time mother presented for 3 follow-up visits within 10 days	Telephone contact at day 3, 4 or 5, 7, 10, 12 days	Each time mother presented for follow-up visit
Method for measuring results	Direct observation with Mother-Baby Assessment tool (see Chapter 7) and maternal self-report of healing	Maternal self-report of nipple pain and dressing comfort; maternal self-report of nipple/areolar condition	Direct observation of nipple/areola by midwife, maternal self-report of nipple pain and dressing comfort

Instrument	Physical assessment with 5-point Likert-type scale, pain behavior scale, self-reports of pain	5-point Likert-type scale to rate maternal perceptions of nipple pain and dressing comfort	5-point Likert-type scale to rate maternal perceptions of nipple pain
Procedure in experimental group	Mothers applied dressing after massaging their own milk onto the nipple; they were instructed to use a new dressing after each feeding	Mothers applied dressing according to manufacturer's instructions, which included directives about hygiene, application and removal of the dressing, and the need for replacing the dressing	Mothers applied dressing according to manufacturer's instructions, which included directives about hygiene, application and removal of the dressing, and the need for replacing the dressing
Teaching	Teaching for proper latch-on	Teaching for proper latch-on	Teaching for proper latch-on
Results	In both groups, the sum of adverse nipple attributes significantly decreased at time of follow-up; hydrogel group had higher adverse nipple attribute scores, but not statistically significant; degree of healing significantly higher in lanolin group	Results were reported in terms of actual pair level (not degree of improvement); when compared with baseline, reported pain ratings during the 12-day period were significantly improved in the hydrogel pad group, but not in the lanolin group	Preliminary results of pain were reported in relative terms (i.e., in degree of improvement) from before treatment to after treatment; reported pain ratings were reduced by 1.76 points in the hydrogel group compared with 1.1 points in the lanolin group; healing was about the same in both groups; dressing improved maternal satisfaction
Untoward effects noted	Bacterial growth noted in 9 of the 42 subjects (7 in dressing group and 2 in lanolin group)	No bacterial growth noted in the MaterniMates group; bacterial growth noted in 8 subjects in the lanolin-cream group	No increased risk of infection
Comments	Investigators did not specify directions for hygiene precautions, which may explain the high rate of bacterial growth	Abstract explicitly describes hygiene instructions for the hydrogel group, but not for the lanolin group where bacterial growth occurred	Inferences about this segment of the study are limited to results reported in these 30 subjects; data analysis of all 90 subjects is incomplete

*Results of 30 reported in the abstract; data analysis of the other 2 groups of 30 are underway.

RESEARCH HIGHLIGHT

Mastitis: New Evidence for Old and Recurring Problem

Citation: Foxman B, D'Arcy H, Gillespie B et al. Lactation mastitis: occurrence and medical management among 946 breastfeeding women in the United States. *Am J Epidemiol* 2002;155:103-114; and Riordan JM, Nichols FH. A descriptive study of lactation mastitis in long-term breastfeeding women. *J Hum Lact* 1990;6:53-58.

FOCUS

Foxman and colleagues followed 946 breastfeeding women in a prospective, longitudinal study from birth until 3 months postpartum, or until they stopped breastfeeding. The subjects were recruited from a birthing center in Michigan and from a large company where they worked in Nebraska. The study was conducted over a 4-year period, so some women who gave birth more than once during the study period entered the study more than once.

The investigators conducted interviews at 3, 6, 9, and 12 weeks postpartum, or until they weaned. The interview consisted of questions about the current physical aspect of breastfeeding (e.g., how often the breast was offered, breast-related symptoms, sleeping, smoking), as well as the past history of mastitis, medical history, and sociodemographic information. Mastitis was defined "by self report of mastitis diagnosed by a health care provider."

INCIDENCE

During the 12-week study period, 8.1% of the subjects reported one episode of mastitis, 1.3% reported two episodes, and 0.1% reported three episodes. Overall, 9.5% of the subjects had mastitis during the first 12 weeks. Mastitis incidence was highest in the first few weeks postpartum and declined thereafter. The incidence reported here was higher than that in previous studies.

DIAGNOSIS, SYMPTOMS, AND CHANGE IN HABITS

Most women were diagnosed by telephone; the most common symptoms they reported were breast tenderness (98%), fever (82%), malaise (87%), chills (78%), redness (78%), and a hot spot of tenderness on the breast (62%). Almost half of the women changed their breastfeeding habits as a result of the symptoms; 36% fed more often, whereas 11% fed less often overall. A variation was that 49% fed on the affected breast more often, whereas 8% fed on the affected breast less often. With the onset of mastitis, 33% of the women changed the nursing hold they were using, 12% tried a different hold, and 12% tried or a new hold.

TREATMENTS

Antibiotics were prescribed for 86% of the women; cephalexin was usually given, but amoxicillin, ampicillin, or augmentin were occasionally prescribed also. None of the providers ordered cultures, but the vast majority recommended warm compresses and more frequent feeding; a little less than half suggested different nursing positions.

ASSOCIATIONS

Previous breastfeeding experience was associated with an increased risk for mastitis. The incidence of mastitis was higher among women who had breastfed previously (10.8%) compared with those who had never breastfed (7.3%). Similarly, a history of mastitis appears to be a risk factor for future episodes; women who had previously experienced mastitis were more at risk for repeated episodes (23.9%) compared with first-time mothers (8.3%).

Cracks and nipple soreness are associated with mastitis. Women with a history of mastitis were more likely to report cracks and soreness of their nipples. If women had *no* history of mastitis but experienced nipple cracks or sores, they were six times more likely to get mastitis during the week that the cracks were present. If women *did* have a history of mastitis and experienced nipple cracks or sores, they were three times more likely to get mastitis during the week that the cracks or sores were present. More than one third of the women reported cracks during the first week postpartum.

RESEARCH HIGHLIGHT—cont'd

Feeding frequency, but not duration, was associated with mastitis; mastitis was more likely to occur when the number of feedings was greater than usual. Breast pain was associated with mastitis, but only if it occurred less than 1 week before the mastitis was reported. This suggests that the breast pain is more of symptom than a predisposing factor. Similarly, women who took naps had higher rates of mastitis, but researchers could not determine whether fatigue made the woman more vulnerable to mastitis or if it was merely a symptom of mastitis.

A hand-operated breast pump was significantly associated with mastitis, but only for women who had no history of mastitis. The investigators did not describe the specific pump or pumps that the subjects used.

STRENGTHS, LIMITATIONS OF THE STUDY

A major strength of the study was that there were 946 subjects who participated, beginning in pregnancy, thus enabling the researchers to conduct a prospective study. In addition to the shear volume of subjects, it is also notable that only 11 of those who were contacted refused to participate, which dramatically reduces the possibility of sampling error. A weakness of the study is that the authors do not describe the effect of mastitis on weaning, which has been reported in other literature.[56] Another limitation is that only 74% of the women were reportedly diagnosed with mastitis by a doctor or a nurse; it is unclear who diagnosed the remaining 36% of the women in the study, and hence, the definition of mastitis may have jeopardized the validity of the study. Nonetheless, this study makes a major contribution to the existing literature on the topic.

CLINICAL APPLICATION

Several points are noteworthy for clinical application. First, mastitis does occur in nearly 10% of the healthy population, and sociodemographic factors are not significant risk factors. It is likely that women need more help with achieving optimal positioning, because cracks on the nipple occurred in one third of the study group and were significantly associated with the development of mastitis.

Reprinted from Biancuzzo M. *Breastfeeding Outlook* 2002;3:1, 4.

Pathologic Engorgement. Pathologic engorgement occurs when the amount of tissue distention is preventable, extreme, or the result of some unphysiologic cause. In most circumstances, pathologic engorgement is preventable. There is a strong correlation between pathologic engorgement and delayed initiation of the first feeding(s), infrequent feedings, severely limited-time feedings, and supplementation.[44] Therefore avoiding these practices, as described in Chapters 7 and 8, is likely to prevent most episodes of pathologic engorgement.

Clinical Manifestations

Breast assessment should *always* be included as part of the overall postpartum assessment. Beyond the objective physical assessment, it is helpful to ask the woman about her subjective sensations of breast fullness. Some women report that they feel a sudden, unmistakable "coming-in" of milk, whereas others report a more gradual onset and are less aware of the "coming-in." Engorgement happens sooner and more dramatically in second-time breastfeeding mothers than in those who have never lactated before.[45] When her milk supply starts to become copious, the woman may have a slight fever and general malaise. She may become tearful. She is usually less frustrated if she is warned well ahead of time that the sensation of engorgement that occurs around day 3 is caused by swelling of the *tissue*. Although the swelling goes away, this does not mean that the *milk* has gone away!

There are several signs and symptoms of engorgement. Some of those associated with pathologic engorgement are present with physiologic

Table **12-3** Causes and Clinical Strategies for Sore Nipples

Causes	Possible Contributing Factors	Prevention and Goals	Clinical Strategies
Simple mismanagement of breastfeeding	Improper positioning and latch-on	Achieve proper latch-on	As described in Chapter 7
	Unrelieved negative pressure when milk is not yet abundant; Not breaking suction before removing infant from breast	Minimize unrelieved negative pressure	Encourage use of both breasts at each feeding to minimize unrelieved negative pressure; Teach mother to break suction by using her finger if she needs to take the infant off the breast
Deviations from normal	Flat or retracted nipples	Achieve good latch-on	Listen for audible swallowing
	Pathologic engorgement	Prevent milk stasis	Avoid pathologic engorgement by early, frequent, and effective feeding (i.e., milk transfer)
	Breast infections	Prevent milk stasis	Assess for breast infections and initiate treatment if indicated
Improper use of apparatus/products	Improper use of breast pumps	Demonstrate and explain proper use of equipment	Decrease intensity of suction and increase number of suction cycles
	Prolonged exposure to moist breast pads	Allow air to circulate to nipple	Change pads frequently; Use no pads or disposable pads if infection is present (e.g., candidiasis) because this provides medium for growth
	Allergies to creams and ointments	Avoid contact with potential allergens	Discontinue use
	Use of nipple shields	Avoid trauma to nipple tissue	Discontinue use
	Use of cutoff syringe to evert nipples	Avoid trauma to nipple tissue	Use devices designed for everting nipples

Box **12-4** AREOLAR VERSUS PERIPHERAL ENGORGEMENT

AREOLAR ENGORGEMENT

Obliterates nipple; difficult for infant to properly grasp areola. Collecting ducts will not be milked and therefore do not empty.

May occur alone or in conjunction with peripheral engorgement

More likely to occur during physiologic engorgement.

Treatment:

- Hand expression to soften the areola so that the infant can get a good grasp of the nipple and areola

PERIPHERAL ENGORGEMENT

Initially, engorgement is vascular; therefore-pumping is not productive and may be traumatic. reasts are full, hard, tender; swelling starts at the clavicle and goes to the lower ribcage and from the midaxillary line to the midsternum. Most likely to occur with areolar engorgement.

More likely to occur during pathologic engorgement.

Treatment:

- Frequent breastfeeding around the clock! Relief is based on establishment of milk flow
- Wear supportive bra 24 hours a day
- Warm showers and warm packs help release accumulation of milk
- Cold packs *after* breastfeeding to decrease congestion
- If ordered, administer analgesic immediately before breastfeeding; drug will not reach milk for at least 20-30 minutes (aspirin, acetaminophen, codeine, short-acting barbiturates)
- Manual expression and massage

Data derived from Lawrence RA, Lawrence RM. *Breastfeeding: a guide for the medical profession.* 5th ed. St. Louis: Mosby; 1999.

engorgement, but to a greater degree. The signs and symptoms of engorgement may involve only the areola, only the body of the breast (peripheral engorgement), or both. Box 12-4 compares and contrasts clinical manifestations.

Areolar Engorgement. Areolar engorgement is distention of the areolar tissue only. The areola may become distended to the extent that the nipple is shortened and may virtually disappear. This creates a snowballing problem: The infant is unable to latch on and effectively empty the breast; milk then accumulates, and the engorgement becomes more severe and more painful.

Peripheral Engorgement. Peripheral engorgement is likely to occur in the presence of areolar engorgement. Peripheral engorgement includes the "body" of the breast and is more likely to be a sign of pathologic rather than physiologic engorgement.

Treatments Strategies

Engorgement can and should be prevented as described earlier. The aim of treatment is to decrease the overdistention of the ducts. Ductal distention is minimized if accumulation of milk can be reduced or if vascular congestion can be reduced. Although the infant provides the best relief for engorgement, other interventions that achieve this aim are also helpful. Warm showers, warm compresses, or leaning over a basin of warm water reduces the accumulation of milk in the ducts. Applying cold packs after breastfeeding causes vasoconstriction, thereby reducing vasocongestion and discomfort. (Cold packs on or near the nipples before feedings can interfere with the milk-ejection reflex.) Perhaps the most convenient and accessible cold pack is a bag of frozen vegetables. Frozen peas work especially well because their shape and size allow the bag to be flexible. Ice packs are certainly acceptable, but they are more rigid when frozen, and they make a watery mess as they melt. Commercially available warm/cold packs, including those that are specifically designed for breastfeeding women,* have been noted, anecdotally, to provide excellent relief.

Breast-Nurse is available through Thermal Therapeutic Supplies at 800-752-5797.

Historical Highlight

Sore Nipples

Citation: Gunther M. Sore nipples, causes and prevention. *Lancet* 1945;249:590-593.

A descriptive study was conducted on a total of 114 primiparae and multiparae from their first to eleventh postpartum day. All mothers were healthy and had average-weight, healthy newborns. Dr. Gunther identified two types of lesions that differed in nature, position, and time of incidence: the petechial (erosive) lesion and the ulcerative lesion (i.e., fissure). About 62% had the erosive type of lesion, and about 4% had the ulcerative type of lesion; three women had both types.

Gunther described four grades of soreness: (1) soreness but no visible change; (2) edema of papillae visible; (3) petechiae, separated; (4) petechiae, merged to form a transverse crescent. The petechial lesions were small and almost always preceded by translucent edema. The most extensive petechiae merged to form a red, crescent-shaped lesion across the nipple. Erosion of the epithelium from a ruptured blister was also noted. Gunther emphasized that the line of merged petechiae across the nipple corresponded to where the infant exerted the most pressure.

Unlike the erosive type, the onset of ulcerative lesions was noted after a few days.

Gunther further explained that nipple soreness was related to lack of swallowing and that soreness was not reported as frequently when the infant could be heard swallowing. Negative pressure was measured, and it was shown that the infant exerted greater negative pressures on the breast when there was very little milk to be obtained (either because it was shortly after birth, or at the end of feeding when very little milk was left). The infant used high continuous negative pressure, but the pressure was relieved when the infant swallowed.

Infants in this study were limited in the amount of time they suckled. Obviously this did not prevent the sore nipples. Furthermore, there was no attempt to correct their positioning at the breast, and one might wonder if negative pressure would have been so high if the infants had been positioned differently. Nonetheless, today's nurse has much to learn from this study in terms of points to look for in assessing the breasts, the futility of limiting suckling time in an attempt to prevent sore nipples, and the need to evaluate milk transfer as evidenced by audible swallowing.

Hand expression is the treatment of choice for areolar engorgement. (It may give some relief for peripheral engorgement as well.) Assist the mother to express a little milk—just enough to soften the nipple/areola complex. Softening usually can be accomplished by expressing less than 15 ml. This enables the infant to attach properly and is the start of problem resolution. Using an electric breast pump, although acceptable, is a less desirable strategy because the negative pressure exerted and the pump's flange are more likely to cause trauma to tissue that is already taut and distended.

If the degree of engorgement is already causing the mother pain, initiate measures to reduce the pain and solve the problem. Usually, a variety of analgesics are ordered for the discomforts associated with the postpartum recovery. A mild analgesic (such as acetaminophen) typically is sufficient to relieve the discomfort associated with breast engorgement, but if it is not, stronger analgesics are appropriate.

Cool cabbage leaves have been used to relieve engorgement.[46-48] Anecdotal reports of such use have not demonstrated efficacy of the leaves for relieving engorgement. One study suggested that maternal confidence and reassurance seemed to be as effective as the cabbage leaves, and another showed that the cabbage leaves were no more effective than cold gel packs.[47]

LATER PROBLEMS

Breast and nipple problems can occur at any time, but usually, the problems that occur later include plugged ducts, mastitis, breast abscess, and candidiasis.

Plugged Duct

A plugged duct is a duct that has, for whatever reason, not drained well. Frequently, it is caused by inadequate emptying of the breast (e.g., when an infant has an inadequate suck). It could also be the result of other causes, such as a bra that is too tight or a cream that has been used on the nipple. The plugged duct is not a problem per se, but it can result in mastitis if it is not corrected (see section on mastitis).

Clinical Manifestations

Typically, the woman who presents with a plugged duct complains of a tender, sore lump that is not accompanied by a fever or other signs of infection. It may feel hot to the touch. Often, she will report that she is feeding less frequently (e.g., eliminated night feedings) or had a change in the feeding pattern.

Prevention and Treatment Strategies

Plugged ducts can often be prevented by frequent nursing. If a plugged duct is suspected, alternating the position of the infant can improve drainage in all of the ducts. If necessary, a more unusual position can be used to drain the ducts, such as the modified side-lying position, shown in Fig. 12-5, which may be used in addition to the more common cradle, side-lying, and football holds. If the infant is unable to suckle, suggest a pump, or better still teach hand expression (see Chapter 14). Hand expression works well, along with warm, moist heat. It is helpful for the woman to express milk by hand while she leans over a basin of warm water. In this way, her fingers can "milk" the ducts, while the heat causes vasodilation and the leaning over allows gravity to enhance drainage.

Mastitis

Description and Etiology

Mastitis is a fairly common problem; it is reported that up to 23% of women have had one or more episodes of mastitis.[49] The highest incidence of mastitis occurs around 6[50] to 7 weeks[51] and declines thereafter.

There are two types of mastitis: inflammatory and infectious. Both occur in the breast's ductal system and are associated with milk stasis. Milk stasis is problematic because the mammary gland is designed to secrete and transport milk, but not to store milk. Any mother with milk stasis is at high risk for a plugged duct, engorgement, mastitis, or all three. Table 12-4 compares and contrasts these conditions.

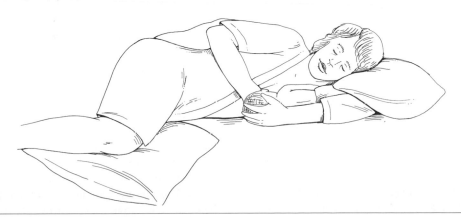

FIGURE **12-5** Modified side-lying position.

Table **12-4** COMPARISON OF FINDINGS OF ENGORGEMENT, PLUGGED DUCT, AND MASTITIS

Characteristics	Engorgement	Plugged Duct	Mastitis
Onset	Gradual, immediately postpartum	Gradual, after feedings	Sudden, after 10 days
Site	Bilateral	Unilateral	Usually unilateral
Swelling and heat	Generalized	May shift a little or no	Localized, red, hot, and swollen
Pain	Generalized	heat Mild but localized	Intense but localized
Body temperature	<38.4° C	<38.4° C	>38.4° C
Systemic symptoms	Feels well	Feels well	Flulike symptoms

From Lawrence RA, Lawrence RM. *Breastfeeding: a guide for the medical profession.* 5th ed. St. Louis: Mosby; 1999.

Risk factors

Milk stasis and nipple trauma predispose the ductal system to bacterial invasion. Milk stasis often occurs when the mother has an oversupply of milk.[51] For example, women who are breastfeeding multiples are probably more at risk because they produce about twice the amount of milk as mothers of singletons.[52] It can also occur when there is an abrupt change in the feeding pattern (for example, when the infant begins to sleep through the night). Contributing factors include tight bras, a missed feeding, or plugged ducts. Although it is difficult to explain why, women who have had previous breastfeeding experience are more at risk for mastitis.[92] A history of mastitis also appears to be a risk factor for future episodes.[92]

Women who have sore nipples are more at risk for mastitis.[53,54,92] If women have no history of mastitis but experience nipple cracks or sores, they are six times more likely to have mastitis during the week that the cracks are present.[92] A likely explanation is that the woman who has sore nipples has not had complete removal of milk from her breast on a regular basis. In addition, if the nipple skin is no longer intact, it can become a portal of entry for the invading bacteria.

Other factors have been identified as risk factors for mastitis. Women who have had mastitis while lactating for previous children tend to suffer from mastitis with subsequent children.[54,55] Mothers who have been exposed to the bacterial organism or those with lowered body defenses or extreme fatigue or stress are vulnerable.[56] Also, daily pacifier use has been associated with greater incidence of mastitis.[49]

Some factors, commonly thought to be risk factors, apparently are not. There is no evidence to support the commonly held belief that suckling on only one side at a feeding increases the risk for mastitis.[57] Parity does not seem to be a risk factor for mastitis.[53,58]

Clinical Manifestations

Milk stasis frequently causes a duct to be obstructed, resulting in the first sign of serious trouble: a small, hard, warm, tender lump. Within about 12 to 24 hours of ductal obstruction, "inflammatory mastitis" begins. As the "-itis" suffix implies, the internal ducts and ductules become inflamed causing further local effects: a breast that is swollen, hard, tender, and hot.[59] These signs and symptoms—subtle at first—often (but not always) appear in the upper outer quadrant of the breast, as shown in Fig. 12-6, where the glandular tissue is most dense; they then progressively intensify, and red streaking also appears. Often, it is the upper outer quadrant because this is the location of the largest amount of glandular tissue. At this point, the white blood cell count in the milk increases—a normal response to inflammation—but the bacterial count remains largely unchanged. If the obstructed duct is not treated, however, the inflammation is followed by "infectious mastitis" within about 24 to 48 hours, and the bacterial count is elevated along with the white blood cell count. Systemic effects of infectious mastitis—fever, chills, flulike symptoms and malaise—occur when the inflamed tissue becomes infected by bacteria. Most frequently, the invading organism is *Staphylococcus aureus*,[60] but sometimes *Escherichia*

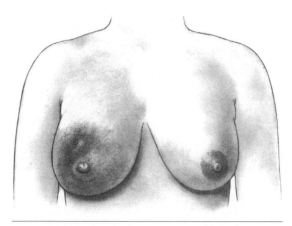

FIGURE **12-6** Mastitis. *(From Lawrence RA, Lawrence RM. Breastfeeding: a guide for the medical profession. 5th ed. St. Louis: Mosby; 1999.)*

coli and, more rarely, *Streptococcus* are the causative organisms.

Prevention and Treatment Strategies

Prevention is certainly possible. Some papers suggest that inflammatory mastitis can perhaps be prevented by improving the maternal ingestion of micronutrients,[61,62] particularly vitamin E–rich sunflower oil.[63] Inflammatory mastitis may be prevented with frequent breast emptying.[64,65] Infants may react to the taste of the milk, however, because increased sodium levels in the milk have been associated with mastitis.[66]

Antibiotic therapy is required and usually results in rapid relief.[5] Most clinicians recommend a full round of antibiotics, even when the infectious signs are not present.

The most important teaching points about mastitis are related to stress and fatigue.[56] Suggest to the woman that she take the infant to bed with her and discourage well-meaning visitors who deprive her of rest; women who take afternoon naps appear to be less vulnerable to mastitis.[55] Encourage the woman to seek help from friends or relatives who would be willing to perform household chores so that she can take care of herself and her infant. Other priorities for care are listed in Box 12-5.

Sometimes, mastitis is difficult to cure.[67] Recurrent mastitis is likely to occur when mothers have milk stasis, or an oversupply of milk.[68] The most likely cause for recurrent mastitis is that the mother did not finish the prescribed round of antibiotics, or she may not have had enough rest to fortify her body's natural defenses. Occasionally, however, the mother may have a chronic bacterial infection, a secondary fungal infection (e.g., *Candida albicans*), or some more serious underlying disease.

Differentiating infective from noninfective (inflammatory) mastitis can be difficult.[69] Fetherston suggests that there should be a greater emphasis on determining the causative organism associated with individual cases of mastitis and that women need more information about those possible causes and the gamut of possible treatment options.[70] Homeopathic treatments have been reported for the treatment of mastitis,[71] but this has not yet been shown as an evidence-based practice.

Mastitis is commonly cited as the reason for weaning.[72] Unfortunately, discontinuation of breastfeeding only worsens the situation. The milk becomes "backed up" in the ducts, and milk stasis provides food for the invading organism. Mastitic milk is not harmful to the infant; it contains the same antiinflammatory components as normal milk.[73] Furthermore, it appears that the milk protects the infant against infections of the gastrointestinal tract.[74] Some recent speculation suggests that the presence of mastitis increases the chances of vertical transmission of HIV,[75] but this idea has not yet been well substantiated.

Breast Abscess

An abscess can occur anywhere on the body. Typically, it is a pus-filled cavity that is surrounded by inflamed tissue. The inflammation is a localized infection, usually staphylococcal. Less frequently, it may be caused by *Streptococcus*.[76] Breast abscesses are more common among smokers.[77]

Box 12-5   Priorities for Care: Mastitis

- Identify patients who are at risk for developing mastitis and initiate teaching to reduce the likelihood of mastitis developing. Women with plugged ducts are among the most likely candidates for developing mastitis. Women with an oversupply of milk are also likely to develop mastitis.[51]
- For telephone inquiries, advise the woman to get immediate in-person evaluation and, if indicated, treatment. Antibiotics usually provide swift relief.
- For in-person assessments, use inspection, palpation, and good interview skills to recognize the presence of an invading organism; refer to physician immediately. Early antibiotic therapy is ideal.
- Encourage frequent, regular breastfeeding with complete emptying of each breast! If the infant is unable to completely empty the breast, initiate pumping.
- Instruct the mother to start the infant on the unaffected side first. Then, when the infant comes to the affected side, suckling will be

less vigorous and the mother will have already experienced a let-down, thereby making the experience less painful. Explain the importance of complete emptying of the breast.
- Review steps to overcome any infection, including increasing fluids, maintaining bedrest, and taking prescribed antibiotics on time and for the full course.
- Reassure the mother that the prescribed antibiotic is compatible with breastfeeding (see Chapter 13).
- Suggest comfort measures: warm packs promote drainage of the ductal system, but ice packs cause vasoconstriction and increase comfort. Either may be used. A bra may be worn to promote comfort, but be cautious in this recommendation; sometimes the bra the mother owns is too tight and caused the problem in the first place. If a mild analgesic has been prescribed, encourage her to take it because breast emptying is more likely to occur if her pain level is more tolerable.

Clinical Manifestations

Upon inspection, there is redness as a result of the accumulation of blood at the site where the inflammatory process occurs. The formation of pus causes the swelling. Women usually report pain because of the pressure of the pus against the nerve tissue. The presence of the abscess can be determined with ultrasound.[78]

Prevention and Treatment Strategies

Manual stripping of pus among women with mastitis seems to prevent abscess formation.[79] For healing to occur, the abscess must drain. Surgical drainage has been the traditional treatment.[76] Sometimes, a surgical drain is put in to get adequate drainage. In such cases breastfeeding can probably continue. The caveat here is that the drain must be far enough away that it is not involved in the feeding process. Whether or not the infant breastfeeds, the important thing is to drain the ductal system as completely as possible when the breasts feel full. A more recent alternative to a surgical drain is an ultrasound percutaneous catheter.[80]

Encourage the woman to continue breastfeeding frequently because emptying the ducts expedites the drainage. The milk is "clean" unless the abscess ruptures into the ducts.[5] Watch for signs and symptoms of infection in the infant, and refer him for medical treatment if indicated. In most cases, antibiotics are prescribed for the woman (and for the infant, if indicated). Other interventions may be needed as well.

If the physician orders cultures of the mother's milk, instruct her on the correct way to obtain a midstream "clean-catch" specimen. This process is fairly simple, with steps similar to those used to obtain a clean-catch specimen of urine. Instruct the woman to wash her hands vigorously with soap and water, then to rinse her breasts with plain water. Suggest that she initiate hand expression, then discard the first 3 to 5 ml of milk, and express a small sample into a sterile container. Emphasize to her the importance of keeping her nipple well away from the cup so that sterility can be maintained. The specimen should then be capped (touching only the outside of the cap), labeled, and taken to the laboratory immediately.

Candidiasis/Thrush

Candida is a fungal organism that normally inhabits the mouth, vagina, and intestines. An overgrowth of *Candida* can occur, however, leading to the infection known as *candidiasis,* more commonly known as *thrush* or *yeast* (and formerly called *monilia*). Candidiasis can occur on the lactating woman's nipples ("yeast") and the inside of her infant's mouth (oral "thrush"), as well as on the infant's diaper area (diaper rash) and in the mother's vagina. The discussion here is limited to an overgrowth of *Candida* on the mother's nipples or in the infant's mouth. When the infection is present at one site, however, there is a high likelihood that it will affect another as well.

Women who breastfeed are at risk for developing candidiasis because, like other fungi, *C. albicans* typically thrives on carbohydrates, so the lactose in milk provides the ideal food for the organism's growth. As described earlier, having mastitis predisposes the woman to future candidiasis infections. Other factors have been identified as risk factors for the development of breast candidiasis, including vaginal candidiasis, nipple trauma, and previous antibiotic use.[81] Daily pacifier use has been associated with greater incidence of candidiasis.[82,83] Antibiotics destroy the normal flora that would otherwise oppose the overgrowth of *Candida.* Having prior nipple damage makes the nipple vulnerable to growth of *Candida.* Diabetic persons with suppressed immune systems and anemic women are at increased risk for candidiasis.

Clinical Manifestations

Physical assessment may reveal one or more signs and symptoms in the infant, the mother, or the mother's partner. Clinical experts have clearly delineated the signs and symptoms for the lactating mother, breastfeeding infant, and the mother's partner, which are summarized and augmented here.[84] Typically, the infant has white patches in the mouth that are easily mistaken for milk. If a white patch clings to the infant's tongue when rubbed with a clean finger or cotton-tipped swab, it is likely to be thrush; rubbing a white patch leaves a red or bleeding spot. In addition, the oral sign is commonly accompanied by a bright red rash extending from the infant's anus outward. The infant may be feeding poorly or may refuse to eat. He may also be restless and irritable.

Inspect the color of the mother's nipples; they may be bright red or purple. Sometimes the bright red nipples are in sharp contrast to the paler areola—the nipple looks almost like a raspberry atop the areola. Inspect for lesions; on rare occasions, the white plaque can be seen, but in most cases it cannot be observed on light-skinned women. Even if it is visible, it may be dismissed on the assumption that it is only milk on the nipple. Often, the woman's partner is asymptomatic, but if he has engaged in any oral contact with her breast, he may have white patches in his mouth. He also may have a red rash on his penis and may complain of itching and burning.

The mother is likely to complain of pain. A very precise description of the pain can help determine its cause. Women with candidiasis generally complain of a severe burning sensation, or they may say it feels as if their milk is on fire. Some say it is worse immediately after the feeding; others say that their nipple feels as if it has broken glass in it. Some report a shooting pain.[85] *Candida* in the ducts is usually described as a "deep" pain, whereas an overgrowth of *Candida* can be on the nipples only and generally occurs without the deep pain.[86] All of these descriptions require further follow-up.

Prevention and Treatments Strategies

When the mother reports discomfort associated with candidiasis, refer both her and her infant for prompt treatment. If the mother is breastfeeding more than one infant, the entire group must be treated. Candidiasis is easily passed back and forth from the infant's mouth to the mother's breast and therefore can be extremely difficult to eradicate without prompt, thorough treatment of all the involved parties, including the woman's partner.

Treatment for candidiasis is best carried out with a simple understanding of how yeast thrives. Yeast flourishes in a warm, moist, dark place such as inside the vagina, bra, bra pads, folds of the skin, and the diaper; therefore these are likely environments for growth. (Reused breast pads promote the growth of *Candida;* if they are used, breast pads should be disposable.)

Once the diagnosis of candidiasis has been established, initiate some simple measures and reinforce the prescribed treatment regimen.

- Explain to the woman that the warm, moist, dark environment is created when the lactating nipples are constantly inside the bra. In addition, the fungus thrives on the milk.
- Suggest that she rinse her nipples and air-dry them after feeding, and encourage her to spend at least a few minutes during the day with the bra flaps down and the nipples exposed to the light.
- Rinse nipples with vinegar water (1 tablespoon of vinegar to 1 cup of water) and air-dry the nipples before applying topical medication.
- Recommend washing the bedding, towels, bra, and diapers with hot water with 1 cup of distilled vinegar added to the rinse. (If the mother uses breast pads, encourage the disposable type.)
- If the mother expresses her milk while she is experiencing candidiasis, explain that she may feed it to the infant during that time but should not freeze it for later use. (This is somewhat controversial, but still recommended.[5]) Boil for 20 minutes all parts of the breast pump that come in contact with the milk, as well as nipples or pacifiers, at least once a day.
- Discourage use of pacifiers because they become just one more medium that can transfer the organism.
- It may be helpful for the mother to avoid consuming refined sugar in her diet, also.

Medications may be prescribed for the mother, the infant, or the mother's partner; which drug is prescribed usually depends on the severity of the infection and whether the candidiasis is primarily oral, genital, or gastrointestinal. The discussion here is limited to those drugs used for oral candidiasis.

Topical treatments are usually used for oral thrush and generally fall into two categories: corticosteroids and antifungal (or antiinfective) drugs. A nonsystemic (topical) antifungal agent, such as nystatin, is the recommended therapy for oral thrush. Several agents are listed in Table 12-5. Some preparations are combination products, containing both an antifungal agent (e.g., nystatin) and triamcinolone (a corticosteroid). Frequently, combination products (e.g., Mycolog II, Myconel, Mytrex F) are recommended during the first 3 days or so when the pain is most severe. After the pain has subsided, the woman and her infant complete the 14-day treatment with the noncortisone preparation (e.g., nystatin only). Clotrimazole has also been used successfully.[87] Emphasize to the woman the importance of completing the treatment for herself and her infant; the symptoms may disappear in 2 to 3 days, but treatment must be continued even after the symptoms have diminished or disappeared.

Instruct the mother to apply topical agents to the nipple and areola and to the infant's oral area as described in Table 12-5. It is not necessary to remove the cream before breastfeeding. Antifungals or antiinfective creams (or lotions) are not absorbed through the mucous membranes. Furthermore, these same drugs are safe for and prescribed for infants. Corticosteroid preparations may be slightly absorbed, but these do not need to be removed before feeding either. Advise the mother that she may apply an antifungal cream to the infant's diaper area with her fingers after each diaper change. She must, however, wash her hands thoroughly after touching the infected area.

In the United States a less common but increasingly popular treatment is gentian violet, a purple dye that can be applied using a cotton swab to "paint" the inside of the infant's mouth and the nipple/areola complex. Or, the infant can simply suckle the breast after his mouth has been painted, thereby painting the breast as well. Administered once a day, this treatment (ideally done before bedtime so that the nipples can be exposed rather than covered with clothing afterwards) has not been approved for use in this way. However, relief is often noted within a few hours; if there is no relief within 3 days, it should be discontinued and medical help sought.

Systemic treatments, such as fluconazole (Diflucan), are generally prescribed when candidiasis has been resistant to topical medications. Although the safety of the concentration of this

Table 12-5 COMMON TREATMENTS FOR CANDIDIASIS ASSOCIATED WITH BREASTFEEDING*

Drug	How Supplied	Dosage Range and/or Frequency	Medication Administration and Teaching Responsibilities
Gentian violet	Solution (OTC)	Mother: Use 0.5% or 1% solution Infant: Use 0.5% or 1% solution qd × 3 days	• Caution that using a solution stronger than 1% or too-frequent applications can irritate or ulcerate the infant's oral mucosa or mother's nipple/areolar skin. • Stains skin and clothing. • Suggest disposable breast pads to avoid clothing stains.
Nystatin (Nilstat)	Oral Suspension (Rx)	Infant: Apply as directed, usually 1 ml qid *(For persistent cases, half-doses can be applied twice as often, i.e., ½ ml 8 times daily)*	• Shake well before using. • Apply oral suspensions to infant's cheeks, gumline, and tongue of the baby's mouth; make sure all oral surfaces are covered. • Hold infant snuggly while applying medicine because it creates initial discomfort in the oral mucosa. • Use one cotton-tipped applicator for one side of the mouth. Do *not* reinsert the applicator into the bottle; get a clean applicator to apply the medication to the other side.
Nystatin (Mycostatin)	Cream (Rx)	Mother: Apply liberally to nipple/areolar area bid to tid after breastfeeding	• Wait at least 10 minutes before replacing bra. • Oral absorption of this topical cream is poor, so it s not necessary to remove this from nipples before the infant breastfeeds.
Clotrimazole (Lotrimin†)	Cream, lotion, topical solution (OTC)	Mother: 1%; apply liberally to nipple/areolar area bid after breastfeeding	• Emphasize the importance of continuing this antifungal for total of 14 days; reassess mother and infant after 4 weeks. • Very limited oral absorption of topical preparation, so it is not necessary to remove this from nipples before the infant breastfeeds.
Miconazole (Monistat-Derm)	Cream (OTC)	Mother: Apply in a thin coat‡ to nipple/areolar area bid after breastfeeding	• Emphasize the importance of continuing this antifungal for the prescribed treatment period. • Oral absorption of this topical cream is poor, so it is not necessary to remove this from nipples before the infant breastfeeds.

Continued

Table 12-5 COMMON TREATMENTS FOR CANDIDIASIS ASSOCIATED WITH BREASTFEEDING*—CONT'D

Drug	How Supplied	Dosage Range and/or Frequency	Medication Administration and Teaching Responsibilities
Nystatin and triamcinolone (Mycolog II)	Cream (Rx)	Mother: Apply in a thin coat to nipple/areolar area bid to qid or tid after breastfeeding	• Indicated for severe pain. This product is usually used for about 3 days; the therapy continues with nystatin only (14 days total). • It is not necessary to remove this from nipples before the infant breastfeeds.
Clotrimazole and betamethasone (Lotrisone)	Cream (Rx)	Mother: Apply in a thin coat to nipple/areolar area bid after breastfeeding	• Indicated for severe pain. This product is usually used for the first 3 days; the therapy continues with clotrimazole only (14 days total). • It is not necessary to remove this from nipples before the infant breastfeeds.
Fluconazole (Diflucan)	Tablet (Rx)	As directed; typically, 200 mg PO on day 1, followed by 100 mg × 10 days thereafter (One or two single doses, as prescribed for treatment of vaginal yeast, are ineffective for treating nipple candidiasis.)	• This does pass into mother's milk, but amount in milk is still less than the amount that would be prescribed for an infant. • Emphasize to the mother that she should tell the pediatrician if she is taking Diflucan so that he or she can adjust the infant dosage accordingly. Mothers who have heard that Diflucan is contraindicated during lactation will question its safety. Explain that package inserts are written by the manufacturer, and reassure mothers that like other medications prescribed for pediatric use on the merits of scientific research, this medication is safe for breastfeeding mothers.
Fluconazole (Diflucan)	Oral suspension (Rx)	5-6 mg/kg first day; 3 mg/kg thereafter 5 for period of at least 2 wk	• May be given to the infant via dropper.

OTC, Over-the-counter; *Rx*, prescription.
*If the mother also has a vaginal yeast infection, she should also seek treatment.
†Not to be confused with Lotrimin AF 2%, which is supplied as a spray; its active ingredient is miconazole.
‡Many pharmacists discourage applying products containing corticosteroids (e.g., triamcinolone, betamethasone) to any open wound (e.g., cracked nipple) or "liberal" application of these to avoid systemic absorption.

drug in the milk has been questioned,[88] the dosage that the infant would receive from the mother's milk is less than what would be prescribed for the infant.

Do not assume that the problem is resolved just because the therapy has begun; all parties must be reevaluated to ensure that signs and symptoms do not persist after therapy has begun. Sometimes, a medication that was initially effective or that was effective during the first episode loses its effectiveness with subsequent episodes. The goal is to conquer the fungus by prompt, simultaneous treatment of all parties involved.

Pain medication is often needed. Over-the-counter analgesics are not always effective in pain management.[51]

Other

Galactocele

A galactocele is a closed sac in or under the skin that is lined with epithelium and contains fluid or semisolid material. These are fairly uncommon and are believed to be caused by the blockage of a milk duct.[5] Women who have galactoceles report breast pain and a mass can be palpated.[89] Inspection reveals a smooth, rounded, raised area; compressing the sac produces some milky fluid. The exact cause of a galactocele is unknown, but sometimes it can follow breast reduction surgery[90] or augmentation.[91]

SUMMARY

Several breast and nipple problems can occur. Some problems are present before pregnancy; others occur in relation to lactation. Few, if any, preclude successful breastfeeding. Many problems can be prevented; others can be corrected with relatively simple strategies. Ongoing assessment and evaluation are often required.

REFERENCES

1. Hytten FE. Clinical and chemical studies in human lactation. *BMJ* 1954;175-182.
2. Terrill PJ, Stapleton MJ. The inverted nipple: to cut the ducts or not? *Br J Plast Surg* 1991;44:372-377.
3. Alexander JM, Grant AM, Campbell MJ. Randomised controlled trial of breast shells and Hoffman's exercises for inverted and non-protractile nipples. *BMJ* 1992;304:1030-1032.
4. The MAIN Trial Collaborative Group. Preparing for breast feeding: treatment of inverted and non-protractile nipples in pregnancy. *Midwifery* 1994;10:200-214.
5. Lawrence RA, Lawrence RM. *Breastfeeding: a guide for the medical profession.* 5th ed. St. Louis: Mosby; 1999.
6. Clum D, Primomo J. Use of a silicone nipple shield with premature infants. *J Hum Lact* 1996;12:287-290.
7. Brigham M. Mothers' reports of the outcome of nipple shield use. *J Hum Lact* 1996;12:291-297.
8. Bodley V, Powers D. Long-term nipple shield use—a positive perspective. *J Hum Lact* 1996;12:301-304.
9. Wilson-Clay B. Clinical use of silicone nipple shields. *J Hum Lact* 1996;12:279-285.
10. Woolridge MW, Baum JD, Drewett RF. Effect of a traditional and of a new nipple shield on sucking patterns and milk flow. *Early Hum Dev* 1980;4:357-364.
11. Jackson DA, Woolridge MW, Imong SM, et al. The automatic sampling shield: a device for sampling suckled breast milk. *Early Hum Dev* 1987;15:295-306.
12. Auerbach KG. The effect of nipple shields on maternal milk volume. *J Obstet Gynecol Neonatal Nurs* 1990;19:419-427.
13. Bocar DL. *Breastfeeding educator program resource notebook.* Oklahoma City: Lactation Consultant Services; 1997.
14. Hoffman JB. A suggested treatment for inverted nipples. *Am J Obstet Gynecol* 1953;66:346-348.
15. Bremme K, Eneroth P, Kindahl H. 15-Keto-13, 14-dihydroprostaglandin F2a, and prostaglandin E2 or oxytocin therapy for labor induction. *J Perinat Med* 1987;15:143-151.
16. Kesaree N, Banapurmath CR, Banapurmath S et al. Treatment of inverted nipples using a disposable syringe. *J Hum Lact* 1993;9:27-29.
17. Graffy JP. Mothers' attitudes to and experience of breast feeding: a primary care study. *Br J Gen Pract* 1992;42:61-64.
18. Ziemer MM, Paone JP, Schupay J et al. Methods to prevent and manage nipple pain in breastfeeding women. *West J Nurs Res* 1990;12:732-743.
19. Newton NR, Newton M. Relationship of ability to breastfeed and maternal attitudes toward breast feeding. *Pediatrics* 1950;5:869-875.
20. Newton N, Lansdowne PA. Nipple pain and nipple damage. *J Pediatrics* 1952;4:411-423.
21. Ziemer MM, Pigeon JG. Skin changes and pain in the nipple during the 1st week of lactation. *J Obstet Gynecol Neonatal Nurs* 1993;22:247-256.
22. Biancuzzo M. *Sore nipples: prevention and problem solving.* Herndon VA: WMC Worldwide; 2000. Available at http://www.wmc-worldwide.com/modules/Sore Nipples.html.
23. Gunther M. Sore nipples, causes and prevention. *Lancet* 1945;249:590-593.

24. Medoff-Cooper B, Weininger S, Zukowsky K. Neonatal sucking and clinical assessment tool: preliminary findings. *Nurs Res* 1989;38:162-165.

25. Woolridge MW. Aetiology of sore nipples. *Midwifery* 1986;2:172-176.

26. Hewat RJ, Ellis DJ. A comparison of the effectiveness of two methods of nipple care. *Birth* 1987;14:41-45.

27. Righard L. Are breastfeeding problems related to incorrect breastfeeding technique and the use of pacifiers and bottles? *Birth* 1998;25:40-44.

28. Messner AH, Lalakea ML, Aby J et al. Ankyloglossia: incidence and associated feeding difficulties. *Arch Otolaryngol Head Neck Surg* 2000;126:36-39.

29. DeCarvalho M, Robertson S, Klaus MH. Does the duration and frequency of early breastfeeding affect nipple pain? *Birth* 1984;11:81-84.

30. Gosha JL, Tichy AM. Effect of a breast shell on postpartum nipple pain: an exploratory study. *J Nurse Midwifery* 1988;33:74-77.

31. Kearney MH, Cronenwett LR, Barrett JA. Breast-feeding problems in the first week postpartum. *Nurs Res* 1990;39:90-95.

32. L'Esperance C. Pain or pleasure: the dilemma of early breastfeeding. *Birth Fam J* 1980;7:21-25.

33. Storr GB. Prevention of nipple tenderness and breast engorgement in the postpartal period. *J Obstet Gynecol Neonatal Nurs* 1988;17:203-209.

34. L'Esperance C, Frantz K. Time limitation for early breastfeeding. *J Obstet Gynecol Neonatal Nurs* 1985;14:114-118.

35. Renfrew MJ, Lang S, Martin L et al. Feeding schedules in hospitals for newborn infants. *Cochrane Database Syst Rev* 2000:CD000090.

36. Spangler A, Hildebrandt E. The effect of modified lanolin on nipple pain/damage during the first ten days of breastfeeding. *Int J Childbirth Ed* 1993;8:15-19.

37. Brent N, Rudy SJ, Redd B et al. Sore nipples in breast-feeding women: a clinical trial of wound dressings vs conventional care. *Arch Pediatr Adolesc Med* 1998;152:1077-1082.

38. Pugh LC, Buchko BL, Bishop BA et al. A comparison of topical agents to relieve nipple pain and enhance breastfeeding. *Birth* 1996;23:88-93.

39. Buchko BL, Pugh LC, Bishop BA et al. Comfort measures in breastfeeding, primiparous women. *J Obstet Gynecol Neonatal Nurs* 1994;23:46-52.

40. Lavergne NA. Does application of tea bags to sore nipples while breastfeeding provide effective relief? *J Obstet Gynecol Neonatal Nurs* 1997;26:53-58.

41. Dodd VA, Chalmers C. A comparative study of the use of the MaterniMates(tm) gel disc dressing versus Lansinoh® lanolin cream with lactating mothers. (Abstract). 2001.

42. Cadwell K. A comparison of treatment modalities for sore nipples in nursing mothers: the use of Soothies™ glycerin gel therapy and the use of breast shells with Lansinoh® Lanolin Cream, preliminary results. (Abstract). 2001.

43. Newton M, Newton N. Postpartum engorgement of the breast. *Am J Obstet Gynecol* 1951;61:664-667.

44. Moon JL, Humenick SS. Breast engorgement: contributing variables and variables amenable to nursing intervention. *J Obstet Gynecol Neonatal Nurs* 1989;18:309-315.

45. Hill PD, Humenick SS. The occurrence of breast engorgement. *J Hum Lact* 1994;10:79-86.

46. Corrieri D. Cabbage leaves: an effective treatment for swollen tissues. *J Hum Lact* 1992;8:126-127.

47. Nikodem VC, Danziger D, Gebka N et al. Do cabbage leaves prevent breast engorgement? A randomized, controlled study. *Birth* 1993;20:61-64.

48. Roberts KL. A comparison of chilled cabbage leaves and chilled gelpaks in reducing breast engorgement. *J Hum Lact* 1995;11:17-20.

49. Vogel A, Hutchison BL, Mitchell EA. Mastitis in the first year postpartum. *Birth* 1999;26:218-225.

50. Kinlay JR, O'Connell DL, Kinlay S. Incidence of mastitis in breastfeeding women during the six months after delivery: a prospective cohort study. *Med J Aust* 1998;169:310-312.

51. Bodley V, Powers D. Long-term treatment of a breastfeeding mother with fluconazole-resolved nipple pain caused by yeast: a case study. *J Hum Lact* 1997;13:307-311.

52. Hartmann PE, Prosser CG. Physiological basis of longitudinal changes in human milk yield and composition. *Fed Proc* 1984;43:2448-2453.

53. Jonsson S, Pulkkinen MO. Mastitis today: incidence, prevention and treatment. *Ann Chir Gynaecol Suppl* 1994;208:84-87.

54. Kinlay JR, O'Connell DL, Kinlay S. Risk factors for mastitis in breastfeeding women: results of a prospective cohort study. *Aust NZ J Public Health* 2001;25:115-120.

55. Foxman B, Schwartz K, Looman SJ. Breastfeeding practices and lactation mastitis. *Soc Sci Med* 1994;38:755-761.

56. Riordan JM, Nichols FH. A descriptive study of lactation mastitis in long-term breastfeeding women. *J Hum Lact* 1990;6:53-58.

57. Evans K, Evans R, Simmer K. Effect of the method of breast feeding on breast engorgement, mastitis and infantile colic. *Acta Paediatr* 1995;84:849-852.

58. Kaufmann R, Foxman B. Mastitis among lactating women: occurrence and risk factors. *Soc Sci Med* 1991;33:701-705.

59. Biancuzzo M. Mastitis: painful and preventable. *Childbirth Instructor* 1998:10-12.

60. Osterman KL, Rahm VA. Lactation mastitis: bacterial cultivation of breast milk, symptoms, treatment, and outcome. *J Hum Lact* 2000;16:297-302.

61. Semba RD. Mastitis and transmission of human immunodeficiency virus through breast milk. *Ann NY Acad Sci* 2000;918:156-162.

62. Semba RD, Neville MC. Breast-feeding, mastitis, and HIV transmission: nutritional implications. *Nutr Rev* 1999;57:146-153.

63. Filteau SM, Lietz G, Mulokozi G et al. Milk cytokines and subclinical breast inflammation in Tanzanian women: effects of dietary red palm oil or sunflower oil supplementation. *Immunology* 1999;97:595-600.

64. Olsen CG, Gordon RE Jr. Breast disorders in nursing mothers. *Am Fam Physician* 1990;41:1509-1516.

65. Semba RD, Kumwenda N, Hoover DR, et al. Human immunodeficiency virus load in breast milk, mastitis, and mother-to-child transmission of human immunodeficiency virus type 1. *J Infect Dis* 1999;180:93-98.

66. Semba RD, Kumwenda N, Taha TE et al. Mastitis and immunological factors in breast milk of lactating women in Malawi. *Clin Diagn Lab Immunol* 1999;6:671-674.

67. Lawrence RA. A 35-year-old woman experiencing difficulty with breastfeeding. *JAMA* 2001;285:73-80.

68. Bodley V, Powers D. Case management of a breastfeeding mother with persistent oversupply and recurrent breast infections. *J Hum Lact* 2000;16:221-225.

69. Fetherston C. Mastitis in lactating women: physiology or pathology? *Breastfeed Rev* 2001;9:5-12.

70. Fetherston C. Management of lactation mastitis in a Western Australian cohort. *Breastfeed Rev* 1997;5:13-19.

71. Castro M. Homeopathy. A theoretical framework and clinical application. *J Nurse Midwifery* 1999;44:280-290.

72. Fetherston C. Characteristics of lactation mastitis in a Western Australian cohort. *Breastfeed Rev* 1997;5:5-11.

73. Buescher ES, Hair PS. Human milk anti-inflammatory component contents during acute mastitis. *Cell Immunol* 2001;210:87-95.

74. Goldman AS, Thorpe LW, Goldblum RM et al. Anti-inflammatory properties of human milk. *Acta Paediatr Scand* 1986;75:689-695.

75. John GC, Nduati RW, Mbori-Ngacha DA et al. Correlates of mother-to-child human immunodeficiency virus type 1 (HIV-1) transmission: association with maternal plasma HIV-1 RNA load, genital HIV-1 DNA shedding, and breast infections. *J Infect Dis* 2001;183:206-212.

76. Rench MA, Baker CJ. Group B streptococcal breast abscess in a mother and mastitis in her infant. *Obstet Gynecol* 1989;73:875-877.

77. Bundred NJ, Dover MS, Coley S et al. Breast abscesses and cigarette smoking. *Br J Surg* 1992;79:58-59.

78. Hayes R, Michell M, Nunnerley HB. Acute inflammation of the breast—the role of breast ultrasound in diagnosis and management. *Clin Radiol* 1991;44:253-256.

79. Bertrand H, Rosenblood LK. Stripping out pus in lactational mastitis: a means of preventing breast abscess. *Can Med Assoc J* 1991;145:299-306.

80. Berna JD, Garcia Medina V, Madrigal M et al. Percutaneous catheter drainage of breast abscesses. *Eur J Radiol* 1996;21:217-219.

81. Tanguay KE, McBean MR, Jain E. Nipple candidiasis among breastfeeding mothers. Case-control study of predisposing factors. *Can Fam Physician* 1994;40:1407-1413.

82. Darwazeh AM, al Bashir A. Oral candidal flora in healthy infants. *J Oral Pathol Med* 1995;24:361-364.

83. Mattos-Graner RO, de Moraes AB, Rontani RM et al. Relation of oral yeast infection in Brazilian infants and use of a pacifier. *ASDC J Dent Child* 2001;68:33-36, 10.

84. Hancock KF, Spangler AK. There's a fungus among us! *J Hum Lact* 1993;9:179-180.

85. Amir LH. Candida and the lactating breast: predisposing factors. *J Hum Lact* 1991;7:177-181.

86. Thomassen P, Johansson VA, Wassberg C et al. Breast-feeding, pain and infection. *Gynecol Obstet Invest* 1998;46:73-74.

87. Johnstone HA, Marcinak JF. Candidiasis in the breastfeeding mother and infant. *J Obstet Gynecol Neonatal Nurs* 1990;19:171-173.

88. Force RW. Fluconazole concentrations in breast milk. *Pediatr Infect Dis J* 1995;14:235-236.

89. Makanjuola D. A clinico-radiological correlation of breast diseases during lactation and the significance of unilateral failure of lactation. *West Afr J Med* 1998;17:217-223.

90. Bronson DL. Galactorrhea after reduction mammaplasty. *Plast Reconstr Surg* 1989;83:580.

91. Deloach ED, Lord SA, Ruf LE. Unilateral galactocele following augmentation mammoplasty. *Ann Plast Surg* 1994;33:68-71.

92. Foxman B, D'Arcy H, Gillespie B et al. Lactation mastitis: occurrence and medical management among 946 breastfeeding women in the United States. *Am J Epidemiol* 2002;155:103-114.

13

Disease Implications and Risks-Benefits of Pharmacologic and Herbal Therapies

Usually, breastfeeding is best for both the mother and the infant. In relatively few circumstances the primary health care provider may determine that breastfeeding poses a safety threat. Occasionally, a disease state makes it unsafe for the infant to breastfeed. More often, the pathologic condition itself does not contraindicate breastfeeding, but the medications for the disease can contraindicate or temporarily interrupt breastfeeding. In either case, the nurse is often in a precarious situation. As a breastfeeding advocate, she may find herself wondering if the disease or medication truly contraindicates breastfeeding and if so, whether such a contraindication is permanent or only temporary. With respect to the pharmacologic issues, she may find herself in a situation in which she simply cannot make the final decision; most nurses do not have prescriptive privileges.

The purpose of this chapter is to help the nurse who does not have prescriptive privileges to provide care within her scope of practice in situations that could potentially contraindicate breastfeeding. (Nurses who do have prescriptive privileges should refer to other sources[1-4] or obtain information from an authoritative source.*) Pertinent situations include presence of disease, pharmacologic therapy, alternative therapies, and environmental hazards.

DISEASE AND IMPLICATIONS FOR BREASTFEEDING

The presence of disease in the mother does not necessarily preclude breastfeeding, as described in Chapter 6. The presence of disease does, however,

*University of Rochester Lactation Studies Center, 585-275-0088.

require consideration in terms of how or if it will affect the breastfed infant. In some cases breastfeeding is absolutely contraindicated; in other cases it is only temporarily contraindicated.

Infectious Diseases

Whether or not infectious disease contraindicates breastfeeding depends on two factors: transmission and associated medication. Infectious diseases are often presumed to contraindicate breastfeeding, but again, these require careful consideration by the primary health care provider. Lawrence states that "For common infections, infants have already been exposed by maternal contact during the prodromal period, and to interrupt breastfeeding at a time that antibodies and other anti-inflammatory and immunomodulating substances are being provided by breastfeeding is counterproductive" (p. 236).[5]

There are five classes of infectious organisms: (1) bacteria, (2) viruses, (3) fungi, (4) protozoa, and (5) helminths. Common infections and their relationship to the perinatal period are outlined briefly in the following sections.

Bacteria

Signs and symptoms of bacterial infections should be noted promptly. When assessing the mother for signs and symptoms of infection during the first few days after delivery, however, the nurse must recognize that an otherwise unexplained low-grade fever is not necessarily the result of an infection; it may be associated with physiologic engorgement. If maternal fever is greater than 38° C twice, artificially fed infants should be isolated from the mother, but breastfed infants should be with their mothers, who should initiate and continue breastfeeding while the origin of the maternal fever is being identified.

If a bacterial infection is confirmed, antibiotic therapy is started. Some hospital policies may require that the mother have therapeutic serum levels of the medication for at least 12 hours before the infant is allowed to go to the breast. Policies that require a greater number of hours are based on the needs of artificially fed infants, who do not have the advantage of immunities from their mothers, as do the breastfed infants. Even if the severity of the infection is such that the mother needs to be isolated from other patients, she and her infant can usually remain together.

Staphylococcal and streptococcal infections are very common during the perinatal period. In general, staphylococcal and streptococcal infections do not preclude breastfeeding. Mothers whose membranes have been ruptured for more than 24 hours are especially vulnerable to infection. However, their infants should begin breastfeeding and continue uninterrupted. Furthermore, not all staphylococcal bacteria are pathogenic; staphylococci are frequently found on the nipples.

Streptococcal infections can occur in postoperative wounds. Drainage or red streaking on the incision is likely to indicate a streptococcal infection, which requires medical management. Generally, these mothers are treated with antibiotics, and isolation from the infant is not indicated. However, strict handwashing by health care personnel and the mother is imperative.

Group B streptococcus (GBS) can occur in maternal endometritis, amnionitis, and urinary tract infection. Generally, penicillin is the recommended therapy. If the infant becomes infected, cultures of the milk are usually ordered, and a sample can be collected (see Chapter 12).

Escherichia coli is the usual culprit in urinary tract infections, which are common in perinatal patients. These infections are self-contained; breastfeeding should be initiated and continue uninterrupted. Usually, antibiotics that are safe for pediatric use are prescribed for the mother. Antibiotics for the mother work well but may cause diarrhea in the breastfeeding infant. Although increased fluid

intake is required for anyone who has a urinary tract infection, it is especially important with the lactating mother because fluids are lost through breastfeeding. Offering cranberry juice to the mother to acidify her urine has been shown to be helpful.[6]

Breastfeeding is contraindicated if the mother has active tuberculosis (TB). Caused by *Mycobacterium,* active tuberculosis can be treated with a combination of several drugs (most frequently isoniazid plus two to three others), usually for 6 to 9 months. Breastfeeding may be initiated or resumed after treatment has been established.[7]

Postpartum maternal Lyme disease is caused by a spirochete infection. Breastfeeding may resume after the mother has been treated, but because her milk may contain the organism, the newborn should also be treated.

Viruses

More than other infectious diseases, viral infectious diseases place infants more at risk during breastfeeding. Sometimes, such risk may contraindicate breastfeeding or require a temporary cessation of breastfeeding.[5]

Herpes. Four types of herpes viruses exist: cytomegalovirus (CMV), herpes simplex virus (HSV), herpes varicella-zoster virus (VZV), and Epstein-Barr virus. Implications related to breastfeeding are found in Table 13-1.

CMV may result in serious injury to the fetus if the mother has primary CMV; those who are exposed to recurrent or reactivated CMV infections during delivery or breastfeeding generally have a low risk of serious injury.[8] Lactoferrin, present in human milk, appears to inhibit the growth of CMV.[9,10]

If the mother has CMV, breastfeeding may pose a greater risk for postnatal preterm infants than has previously been thought.[11] Infants who are very premature have the greatest risk for acquiring an early and symptomatic CMV infection.[12]

Concurrent problems should also be considered carefully when evaluating the risk-benefit of breastfeeding in CMV situations. If infants with immunodeficiency syndromes concurrently have a CMV infection, a fatal outcome can occur.[13] Breastfeeding increases the risk of combined

Table **13-1**   TYPES OF INFECTIONS AND BREASTFEEDING SAFETY RECOMMENDATIONS

Type of Infection	Example/Problem	OK to Breastfeed in the U.S.?	Conditions/Comments
Bacterial	Acute infectious process, including premature rupture of membranes; >24 hr without fever and delivery of term or preterm infant	Yes	Respiratory, reproductive, gastrointestinal infections
	Maternal fever >38° C twice, 4 hr apart, 24 hr before to 24 hr after delivery, or endometriosis; term or preterm infant	Yes	Infant should be treated with antibiotics
	Salmonella infection	Yes	Infant should be treated with antibiotics
	Shigella	Yes	If culture is negative
	Tuberculosis		
	• Mother with inactive disease	Yes	
	• Mother with active disease	No	No *until treatment is established*
Viral	HIV	No	Recommendation from Centers for Disease Control and Prevention and American Academy of Pediatrics
	Hepatitis		
	• Hepatitis A	Yes	As soon as mother receives gamma globulin
	• Hepatitis B	Yes	After infant receives HBIG, first dose of hepatitis B vaccine should be given before hospital discharge
	• Hepatitis C	Yes	If no coinfections (e.g., HIV)
	Venereal warts	Yes	Venereal warts have not been reported to occur on the breast; genital warts do not contraindicate breastfeeding
	Herpes viruses		
	• Cytomegalovirus	Yes	Passively transferred maternal antibodies in human milk make breastfeeding safe
	• Herpes simplex	Yes	Except if lesion is on breast
	• Varicella-zoster (chicken pox)	Yes	As soon as mother becomes noninfectious
	• Epstein-Barr	Yes	
	Human T-cell leukemia virus type I	No	
Fungus	Candidiasis	Yes	Treatment for all parties is imperative
Protozoa	Toxoplasmosis	Yes	

Adapted from Lawrence RA. *A review of medical benefits and contraindications to breastfeeding in the United States (Maternal and Child Health Technical Information Bulletin).* Arlington, VA: National Center for Education in Maternal and Child Health; 1997.
HBIG, Hepatitis B immune globulin.

Pneumocystis carinii pneumonia (PCP) and CMV infection, which is associated with infants with human immunodeficiency virus (HIV).[14]

Herpes simplex can be fatal to the neonate if transmitted intrauterine or intrapartum. However, breastfeeding is a different matter. Mothers may breastfeed *unless a herpes lesion is on the breast.* If the lesion is present on the breast, the mother should express and discard her milk until it has cleared. (Good handwashing technique is essential.) Maternal VZV, also called chicken pox, requires temporary isolation of the mother from her infant, regardless of the mode of feeding. When no VZV lesions are on the breast, expressed milk may be given to the infant who has received varicella-zoster immunoglobulin (VZIG). Breastfeeding is permissible "when the mother is no longer infectious, no new lesions have developed after 72 hours, and crusting of the existing lesions has occured, usually 6-10 days after the onset of the rash. Maternal VZV infection after 1 month postpartum probably requires no suspension of breastfeeding, especially if an infant received VZIG in a timely fashion."

Hepatitis. There are several types of hepatitis; all are viral, but they differ in route of transmission, clinical course, and treatment. The three most common types are hepatitis A, B, and C. Hepatitis types D and E have been recognized more recently and are less well understood.

Hepatitis A is rarely transmitted vertically. (*Vertical transmission* means transfer from one generation to the next, through either the mother's milk or the placenta; *horizontal transmission* is the spread of infection by contact from one person to another, usually through contact with contaminated material.) Hepatitis A has a short incubation period and in most cases requires little special care for the infant. Breastfeeding should be initiated and continue uninterrupted.

Hepatitis B can be transmitted vertically. If a woman has active hepatitis during the third trimester or at delivery, her infant should immediately receive hepatitis B immune globulin (HBIG) at delivery. Rooming-in is in the best interest of all the patients on the unit because this mother should not visit the nursery. She may, however, breastfeed the infant after he has been immunized with HBIG.

Hepatitis types C, D, and E are not as well understood as hepatitis types A and B. Currently, most experts agree that mothers with hepatitis C may breastfeed[15,16]; infants infected with hepatitis D and E should not.

HIV and AIDS. Citing statements by the World Health Organization,[17,18] the American Academy of Pediatrics (AAP),[19] and clinical investigations,[20] Lawrence and Lawrence assert that "the one infectious disease, when it occurs in industrialized countries, that is a clear contraindication to breastfeeding is maternal HIV infection."[7] They emphasize, however, that the risk-benefit is different in developing countries.

There has been and continues to be a raging controversy over this recommendation.[21,22] However, it is clear that HIV type I can be transmitted through human milk.[23] The varying rates of such transmission by human milk have been reported in numerous studies.[20,24-27] Rates of transmission are often affected by a host of other coexisting factors, such as the viral load, the duration of breastfeeding, and the presence of mastitis.[28] It is clear, however, that transmission of the virus is more likely in breastfed infants than in formula-fed infants in developing countries.[27,29] Furthermore, maternal morbidity is greater among breastfeeding than nonbreastfeeding mothers.[30]

Women in the United States who are HIV positive should not be encouraged to breastfeed.[19] However, those who are merely thought to be HIV positive or those who have a history of risk factors that have since been resolved should not be dissuaded from breastfeeding. In underdeveloped countries, breastfeeding may represent more benefit than risk for the infant.

Women need to understand their rights and know their options.[31] Options for HIV-positive women living in the United States are twofold. Most elect to use artificial milk. However, all mothers should be informed that donor milk is an excellent choice. Bringing the mother's own milk to a boil may be effective in reducing infectivity.[32] In clinical practice, however, it may be too early to write broad protocols based on one study; assessment of concomitant risk factors to specific individuals should also be considered.

Fungi. The main fungal infection encountered in breastfeeding mothers is candidiasis. Oral candidiasis—an overgrowth of *Candida* in the infant's mouth or on the mother's nipples—is a common problem among breastfeeding mothers and is discussed further in Chapter 12. There is no need to isolate the infant from an infected mother if candidiasis is present; she may initiate and continue breastfeeding uninterrupted.

Protozoa

Toxoplasmosis is the most common protozoan affecting pregnant women. There is no need to isolate the infant from the mother; she may initiate and continue breastfeeding uninterrupted.

Nutritional Risks for Breastfeeding

Special consideration should be given to the infant who has a unique nutritional need or the mother who has a metabolic disease. For example, infants who have galactosemia have a unique nutritional need. According to Lawrence and Lawerence[5] breastfeeding is contraindicated for infants with the classic variant of galactosemia because they are lactose intolerant, whereas infants with the milder version may, under the right circumstances, be partially breastfed. Infants with inborn errors of metabolism that result in amino aciduria, such as phenylketonuria (PKU), require special management. Infants with PKU may be partially breastfed.

Maternal metabolic diseases may pose a problem. For example, women with Wilson's disease (associated with excessive copper intake) should not breastfeed because of the treatment for the disease.[5]

Clinical Management When Breastfeeding Is Contraindicated or Interrupted

Breastfeeding usually can be initiated and continue uninterrupted for most cases, as shown in Table 13-1. Recommendations in relation to breastfeeding and/or isolation are based on Lawrence[7] and the AAP's *Red Book*.[16] These directives should be incorporated into the hospital's infection control policy and/or unit policy or protocol because a written document helps ensure an uninterrupted breastfeeding experience.

Certainly, if a woman's health history includes factors known to contraindicate breastfeeding, she should be advised of alternatives (including the use of donor human milk). However, it is important to be certain that these factors actually exist; as Schanler and colleagues note, sometimes "Reasons given for not recommending breastfeeding included medical conditions with known treatments that did not preclude breastfeeding."[33] To make an informed decision, the mother should also be advised of Lawrence's strong position that "Breastmilk should not be withheld from any infant unless absolutely necessary"[7] (p. 32).

Sometimes, breastfeeding is contraindicated because of a particular clinical condition or the medical therapy required to treat it, as described throughout this chapter. With the vast number of medications, however, the benefits of breastfeeding outweigh the possible risks.[34] Box 13-1 lists priorities for care when breastfeeding is contraindicated.

Some conditions may require a temporary interruption of breastfeeding. However, teaching programs should not require women to list those specific conditions. Rather, they should recognize that very few conditions require breastfeeding to be interrupted and that individuals can question any health care provider who recommends breastfeeding interruption, except in some very unusual situations, for example, treatment with radiopharmaceuticals.[7,35] Women need to identify sources of personal, professional, and community support mechanisms if the need for temporary cessation of breastfeeding should arise.

PHARMACOLOGIC THERAPY DURING BREASTFEEDING AND LACTATION

A full discussion of pharmacologic therapy during breastfeeding and lactation is beyond the scope of this book. This brief section addresses the nurse's role in medical therapy, the safety of a particular medication, medications commonly used during lactation, and strategies to minimize risk or exposure.

The Nurse's Role in Medication Therapy during Breastfeeding and Lactation

The nurse's primary responsibility for medications focuses on patient advocacy, patient teaching, and

Box 13-1   Goals and Priorities for Care: When Breastfeeding Is Contraindicated or Temporarily Halted

- When in doubt, allow the infant to suckle, at least until the condition in question is confirmed as a strict contraindication to breastfeeding.
- Clarify any misunderstandings between the patient, her physician, and the staff about whether breastfeeding is truly contraindicated.
- In very few circumstances, breastfeeding is strictly prohibited (see Table 13-1). In most situations, cessation of breastfeeding, if ordered, is only temporary.
- Explain to the mother, in simple terms, why breastfeeding is contraindicated at this time. Focus on the infant's safety and avoid any implication that her milk is "dirty" or that she has done something "bad."
- Initiate and update information about when breastfeeding may resume.
- Advocate rooming-in. Isolation of the mother or the infant is seldom indicated and should be based on current research that supports the agency's infection control policy.
- Collaborate with the mother and the physician to develop a plan for adequate infant nutrition for both the long and the short term; in most cases, expressed milk is best (mother's own milk or banked donor milk), while in a few cases artificial milk may be required.

administration of the medication in a way that achieves optimal therapeutic and minimal adverse effects.

Patient Advocacy

One of two situations exists when the nurse needs to become an advocate for the breastfeeding mother. The first situation occurs when a medication that will interfere with breastfeeding or cause potential harm for the infant has been or is likely to be prescribed for the lactating mother. This often occurs in major medical centers where multiple specialists may be involved in the woman's care and some may be unaware that she is breastfeeding. Making a notation in a conspicuous place—for example, on the front of the mother's medical record—that she is breastfeeding helps avoid the problem.

More commonly, however, the reverse situation occurs. Medications are often withheld or breastfeeding is interrupted by some member of the interdisciplinary team who is well intentioned but unaware of the risk-benefit that the situation poses. In this case the nurse needs to provide data that show that the medication can be given safely during breastfeeding. The common approach of "the medication might be harmful so let's stop breastfeeding" is unacceptable. The nurse needs to become an advocate for helping the woman get the medication she needs and continue breastfeeding until it has been shown that the risk outweighs the benefit, which in most cases it does not.

Patient Teaching

Perhaps the first and foremost teaching responsibility is to assure lactating mothers that a medication has not been prescribed without careful thought and consideration of the risks and benefits involved. Furthermore, although nearly all medications enter the milk, the quantity is usually very small. Hence, there may be little, if any, adverse effect on the infant, and the number of medications generally recognized as safe during lactation far outnumber those that are associated with adverse outcomes. The mother needs to be informed of other effects the medication may have.

Effects of the Medication on Milk Production. Although some medications may not be "harmful" to the infant, they may cause the mother's milk to decrease in volume. If the mother takes these medications during lactation, the infant should be monitored carefully for sufficient weight gain.

Smoking is no longer a contraindication to breastfeeding.[2] However, smoking reduces milk volume and has other harmful effects for both the mother and the infant. Counseling during the prenatal period should be aimed at helping the pregnant woman quit smoking.

Some medications decrease prolactin levels and therefore decrease milk production. Examples include alcohol (in excessive amounts), antihistamines, barbiturates,[36] bromocriptine, estrogens, and others. If these or other prolactin-inhibiting medications are prescribed, the mother should be informed of their effects. She may need to understand that her supply may be so severely curtailed that she may be forced to stop breastfeeding earlier than she had planned.

Lactating women may wish to resume their use of oral contraceptives. For the most part, oral contraceptives do not affect milk supply. Traditional birth control pills (i.e., estrogen-progestin combination) should not be used while lactating, but the progestin-only pill has not been shown to have ill effects on lactation. Table 13-2 describes the effects of contraceptive agents on milk supply.

Medications that have anticholinergic properties block parasympathetic neural activity, causing decreased bodily secretions, most notably saliva. Similarly, these medications can also decrease milk secretion. For example, antihistamines, such as diphenhydramine (Benadryl), that are available as OTC preparations can reduce milk supply. Similarly, if used in excess, preparations for the common cold or allergies contain antihistamines that reduce bodily secretions, including maternal milk. Medications that act as sympathomimetic vasoconstrictors (e.g., pseudoephedrine [Sudafed]) have anecdotally been reported to decrease milk supply.[37]

Adverse Effects on the Infant. Often, women who are pregnant or who have just delivered ask the nurse whether medications that are prescribed for medical or obstetric conditions are harmful to the infant. Ideally, the physician should answer this question, but often the nurse is called upon to respond. In most cases, however, the woman can be reassured that medications used for conditions that occur during pregnancy or parturition do not preclude breastfeeding. For example, magnesium sulfate, which may be given to arrest preterm labor or for maternal hypertension during pregnancy, delivery, or immediately postpartum, is generally recognized as safe for breastfeeding infants.[38,39] The medication is nearly always given intravenously to the mother, but it is poorly absorbed in the infant's gastrointestinal tract; hence, safety is not an issue. The medication may have undesirable effects on the newborn, however. When compared with infants who have not been exposed to magnesium sulfate in utero, serum levels

Table **13-2** EFFECTS OF CONTRACEPTIVE AGENTS ON MILK YIELD AND INFANT DEVELOPMENT

Agent	Milk Yield	Effect on Infant
Combined estrogen/progestin	Moderate inhibitory effect Shorter breastfeeding Milk concentration unchanged Small amount of steroid in milk	Slower weight gain No long-term effects
Progestin only Minipill (norethindrone [Micronor, Nor-QD])	No effect on volume No effect on duration	No effect on weight gain No reported long-term effects
Other products Injectable depot medroxyprogesterone acetate (DMPA), Depo-Provera, and norethindrone enanthate (NET-ED, NORISTERAT)	Breastfeeding lasts longer ? change in milk: protein increased, fat decreased Steroid present in milk	No long-term effects
Levonorgestrel (Norplant System)	No effect Small amount of steroid in milk	Normal growth No long-term effects
Vaginal rings containing natural hormone progesterone	No significant differences	No effects on growth Long-term effects under study

In Howard CR, Lawrence RA. *Pediatr Clin North Am* 2001;48:485-504. Modified from Winikoff B, Smeraro P, Zimmerman M: *Contraception during breastfeeding: a clinician's source book.* New York: Population Council; 1987.

return to baseline by 48 hours after birth. Terbutaline, also used recently to arrest preterm labor or more classically for maternal respiratory difficulty, is also considered compatible with breastfeeding[2] and has no significant effect on the breastfed infant.[40] The effects of intrapartum analgesia and anesthesia on breastfeeding continue to be a controversial issue. There are numerous reports but no consensus about whether epidural anesthesia contributes to the infant's ability to suckle[41] (Box 13-2). Beyond the ability to suckle, related questions include the newborn's general

Box 13-2   DOES AN EPIDURAL INFUSION AFFECT NEWBORN SUCKLING?

Suckling is one of many neurologic behaviors that a newborn must accomplish. One measure of newborn neurologic status is his performance on the Neonatal Behavioral Assessment Scale (NBAS). Sepkoski[42] studied the effects of intrapartum epidural analgesia on the NBAS, administering the test on days 1, 3, 7, and 28 after birth. Here, the 20 healthy newborns exposed to epidural analgesia showed poorer performance on the orientation and motor clusters during the first month of life when compared with 20 cohorts who were not exposed to any epidural analgesia. This is one of the few studies in which one group was exposed to intrapartum analgesia and the control group received no medication whatsoever. A limitation, however, is that although the NBAS measures neurologic status in general, it does not measure suckling behavior specifically. It is also notable that although Sepkoski's study shows poorer neurologic performance at 28 days, another study that looked at long-term effects[43] showed no correlation between breastfeeding success at 6 to 8 weeks and labor analgesia.

A few investigators studied the possible effects of epidural analgesia or anesthesia on suckling effectiveness, intake, and/or weight gain. One study[44] looked at 181 subjects who experienced either spontaneous or cesarean births. Before hospital discharge, data were gathered from maternal reports of how well the infant was suckling. Compared with mothers who did not receive epidural infusions, those born to mothers who had epidural analgesia or anesthesia showed no difference in weight loss, quality of feeding, alertness, or ability to learn to feed. Some mothers in this study also received intrapartum Nubain, which may have influenced the study results.

Righard's[45] 1990 study, frequently quoted in the literature, reported that suckling was delayed for more than 2 hours after birth in infants whose mothers had had epidural infusions. In closely examining the study, however, one wonders if the administration of inhalation analgesia and intramuscular analgesia to some mothers may have been part of the problem while analgesia via the epidural route has become the commonly identified culprit.

Riordan's[46] study looked at scores on the Infant Breastfeeding Assessment Tool (IBFAT), which measures a newborn's readiness to feed, rooting, fixing (latching-on), and suckling pattern (see Chapter 7). IBFAT scores were compared between groups (medicated vs. unmedicated mothers during labor) and within the group (epidural analgesia vs. intravenous analgesia during labor). Newborns whose mothers did not have any labor analgesia achieved higher IBFAT scores compared with those whose mothers were medicated. IBFAT scores were similar regardless of the route of medication administration, but scores were lower if medication administration occurred by both routes.

It is difficult to come to any meaningful conclusions when the existing studies show such conflicting results. Rather than waiting for a cause-and-effect relationship to be established—which may present an insurmountable investigative challenge—a few things can help as we deliver care to mothers who have had intrapartum analgesia or anesthesia.

• Put the infant to the breast. The medications used for intrapartum pain relief have not been identified as contraindications to breastfeeding.
• Recognize that the medications administered by the epidural route may not be the culprits. Typically, women are "bolused" with large volumes of fluid before the beginning of the epidural infusion. These women often experience extreme fluid retention in their bodily tissues, including their nipple/areolar tissue. The edematous tissue can make it especially

Box **13-2** DOES AN EPIDURAL INFUSION AFFECT NEWBORN SUCKLING?—CONT'D

difficult for newborns to latch on. Suggest to the mother than she "redistribute" this excess fluid. She can do this by first placing digital pressure on the areola, close to the nipple and pushing straight in toward the ribs for about a minute. (Alternatively, a breast shell worn for about 20 minutes before the feeding accomplishes the same thing.) She may then wish to rhythmically open and close her fingertips over her areola (which may elicit a milk-ejection reflex). This redistributes the fluid away from the nipple so that the infant can better grasp it.[108]

- Work with the anesthesia department to advise mothers of the potential risks involved. Health care providers have an ethical responsibility to advise patients of potentially adverse outcomes; this is part of informed consent.
- Collaborate with labor/delivery nurses, doulas, midwives, childbirth educators, and others in a way that will enhance the mother's ability to use nonpharmacologic means to cope with labor.
- Teach parents subtle signs of hunger.

Reprinted from Biancuzzo M. *Breastfeeding Outlook* 2001;3:1, 2, 7.

 # RESEARCH HIGHLIGHT

Short-Term Use of Commonly Prescribed Medications Poses Little Risk to Breastfed Infants

Citation: Ito S, Blajchman A, Stephenson M et al. Prospective follow-up of adverse reactions in breastfed infants exposed to maternal medication. *Am J Obstet Gynecol* 1993;168:1393-1399.

FOCUS

This prospective study was designed to identify adverse effects of groups of medications—antibiotics, analgesics, antihistamines, sedatives, antidepressants, and antiepileptics—on healthy infants. A total of 838 breastfed infants were observed for adverse effects when their mothers took at least one medication.

RESULTS

Of the 838 subjects, only 94 women (11%) reported minor adverse effects in their infants that were associated with the drug therapy: antibiotics, 19.3% (32/166); analgesics or narcotics, 11.2% (22/196); antihistamines, 9.4% (8/85); antidepressants or antiepileptics, 7.1% (3/42). Most commonly, antibiotics caused diarrhea, analgesics caused drowsiness, antihistamines caused irritability, and antidepressants and antiepileptics caused drowsiness. However, none of the adverse drug reactions was severe enough to require medical attention.

STRENGTHS, LIMITATIONS OF THE STUDY

The large sample size and the prospective design strengthen the findings of this study. Some limitations include the fact that data were collected from mothers' self-reports, and the fact that they were counseled to look for the anticipated side effects. The time of the medication administration was not noted in relation to the time the infant fed or the observation of symptoms, and hence may influence the results.

CLINICAL APPLICATION

These data add to what has been reported anecdotally in many published single-case reports and in clinical practice, as well as some controlled studies. The small number of infants who reportedly experienced an adverse effect and the mild nature of the effects should help clinicians encourage continuation of breastfeeding and give anticipatory guidance about possible adverse effects. The short-term effects of maternal medication on breastfed infants pose little risk for infants, and breastfeeding should be continued unless data show that the risks of maternal medication passed to the infant outweigh the benefits of continued breastfeeding.

neurologic status, weight gain patterns, and the overall continuation of breastfeeding. Furthermore, in scrutinizing the existing studies, it is important to recognize that *epidural* simply refers to the route by which analgesia or anesthesia is administered; whether the infusion is given during labor or delivery or postpartum—or all three—is important when interpreting and applying results. A host of factors are to be considered when using the existing literature as a basis for clinical management.

Postpartum patients commonly raise questions about whether prescribed analgesics are harmful to the infant. In most cases they are not. Ibuprofen is perhaps the most commonly prescribed analgesic for the postpartum woman, and its use has not been shown to be detrimental[47]; the AAP considers its use compatible with breastfeeding. Another medication that often is given for postpartum pain is oxycodone with acetaminophen (Percocet). Quoting Marx and colleagues, one source[4] reports that this medication has no apparent effects on the breastfeeding newborn, and peak milk concentrations occur 1½ to 2 hours after the first dose and are variable thereafter. The AAP[2] does not give guidelines with respect to this medication, and one expert[48] offers a caution without citing a study or even a report. Tylenol #3, a combination of codeine and acetaminophen, is another commonly prescribed narcotic analgesic. Acetaminophen is compatible with breastfeeding, as described later in this chapter, and codeine has been shown to have no significant effects on infants in studies conducted as early as 1947[49] and later.[50,51] Therefore Tylenol #3 can be given with confidence that it will adequately relieve the mother's pain without detrimental effects to the newborn.

Teaching about potential side effects for the infant as a result of medications that have been prescribed for the mother (Box 13-3) is the nurse's responsibility. Behavioral changes in the infant may be seen after the administration of a narcotic analgesic, or gastrointestinal symptoms may be seen after the mother has ingested antibiotics. Skin rashes can also be observed after the mother has taken antibiotics.

After women are discharged from the hospital, they often raise questions about nontherapeutic substances. Mothers often ask about alcohol. Beer,

Box 13-3   Signs and Symptoms of Infant Response to Medication

BEHAVIORAL CHANGES
- Alertness
- Neuromuscular irritability/flaccidity
- Sleep patterns

GASTROINTESTINAL ALTERATIONS
- Feeding behaviors
- Diarrhea, constipation
- Weight loss

SKIN RASHES

in particular, raises questions for mothers who have heard that it is strictly contraindicated, whereas others have heard that it has been "prescribed" for improved milk supply. Beer consumption has been significantly correlated with increased prolactin levels in nonlactating subjects.[52,53] Even more interesting is that subjects who drank nonalcoholic beer[53] experienced the rises in prolactin levels. (It may be that a polysaccharide from barley is the agent that elevates the prolactin levels.[54]) Nonetheless, reports that it has special effects on breastfeeding[55] are as yet unproven. However, infants achieve a greater number of sucks but a lower overall milk intake when their mothers consumed orange juice mixed with ethanol as compared with when they consumed orange juice only.[56]

Alcohol is not contraindicated for lactating mothers, but it should be consumed in moderation. The Subcommittee on Nutrition[58] has determined that consumption of more than 0.5 g of alcohol per kilogram of maternal body weight may impair the milk-ejection reflex. (For a woman who weighs 132 pounds, this translates to approximately 2 to 2.5 oz of liquor, 8 oz of table wine, or 24 oz of beer per day.) Although this may seem surprising to some, the aversion to alcohol for breastfeeding mothers is culturally biased. In other cultures women regularly consume this amount of alcohol, often in the form of wine, and no deleterious effects have been shown, as described in Chapter 5.

Caffeine may cause infants to be wakeful and cranky. Consumption should be limited to 1 to 2

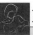

RESEARCH HIGHLIGHT

Very Little PCA Morphine in Colostrum

Citation: Baka NE, Bayoumeu F, Boutroy MJ et al. Colostrum morphine concentrations during postcesarean intravenous patient-controlled analgesia. *Anesth Analg* 2002;94:184-187.

Baka and colleagues conducted a study to describe how morphine and its active metabolite, morphine-6 glucuronide (M6G), were transferred to maternal plasma and colostrum. Specifically, they looked at the transfer when these substances were administered intravenously in a patient-controlled analgesia (PCA) situation. Women who were scheduled for a cesarean delivery in the investigators' facility in Nancy, France, were eligible for the study if they intended to breastfeed. Women were excluded if they had been given epidural analgesia for postoperative pain management or if they had significant health problems.

Seven women, whose average age was 30.2 years and average weight was 67.5 kg, delivered singletons at an average of 31 weeks of gestation. After delivery, blood (5 ml) and milk (2 ml or greater) samples were obtained at the time of initial titration and at 12, 24, 36, and 48 hours after delivery. Initially, women were given 4 mg of intravenous (IV) morphine, and followed by 1 mg every 10 minutes until they reported pain levels of 3 or less on a 10-point visual analog scale. Then, IV-PCA morphine sulfate (1 mg/ml) was available in 1-mg incremental doses with a 10-minute lockout and a 20-mg maximal cumulative load per 4 hours. The PCA was discontinued after 48 hours. The infants, who were all preterm and often

experiencing other problems, did not suckle during the study period.

All women used their pumps, and an average cumulative dose of 0.58 mg/kg during the first 24 hours and 0.17 mg/kg was required to achieve satisfactory pain relief during the following 24-hour period.

In the maternal plasma, morphine concentrations ranged from less than 1 to 170 ng/ml in the first 24-hour period and from less than 1 to 274 ng/ml in the following 24-hour period. M6G concentrations were less than 5 to 559 ng/ml and less than 5 to 974 ng/ml in the following 24-hour period. In the colostrum, morphine concentrations ranged from less than 1 to 37 ng/ml in the first 24 hours and from less than 1 to 48 ng/ml in the following 24-hour period, and M6G was less than 5 to 1084 ng/ml and less than 5 to 816 ng/ml. Hence, the morphine concentrations were always smaller in colostrum than in plasma. In contrast, the M6G concentrations were always larger in colostrum than in plasma.

The authors state, "According to the largest concentration values observed among all patients, the drug amounts likely to be transferred to the infant [if he had consumed the colostrum] were 0.0048 mg/100 mL for morphine and 0.1 mg/100 mL of milk for M6G." They also explained that oral bioavailability is only 20% to 30%, which further reduces the risks for newborns. The authors conclude that if mothers are receiving routine doses of morphine via IV-PCA, they should be allowed to breastfeed.

Modified from Biancuzzo M. *Breastfeeding Outlook,* 2002;1:7.

cups of caffeinated beverages per day. Although most mothers usually associate caffeine with coffee, it is also contained in soft drinks, chocolate, tea, and other products. Caffeine is a drug; like other drugs, it should be consumed with caution.

Nontherapeutic substances are indeed that—they provide no therapeutic value. The risk of ingesting these, by definition, outweighs any potential benefit. An excellent discussion of nontherapeutic and illicit substances is found elsewhere.[59]

Over-the-Counter Medications. Ideally, all women would check with their physician or other primary health care provider before taking OTC medications. When this does not happen, however, the nurse may be put in the position of giving the advice. In today's society, it is often difficult to give advice about OTC and other medications. On one hand, telling women never to take any OTC products while lactating may only be a deterrent to breastfeeding. On the other hand, women should not be self-medicating unless they understand that the medication may affect their ability to produce milk or their infant's safety. The nurse, then, may face some practical questions about OTC medications. A useful summary of the effects of OTC products is found elsewhere.[60]

Approximately 3000 OTC products are available in the United States today, but only about 700 active ingredients are in those products. This is because the active ingredients are found in many different combination products. An important clinical consideration, therefore, is, does the woman really need the combination product, or would a single-entity product provide the relief she needs? When possible, a combination product should be avoided. Similarly, sometimes nonpharmacologic remedies relieve the woman of her symptoms, and these should be used when possible (see discussion later in this chapter).

Administration Responsibilities

This next section explains how the prescriber decides whether a medication is safe. However, the nurse must make several determinations after the medication has been prescribed: (1) Is the medication contraindicated during lactation? (2) Who should recommend cessation of breastfeeding, and why? (3) When should the dose be given? and (4) Which as-needed (prn) analgesic should be offered to the woman when ordered?

Is the Medication Contraindicated during Lactation? Contrary to popular myth, very few medications are strictly contraindicated during lactation. As a general rule, any medication that is prescribed for infants is not contraindicated during breastfeeding. More specifically, the AAP position statement[2] includes seven tables that classify medication and other chemicals based on their compatibility with breastfeeding, as shown in Box 13-4. The AAP states that "Most drugs likely to be prescribed to the nursing mother should have no effect on milk supply or on infant well-being," but certainly, some substances have been shown to have adverse effects. Some require temporary cessation of breastfeeding. Interested readers can access the tables,[2] free of charge on the web (http://www.aap.org/policy/0063.html).

Who Should Recommend Cessation of Breastfeeding, and Why? Breastfeeding should not be automatically discontinued just because a woman has started to receive a medication that the nurse thinks may be unsafe. Except for radioactive metabolites, it is not harmful to give one dose of a prescribed medication while pursuing its safety with the prescriber.[1] In the meanwhile, therefore, the prescribed dose of medication should continue to be administered and breastfeeding should continue uninterrupted unless otherwise indicated.

Sometimes, overzealous staff members mistakenly forbid breastfeeding for medications that require only a temporary cessation of breastfeeding, such as metronidazole (Flagyl)[61] and radiopharmaceuticals. In this case the nurse needs to be an advocate, assuring both the staff and the mother that this situation requires a temporary interruption of breastfeeding but is not a reason to wean. Furthermore, the nurse will need to initiate a

Box **13-4** AAP Tables Describing the Transfer of Drugs and Other Chemicals into Human Milk[2]

Table 1	Cytotoxic Drugs That May Interfere with Cellular Metabolism of the Nursing Infant
Table 2	Drugs of Abuse for Which Adverse Effects on the Infant during Breastfeeding Have Been Reported
Table 3	Radioactive Compounds That Require Temporary Cessation of Breastfeeding
Table 4	Drugs for Which the Effect on Nursing Infants Is Unknown but May Be of Concern
Table 5	Drugs That Have Been Associated with Significant Effects on Some Nursing Infants and Should Be Given to Nursing Mothers with Caution
Table 6	Maternal Medication Usually Compatible with Breastfeeding
Table 7	Food and Environmental Agents: Effects on Breastfeeding

"pump and dump" routine with the mother, as described in Chapter 14.

Ultimately, the person who prescribes the medication assesses its risk and benefits during breastfeeding. The mother makes the final decision about ingesting a medication and continuing breastfeeding. As a patient educator and advocate, the nurse can facilitate communication between health care providers that ultimately ensures safety.

When Should the Dose Be Given? Very frequently, nurses find themselves in the position of scheduling the dose if the woman is hospitalized or recommending to the woman when she should take her medications at home. Although there is no one-size-fits-all solution, a few guidelines can be used when determining the optimal time for administration, as shown in Box 13-5. Ideally, the medication should be given so that its serum peak does not coincide with the time of maximal milk secretion. Of course, maximal milk secretion occurs during and right after a feeding. Therefore it is usually, although not always, best to administer the medication toward the end of or immediately after the feeding so that in most cases the peak serum level is reached before the next feeding (peak milk secretion time) occurs. Fig. 13-1 shows the peak serum level of medication at various times relative to a single feeding.

Which prn Analgesic Should Be Offered When Ordered? Often, more than one analgesic is ordered for the postpartum woman. When determining which medication to offer, the first determination should be the extent of her discomfort. A woman who has a forceps delivery today may require acetaminophen with codeine (Tylenol #3), whereas tomorrow she may get adequate relief with 650 mg of acetaminophen (Tylenol) only. In other cases more than one narcotic analgesic may be ordered; the one that has most consistently been generally recognized as safe for lactating women should be given.

It is important to keep in mind that the new mother is taking medications because she herself is experiencing a difficulty. Therefore her efforts to breastfeed should be reinforced and applauded. Priorities for care when the mother is breastfeeding are identified in Box 13-6.

Determining Medication Safety

Only the health care provider who has prescriptive privileges can make the final recommendation about the compatibility of a medication with breastfeeding. To safely administer the medication, support or question the medication order, or reassure the mother of the safety of the medication, the

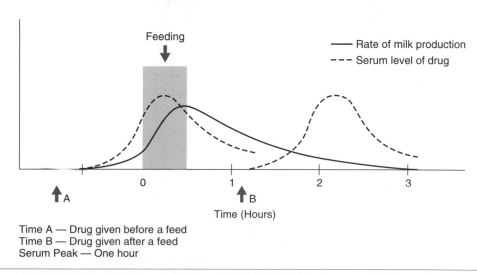

FIGURE **13-1** Peak serum level of medication at various times relative to a single feeding. *(From National Center for Education in Maternal and Child Health.*The art and science of breastfeeding. *Arlington, VA: 1986.)*

Box 13-5 Scheduling Doses of Medication for Lactating Mothers

GENERAL GUIDELINES

- When possible, give the dose of medication immediately after the infant has breastfed. In this way, the peak serum concentration of the drug in the breast milk should be lowest at the time of the next feeding.
- Check the *Physician's Desk Reference* to determine the onset and peak of action. If possible, schedule the dose so that the peak concentration occurs when the infant is not at the breast.

prn ANALGESICS

- If a nonnarcotic medication is being used to relieve postpartum cramps, consider giving the medication approximately 30 minutes before the feeding so that the onset of action coincides with the increased uterine cramps that often accompany the feeding.
- In other cases, give the dose immediately after the infant has breastfed.

DAILY MEDICATIONS

- If appropriate, the dose should be given just before the woman goes to bed or at the beginning of the longest feeding interval. (It would be inappropriate to give a stimulant before bedtime.)

Box 13-6 Goals and Priorities of Care: The Breastfeeding Dyad during Drug Therapy

- Work collaboratively with the mother and the entire health care team to minimize risk and maximize benefits of therapeutic medications.
- Communicate to the entire health care team that the woman is breastfeeding; encourage her to tell *all* of her health care providers.
- Teach the woman to observe for adverse effects of the drug on her ability to lactate or possible responses the infant may exhibit.
- Never make a unilateral decision to discontinue the medication or breastfeeding.
- Be an advocate; suggest that the mother get a second opinion when one health care provider takes a "let's discontinue breastfeeding just to be safe" approach. Remind her that artificial feeding may cause a host of other problems for her and her infant.
- Question an order if the AAP clearly identifies the drug as strictly contraindicated.
- Reassure the mother that the medication that has been prescribed for her is generally recognized as safe for the breastfeeding infant, if indeed that is the case.
- When possible, coordinate administration time of the medication so that peak levels reach the milk when the infant is unlikely to breastfeed.

nurse should have a fundamental understanding of how the medication is determined to be safe during breastfeeding (Box 13-7).

Medication Pharmacokinetics

Pharmacokinetic characteristics describe the *rates* at which medications are absorbed, distributed, metabolized in, and excreted from the body. Specific pharmacokinetic characteristics differ from medication to medication, although similarities may exist among groups of medications. Moreover, these characteristics vary for different patient populations. For example, infants may have very different rates of medication metabolism in the liver compared with rates of older children and adults.

When these pharmacokinetic characteristics are applied to specific patients and the medications they are receiving, we refer to this as *clinical pharmacokinetics*. The clinical pharmacokinetics of a specific medication are considered for both the lactating mother and her infant.

Absorption. Absorption is the process by which a medication moves from its site of administration (extravascular) to the systemic circulation (intravascular). Absorption is dependent on the specific extravascular route used, the size of the molecule, and the dosage form.

BOX 13-7   KEY TERMS RELATED TO TRANSFER OF SUBSTANCES INTO HUMAN MILK

TERM	DEFINITION
Absorption	The process by which a medication moves from its site of administration (extravascular) to the systemic circulation (intravascular).
Dalton	AMU atomic unit mass approximately 1.6605402 E-24 grams.
Distribution	The movement of a medication from the systemic circulation to different tissue sites.
Excretion	Elimination of metabolites of drugs and, in some cases, the active drug itself.
Extravascular	Outside a blood vessel. Extravascular routes of drug administration do not involve direct administration into the blood compartment. Common *extravascular* routes of administration include the oral, dermal, ocular, nasal, intramuscular, intradermal, subcutaneous, rectal, vaginal, intrathecal, and endotrachoal routes.
First-pass effect	The fraction of the oral dose that never reaches the systemic circulation because of hepatic metabolism during absorption; it is responsible for incomplete bioavailability.
Intravascular	Inside a blood vessel. Intravascular routes of drug administration involve direct administration of medication into the blood compartment or systemic circulation. This includes intravenous (IV) and intraarterial routes.
Half-life	The time it takes for the concentration of a medication to decrease by 50%.
Metabolism	The process by which the body inactivates the drug; also called *biotransformation*.
Metabolite	A substance produced by metabolic action. Metabolites may or may not be pharmacologically active.
M/P ratio	The ratio of the concentration of a substance in the milk to the ratio of the same substance in the maternal plasma.
Peak plasma concentration	A commonly used indicator for determining the *extent* of the absorption.
Pharmacokinetic	Pharmacokinetic characteristics describe the *rates* at which medications are absorbed, distributed, metabolized in, and eliminated from the body.
Routes of administration	There are two routes of administration; intravascular and extravascular, as described above.
Toxic	Of, or pertaining to, a poison.

Medications that are administered intravascularly—most commonly through the intravenous route—do not go through an absorption phase because they are introduced directly into the systemic circulation and therefore are 100% absorbed. Conversely, medications that are administered extravascularly (e.g., orally, rectally) need to be absorbed into the systemic circulation. Medications cannot enter the mother's milk until they are in the systemic circulation.

When one is choosing an appropriate route of administration for the lactating woman, the primary considerations are the *extent* and the *rate* of absorption.

Peak maternal plasma concentration is a commonly used indicator for determining the *extent* of the absorption. As an example, after a 500-mg dose of acetaminophen (Tylenol), a peak maternal plasma concentration of 2 µg/ml is expected within 60 minutes after administering the dose.

Time to peak plasma concentration is an indicator of the *rate* of absorption. Rates of absorption vary for different medications and for different routes of administration. For example, a medication that can be administered orally or intramuscularly must go through an absorption phase before it can move to the systemic circulation. The rate of absorption following oral administration may differ significantly from the intramuscular absorption rate. Furthermore, intramuscular absorption rates can vary, depending on the size of the muscle used for medication administration and the amount of blood flow to the muscle. Rates of absorption also depend on the dosage form that is used for medication delivery. Sustained-release oral, transdermal, and intramuscular dosage forms exist. The sustained-release nature of these forms dictates that their absorption is prolonged.

Rate and extent of absorption are considered when determining whether a medication can be used safely during breastfeeding. Some medications are simply not absorbed in the gastrointestinal tract. These absorption characteristics apply to both the mother and the infant. If a medication is not absorbed following oral administration to the mother, it will not appear in her milk. If a mother has received an intravenous medication that is not orally absorbed, that medication will not be absorbed in her infant's gastrointestinal tract, even though it may be present in the milk.

Vancomycin can be used to illustrate several of these points. Vancomycin is a large molecule that has minimal systemic absorption following oral administration. If a woman is taking *oral* vancomycin, very little, if any, of the medication would be found in her milk because it is not absorbed orally. However, if the woman is taking vancomycin *intravenously,* the medication would be found in her milk. Because the medication is not absorbed orally, however, her infant—who would ingest it orally—will have little systemic exposure to it.

Distribution. Distribution is the movement of a medication from the systemic circulation to different tissue sites. When determining the risk-benefit ratio of a medication during breastfeeding, several factors are considered, including lipophilic or hydrophilic characteristics, molecular weight, plasma protein binding, ionization, and volume of distribution. Each of these factors can have a significant effect on the presence of a medication in human milk.

Lipophilic or Hydrophilic Characteristics. Medications that are lipophilic are more soluble in fat than they are in water. Conversely, hydrophilic medications are more soluble in water than in fat. Therefore more lipophilic medications are more likely to be well distributed to tissue sites in the body, including the breast. This is because the alveolar epithelium of the breast is a lipid layer. Subsequently, lipophilic medications are more likely than hydrophilic medications to be concentrated in human milk. Small amounts of hydrophilic medications can be distributed into the milk via pores in the basement membranes and intercellular spaces.

In term infants, body fat accounts for approximately 12% of body weight. In preterm infants, the body fat concentration may be as low as 3%. In preterm infants with less body fat, larger amounts of lipophilic medications may be distributed to the brain when compared to term infants. Therefore lipophilic medications that have sedating effects on the central nervous system have more profound effects on preterm infants.

The fat content of milk itself must also be considered. This may be difficult because fat is the most variable component of milk. It is especially important to note that the fat content of the milk is greatest at the end of the feed.

Molecular Weight. Molecular weight was discussed early in regard to absorption. Similar to absorption, distribution of medications to human milk is limited by the molecular weight of the medication. More simply stated, the size of a medication influences its distribution; the smaller the molecular weight, the more likely it is to cross the membrane and enter the maternal milk. Most medications have a molecular weight between 100 and 300 daltons. Different investigators suggest different parameters, but most agree that those with molecular weights less than 300 daltons can be passed into the maternal milk. Some medications have extremely high molecular weights; for example, insulin and heparin have molecular weights of greater than 1000, and these are too large to cross the membrane and therefore are never passed into the maternal milk.

Plasma Protein Binding. Medications in the plasma can be either free or bound to protein, and the degree of protein binding ranges from minimal to extensive. The percentage of the medication that is bound to protein is not freely available, and diffusion across the cell membrane is unlikely for the protein-bound percentage, as shown in Fig. 13-2. Therefore there is no pharmacologic effect from this protein-bound portion. Warfarin, for example, which is more than 97% plasma protein bound, is not found in human milk in significant amounts. It is considered safe for breastfeeding mothers.[62] Conversely, the percentage of medication that is free (not protein bound) can easily diffuse across the cell membrane and is then distributed in human milk. Lithium, for example, is not bound at all to plasma proteins and is found in human milk, which explains why adverse effects have been reported in breastfed infants exposed to it.[63]

The same principles regarding protein binding can be applied to the breastfeeding infant. In newborns, protein accounts for 12% of body weight. In preterm infants with a significantly lower birth weight, the total amount of available protein is significantly lower. If total protein is decreased, the number of protein binding sites also is decreased. As a result, more medication that is not bound to plasma protein is available for both pharmacologic and toxicologic effects.

Medications that have high protein binding can have significant effects on the infant during the first 7 days of life. Bilirubin is bound to plasma proteins, and thus medications that are also bound to plasma proteins can displace bilirubin. The result is an increase in free bilirubin and possible kernicterus in the newborn whose serum bilirubin levels are considerably less than 20 mg/dl.

Ionization. Substances that are ionized have an electrical charge, and ionization is a pH-dependent characteristic. The pH of a medication or body fluid indicates whether it is an acid or base; a pH of 7 is considered neutral. The pH of human plasma is 7.4 (i.e., slightly basic). The pH of human milk ranges from 6.8 to 7.3 (i.e., slightly acidic to basic).

When an acidic medication appears in an acidic body fluid, the medication is un-ionized. An un-ionized medication is readily distributed to tissue. However, if that same medication is found in a more basic body fluid, it is ionized. Ionized medications, which have an electrical charge, are not well distributed to tissue. Different molecules are ionized at different pH levels. The molecules may be ionized in the blood or in the milk, but if a medication is ionized in the bloodstream, it tends to stay ionized in the bloodstream; hence, it diffuses more slowly across the membrane, as shown in Fig. 13-3.

Medications that are weak acids have higher concentrations in maternal plasma than in milk. Medications that are weak bases have equal or higher concentrations in milk when compared with plasma. For example, amphetamine, which is a weak base, is un-ionized in the basic pH of plasma and is found in high concentrations in human milk.

Volume of Distribution. Following absorption, medications are distributed from the plasma compartment to tissue sites. The degree of distribution is often described as the *volume of distribution.* Medications with volumes of distribution less than 1 L/kg are described as having a low volume of distribution. A good example is caffeine, which has a volume of distribution of about 0.5 L/kg, and easily passes into the milk. Conversely, volumes of

Plasma   **Milk**

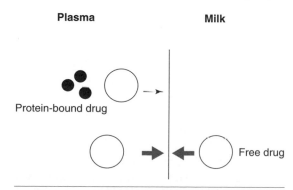

Protein-bound drug

Free drug

FIGURE **13-2** Diffusion of a protein-bound medication. *(From National Center for Education in Maternal and Child Health.* The art and science of breastfeeding. *Arlington, VA: 1986.)*

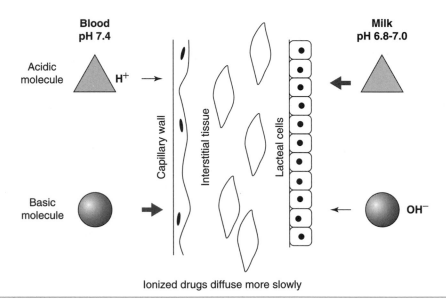

Ionized drugs diffuse more slowly

FIGURE **13-3** Diffusion of ionized molecules. *(From National Center for Education in Maternal and Child Health. The art and science of breastfeeding. Arlington, VA: 1986.)*

distribution greater than 3 L/kg are considered high. A good example is digoxin, which has a volume distribution of about 5.0 L/kg, and little gets into the milk.

Metabolism. Metabolism, also called *biotransformation*, is the process by which the body inactivates the medication. Metabolism of medications occurs primarily in the liver, but it can also occur in other areas, including the blood, kidneys, and stomach. Metabolites, produced as a result of metabolism, may have pharmacologic and toxicologic effects. The mother's and the infant's ability to metabolize the medication influences the medication's effect during breastfeeding.

The antidepressant imipramine (Tofranil) is an example of how metabolism influences breastfeeding. Imipramine is metabolized in the liver to the antidepressant desipramine. Both imipramine and desipramine can be found in human milk. Subsequently, the infant who is breastfeeding could experience some of the central nervous system effects of these antidepressants.

Acetaminophen use is generally recognized as safe during lactation. Fig. 13-4 shows how an adult metabolizes and excretes the medication. About 90% of acetaminophen is conjugated with sulfate

and glucuronide in the liver. Approximately 4% of acetaminophen is metabolized via the hepatic P-450 system to a toxic intermediate, NAPQI. Following therapeutic doses of acetaminophen, however, this toxic metabolite is quickly detoxified by hepatic glutathione. (The metabolite of a medication may or may not be pharmacologically active.)

Excretion. After a medication is metabolized, it must be excreted. It may be excreted as a metabolite or as active medication. Excretion occurs primarily through the kidneys and the gastrointestinal tract following hepatic metabolism. Renal clearance of unchanged medications and of metabolites of medications is a major route of medication elimination from the body. In preterm infants, renal clearance will probably be prolonged. Cocaine, for example, is metabolized in the plasma and the liver. Both unchanged cocaine and its metabolites are then excreted into the urine. Cocaine is distributed to human milk, and it can be absorbed, to some degree, in the breastfed infant's gastrointestinal tract. The breastfed infant's urine analysis will reveal cocaine and its metabolites after this exposure.

Elimination is accomplished by metabolism and excretion. Half-life, which is the time it takes for the concentration of a medication to decrease

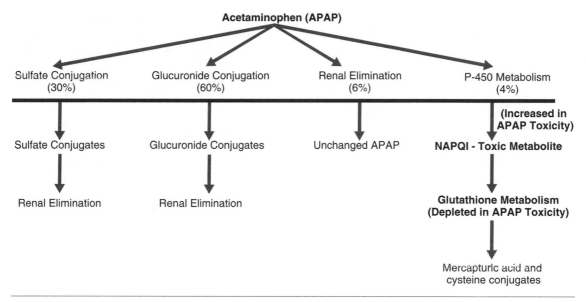

FIGURE 13-4 Metabolism and elimination of acetaminophen. Acetaminophen is known to be safe during lactation. This diagram shows how an adult metabolizes the drug and excretes it. Notice that there are several pathways by which to break it down and that the metabolites are excreted in the urine. The infant also handles acetaminophen well but differently via the sulfate conjunction pathway, which does not lead to toxic metabolites. This elaborate diagram illustrates the complexity of pharmacokinetics and is a reminder that the question of drugs in human milk is not a simple one.

by 50%, is used to characterize the rate of elimination of medications from the body. For example, the medication theophylline has a mean half-life of 8 hours in a healthy adult patient. If the patient has a therapeutic plasma concentration of 16 µg/ml at noon, she will have a plasma concentration of 8 µg/ml at 8 PM, based on an 8-hour half-life. After 4 to 5 half-lives, a medication will have been virtually eliminated from the adult body.

The concept of half-life forms the basis for the AAP's recommendation to take a dose of medication immediately after breastfeeding. If the medication has a relatively short half-life, a significant amount or possibly all of it will have been eliminated by the time of the next feeding.

Medications with a particularly short half-life are preferable to those with a relatively long half-life. For example, cephalexin HCl (Keflex), which may be given for postpartum infections, and ibuprofen, which is very commonly given for postpartum "cramps" and other discomforts, have short half-lives.

Maternal and Infant Health and Physiology

As mentioned earlier, the mother's ability to metabolize and excrete the medication is important. Therefore the nurse should be alert to any maternal history of renal or hepatic insufficiency and to any clinical signs that suggest this might be a problem. Similarly, weight and gestational age can influence the infant's ability to safely handle a medication. Therefore, when administering a medication to a mother who is breastfeeding a low-birth-weight or preterm infant, the nurse should proceed cautiously and be especially alert for adverse effects.

As explained earlier, medications enter the circulation as either protein bound or free. Usually, more medication is found in the plasma than in the milk because only a small free fraction of medication can cross the biologic membrane. During the first 5 to 7 days of lactation, however, the free fraction increases. Therefore some medications, such as salicylates, phenytoin, and diazepam, more readily cross into the milk.[1] Furthermore, the spaces between alveolar cells are more "open" at delivery and gradually "tighten" after the first few days. Hence, the amount of medication that passes into the milk is greater during the first few days. On the other hand, a relatively small amount of milk is present for the infant to consume on those first few days, so this should not present a problem in most cases.

A complete explanation of the infant's health in relation to his ability to metabolize and excrete the medication is presented by Lawrence.[1] Briefly, the infant's ability to metabolize and excrete the medication is of paramount importance. The infant's age is also especially important; preterm infants have more immature systems and have less ability to adequately detoxify and excrete the medication.

The Breast: A Selective Organ

As described earlier, the breast is not a sieve; through pharmacokinetics, the amount of medication that reaches the mother's systemic circulation is considerably less than what she initially ingested. Furthermore, all of the medication that is in the mother's bloodstream does not necessarily go into the milk. The parenchyma (organ tissue) is separated from the blood, and this prevents or slows the passage of medication from the maternal circulation to the milk. The milk, of course, is secreted by the lacteal cells in the alveoli. The question then becomes, how does the medication pass from the maternal circulation into the cells?

Medications can pass into the alveoli by one of several processes: passive diffusion (from an area of higher concentration to an area of lower concentration), facilitated diffusion (from an area of higher concentration to an area of lower concentration), and active diffusion (from an area of lower concentration to an area of higher concentration). Not unlike the way medications cross membranes in other parts of the body, many medications cross the alveolar membrane primarily by passive diffusion. With passive diffusion, small molecules are excreted through the cytoplasm of the lacteal cells, but they can also enter the alveolus through the intercellular spaces before the closing of the tight junctions in the first few days postpartum. The concentration of the medication in the

milk depends not only on the concentration gradient but also on the lipid solubility, degree of ionization, protein binding, and other factors. Medications that are acidic are not attracted to human milk, which is also acidic. Medications bound to albumin in the plasma are not available to pass into milk.

The milk-to-plasma (M/P) ratio is an important consideration; it is the ratio of the concentration of a substance in the milk to the concentration of the same substance in the *maternal* plasma at the same time. However, it is impossible to determine the safety of a medication on the basis of M/P ratio only. First, the M/P ratio is one of several factors that must be considered. Second, the reported "textbook" values for an agent's M/P ratio are not necessarily the actual M/P ratio that might be obtained in any one mother's milk, or at all of the times when she is secreting milk.

The M/P ratio is affected by the fact that medications move back and forth between the maternal systemic circulation and the milk. When milk is being actively produced during a feeding, the medication in the plasma at that time is available to pass into the milk. This is why the level in maternal plasma during a feeding is significant.

A milk-to-plasma measurement is also related to time: time after dosing and peak plasma time. If passive diffusion occurred continuously, unrestrained by binding and other factors over an indefinite period, the M/P ratio would be 1. However, because the properties of the medication slow down the diffusion process, the M/P ratio is usually much less than 1. A typical M/P ratio for many medications of medium molecular size is .005 to .05.

The number of doses administered can also affect the M/P ratio. The M/P ratio would be lower, for example, if the mother had received one "stat" dose of a medication, rather than multiple regular doses over time. Also, the textbook M/P ratio may not be the same as the M/P ratio in an individual mother. The textbook M/P ratio may have been determined at any point during the dosing interval; an M/P value determined at the time of peak concentration would be very different from the M/P ratio at some other point in the dosing interval.

Similarly, an M/P ratio reported in the literature may be determined by obtaining and averaging several values or as the result of only one data point. Therefore it is difficult to extrapolate data from a published report to an actual clinical case.

There is an important distinction between the M/P ratio and the total amount passed into milk. For example, if the M/P ratio is .03, that does *not* mean that 3% of the medication is passed into the milk. The total amount passed into milk depends on the pharmacokinetics described earlier and the rate of milk secretion. Furthermore, the mother's blood volume is about 10 times greater than the volume of milk she secretes, so in general, the percentage of medication passed into the milk is much lower. (Methods of estimating drug exposure for infants are described in Box 13-8.)

Medications Used during Breastfeeding

Most medications are safe for use during breastfeeding. Adverse effects can and do occur, however, as shown in Table 13-3.[105] The reader should keep in mind, however, that like other tables and lists, *this one should not be used as the sole resource or criterion for determining the risk-benefit ratio of a specific medication.*

A few medications—antidepressants,[64] antipsychotics, mood stabilizers, and benzodiazepines—deserve special mention because they have received so much attention in the popular press and because the AAP has created a special category for these.[2] Interestingly, however, most of the professional literature consists mainly of single case reports rather than controlled, longitudinal investigations.[65,66]

Box **13-8** Methods of Estimating Drug Exposure for Infants

Infant dose = (drug concentration in milk) × (milk volume consumed)

M/P ratio = (unbound drug in milk) ÷ (drug in maternal plasma)

Drug concentration in milk = (maternal plasma concentration) × (M/P ratio)

Data from Howard CR, Lawrence RA. *Pediatr Clin North Am* 2001;48:485-504.

Nonetheless, Briggs cautions that "psychotropic agents change the brain chemistry of the mother and may [do] so in a nursing infant. That this may occur during a rapidly changing and very vulnerable period of infant neurodevelopment heightens the concern"[105] (p. 19).

Antidepressants, including tricyclics and serotonin selective reuptake inhibitors (SSRIs), are generally not contraindicated if the infant is healthy; Yoshida and colleagues have pointed out that the benefits of breastfeeding usually outweigh the possible risks.[65] The antidepressive medication fluoxetine (Prozac) may be associated with poor weight gain in situations in which the infant is already at risk for insufficient weight gain.[67] Fluoxetine toxicity has been reported.[106] And, the effects of another popular SSRI, paroxetine (Paxil), have also been studied. When the mother is taking the medication, breastfed infants have low concentrations of paroxetine, and they do not exhibit adverse effects.[68]

Antipsychotics, including chlorpromazine, perphenazine, haloperidol, and clozapine, are probably safe if the mother requires fewer than two antipsychotic medications and is at the lower end of the dosage range.[69] Mood stabilizers, including lithium,[70,71] carbamazepine,[72] and benzodiazepines,[73] require careful, individualized assessment.

Strategies to Minimize Medication Exposure and Risk during Breastfeeding

Wellstart International has developed strategies designed to minimize the harmful effects of medication therapy during breastfeeding and lactation. Based on Wellstart's principles,[74] a series of questions follows. Although the person prescribing the medication assumes the greatest amount of responsibility, there are clear implications for the nurse, particularly the hospital staff nurse or visiting nurse who cares for the mother and newborn.

Is Medication Essential? Very often, medications are used when other remedies may work just as well. This is especially true with OTC products. For example, if the woman is tempted to buy an OTC expectorant, she should be first advised to drink large quantities of water; water is an excellent

Table **13-3**   ADVERSE EFFECTS IN THE BREASTFEEDING INFANT FROM DRUGS IN MILK

Drug	Use in Nursing	Toxicity
Acebutolol	RT	Accumulates in milk (ion trapping); β-adrenergic blockade (hypotension, bradycardia, transient tachypnea); see also atenolol
Alprazolam	RT	Withdrawal—irritability, crying, and sleep disturbances (after 9 months of exposure when mother weaned herself off the medication)
Amantadine	PT	Potential for urinary retention, vomiting, and skin rash
Amiodarone	PT	High iodine content, potential for accumulation
Amitriptyline	PT*	Potential for short- and long-term CNS toxicity
Amoxapine	PT*	Potential for short- and long-term CNS toxicity
Amphetamines	C*	Concentrated in milk; no adverse effects reported but potential for serious toxicity
Aspirin	RT*	Severe salicylate intoxication, metabolic acidosis (1 case)
Atenolol	RT*	Accumulates in milk (ion trapping); β-adrenergic blockade (cyanosis, hypothermia, bradycardia); see also acebutolol
Antineoplastics (All)	C	Cytotoxic; may suppress immune function; may cause neutropenia; unknown association with carcinogenesis or growth; doxorubicin is concentrated in milk (AAP considers only cyclophosphamide, doxorubicin, and methotrexate as contraindicated)[2]
Azathioprine	PT	See cyclosporine
β-Adrenergic blockers	PT	β-Adrenergic blockade in the nursing infant is a potential complication of all agents in this class; occasional reports of this adverse effect have appeared (see acebutolol and atenolol); these agents, however, are considered to be compatible with breastfeeding by the AAP
Bromocriptine	C	Suppresses lactation
Brompheniramine	RT	Irritability, excessive crying, sleep disturbance (in combination with isoephedrine) (1 case)
Bupropion	PT	Potential for short- and long-term CNS toxicity
Buspirone	PT	Potential for short- and long-term CNS toxicity
Carisoprodol	PT	Concentrated in milk, possible sedation
Chloramphenicol	PT*	Possible idiosyncratic bone marrow depression
Chlordiazepoxide	PT	Potential for short- and long-term CNS toxicity
Chlorpromazine	PT*	Drowsiness and lethargy (1 case); potential for short- and long-term CNS toxicity
Chlorpropamide	PT	Potential for hypoglycemia
Ciprofloxacin	PT	Potential for arthropathy; phototoxicity
Clemastine	RT*	Drowsiness, irritability, refusal to feed, neck stiffness, and high-pitched cry (1 case)
Clindamycin	RT	Bloody stools (1 case)
Clofazimine	RT	Pigmentation of infant's skin (1 case)
Clonazepam	RT	Persistent apneic spells (1 case); measurement of serum levels suggested
Clozapine	PT	Concentrated in milk; potential for short- and long-term CNS toxicity
Cocaine	C*	Cocaine poisoning, irritability, vomiting, diarrhea, tremors, increased startle response, hyperactive Moro reaction, increased symmetric deep tendon reflexes with bilateral ankle clonus, marked lability of mood (1 case)

Table **13-3**   ADVERSE EFFECTS IN THE BREASTFEEDING INFANT FROM DRUGS IN MILK—CONT'D

Drug	Use in Nursing	Toxicity
Cyclosporine	C*	Possible immune suppression; unknown effect on growth and carcinogenesis; renal damage
Dapsone	RT	Hemolytic anemia (1 case)
Desipramine	PT*	Potential for short- and long-term CNS toxicity
Dexfenfluramine	PT	Potential for short- and long-term CNS toxicity
Diazepam	PT*	Potential for short- and long-term CNS toxicity
Doxepin	RT*	One infant was pale, hypotonic, and near respiratory arrest
Ergotamine	C^x	Vomiting, diarrhea, convulsions with doses used in migraine therapy (based on 1934 study): ergot alkaloids may also suppress lactation
Estrogens	PT	May decrease milk volume
Ethanol	RT	Chronic exposure may inhibit psychomotor development
Felbamate	PT	Potential for aplastic anemia and acute liver failure
Fenfluramine	C	Potential for accumulation (long plasma half-life) and neurotoxicity
Fluorescein sodium	PT	Potential for phototoxic reaction when high doses given to mother (severe bullous skin eruption)
Fluoroquinolones	PT	See ciprofloxacin
Fluoxetine	RT	Colicky symptoms consisting of increased crying, irritability, decreased sleep, vomiting, watery diarrhea (1 case)
Fluvoxamine	PT*	Potential for short- and long-term CNS toxicity
Gold sodium thiomalate	PT	Although the AAP considers gold salts to be compatible with breastfeeding, gold absorption by the nursing infant has been documented and the prolonged excretion of gold into milk may allow a nursing infant to accumulate the drug, resulting in potential toxicity
Haloperidol	PT*	Potential for short- and long-term CNS toxicity
Heroin	C*	Excreted in sufficient amounts to cause addiction in the nursing infant; withdrawal symptoms have been reported
Imipramine	PT*	Potential for short- and long-term CNS toxicity
Iodine	RT	Goiter; considered compatible with breastfeeding by the AAP
Itraconazole	PT	Potential for tissue accumulation in the nursing infant from chronic exposure
Lithium	C	Blood levels in infants are one third to one half therapeutic levels; toxicity possible
Lorazepam	PT*	Potential for short- and long-term CNS toxicity
Marijuana	C*	No adverse effects reported in two infants, but AAP considered marijuana contraindicated because of its potential adverse effects on the health of the mother and infant
Meperidine	RT	Neurobehavior depression
Mesalamine	RT*	Diarrhea (possible allergic reaction) (1 case)
Metoclopramide	PT*	Potential for short- and long-term CNS toxicity
Metronidazole	PT*	In vitro mutagen; hold breastfeeding for 12 to 24 hours after single 2-g dose therapy

Continued

Table **13-3**   ADVERSE EFFECTS IN THE BREASTFEEDING INFANT FROM DRUGS IN MILK—CONT'D

Drug	Use in Nursing	Toxicity
Midazolam	PT*	Potential for short- and long-term CNS toxicity
Nefazodone	RT	Drowsiness, lethargy, hypothermia, poor feeding (1 case)
Oxycodone	PT	Relatively high levels in milk; use alternative agents if frequent dosing
Paroxetine	PT*	Potential for short- and long-term CNS toxicity
Perphenazine	PT*	Potential for short- and long-term CNS toxicity
Phencyclidine (PCP)	C*	Potential for severe toxicity
Phenobarbital	RT*	Accumulation in infant may occur; sedation; withdrawal may occur when breastfeeding stopped; methemoglobinemia (1 case); measure infant serum levels during chronic maternal therapy
Phentermine	C	Potential for CNS stimulation, decreased appetite
Primidone	RT*	Sedation, feeding problems
Radiopharmaceuticals	C*	Hold breastfeeding until radioactivity no longer in milk
Sertraline	PT	Potential for short- and long-term CNS toxicity
Sulfonamides	PT	Avoid in ill, stressed, or premature infants and in infants with hyperbilirubinemia or glucose-6-phosphate dehydrogenase deficiency
Tamoxifen	C	Inhibits lactation; potential for serious toxicity
Temazepam	PT*	Potential for short- and long-term CNS toxicity
Theophylline	RT	Irritability in one infant when mother took a rapidly absorbed oral liquid dose of aminophylline
Tolbutamide	PT	Potential for hypoglycemia
Trazodone	PT*	Potential for short- and long-term CNS toxicity
Trifluoperazine	PT*	Potential for short- and long-term CNS toxicity
Zuclopenthixol	PT	Potential for short- and long-term CNS toxicity

Data from American Academy of Pediatrics Committee on Drugs. *Pediatrics* 2001;108:776-789; Ito S. *N Engl J Med* 2000;343: 118-126; Briggs GG, Freeman RK, Yaffe SJ. *Drugs in pregnancy and lactation: a reference guide to fetal and neonatal risk.* 6th ed. Baltimore: Williams & Wilkins; 2001. In Briggs GG. *Clin Obstet Gynecol* 2002;45:6-21.
AAP, American Academy of Pediatrics; *C,* contraindicated; *CNS,* central nervous system; *PT,* unknown toxicity but potentially serious; use with caution; *RT,* toxicity has been reported; use alternative agents if available.
*Listed this way according to the AAP.

expectorant and often works better than the commonly used OTC product guaifenesin. Similarly, the woman who complains of sinus congestion may be tempted to self-medicate. Instead, suggest that she use a humidifier, which is very effective in relieving head congestion.

Dissuade the woman from using combination OTC products, as mentioned earlier. Similarly, suggest a topical product rather than a systemic product if that is a reasonable alternative. For example, Afrin Nasal Spray nose drops are a better choice than pseudoephedrine tablets.

Can Therapy Be Delayed? Sometimes medication administration or therapy that may result in

medication administration can be delayed. For example, hormonal birth control pills can be used, but it is better if the woman can delay using the progestin-only oral contraceptive until around 6 weeks. In this way, breastfeeding can be well established before the hormone is used. Meanwhile, nonhormonal barrier methods or natural methods of birth control may be used. Similarly, help the woman determine whether an elective surgery that will require postoperative medication administration can be delayed. The same may hold true for complicated dental procedures.

Should Breastfeeding Be Temporarily Delayed? Sometimes a medication that provides a needed benefit for the mother poses a potential risk to the infant. If so, plan for the interruption and use the strategies suggested in Chapter 14 to facilitate breastfeeding when the mother and infant are separated.

Can Only Medications with Established History Be Used? For some medications—especially new medications—there is little or no information available in terms of their effect on lactation or the breastfeeding infant. If possible, persuade the mother and her physicians to explore other choices.

Can Only Medications with Known Poor Passage into Milk Be Used? Medications that do not pass readily into mothers' milk are preferable to those that do. In the hospital setting, it may be helpful to make a list of medications that are commonly prescribed on the unit, separating them into columns: those that easily pass into milk and those that do not. Although this should not provide the sole criteria for whether the medication can be prescribed, it should help nurses feel safe administering medications that do not readily pass into milk.

Can Alternative Routes of Administration Be Used? Using a different route of administration may decrease the amount of medication in the mother's milk. Of course, the nurse cannot change the route of administration without a written order, but she can become an advocate for the woman. For example, an inhaled bronchodilator would be preferable to an oral agent for asthma because the inhaled medication would minimize the amount of the medication that gets into the milk.

HERBAL THERAPIES

Plants have been the basis for treatment for centuries; even the Bible mentions plants as having medicinal uses. Although often presumed to be harmless, plants can have potentially toxic effects. Hypocrites, the father of Medicine (460-370 BC) used only botanical medicines, not modern pharmaceutical medications, when he said, "Primum non nocere" (Latin for "First, do no harm"). Even today, one fourth of the medications dispensed in the United States are created from plants, and some,

including digitalis (derived from the foxglove plant), can be toxic. Therefore those who use or prescribe botanical medicines should be aware that like pharmaceutical medicines, therapeutic or toxic effects *can* occur, whether or not they do.

About one third to one half of adults in the United States, Canada, and Australia use alternative therapies, including herbal remedies.[75,76] Certainly, the use of herbal medicine has been documented for centuries, but the safety and efficacy of herbs have not been proven in rigorously controlled trials. In most cases, therefore, recommendations about herbs for adult use are usually limited to case reports and the experience of individual practitioners. There is even less information about the safety and efficacy of herbal medicines for the pregnant or lactating woman. However, in general, the U.S. Food and Drug Administration (FDA) categorizes approximately 250 herbs—including chamomile, garlic, ginger, ginseng, and valerian—as safe.[77] Some herbs, however, have been determined to be contraindicated[82] during lactation and are shown in Box 13-9.

A problem with herbal medicine in the United States is that unlike FDA-approved medications, doses for herbal therapies are not necessarily

---

Box 13-9 Herbs That Are Contraindicated for Lactating Women[82]*

Aloe *(aloe vera)* (dried juice is contra-indicated for internal use)
Buckthorn bark and berry *(Rhamnus cathartica)*
Cascara Sagrada bark *(Rhamnus purshiana)*
Coltsfoot leaf *(Tussilago farfara)*
Fixed combinations of Senna leaf, Peppermint oil, and Caraway oil
Indian snakeroot *(Rauwolfia serpentia)*
Kava Kava root *(Piper methysticum)*
Petasites root *(Petasites hybridus)*
Rhubarb root *(Rheum palmatum)*
Senna leaf *(Saccia senna)*
Uva-ursi *(Arctostaphylos uva-ursi)*

*Inclusion here does not necessarily mean that the herb cannot be used topically or in food.

standardized by content of active ingredients, which are often unknown.[77] And, unlike FDA-approved medications, herbal therapies have no requirement for proof of purity, some of the plants used in a preparation can be misidentified at the time of harvesting, and no quality control is required.[77] At the same time, there is no mechanism in the United States for reporting adverse effects of the herbal therapies because they are not classified as drugs. Hence, with so many potentially unknown factors and inconsistencies, it is difficult, if not impossible, to consistently control or predict either the therapeutic or the adverse effects of herbal medicine.

The safety and efficacy of herbal therapy are further clouded by other issues. Consumers and providers are often confused because some sources say an herbal remedy is safe and effective, whereas other sources say it is not. It is sometimes helpful to understand why these apparent discrepancies arise. First, some sources are referring to use of one part of the plant (e.g., the seeds, or sometimes called the *fruit*), and another source is talking about use of a different part of the plant (e.g., the leaves). Often, lists of contraindications "during pregnancy and lactation" are lumped together without sufficient realization that the absorption, metabolism, and excretion of any substance differ during pregnancy than during lactation. Part of this can be attributed to the fact that funding for herbal therapy is limited and studies are often flawed.[78] Criteria for evaluating reports of herbal toxicity include the following[79]: (1) What is the basis of the report (e.g., animal or human subjects and the possibility for contamination in case reports)? (2) What part of the plant was used, in what form, and by what route was it given? (3) What was the dose and duration of usage? (4) Were other possible causes of the effect ruled out? (5) What is the risk-benefit ratio?

Some herbs are strictly contraindicated in lactation,[80-82] and others have adverse effects that warrant their inclusion on the list of contraindications. For example, goldenseal has been associated with newborn jaundice.[77] Nurses have a responsibility to advise mothers of these. Advice-giving that is limited to responding to the mother's questions may be

prudent; "recommending" herbs as a medical treatment is likely to be beyond the scope of practice for those who have not had extensive training and experience in botanical medicines. As with conventional medications, the mother should be referred to someone who has special knowledge in this field.

Nurses and other health care providers should have handy a few authoritative sources for determining the safety of the herbal treatment. In the United States, a useful list, originally developed by the FDA in 1962 and updated frequently, is the Generally Recognized as Safe (GRAS) list. Inclusion on this list is reassuring, but some herbal medications that are listed as safe by other national agencies do not appear on the GRAS list. In Germany, authorities have devised and enforced a system for reporting adverse effects of herbal therapies since 1978. Hence, they have developed a book that is arguably the most authoritative resource for the safety and efficacy of herbal medicine in the modern world. It has now been translated into English.[82] Similarly, a compendium to the *Pharmacopeia* exists in the UK, and this resource is also extremely helpful.[83] Parents can be directed to sources that are easily understood and written by authoritative sources.[84] Nurses are in an ideal situation to provide information to consumers to allow them to make choices based on sound principles, as outlined in Box 13-10.

The complexities of herbal therapies are beyond the scope of this text, but readers are encouraged to pursue literature that explains that herbal therapies, although perhaps safe and effective, can be unsafe or ineffective in some cases. Other sources may be helpful.[76,77,79,85-92] Table 13-4 lists herbs that lactating women commonly ask about, but this table should be used with discretion and attention to the individual's needs.

Products advertised as "mother's milk tea" are often assumed to be harmless, or even beneficial. Certainly, some teas, including chicory, orange spice, peppermint, raspberry, red bush tea, and rose hips, are considered safe.[1] However, consumers and providers should be aware of the ingredients in teas; toxicity is possible from some teas.[93]

Box 13-10   PRINCIPLES FOR SAFE USE
OF HERBAL THERAPY

Be certain that a specific diagnosis has been determined. As with conventional medications, herbs should be used for their intended purpose, not as a result of self-diagnosing. Similarly, herbal therapy should be used in conjunction with other problem-solving techniques. For example, if a woman does not have enough milk, she should first receive a thorough assessment and simple interventions.

Scrutinize qualifications of the person who is recommending the herbal therapy. Because herbs are not classified as drugs, qualifications of those who recommend or prescribe them varies tremendously both in the United States and abroad.[94] If parents inquire about the use of herbs, be prepared to suggest names of herbalists who have had extensive training and experience in the field.

Buy herbs from a reputable source. Herbal preparations may not contain a therapeutic level of the active component, or the preparation may be contaminated. Therefore it is imperative to purchase the herb from a reputable source.

Evaluate studies carefully. Parents as well as colleagues may have difficulty sorting through all of the information that is available. Using evaluation criteria, as described earlier,[79] helps the reader come to reasoned conclusions.

Look for reputable sources of information. Medical libraries have many of the resources suggested here; community libraries generally have good resources for parents.

ENVIRONMENTAL AND FOOD HAZARDS

Some environmental conditions or food hazards could present a threat to breastfeeding infants and should be evaluated on a case-by-case basis, although the risk in most situations is low. A brief discussion of herbicides, pesticides, and heavy metals follows, but readers are referred to more authoritative sources for details.[7]

Herbicides and Pesticides

Herbicides and pesticides are not usually a problem for women in the United States, although they may be a problem elsewhere. For the most part, exposure to environmental contaminants such as herbicides and pesticides usually does not preclude breastfeeding.

Heavy Metals

Lawrence and Howard[95] point out that heavy metal exposure usually occurs through the water supply, and even through infant formula. Therefore "[T]he breastfed infant is exposed to lower levels through human milk in geographic areas where levels are high"[95] (p. 485). However, lead exposure, particularly in low-income or older housing, constitutes a potential problem for the family, and if one family member has a problem, each member should be assessed. Generally, however, the breastfed infant who was exposed to lead in utero loses lead after birth if the amount in the maternal milk is 5 µg/dl/day or less.[96] If the mother's blood level of lead is 40 µg/dl or less, breastfeeding is *not* contraindicated because the lead levels in her milk are very low or undetectable.[5]

Mercury exposure can happen in peoples throughout the world, usually as the result of industrial waste.[95] Individuals can get mercury poisoning by eating contaminated fish. However, there appears to be no correlation between the maternal blood levels of mercury and her infant's development, except in extreme cases.[97] Cadmium exposure from industrial waste poses a threat in Japan but rarely is reported in the United States. Radionuclides—a specific type of atom that exhibits radioactivity (e.g., carbon 14)—deserve careful consideration. However, research conducted after the Chernobyl accident showed that radioactivity in human milk posed less of a threat to infants than bottle-feeding.[98,99]

Although environmental contaminants in maternal milk may seem worrisome, the Chernobyl accident demonstrates a principle that may be useful in understanding the broader context of the infant's exposure. That is, the infant is exposed to the environment where not only his mother but also he lives. Lawrence concludes that "breastfeeding is not

Table 13-4 HERBS THAT LACTATING WOMEN COMMONLY INQUIRE ABOUT

Common Name, Scientific Name, Part Used	Common Use	Safety	Possible Side Effects	Administration	Contraindications	Implications
Fenugreek *Trigonella foenum-graecum* Seeds	To relieve gastrointestinal (GI) upset and constipation. Lowers blood glucose levels, especially in those with type 2 diabetes. Also used to improve milk supply.	In USA, on GRAS list. German and British authorities consider it acceptable for use.	Hypersensitivity. Seeds have demonstrated uterine stimulant effects.[81] Hypocholesteremic effect. Well known for hypoglycemic effects in animal studies.	Capsules typically contain either 580 or 610 mg. (Lactating mothers should not exceed this dosage.[81])	Contraindicated in pregnancy because it can cause mild uterine cramps. Because the herb is related to peanuts, those with allergies to peanuts may be hypersensitive to fenugreek also.	Controlled studies, if available, have not demonstrated safety and efficacy in lactating humans (Trials are currently under way.[81]) When consumed in large doses, the breast-feeding infant's urine will smell like maple syrup, which may prompt the pediatrician to assess for presence of maple syrup disease. Also has hypoglycemic effects. Tea has bitter taste.
Fennel seed *Foeniculum vulgare* Seeds	To reduce flatulence, stomach cramps, bloating, indigestion, and infant colic.[81] Many cultures use as galactagogue.	In USA, on GRAS list. German and British authorities consider it acceptable for use.	No side effects reported.	½ teaspoon of powdered fennel seed in a cup with water may be drunk several times a day.[81]	Many textbooks identify this as contraindicated during lactation, but herbal experts[81] disagree.	Controlled studies, if available, have not demonstrated safety and efficacy in lactating humans. Commonly used along with catnip in remedies to alleviate infantile colic in England.

Goat's rue *Galega officinalis* Seeds	For diuresis and diabetic control. In other cultures, seeds have been used as a galactagogue for centuries (not whole plant).	Not on GRAS list in USA. Not on "approved" list of herbs by German standards, but not on their contraindicated list either. Not contraindicated by British standards.	No side effects reported in humans in Europe, where it has been used as a galactagogue for 10 centuries.[81]	1 cup of boiling water poured over 1 teaspoon of herb; limit to 2 cups per day.[81]	Many sources strongly discourage during lactation, presumably because toxicity occurred in animal study. Experts disagree with this contraindication.[81]	Controlled studies, if available, have not demonstrated safety and efficacy in lactating humans. Large oral doses of the plant have been associated with lethal poisoning in sheep. (Such toxicity would be highly unlikely to occur with normal doses in humans.) Still used in veterinary medicine as galactagogue. Also has known hypoglycemic effects.
Milk thistle *Silybum marianum* Seeds	Used for liver disorders. In other cultures, seeds (not whole plant) have been used as galactagogue.	Not on GRAS list in USA. Not on German list of approved herbs, but not listed as being contraindicated during lactation.	Toxic effects noted in animal reports.[107] In humans, seeds are completely nontoxic and can be crushed and used in bread recipes.[81]	Steep 1 teaspoon of crushed seeds; tea can be consumed several times a day.	Not contraindicated during lactation in Europe.	Controlled studies, if available, have not demonstrated safety and efficacy in lactating humans. However, women have used this for centuries.[81] (Not to be confused with blessed thistle *[Cnicus benedictus].)* The white "veins" of the milk thistle were thought to represent milk used by the Virgin Mary to suckle Jesus.
Chamomile *Matricaria recutita, Chamaemelum nobile,* and other names Dried flowers	Used for insomnia, anxiety, spasms, digestive irritation, inflammation.	In USA, on GRAS list. Generally considered acceptable for use by German and British authorities.	Hypersensitivity. No serious side effects known.	Steep dried flowers in 1 cup water (1 tsp of chamomile flowers ≈1000 mg). Take as tea as necessary. Use dried flowers only, not the whole plant.	Individuals who are sensitive to sunflowers, ragweed, or members of the aster family (echinacea, feverfew, milk thistle) may have cross-sensitivity to chamomile.	Controlled studies, if available, have not demonstrated safety and efficacy in lactating. May interfere with anticoagulants and concurrent use of sedative.

Continued

Table 13-4 HERBS THAT LACTATING WOMEN COMMONLY INQUIRE ABOUT—CONT'D

Common Name, Scientific Name, Part Used	Common Use	Safety	Possible Side Effects	Administration	Contraindications	Implications
Echinacea *Echinacea purpurea* Leaf, stalk, root	Antiinfective agent. Used for acute and chronic infections of the upper and lower respiratory tract.	Not on GRAS list. Considered acceptable for use by German and British authorities.	When taken orally for duration of up to 12 wk, no adverse effects reported. Sensitive individuals may experience dermatitis.	Steep 1 g root in 1 cup of boiling water 5-10 min; may be taken up to three times daily.	Hypersensitivity. People who are allergic to ragweed and chrysanthemum may be hypersensitive to echinacea.	Controlled studies, if available, have not demonstrated safety and efficacy in lactating humans.
Garlic cloves *Allium sativum* Cloves, root	Used for hypertension; also used as antioxidant and anti-microbial.	On GRAS list, including a specification that it is safe for use during pregnancy and lactation. Considered acceptable for use by German and British authorities.	No serious side effects; halitosis, GI disturbance.	Take ½ to 1 fresh clove per day.	Contraindicated if GI inflammation is present.	Controlled studies, if available, have not demonstrated safety and efficacy in lactating humans. Increases clotting time.
Ginger root *Zingiber officinale* Root	Used for prevention of nausea and vomiting and dyspepsia.	On GRAS list in USA, including a specification that it is safe for use during pregnancy and lactation. Considered acceptable for use by German and British authorities.	GI and skin hypersensitivity.	For tea, steep 1 teaspoon powder or 2 teaspoons of grated fresh root in boiling water. (Steep 10 minutes for the fresh root.)	Cholelithiasis.	Controlled studies, if available, have not demonstrated safety and efficacy in lactating humans.

contraindicated in association with environmental hazards in the United States under ordinary circumstances. Special circumstances of exposure should be assessed on an individual basis"[1] (p. 487).

Silicone

Silicone is present in breast implants, and because so many women of childbearing age have breast implants, nurses and other care providers frequently wonder if the situation contraindicates breastfeeding. Only one study assayed the milk of women with implants; the concentrations were not significantly elevated over control samples.[100] The question then becomes, what are the clinical outcomes?

Early reports described esophageal dysfunction in 11 children who were breastfed by mothers with silicone implants.[101,102] Later reports have shown that there are no clinical problems among children breastfed by mothers who have the implants.[103,104] Interestingly, it appears that there is more silicone in artificial milk than in human milk, and hence the AAP has determined that breast implants are not a contraindication to breastfeeding.[2]

SUMMARY

Like all recommendations during the perinatal period, nurses and other health care professionals should make recommendations about breastfeeding after critically appraising the available evidence and considering the cost-benefit. In nearly all cases the benefits of breastfeeding far exceed any possible risks. Certainly, the family should have informed consent, and the mother should be regarded as the final decision maker. In the case of disease or pharmacologic therapy, modifications or a temporary cessation of breastfeeding with later resumption may be indicated. Because mothers frequently initiate herbal therapy without the advice of a professional, the nurse must be prepared to work within her scope of practice to help mothers recognize both the potential benefits and known risks of herbal therapy. The nurse has a responsibility to minimize the possible adverse effects of disease, pharmacologic therapy, or herbal therapies. Most important, the nurse has a responsibility to become an advocate for maintaining the breastfeeding relationship.

REFERENCES

1. Lawrence RA, Lawrence RM. *Breastfeeding: a guide for the medical profession.* 5th ed. St. Louis: Mosby; 1999.
2. American Academy of Pediatrics Committee on Drugs. Transfer of drugs and other chemicals into human milk. *Pediatrics* 2001;108:776-789.
3. Hale T. *Medications & mothers' milk: a manual of lactational pharmacology.* 10th ed. Amarillo, TX: Pharmasoft Publishing; 2002.
4. Briggs GG, Freeman RK, Yaffe SJ. *Drugs in pregnancy and lactation: a reference guide to fetal and neonatal risk.* 6th ed. Baltimore: Williams & Wilkins; 2001.
5. Lawrence RM, Lawrence RA. Given the benefits of breastfeeding, what contraindications exist? *Pediatr Clin North Am* 2001;48:235-251.
6. Kontiokari T, Sundqvist K, Nuutinen M et al. Randomised trial of cranberry-lingonberry juice and lactobacillus GG drink for the prevention of urinary tract infections in women. *BMJ* 2001;322:1571.
7. Lawrence RA. *A review of the medical benefits and contraindications to breastfeeding in the United States (Maternal and Child Health Technical Information Bulletin).* Arlington VA: National Center for Education in Maternal and Child Health; 1997.
8. Brown HL, Abernathy MP. Cytomegalovirus infection. *Semin Perinatol* 1998;22:260-266.
9. Clarke NM, May JT. Effect of antimicrobial factors in human milk on rhinoviruses and milk-borne cytomegalovirus in vitro. *J Med Microbiol* 2000;49:719-723.
10. van der Strate BW, Harmsen MC, Schafer P et al. Viral load in breast milk correlates with transmission of human cytomegalovirus to preterm neonates, but lactoferrin concentrations do not. *Clin Diagn Lab Immunol* 2001;8:818-821.
11. Hamprecht K, Maschmann J, Vochem M et al. Epidemiology of transmission of cytomegalovirus from mother to preterm infant by breastfeeding. *Lancet* 2001;357:513-518.
12. Vochem M, Hamprecht K, Jahn G et al. Transmission of cytomegalovirus to preterm infants through breast milk. *Pediatr Infect Dis J* 1998;17:53-58.
13. Richter D, Hampl W, Pohlandt F. Vertical transmission of cytomegalovirus, most probably by breast milk, to an infant with Wiskott-Aldrich syndrome with fatal outcome. *Eur J Pediatr* 1997;156:854-855.
14. Williams AJ, Duong T, McNally LM et al. Pneumocystis carinii pneumonia and cytomegalovirus infection in children with vertically acquired HIV infection. *AIDS* 2001;15:335-339.
15. Zanetti AR, Tanzi E, Newell ML. Mother-to-infant transmission of hepatitis C virus. *J Hepatol* 1999;31(Suppl 1):96-100.
16. AAP Committee on Infectious Disease. *Red book.* Elk Grove Village: American Academy of Pediatrics; 1997.
17. WHO/UNAIDS/UNICEF. HIV and infant feeding. Guidelines for decision-makers. 1998. Retrieved from

http://www.unaids.org/publications/documents/mtct/infantpolicy.html.

18. World Health Organization. *HIV and infant feeding: guidelines for health care managers and supervisors.* Geneva: World Health Organization; 1998.

19. American Academy of Pediatrics Committee on Pediatric AIDS. Human milk, breastfeeding, and transmission of human immunodeficiency virus in the United States. *Pediatrics* 1995;96:977-979.

20. Weinberg GA. The dilemma of postnatal mother-to-child transmission of HIV: to breastfeed or not? *Birth* 2000;27:199-205.

21. Greiner T, Sachs M, Morrison P. The choice by HIV-positive women to exclusively breastfeed should be supported. *Arch Pediatr Adolesc Med* 2002;156:87-88.

22. McIntyre J, Gray G. What can we do to reduce mother to child transmission of HIV? *BMJ* 2002;324:218-221.

23. Ruff AJ. Breastmilk, breastfeeding, and transmission of viruses to the neonate. *Semin-Perinatol* 1994;18:510-516.

24. Leroy V, Newell ML, Dabis F et al. International multicentre pooled analysis of late postnatal mother-to-child transmission of HIV-1 infection. Ghent International Working Group on Mother-to-Child Transmission of HIV. *Lancet* 1998;352:597-600.

25. Karlsson K, Massawe A, Urassa E et al. Late postnatal transmission of human immunodeficiency virus type 1 infection from mothers to infants in Dar es Salaam, Tanzania. *Pediatr Infect Dis J* 1997;16:963-967.

26. Miotti PG, Taha TE, Kumwenda NI et al. HIV transmission through breastfeeding: a study in Malawi. *JAMA* 1999;282:744-749.

27. Nduati R, John G, Mbori-Ngacha D et al. Effect of breastfeeding and formula feeding on transmission of HIV-1: a randomized clinical trial. *JAMA* 2000;283:1167-1174.

28. Nduati R. Breastfeeding and HIV-1 infection. A review of current literature. *Adv Exp Med Biol* 2000;478:201-210.

29. Coutsoudis A, Pillay K, Kuhn L et al. Method of feeding and transmission of HIV-1 from mothers to children by 15 months of age: prospective cohort study from Durban, South Africa. *AIDS* 2001;15:379-387.

30. Nduati R, Richardson BA, John G et al. Effect of breastfeeding on mortality among HIV-1 infected women: a randomised trial. *Lancet* 2001;357:1651-1655.

31. United States Breastfeeding Committee. Position statement on HIV. 2000. Retrieved from http://www.usbreastfeeding.org.

32. Chantry CJ, Morrison P, Panchula J et al. Effects of lipolysis or heat treatment on HIV-1 provirus in breast milk. *J Acquir Immune Defic Syndr* 2000;24:325-329.

33. Schanler RJ, O'Connor KG, Lawrence RA. Pediatricians' practices and attitudes regarding breastfeeding promotion. *Pediatrics* 1999;103:E35.

34. Howard CR, Lawrence RA. Drugs and breastfeeding. *Clin Perinatol* 1999;26:447-478.

35. Stabin MG. Health concerns related to radiation exposure of the female nuclear medicine patient. *Environ Health Perspect* 1997;105(Suppl 6):1403-1409.

36. Howard CR, Lawrence RA. Xenobiotics and breastfeeding. *Pediatr Clin North Am* 2001;48:485-504.

37. Sylvia L. Personal communication, 2001.

38. Cruikshank DP, Varner MW, Pitkin RM. Breast milk magnesium and calcium concentrations following magnesium sulfate treatment. *Am J Obstet Gynecol* 1982;143:685-688.

39. Idama TO, Lindow SW. Magnesium sulphate: a review of clinical pharmacology applied to obstetrics. *Br J Obstet Gynaecol* 1998;105:260-268.

40. Lindberg C, Boreus LO, de Chateau P et al. Transfer of terbutaline into breast milk. *Eur J Respir Dis Suppl* 1984;134:87-91.

41. Biancuzzo M. Does an epidural infusion affect newborn suckling? *Breastfeeding Outlook* 2001;2:1, 2, 7.

42. Sepkoski CM, Lester BM, Ostheimer GW et al. The effects of maternal epidural anesthesia on neonatal behavior during the first month. *Dev Med Child Neurol* 1992;34:1072-1080.

43. Halpern SH, Levine T, Wilson DB et al. Effect of labor analgesia on breastfeeding success. *Birth* 1999;26:83-88.

44. Rosen AR, Lawrence RA. The effect of epidural anesthesia on infant feeding. *J University of Rochester Medical Center* 1994;6:3-7.

45. Righard L, Alade MO. Effect of delivery room routines on success of first breast-feed. *Lancet* 1990;336:1105-1107.

46. Riordan J. The effect of labor pain relief medication on neonatal suckling and breastfeeding duration. *J Hum Lact* 2000;16:7-12.

47. Townsend RJ, Benedetti TJ, Erickson SH et al. Excretion of ibuprofen into breast milk. *Am J Obstet Gynecol* 1984;149:184-186.

48. Ito S. Drug therapy for breast-feeding women. *N Engl J Med* 2000;343:118-126.

49. Sapeika N. The excretion of drugs in human milk—a review. *J Obstet Gynaecol Br Empire* 1947;54:426.

50. Findlay JW, DeAngelis RL, Kearney MF et al. Analgesic drugs in breast milk and plasma. *Clin Pharmacol Ther* 1981;29:625-633.

51. Meny RG, Naumburg EG, Alger LS et al. Codeine and the breastfed neonate. *J Hum Lact* 1993;9:237-240.

52. De Rosa G, Corsello SM, Ruffilli MP et al. Prolactin secretion after beer. *Lancet* 1981;2:934.

53. Carlson HE, Wasser HL, Reidelberger RD. Beer-induced prolactin secretion: a clinical and laboratory study of the role of salsolinol. *J Clin Endocrinol Metab* 1985;60:673-677.

54. Koletzko B, Lehner F. Beer and breastfeeding. *Adv Exp Med Biol* 2000;478:23-28.

55. Grossman ER. Beer, breast-feeding, and the wisdom of old wives. *JAMA* 1988;259:1016.

56. Mennella JA, Beauchamp GK. The transfer of alcohol to human milk. Effects on flavor and the infant's behavior. *N Engl J Med* 1991;325:981-985.

57. Neville MC, Neifert MR, editors. *Lactation: physiology, nutrition and breast-feeding.* New York: Plenum Press; 1983.

58. Institute of Medicine. *Nutrition during lactation.* Washington, DC: National Academy Press; 1991.

59. Howard CR, Lawrence RA. Breast-feeding and drug exposure. *Obstet Gynecol Clin North Am* 1998;25:195-217.

60. Nice FJ, Snyder JL, Kotansky BC. Breastfeeding and over-the-counter medications. *J Hum Lact* 2000;16:319-331.

61. Einarson A, Ho E, Koren G. Can we use metronidazole during pregnancy and breastfeeding? Putting an end to the controversy. *Can Fam Physician* 2000;46:1053-1054.

62. Clark SL, Porter TF, West FG. Coumarin derivatives and breast-feeding. *Obstet Gynecol* 2000;95:938-940.

63. Iqbal MM, Sohhan T, Mahmud SZ. The effects of lithium, valproic acid, and carbamazepine during pregnancy and lactation. *J Toxicol Clin Toxicol* 2001;39:381-392.

64. Wisner KL, Perel JM, Findling RL. Antidepressant treatment during breast-feeding. *Am J Psychiatry* 1996;153:1132-1137.

65. Yoshida K, Smith B, Kumar R. Psychotropic drugs in mothers' milk: a comprehensive review of assay methods, pharmacokinetics and of safety of breast-feeding. *J Psychopharmacol* 1999;13:64-80.

66. Burt VK, Suri R, Altshuler L et al. The use of psychotropic medications during breast-feeding. *Am J Psychiatry* 2001;158:1001-1009.

67. Chambers CD, Anderson PO, Thomas RG et al. Weight gain in infants breastfed by mothers who take fluoxetine. *Pediatrics* 1999;104:e61.

68. Stowe ZN, Cohen LS, Hostetter A et al. Paroxetine in human breast milk and nursing infants. *Am J Psychiatry* 2000;157:185-189.

69. Tenyi T, Csabi G, Trixler M. Antipsychotics and breast-feeding: a review of the literature. *Paediatr Drugs* 2000;2:23-28.

70. Llewellyn A, Stowe ZN, Strader JR Jr. The use of lithium and management of women with bipolar disorder during pregnancy and lactation. *J Clin Psychiatry* 1998;59(Suppl 6):57-64.

71. Iqbal MM, Gundlapalli SP, Ryan WG et al. Effects of antimanic mood-stabilizing drugs on fetuses, neonates, and nursing infants. *South Med J* 2001;94:304-322.

72. Brent NB, Wisner KL. Fluoxetine and carbamazepine concentrations in a nursing mother/infant pair. *Clin Pediatr* 1998;37:41-44.

73. Birnbaum CS, Cohen LS, Bailey JW et al. Serum concentrations of antidepressants and benzodiazepines in nursing infants: a case series. *Pediatrics* 1999;104:e11.

74. Woodward-Lopez G, Creer AE, editors. *Lactational management curriculum: a faculty guide for schools of medicine, nursing and nutrition.* San Diego, CA: Wellstart International; 1994.

75. Eisenberg DM, Davis RB, Ettner SL et al. Trends in alternative medicine use in the United States, 1990-1997: results of a follow-up national survey. *JAMA* 1998;280:1569-1575.

76. Kemper KJ, Cassileth B, Ferris T. Holistic pediatrics: a research agenda. *Pediatrics* 1999;103:902-909.

77. O'Hara M, Kiefer D, Farrell K et al. A review of 12 commonly used medicinal herbs. *Arch Fam Med* 1998;7:523-536.

78. Nahin RL, Straus SE. Research into complementary and alternative medicine: problems and potential. *BMJ* 2001;322:161-164.

79. Belew C. Herbs and the childbearing woman. Guidelines for midwives. *J Nurse Midwifery* 1999;44:231-252.

80. Low Dog T. Presentation: *The use of herbal medicine during lactation.* ILCA Annual Conference, 1999, Scottsdale, AZ.

81. Low Dog T. *The use of herbal medicines during breastfeeding.* Chapel Hill, NC: Art of Breastfeeding Conference; 2000.

82. German Commission E Monographs. *Monographs: Medicinal plans for human use.* Austin TX: American Botanical Council; 1998.

83. Bradley P. *British herbal compendium.* vol 1. Bournemouth, Dorset; The British Herbal Medicine Association; 1990.

84. Hoffman D. *The herbal handbook: a user's guide to medical herbalism.* Rochester, VT: Healing Arts Press; 1998.

85. Pansatiankul BJ, Mekmanee R. Dicumarol content in alcoholic herb elixirs: one of the factors at risk induced IVKD-I. *Southeast Asian J Trop Med Public Health* 1993;24(Suppl 1):201-203.

86. Zava DT, Dollbaum CM, Blen M. Estrogen and progestin bioactivity of foods, herbs, and spices. *Proc Soc Exp Biol Med* 1998;217:369-378.

87. Blake S. *Alternative remedies* (CD-ROM). St. Louis: Mosby; 1999.

88. Kopec K. Herbal medications and breastfeeding. *J Hum Lact* 1999;15:157-161.

89. Allaire AD, Moos MK, Wells SR. Complementary and alternative medicine in pregnancy: a survey of North Carolina certified nurse-midwives. *Obstet Gynecol* 2000;95:19-23.

90. Einarson A, Lawrimore T, Brand P et al. Attitudes and practices of physicians and naturopaths toward herbal products, including use during pregnancy and lactation. *Can J Clin Pharmacol* 2000;7:45-49.

91. Hardy ML. Herbs of special interest to women. *J Am Pharm Assoc* 2000;40:234-242.

92. McGuffin M, Hobbs C, Upton R et al., editors. *Botanical safety handbook.* Silver Spring, MD: American Herbal Products Association; 1997.

93. Rosti L, Nardini A, Bettinelli ME et al. Toxic effects of a herbal tea mixture in two newborns. *Acta Paediatr* 1994;83:683.

94. Mills SY. Regulation in complementary and alternative medicine. *BMJ* 2001;322:158-160.

95. Lawrence RA, Howard CR. Given the benefits of breast-feeding, are there any contraindications? *Clin Perinatol* 1999;26:479-490.

96. Ong CN, Phoon WO, Law HY et al. Concentrations of lead in maternal blood, cord blood, and breast milk. *Arch Dis Child* 1985;60:756-759.

97. Myers GJ, Marsh DO, Davidson PW et al. Main neurodevelopmental study of Seychellois children following in utero exposure to methylmercury from a maternal fish diet: outcome at six months. *Neurotoxicology* 1995;16:653-664.

98. Gori G, Cama G, Guerresi E et al. Radioactivity in breast milk and placenta after Chernobyl accident. *Am J Obstet Gynecol* 1988;158:1243-1244.

99. Gori G, Cama G, Guerresi E et al. Radioactivity in breast milk and placentas during the year after Chernobyl. *Am J Obstet Gynecol* 1988;159:1232-1234.

100. Berlin CM Jr. Silicone breast implants and breast-feeding. *Pediatrics* 1994;94:547-549.

101. Levine JJ, Ilowite NT. Sclerodermalike esophageal disease in children breast-fed by mothers with silicone breast implants. *JAMA* 1994;271:213-216.

102. Levine JJ, Trachtman H, Gold DM et al. Esophageal dysmotility in children breast-fed by mothers with silicone breast implants. Long-term follow-up and response to treatment. *Dig Dis Sci* 1996;41:1600-1603.

103. Kjoller K, McLaughlin JK, Friis S et al. Health outcomes in offspring of mothers with breast implants. *Pediatrics* 1998;102:1112-1115.

104. Signorello LB, Fryzek JP, Blot WJ et al. Offspring health risk after cosmetic breast implantation in Sweden. *Ann Plast Surg* 2001;46:279-286.

105. Briggs GG. Drug effects on the fetus and breast-fed infant. *Clin Obstet Gynecol* 2002;45:6-21.

106. Hale TW, Shum S, Grossberg M. Fluoxetine toxicity in a breastfed infant. *Clin Pediatr (Phila)* 2001;40:681-684.

107. Flora K, Hahn M, Rosen H et al. Milk thistle *(Silybum marianum)* for the therapy of liver disease. *Am J Gastroenterol* 1998;93:139-143.

108. Cotterman KJ. Reverse pressure softening. Unpublished manuscript, 2002.

Providing Human Milk When Mother and Infant Are Separated

Ideally, the breastfeeding mother and her infant are together 24 hours a day. This situation, allowing the infant unlimited access to his mother's breasts, best facilitates breastfeeding and lactation. Sometimes, however, planned or unplanned circumstances make this impossible or impractical, and separation occurs. Although breastfeeding can be initiated or continued throughout the separation period, the mother may need counseling and support to overcome some barriers that interfere with the breastfeeding relationship.

SEPARATION

Separation of a mother from her child is likely to result in a range of emotions. Depending on the reason for the separation, the new mother may experience any emotion, from being mildly bothered (e.g., if she is going out for the evening) to feeling profound grief (e.g., when the infant is critically ill). Often, mothers will report breastfeeding "problems," but this is a misnomer; such "problems" may be manifestations of her inconvenience, frustration, feelings of inadequacy, or grief.

How greatly the separation affects breastfeeding depends on where in the lactation process the separation occurs, the frequency and duration of the separation, and whether the separation was planned or unplanned. If an infant has been breastfeeding vigorously for at least 1 month, lactation is likely to be well established and the mother usually has relatively little difficulty getting the infant back to the breast and producing enough milk to satisfy his needs when the two are reunited. Being separated before this time, however, is counterproductive to breastfeeding efforts, and it may be relatively difficult to achieve good latch-on and

adequate milk production after the separation. This interferes with the natural supply-and-demand principle; unless the mother is expressing milk, supply diminishes. During the first week, even a few days of separation between the mother and the term infant can result in breastfeeding attrition.[1] "Weaning" begins as soon as the infant has access to anything other than his mother's breasts. For the compromised infant who has never gone to the breast, this critical biologic and psychologic period is gone forever, and some barriers may arise, but unless the infant has a permanently disabling condition, initiation of breastfeeding is entirely possible at any time.

The frequency and duration of the separation, as well as the circumstances, can influence the breastfeeding experience. For example, the mother who wishes to attend her elementary school child's annual concert may be gone for only one feeding on one particular night. A woman who is hospitalized for a cholecystectomy will be unavailable for several consecutive feedings, but after a few days the separation ceases. Other times, the separation continues for many days and occurs on a fairly regular basis, for example, if the woman is employed. If the infant is hospitalized because of a critical illness, the separation may be for 24 hours a day and may continue for months. In all of these situations, the key is to identify the possible barriers to breastfeeding while separated so that helpful strategies can be initiated early on. Multiple problems and concerns arise regardless of the circumstances. These may include inconvenience, negative reactions from others, self-doubts, and keeping up a sufficient milk supply. These potential barriers, along with possible responses, are noted in Table 14-1.

Table **14-1**   Breastfeeding while Separated: Likely Barriers and Responses

Possible Barrier for Mother	Basis for Response
Unnecessary/Unwanted Separation Breastfeeding in public is not an acceptable cultural norm.	Women may feel forced to leave infants at home while they run errands, attend events, and so forth. Help them find ways to breastfeed discreetly.
Inconvenience Not having the infant at the breast is an inconvenience. The woman must express, collect, and store her milk. When carrying out these activities, she may find herself changing her clothing, hauling equipment, and struggling to find privacy.	Help the mother recognize that feeding the infant artificial milk imposes a different set of inconveniences, so she may find that breastfeeding is, in the long run, better for her as well as for her infant.
Negative Reactions from Others Well-meaning relatives, friends, or supervisors may challenge the woman's decision to breastfeed while she is separated from her infant.	Help the woman see that the decision to provide her own milk is a personal decision, driven by values. Give her an opportunity to talk about the reactions of others. Praise her for her choice to give the valuable gift of human milk, which cannot be duplicated in artificial milk. Remind her that is milk artificial not completely hassle-free.
Self-Doubts There are many moments when the woman herself questions, "Why am I doing this?" when artificial milk looks so simple, safe, and convenient.	Reinforce to the woman that only she can provide mother's milk, and that she is capable of doing so. Emphasize that artificial milk is not equivalent to human milk.
Keeping Up Milk Supply This is a primary concern for all mothers, and it is magnified when the infant is not at the breast or is at the breast only minimally.	General suggestions listed in Chapter 7 as well as some specific strategies listed later in this chapter help in establishing and maintaining a milk supply when mother is separated from her infant.

When mothers are separated from their infants, they may need to overcome some or all of the barriers noted here. The purpose of this chapter is to enable the nurse to provide education and support for mothers who must establish and maintain breastfeeding and lactation under both planned and unplanned separations.

Planned Separations

Planned separations are easiest to deal with from an emotional and logistic standpoint. The mother can take control of the situation and implement mechanisms to enhance rather than thwart her breastfeeding efforts. The two most common situations are going out and being employed.

"Going Out" Situations

When mothers say they are going out, this usually means that they plan to be away for a short interval of time and that the event happens irregularly or intermittently. Breastfeeding mothers can and should go out; otherwise, the myth that breastfeeding "ties you down" becomes a reality. Mothers who are going out for a short time—perhaps 2 or 3 hours to run errands, attend events, and so forth—have some simple options.

In many circumstances the mother can take the infant with her. If she is feeling torn between her need to get out and her need to be with her infant, encourage her to bring the infant to a movie theater for her first outing. She may be pleasantly surprised that she can comfortably breastfeed in a public place, and having the first experience in a darkened environment may help her gain the confidence to do it elsewhere.

If she needs to or chooses to be separated from her infant, she must consider the effect of the separation on the breastfeeding experience. The effect varies. For example, there is little effect for the mother who goes out to do errands for a few hours. She can leave her infant with a reliable caregiver and breastfeed just before leaving and just after returning home. This is unlikely to create a problem with breastfeeding.

The mother who is going out to a party may experience a more dramatic effect. The idea of going to a party begs the question of whether the mother intends to consume alcoholic beverages. Mature mothers are likely to consume only a small amount of alcohol, and this will not hurt the infant. (See Chapter 5 for a discussion of safe amounts.) Adolescent mothers sometimes blatantly report that they intend to get drunk. Lecturing about the hazards of alcohol is unlikely to result in a behavioral change. A better approach is to deal with the reality of the situation and help them avoid any harmful effects to the infant. In this case it is better for the mother to express and discard her milk at least until she is no longer feeling the influence of the alcohol.

Maternal Employment

Unquestionably, women can breastfeed after they have resumed employment if they wish. For nurses and other health care providers, the salient questions are related to how employment affects the intention to initiate and continue breastfeeding, how to help the woman develop a plan that fits her circumstances, and the unique problems that arise for the lactating woman who is employed.

Health care professionals often misinterpret employment statistics related to mothering and breastfeeding. They may erroneously presume that statistics show that more than half of the mothers in the United States are employed, but this interpretation is incorrect. The Bureau of Labor shows that more than half of women between the ages 16 and 65 who are available for employment (wish to

be/need to be employed) are actually employed.[2] The percentage of mothers, or even the percentage of women of childbearing age, who are actually employed is less clear.

Breastfeeding attrition can and does occur, however. Studies show that despite intentions to the contrary, once women actually return to the workplace, weaning happens as early as 2 or 3 months postpartum, even after adjusting for demographic variables.[3] Multiple factors, many of which are beyond the woman's control, including travel schedules, result in breastfeeding cessation, even though the woman had originally intended otherwise. Women in professional roles are likely to breastfeed longer than those in clerical positions, most likely because they have greater time flexibility and more control over their work environments.

The intention to breastfeed is also sometimes not clearly understood. The expectation to return to paid employment is not related to the woman's feeding decision.[4] However, planning to return to work before 6 to 8 weeks postpartum does reduce the likelihood that women will initiate breastfeeding.[5] Women in some occupations—for example, those who work on an assembly line—are less likely to choose breastfeeding.[6] Overall, however, the percentage of women who initiate breastfeeding is not substantially different whether they are employed or not.[7]

Continuation of breastfeeding is influenced by the mother's employment status. First, there is a direct relationship between the length of maternity leave and the time weaning[6,8]; the longer the maternity leave, the longer breastfeeding continues. Women who return to work before 6 weeks have more problems and wean earlier than they had intended.[9] Similarly, employed mothers change their minds after they give birth; they wean sooner than they had originally intended to.[10] Women are most likely to quit breastfeeding during the month that they go back to work.[11]

Continuation of breastfeeding for the employed mother is especially related to whether she is working full-time or part-time. Full-time employment is associated with earlier weaning,[12] but part-time employment is not.[13] Working 4 hours or fewer per day does not affect continuation of breastfeeding.[13] Mothers are more likely to continue breastfeeding for 1 year or more if they are working part-time.[14] Overall, maternal employment is not associated with decreased continuation.[3,15]

Employment does not preclude breastfeeding, but the separation requires some adjustments. The key to successful breastfeeding after returning to the workplace depends largely on the education and planning that occur in the prenatal period, in the immediate postnatal period, and before returning to work.

Prenatal Period. As with all mothers, breastfeeding education for the employed mother must begin during the prenatal period. During pregnancy, the focus should be on motivation and decision making, not the how-to of breastfeeding in the work setting.

Women may lack motivation because it seems inconvenient or simply unrealistic to breastfeed while holding a job. The woman may say, "I can't breastfeed because I want to [or need to] return to work," which is tantamount to saying, "It's too difficult for me to combine working with breastfeeding." To explore this further, acknowledge the conflict between work and mothering, and ask open-ended questions that facilitate a discussion about the woman's needs and values. A good response to this statement might be, "Being a mom and an employee can make some difficult demands on us. What do you think would be the hardest thing for you to deal with if you were both working and breastfeeding?" Suggesting ways to overcome

the barrier she identifies may motivate her to breastfeed.

Similarly, the woman's decision to breastfeed may be initially colored by misperceptions that breastfeeding is incompatible with employment.[16] Unlike the barriers discussed in the subsequent sections—barriers that are likely to occur—these misconceptions are usually based more on myth than on reality. She may rethink the breastfeeding decision if the situation is reframed.

Help the woman see that breastfeeding is a benefit to the beleaguered employee. Suckling or expressing her own milk is often less time consuming than purchasing, shelving, preparing, and storing artificial milk; cleaning bottles; and recycling containers. Furthermore, if she is working outside the home because of economic need, the cost of buying artificial milk and medications for a frequently sick infant may seriously gouge her net income. Remind her that breastfed infants have fewer ear infections, upper respiratory infections, and diarrhea—illnesses that are common causes of mothers losing time from work. The idea is to motivate the mother by highlighting what is in it for her. Table 14-2 shows verbatim quotes that the mother is likely to express and a basis for reframing the discussion.

Listening to the perceived barriers and reframing the basic concepts may help the woman choose breastfeeding. However, the woman's needs, goals, and choices—not the nurse's agenda—should drive her decision. An informed decision can be reached by helping the woman explore perceived barriers or

Table **14-2** Objections and Misconceptions about Breastfeeding while Employed

Possible Objection or Misconception	Reframing: Basis for Discussion
"Breastfeeding takes too long."	Breastfeeding may actually take less time.
"Breastfeeding is too much trouble."	Breastfeeding may be more convenient.
"I have a very demanding job."	Women who breastfeed have fewer absences from work than mothers who artificially feed.
"I have a very stressful job; I'll be too nervous to breastfeed."	Breastfeeding provides a connection with the baby and a time for relaxation after work.
"I have too many other things to do."	Money that would be spent on artificial milk could instead be used for household services. Artificial milk costs at least $1200 the first year.

conflicts and discussing options that may minimize or overcome real or perceived barriers.

Identifying Perceived Barriers. The expectant mother may be reluctant to choose breastfeeding because she feels the conflict between work responsibilities and mothering responsibilities and assumes that breastfeeding will intensify that conflict. However, *role conflict or role overload*—not breastfeeding per se—is usually the problem. In addition, although contemporary fathers are often willing to help, the mother is usually the primary caregiver. The woman will be more likely to choose breastfeeding if she can more fully grasp the salient issues.

Help the woman understand that returning to her place of employment will add to her workload and that she will frequently feel the push and pull between the demands on her time as an employee and the demands on her time as a mother. Breastfeeding does not necessarily reduce or intensify the difficulties of balancing motherhood and career responsibilities. These difficulties are magnified for the professional woman, whose employment responsibilities often continue after she leaves the office.

Pregnant mothers may worry about *logistic barriers* that may not actually exist postpartally; other barriers may indeed exist, but the mother may be able to plan for or modify the factors so that breastfeeding becomes a realistic option. For example, one potential problem is finding a caregiver who will support the mother's breastfeeding efforts. A caregiver who does not value the breastfeeding relationship or does not feed the infant in a way that maximizes the mother's efforts is a deterrent to successful breastfeeding. The pregnant woman needs to begin seeking a caregiver who values the breastfeeding relationship and understands the basic biologic and psychologic mechanics of supply and demand. It is helpful for the mother to provide the caregiver with a card that has specific, written instructions that support breastfeeding, as shown in Box 14-1.

Other problems are more related to the *work setting*. In general, problems are related to lack of administrative or peer support, lack of a room furnished with essential equipment, and lack of privacy.

Box 14-1 | **Mother's Instructions to Caregiver**

- Do not underfeed; human milk is easily and quickly digested; the baby will be hungry about every 2 or 3 hours.
- Do not microwave the milk. Put the container of milk in a basin of warm water to thaw.
- Hold the baby during feedings; do not prop the bottle.
- Do not overfeed when mother is expected within the hour; give enough milk to satisfy the baby until mother returns.

Women are likely to experience opposition in the workplace if supervisors or peers cannot see how breastfeeding benefits employee productivity or the company's bottom line. This potential barrier can be minimized with some advanced planning. Encourage the woman to be honest with her supervisor about her plans to breastfeed or express milk during the workday. Arm her with facts that show that doing so will improve her comfort (and hence concentration) during the workday and that breastfeeding is likely to result in fewer absences from work to care for a sick child.[17]

A historical and ongoing problem is lack of a room at the work site where the woman may express her milk; women have had to use the bathroom to express milk because it is often the only place where they can find privacy. This is unfortunate because the bathroom is a place for excretions, not secretions, such as human milk. Ideally, a readily accessible site for expressing milk would include comfortable furnishings, running water and a sink, a small table to hold the pump, another small table to hold related paraphernalia, and an electric pump. Even with a designated room for mothers, lack of privacy can be a problem if the door swings open to a busy corridor. If that is the case, the woman can have anxiety about an intrusion, which may inhibit her milk-ejection reflex. She may need help identifying items that minimize her exposure, such as portable screens, shawls, or other cover-ups.

Overcoming Perceived Barriers, Exploring Options. Even when the gravida recognizes the benefits of initiating breastfeeding, she may think that breastfeeding and being employed are all-or-nothing situations. Part-time breastfeeding is better than no breastfeeding, and part-time employment may be an option to full-time employment. The mother has several options in regard to two issues; the first relates to flexibility within the employment situation, and the second relates to flexibility within the breastfeeding relationship.

During the antepartum period, suggest that the woman set realistic goals within the limitations of her employment responsibilities. Help her sort through her options, including how long she can be on maternity leave and whether she can return on a part-time or flextime basis until gradually resuming full-time employment (if full-time employment is a goal). Suggest that she explore such options as job sharing or contracting with her supervisor to use phone, facsimile, and other telecommunications technology to complete work at home. Emphasize that any amount of breastfeeding is beneficial; initiating breastfeeding but discontinuing after returning to the workplace is not a failure. If the woman wishes to resume work full-time, recommend that she negotiate for a gradual return to a full-time position. Focus on breastfeeding as the best choice and a realistic option.

Part-time breastfeeding is a realistic option. Until the antepartum woman is motivated to breastfeed and sees it as a realistic option within her employment situation, efforts to preach the "how-to" of breastfeeding will fall on deaf ears. Several realistic options can be implemented postpartum but should be discussed as possible options during the antepartum period. These include the following:

- *Feed the infant at the breast on demand.* It is entirely possible for the mother to suckle the infant on demand during the workday. This option is ideal for the self-employed woman, but it can work for others, too. If the mother can reasonably travel from her workplace to the caregiver's location, or if the caregiver can bring the infant to her as often as needed, this option is highly feasible. It is less feasible for a woman who does not have flexible break times or does not work close to the caregiver, or

if her employer objects. The advantage of this option is that breastfeeding can continue with little difference between the stay-at-home situation and the back-to-work situation. This option, which avoids the upset of supply and demand that can occur with supplementation, helps the mother maintain an adequate milk supply. Continuation of exclusive breastfeeding for 6 months is most likely to occur when mothers do not supplement with formula before 4 weeks of age.[18] The disadvantage is that this option can result in unscheduled interruptions that may interfere with the mother's work responsibilities.

- *Express milk while separated from the infant.* Expressing milk during work hours is an option frequently chosen by mothers who work outside the home. This option is likely to be successful when the mother can express milk more or less on demand, and at times when the infant would normally be suckling. The advantage of this option is that the woman is more comfortable after expressing and therefore more able to concentrate on her work. Within this model, she has two other options: She may store and save the milk, or she may discard it. Most women prefer to save it, but some do not. One woman I worked with would stand over a sink and quickly hand express, letting the milk flow into the sink. She worked only part-time, boasted of a plentiful supply, and did not feel any particular need to save and store the milk.

- *Breastfeed only when with the infant.* This is a theme with distinct variations. Most frequently, it entails breastfeeding after work in patterns known as *bunch feeding* or *cluster feeding*. This means that the mother offers numerous feedings to the infant when she is present, in the evening and/or during the weekend. Another variation is reverse-cycle feeding, which entails sleeping with the infant and letting him suckle as often as he pleases during the night. This may be counterproductive for most employed mothers, however, because they may feel completely exhausted in the morning, and fatigue will affect their milk supply. For others, it may work fine.

Teaching everything about breastfeeding during the antepartum period is probably counterproductive. Women do generate a series of questions about the mechanics of expressing and saving milk, but one must wonder if they are asking for how-to instructions or for reassurance that breastfeeding is a realistic option. A general answer is probably better than a detailed discourse because principles of adult education suggest that adults are most likely to retain and use information that is time sensitive.[19] The focus should be on choosing breastfeeding. The woman is more likely to retain the how-to information when it is presented in the later postpartum period.

Immediate Postnatal Period. Unless the woman perceives the initial breastfeeding experience as pleasurable and satisfying, continuation of breastfeeding after returning to work is a moot point. During the immediate postpartum period, she needs to establish lactation and receive support for her choice to initiate and continue breastfeeding.

Presumably, the woman has already considered alternative ways to combine breastfeeding with working. If she made determinations earlier, however, she may have had a change of heart after the birth of her infant. Sometimes, a pregnant woman who is firmly determined to return full-time to the workplace makes a complete turnaround after the infant is born; she may decide to be a full-time mother instead. If this becomes the case, the woman may need help reevaluating the options so that she can confirm a strategy that will best fit her needs and goals.

Before Returning to Work. Before returning to employment, the woman should confirm plans to resume work on a full-time, part-time, or flextime basis. She must also continue to be motivated and receive support for her decision to continue breastfeeding. Motivation is likely to be the most important element in combining breastfeeding and employment. Motivation to continue breastfeeding after returning to work is most likely when early breastfeeding was satisfying and when the woman has adequate information and support for continuation (Table 14-3). Support must come from all factions: from family,

co-workers, employer, and the health care team. Such support should help the woman with the following tasks.

Coping with Problems of Separation. Separation is difficult regardless of whether the mother is lactating. The emotional responses of leaving the infant and the practical aspects of breastfeeding while being employed are not easy. Leaving her infant on the first day back at work is traumatic; the added responsibility of providing milk for the infant may seem like an insurmountable task. Returning on a Thursday or Friday is helpful[20]; a mother is most anxious during the first week back at work, and this allows her to look forward to a weekend that is only a day or two away.

Overcoming Others' Objections. The woman's efforts and motivation may erode with negative responses from others. Help her give up the idea of "converting" relatives, co-workers, or supervisors who are negative about breastfeeding. Rather, suggest that she enlist the support of a few colleagues at work or others who have successfully breastfed. Their encouragement and support will probably outweigh the negative messages given by the naysayers.

Mastering Activities That Promote Success. The woman needs to be well rehearsed and fairly skilled at expressing her milk before she returns to the work setting so that she can accomplish the task in as little time as possible. This is particularly important if she has a fixed and relatively short time for a break.

Expressing milk is a skill to be mastered; teach her this skill by using active learning techniques, which require a return demonstration. The woman should be encouraged to push herself to perform the skill a little faster each day so that she is maximally efficient by the time she returns to work. She should also be encouraged to set up as much of the equipment as possible before she starts work in the morning, if that is possible.

Activating a Transition Plan. Continuation of breastfeeding after returning to work is best accomplished when a transition plan has been developed and initiated before the first day back at work. The nurse has a critical role to play in helping

Table **14-3**   SUGGESTED TEACHING PLAN FOR EMPLOYED MOTHER

	Focus	Content/Activities
Prenatal	Motivate mother to *choose* breastfeeding	**I. Goals of care** 　A. Recognize benefits of breastfeeding for herself and her infant 　B. Recognize that breastfeeding and outside employment are not mutually exclusive **II. Nursing approach** 　A. Discuss barriers and facilitators 　1. How breastfeeding fits with personal and professional needs and values 　2. Perceived barriers to initiating and continuing breastfeeding while employed 　B. Focus on mother's needs, goals, and choices, not on nurse's agenda or values **III. Options** 　A. Explore possible options for continuing breastfeeding after returning to the workplace 　1. Breastfeeding is not necessarily an all-or-nothing endeavor after returning to work 　2. When, whether, and how much to return to work; discuss all possible alternatives 　B. Identify value of breastfeeding for employer
Birth to 4 weeks	Provide support for mother's choice to *initiate* breastfeeding and information to help her gain skills and confidence	**I. Goals of care (woman)** 　A. Achieve affective and psychomotor objectives to carry out effective breastfeeding 　B. Perceive initial breastfeeding experience as successful and enjoyable **II. Nursing approach** 　A. Focus on establishing breastfeeding; avoid the temptation to teach everything the woman ever needs to know about breastfeeding while working; focus on breastfeeding only 　B. Reinforce and praise choice to breastfeed; bolster confidence that breastfeeding is the right choice 　C. Focus on mother's needs, goals, and choices, not on nurse's agenda or values **III. Options** 　A. Reevaluate how or if to continue breastfeeding after returning to work 　B. Revisit expressing and saving as one possibility that is not an all-or-nothing alternative
After 1 month	Facilitate a practical plan to help mother continue breastfeeding in the employment setting	**I. Goals of care** 　A. Determine best option 　1. Whether, how much, and when to return to work 　2. Begin addressing pertinent points of transition plan 　B. Devise a plan that minimizes barriers and maximizes facilitators

Table **14-3** SUGGESTED TEACHING PLAN FOR EMPLOYED MOTHER—CONT'D

Focus	Content/Activities
	II. Nursing approach
	A. Focus on mother's needs, goals, and choices, not on nurse's agenda or values; complete success, by the mother's definition, may never happen, so praise efforts
	B. Discuss concerns (general; talk about impact, not how-to)
	1. Fatigue, role overload
	2. Separation, reluctance to leave infant
	3. Anxiety about caregivers or day care
	C. Identify potential barriers and possible solutions if woman wishes to maintain lactation after returning to the workplace
	1. Insufficient milk supply
	a. Rest—prioritize, and
	b. Allow infant to suckle as often as possible
	• Breastfeeding infant at midday is an option (mother commutes to place where infant is, or someone brings infant to her)
	• In contrast, some mothers do reverse cycle feeding
	• Lots of weekend breastfeeding
	• Strategies to increase milk supply (as described in Chapter 7)
	c. Express (mimic time infant is at breast)
	2. Lack of support from employer/co-workers/family/caregivers
	a. Talk to employer
	b. Talk to co-workers
	c. Caregivers—give practical directives (e.g., when to feed infant)
	3. Time to express milk in the work setting
	4. Difficulty getting infant to take bottle
	D. Suggest possible facilitators
	1. Join support group
	2. Introduce bottle no sooner than 1 month (rationale)
	3. Offer bottle once a week thereafter (rationale: builds parent's confidence that infant will do this) and leave infant—ideally ask someone other than mother to give bottle
	4. Start expressing milk at least 2 weeks ahead (rationale: builds supply and confidence)
	5. Develop an overabundant supply
	III. Options
	Implement transition plan as desired

the woman develop a transition plan that includes issues related to providing supplementation, expressing milk, leaving the infant, and developing an overabundant supply of milk.

When, How, and How Often to Offer Supplementation. Remind the mother that bottles are not the only alternative for delivering milk (see Chapter 16), but they are the most widely accepted among caregivers and may be offered to the infant before the mother returns to work. However, timing is critical. Giving a bottle before lactation is well established undermines breastfeeding efforts; waiting until 4 weeks is preferable[20] because lactation is established then (see Chapter 4). Use of formula in the first month is related to increased risk of weaning.[21] If the first bottle contains warm milk, the infant is more likely to accept it because it contains the sweet milk he is accustomed to. Furthermore, the bottle is more likely to be accepted when it is offered by someone other than the mother; if the infant smells milk in the mother's breasts and the bottle, he will prefer the breasts. Seeing her infant accept the bottle from someone else builds the mother's confidence that he will continue to do so in her absence.

Discourage waiting until 3 months to offer a bottle because the infant is likely to reject the bottle at this time.[22] By this developmental stage, an infant's sucking is more conscious than reflexive, and it may be difficult, if not impossible, to get him to accept the bottle. A cup, dropper, syringe, or another method other than an artificial nipple may be more helpful at this time.

Expressing Milk. Explore with the mother various options for expressing milk. Milk may be expressed by hand (hand expression) or by using a pump (manual, battery, or electric); these are discussed later in this chapter. The type of expression the employed mother uses is often a matter of personal preference and what meets the needs of her situation.

Encourage the mother to start expressing her milk at least 14 days before returning to work. This will accomplish two objectives: First, it will help her develop her own stockpile of frozen milk to be used in her absence; second, it will help minimize the problem of a dwindling supply, which frequently occurs as soon as the woman returns to work.

Leaving the Infant for a Period of Time. Suggest to the mother that she leave her infant with

a trusted caregiver for a brief period before returning to work. This does not necessarily need to be the person who will be the full-time caregiver after she returns to work. The purpose of this first outing is for the mother to have a feeling of confidence that the infant will be safe and content in her absence. Otherwise, her first day back at work may result in multiple panicked phone calls and little ability to concentrate on her work.

Developing an Overabundant Supply of Milk. Strongly encourage the mother to develop an overabundant supply of milk before returning to work. This accomplishes two things: Typically, the milk supply is reduced after the mother returns to work, so if this overabundant supply is reduced, it is likely that the mother will have an adequate amount later. The extra can be put in the freezer in case the infant needs it. Second, it gives the mother confidence that she has plenty of milk or that she can rely on the freezer supply if her own supply dwindles.

After Returning to Work. Several problems have been identified for the employed breastfeeding mother.[23] Few of these problems are specific to the employment situation; most may be experienced by other breastfeeding mothers, particularly those who are separated from their infants. The following common problems can be minimized through good counseling. Fatigue[23] is the most significant problem reported by employed mothers. It is likely to be related to role overload; talking with the woman about her needs, goals, and values will help her develop a routine that is workable for her and her family. Finding enough time to express milk at work can be a real challenge. This problem can be at least partially prevented if the mother masters the skill before returning to work so that she does not waste any time learning the skill on the job. Expressing milk at work can leave clothes looking soggy and disheveled. To minimize this problem, suggest that the woman choose printed designs and washable clothing and that she wear a camisole (to camouflage some of the leaking). Commercial devices for oversupply of milk (described in Chapter 12) are also helpful. Discourage dresses that zip up the back because they wrinkle when the woman is expressing.

Although most mothers worry that they have an insufficient supply of milk, the worry escalates for the working mother who does not have the continuous stimulation of her infant. The most important strategy is to develop an overabundant supply before returning to work. Suggest other strategies that have built-in success features specific to the working mother, including those found in Box 14-2.

The barriers to breastfeeding while employed are many and varied, but so are the potential solutions. The woman must be prepared to overcome the individual, interpersonal, and system problems that occur. A patient education program that focuses on motivation, generation of options, and anticipatory guidance will help the woman overcome many of these problems. The nurse needs to set goals and priorities in accordance with the timeline of the birth as shown in Box 14-3. Most women who successfully combine work and breastfeeding overwhelmingly agree that it is "worth it."[24]

Unique Problems of Employment. The aforementioned comments describe problems more related to the separation experience, rather than to the employment situation only. A few issues, however, seem to be unique to the employed mother. Finding time to express milk at work can be problematic. Similarly, poor staff coverage and insufficient break times figure into the limited time for expressing.[25] Finding quality day care, maintaining job performance, and juggling multiple roles are also concerns that arise for the employed woman.[26]

Legislation has somewhat helped women in the workplace. Links to updated lists of relevant legislation are provided in Appendix D.

Unplanned Separations

Sometimes, unplanned separations occur early in the newborn period. For example, a postpartum mother occasionally may be unable to put the infant to the breast because she is critically ill. The mother may be too weak, or even unconscious, and the nurse may need to be a true advocate for both establishing and maintaining the mother's wish to lactate. In this case the nurse will need to determine whether the woman intended to breastfeed and then proceed accordingly.

During the newborn period, however, separation usually occurs because the infant is ill. This is usually an unplanned event—most mothers expect a healthy infant who will be able to immediately go to the breast—but a plan to deal with the separation must quickly be developed and implemented. Breastfeeding efforts for ill newborns generally constitute a five-step process,[27] including initial education, initiation of nonnutritive time at the breast, progress toward nonnutritive sucking, progress toward nutritive sucking, and transition to breastfeeding. Expanding on that framework, the nurse's responsibility centers on initiating, continuing, and, if necessary, discontinuing breastfeeding efforts.

Initial Education and Maternal Care

No assumptions should be made about the mother's original decision regarding feeding method because this decision may be altered if a newborn is very sick or preterm. Mothers whose infants are

---

BOX 14-2 STRATEGIES FOR MAINTAINING MILK SUPPLY AFTER RETURNING TO THE WORK SETTING

- *Express milk.* Ideally, the working woman should express milk at the times when her infant would normally be hungry.
- *Breastfeed frequently.* Each weekend, the mother should put the infant to the breast very frequently. This will help her to have an overabundant supply each Monday, so if her supply dwindles during the week, she still has enough to satisfy the infant. Breastfeeding frequently during the after-work hours helps too.
- *Rest and relax.* Finding rest or relaxation might be very difficult for the woman who faces the pressures of both job and family. Using relaxation techniques during the times she expresses milk may be helpful (e.g., listening to soft music on a portable tape player). A picture of the infant or something that smells like the infant may also be helpful. Privacy in the workplace is essential to relaxation.

Many other strategies for increasing milk supply are discussed in Chapter 7.

$\mathscr{C}$LINICAL SCENARIO

Employed Mother, Reduced Milk Supply

Your colleague Pat calls and says that she is 5 weeks postpartum and returned to work 2 weeks ago. Now, she says, she thinks she does not have enough milk for her daughter. She is expressing her milk at work, saving it, and bringing it home, but during the day a caregiver provides artificial milk for the baby. The infant "takes it like a champ" but always seems dissatisfied after feeding at the breast. Furthermore, Pat says that she doesn't feel her breasts are very full.

How would you respond to Pat?

POSSIBLE STRATEGIES

First, it is safe to presume that Pat is dissatisfied with the situation as it is, or she would not be calling in the first place. However, it is important to get a clearer picture about what Pat's main objective is and what her life has been like. Since she delivered the newborn, she has taken off only a very short time from work. Some open-ended questions would be good for starters, for example:

"Well, you know, Pat, earlier this morning I was thinking that life gets pretty hairy in this hospital even on quiet days. I really can't imagine how it must be to face a pile of work that's been accumulating for 3 weeks while you're on maternity leave, and then trying to express your milk and take care of your daughter. Seems to me it might be stressful and fatiguing, and often moms don't have as much milk if they're tired or fatigued. Tell me a little about how your day goes, and when you breastfeed Jennifer, and how often you express your milk."

Pat will relate a story of feeding Jennifer when she rises, then getting ready for work and feeding her again just before she leaves. She gets to work around 8 AM; then uses a pump to express around 11:00. She expresses her milk again around 2:00 PM, then picks up Jennifer at the sitter's around 5:00, and sometimes she is not hungry when Pat arrives. She feeds her again around 7:00 and again before they go to bed, and her husband gives the baby a bottle at night. She says she feeds Jennifer about every 3 to 4 hours on the weekend.

Do not skip over the basics. Ask Pat how the feedings go with Jennifer. What signs are reassuring that milk transfer is actually happening? (See Chapter 7.)

Stop her when she says she is using a pump. Inquire what kind of pump she is using and how the session goes—is she able to relax and get plenty of milk? Ask open-ended and closed-ended questions to obtain more information. You will discover several points:

- Pat is using a pump that does not have optimal cycles or suction. Suggest that she rent a large-motor, self-cycling electric pump.
- She finds it difficult to let down to the pump. Suggest that she bring relaxation audio tapes to her office, use warm compresses, or look at a picture of Jennifer to help.
- She has not heard of cluster feedings. Point out that cluster feedings—feeding several times in a short period—may be especially helpful on the weekends.
- She has not identified sleeping with Jennifer as an option. Explore her feelings about night feedings and explain that breastfeeding at night may or may not help—it provides more stimulation to her breasts but may cause her to be more tired in the morning. Sleeping in close proximity to Jennifer (with Jennifer in bed with her mother or in the same room) helps mother and infant synchronize their sleep cycles, and mothers often report feeling more rested.
- Help her to revisit the possibility of part-time employment as an option.

OUTCOME

The most helpful strategy for Pat was finding ways to relax at work, increasing the frequency of breastfeeding after work and on the weekends, and using a more efficient pump at work. She was able to exclusively breastfeed Jennifer for several months, and partially breastfeed thereafter.

less than 33 weeks of gestation are less likely to pursue their initial decision to breastfeed.[28] Therefore the initial counseling session should have both an affective and a psychomotor focus.

Begin with an affective focus. Convey to the mother your awareness of her infant's condition, and give her an opportunity to talk about her feelings, anxieties, and questions. Open a dialogue

Box 14-3   GOALS FOR THE EMPLOYED BREASTFEEDING MOTHER

PRENATAL (NURSING FOCUS: INTENTIONS AND PERCEPTIONS)

- Choose to initiate breastfeeding.
- Identify perceived barriers and explore possible options for combining work and breastfeeding, including how and when to return to work. Ideally, devise a plan to return as late as possible.
- Seek caregiver who values breastfeeding relationship.
- Consider/explore strategies to deal with realities of breastfeeding after returning to work.

IMMEDIATE POSTNATAL (NURSING FOCUS: SUCCESSFUL INITIATION)

- Perceive initial breastfeeding experience as successful and enjoyable.
- Achieve affective and psychomotor objectives to carry out effective breastfeeding.
- Establish full milk supply.
- Establish strong support system.
- Consider/explore/confirm strategies to deal with realities of returning to work.

BEFORE RETURNING TO WORK (NURSING FOCUS: ANTICIPATING REALITIES OF THE CHALLENGE)

- Develop a clear plan to overcome logistic problems of separation, including plan for expressing milk in the work setting (time/location) if appropriate.
- Display confidence to overcome others' objections (legal right, short maternity leave, talk to employer about his or her advantages, talk to co-workers).
- Engage in activities that promote cognitive, affective, and psychomotor learning.
- Successfully implement a transition plan.

AFTER RETURNING TO WORK (NURSING FOCUS: OVERCOMING BARRIERS)

- Review preprinted "how-to" card.
- Identify specific problems encountered and seek appropriate help.
- Muster professional and peer support.

with her by using open-ended questions. For example, it might be appropriate to say, "Mrs. X., I see from the record that you planned to breastfeed Michael. It will probably be several weeks before he is big enough and strong enough to nurse at your breast, but in the meantime, his health could be improved by having your milk fed to him through his tube. Is that something you'd like more information about?"

If the mother decides to lactate for her infant, praise her choice and convey confidence in her ability to express her milk. The mother, who may think that only the doctors and hospital staff can care for her critically ill newborn, should be helped to realize that her milk is as important (or more important) to the infant's well-being or even survival as the technologic advances in the neonatal intensive care unit (NICU). Capitalize on the idea that only she can provide the most life-sustaining nutrients, the first "immunization" and the first "antibiotic." The greatest priority at the initial counseling session is to convey confidence in the woman's ability to provide the most important component of her infant's well-being.

Mothers need to hear a clear and consistent message that they are "doing a good job" with expressing their milk. Often, there is very little volume in the collection device, and this can be discouraging. To overcome this, downplay volume as an indicator of success and consider using a small syringe to hold the milk that is expressed; the volume looks like more when it is in a smaller container.

Later, teach the psychomotor skills involved in expressing. Expressing milk with an electric pump is the preferred method when the infant is very ill, and expression is expected to continue over many days or even months. Media, including videotapes and pamphlets, are helpful for reinforcement (see Appendix B), but there is no substitute for individualized help when the woman first learns. Return demonstrations are ideal because they promote active learning and therefore better knowledge retention.

The initial pumping session should not be delayed, although it often is. Almost half of mothers of low-birth-weight infants do not express milk until 24 hours after giving birth, and nearly one fourth delay past 96 hours.[29] This delay should be

✐ CLINICAL SCENARIO

Handicapped Mother, Preterm Newborn

The wait for the elevator was longer than usual, so I used the stairs. This was not my idea of how to start out a Monday morning, but I walked from the third floor to the eighth floor and found Jeanne, 23 weeks pregnant, in the intensive care unit (ICU). Not only was she in respiratory failure, she was legally blind, and very frightened for herself and her fetus. This had been a long-awaited pregnancy.

I don't remember why I was called for her case that morning—probably to assess her fetus's heart rate. What I remember much more distinctly is climbing and descending many, many flights of stairs between Jeanne's twenty-third and thirty-first week of gestation to respond to complex obstetric concerns. She went from the ICU to the medical unit to the high-risk antepartum unit to the psychiatric unit back to the high-risk antepartum unit to the labor floor and back again. Doctors told her she was risking her life for her fetus; she said she didn't care.

Jeanne finally had a cesarean delivery, and her newborn was admitted to the neonatal intensive care unit. We got her started expressing milk by electric pump within 6 hours of her delivery. This was no small task, because Jeanne could scarcely see what she was doing and she was fragile both physically and emotionally. However, she soon built a good milk supply. She had a slow recovery from her surgery and still suffered many respiratory difficulties.

Eventually, her infant was strong enough to suckle. Jeanne was delighted, and the feeding sessions went well. Jeanne relied completely on how it "felt" when the infant was at the breast. She never experienced sore nipples, and her infant made good weight gains.

Jeanne repeatedly said how important breastfeeding was for her—that she had waited so long to conceive and had had such a difficult pregnancy. She had multiple challenges to overcome for both herself and her infant, but she emphasized that breastfeeding was "the most wonderful, exhilarating experience." She continued exclusive breastfeeding for about 5 months and did not wean for some time thereafter.

---

avoided, primarily because the mother needs early stimulation but also because a delay in initiating pumping increases the bacterial count of the milk.[30] If the mother wishes to breastfeed, instruct her to initiate pumping within 6 hours after birth. There should be a clear, written standard of care that reflects this.

Documentation is essential for comprehensive care of the lactating woman and her newborn.[31] Often, the only thing that is noted on the medical record or Kardex is "patient pumping." This notation does not adequately describe the care required or given by the health care team. Documentation should include when mechanical expression began, when it was initiated, and how often it is being done; amounts obtained (this counts as output on a critically ill mother's intake-output record); the status of the woman's breasts (soft, filling, firm, engorged); and any problems with painful or damaged nipples. There should also be a clear message on the Kardex about what was taught and how much, if any, assistance the mother requires to express her milk.

After the initial counseling session, education and support should continue to reinforce the woman's choice to breastfeed and her efforts to pump. Discharge planning that begins early and a strong social support network are likely to improve breastfeeding efforts.[32]

Initiation of Nonnutritive Sucking

Nonnutritive time at the breast is nipple nuzzling and/or skin-to-skin contact without milk transfer. Nonnutritive time is often a precursor to breastfeeding and is usually used for ill or preterm newborns. For preterm infants, nonnutritive sucking often occurs within the context of *kangaroo mother care.*

Although many professionals use the term *skin-to-skin contact* interchangeably with *kangaroo care,* there is a technical difference. Kirsten and colleagues[33] define *kangaroo care* as "skin-to-skin contact between a mother and her low birth weight infant in a hospital setting" (p. 443). The term *Kangaroo Mother Care* (KMC) was adopted by the First International Workshop on Kangaroo Care.[34,35] The word *mother* was added to emphasize the importance of the mother and her milk. Kirsten and colleagues further specify that there are three essential components of KMC: positioning, feeding, and continuation of the practice after discharge while thriving on mother's milk only. Therefore, using this definition and the components as essential criteria, the skin-to-skin contact that occurs on a spontaneous and irregular basis among term infants, although desirable, is not the same as kangaroo mother care. One is an action; the other is a specific care intervention.

Kirsten and colleagues[33] cite multiple studies on animal subjects showing that separation results in stress behavior; this is common among mammals. This should help explain why when KMC is implemented, both the mother and the infant do well. KMC has multiple benefits (see Research Highlight in Chapter 10), and breastfeeding is only one of the known benefits, as shown in Box 14-4 (also see following Research Highlight box).

Progress Toward Nonnutritive Sucking

Nonnutritive sucking—sucking on an "empty" breast—is the next logical step. While having skin-to-skin contact with the mother, the infant can be encouraged to suckle; whether he obtains milk is not the goal. When infants are at this stage, they may have their mouth on the breast but not latch on or suckle; if they do, they may swallow once or twice, and they frequently fall asleep at the breast.[27] At this point, gastric feeding and maternal pumping continue, but the parents should be taught to observe for infant hunger cues. Nutritive sucking, or direct breastfeeding in which the infant both sucks and swallows, is the next step in the progression.

Progress Toward Nutritive Sucking

At some point the infant will be more able to successfully latch onto and suckle the breast. His skill

---

Box 14-4 Benefits of Kangaroo Care

Kirsten and colleagues[33] have cited evidence for the many benefits of kangaroo mother care.* These include the following:

- Better breastfeeding
  - Longer continuation of breastfeeding[36]
  - More stable milk production[37,38]
  - Greater number of feedings per day[39]
  - Increased confidence[40] competence in breastfeeding[41-43]
  - Greater likelihood of being discharged exclusively breastfeeding.[38,44]
- Physiologic stability
- Maternal confidence and bonding
- Decrease in infections, including necrotizing enterocolitis
- Reduction in costs

*Kirsten and colleagues[33] provided citations for each of these statements.

---

in suckling effectively is usually inconsistent in the beginning. When the infant does effectively coordinate suck-swallow-breathe, however, the first goal is to have one direct breastfeeding per day. The number of breastfeedings is then gradually increased until direct breastfeeding is achieved for all feedings. Although often not the case, ideally, this would occur before discharge.

Direct Breastfeeding; Nutritive Sucking

Delaying direct breastfeeding until the infant has attained a certain weight or gestational age is counterproductive. Furthermore, the infant should not be required to demonstrate successful bottle-feeding before he goes to the breast. Rather, when the infant can coordinate suck, swallow, and breathe, he is ready to start direct breastfeeding. Typically, this occurs as early as 30 weeks (corrected) age,* although it is possible for it to occur sooner or later.

How often the infant feeds depends on his circumstances. An infant who is at or near term but who did not have direct breastfeeding immediately after birth because of illness may feed on demand. Preterm infants are another case. Typically, orders

---

*Corrected age is gestational age at birth plus the number of weeks after birth.

RESEARCH HIGHLIGHT

Skin-to-Skin Effects on Milk Volume

Citation: Hurst NM, Valentine CJ, Renfro L et al. Skin-to-skin holding in the neonatal intensive care unit influences maternal milk volume. *J Perinatol* 1997;17:213-217.

PURPOSE

This study sought to evaluate the effects of skin-to-skin contact on maternal 24-hour milk volume in mothers of preterm infants.

DESIGN AND METHODS

This retrospective study involved 23 mothers (8 in experimental group and 15 in control group). Mothers began expressing within 48 hours using a hospital-grade electric breast pump every 3 hours for at least 15 minutes for a total of six sessions per day. The mean age of the infants was 27.7 weeks of gestation. The skin-to-skin contact began 8 to 26 days after birth (mean, 15 days after birth). The mothers pumped and the volume of milk was measured at 1 (baseline), 2, 3, and 4 weeks.

RESULTS

The average volume for the 24-hour period was 499 ml in the experimental group, compared with 218 ml in the control group. During 2 weeks, the study group had a strong linear increase in milk volume, in contrast to no substantial change in the control group. The number of mothers who quit pumping before discharge was similar in both the study group and the control group. However, of the 6 who dropped out of the control group, *all* had low milk volume (range, 90-360 ml/24 hr), and all expressed feelings of inadequacy that they were unable to provide 100% of their infant's milk.

CRITICAL COMMENT AND CLINICAL APPLICATION

Skin-to-skin contact has many physiologic and psychologic benefits, as documented in the literature over the last two decades. This simple intervention has no apparent disadvantage and costs nothing. The results of this study should be replicated with larger samples because it appears to help mothers of preterm infants attain milk volumes more similar to those found in term infants.

---

are written for preterm infants to feed about every 2 or 3 hours. Such a schedule works well at first because the infants are often in a semidrowsy state and need to be awakened for feedings. It is important, however, to observe and record when the infant starts to exhibit feeding cues. Ideally, the infant should move to cue-based rather than scheduled feedings before discharge.

Discontinuing Lactation, if Necessary

Sometimes a mother may say that she no longer wants to express milk for her compromised newborn. This is not at all uncommon. The nurse's reaction to this decision is critical. On one hand, there must not be a message that implies the nurse is indifferent or unwilling to help the mother suc-ceed with pumping. On the other hand, the woman's statement should not be interpreted as a final decision. When a mother says that she is unwilling to continue, respond with an acknowledgment of her feelings and decision, and an open-ended question about what drove the decision. One appropriate example might be, "Oh heavens. I was thinking that things were going very well with your pumping. I'm wondering if you have truly made a final decision, or if maybe you are having some difficulties and need more help and support from the staff and your family." In this way, if she has truly made up her mind, she can gracefully say, "No, I've really made up my mind." If, on the other hand, she is discouraged at the moment, she has the option to reveal what she thinks is not going well or what kind of support she needs. If she needs more help, provide it. If she has truly made up her mind, respond by reassuring her that revisiting her prior decision is okay and that you are still there to help her. Acknowledge that she is the best judge of her own feelings and capabilities and that you are confident that she is a good mother. Help her verbalize any feelings of failure, but focus on all of the strategies that she has used to succeed and reinforce the goodness of any amount of human milk that the infant has received. Optimize her interaction with the infant and teach her good bottle-feeding skills.

Sometimes a mother needs to discontinue her efforts to breastfeed because her infant dies. This is very traumatic, because the milk she has expressed for her infant was done in the hopes that he would survive. All of the physical feelings of nourishing an infant are still present in her breasts, but there is no infant in her arms. Some mothers want to donate their milk to other infants; this is best accomplished by contacting the Human Milk Banking Association of North America (HMBANA) (see Appendix A). Donating to a milk bank may make the bereaved mother feel as though she has at least helped another child. (Discourage any informal sharing of milk between individual mothers because this can be a liability issue.) Above all, praise the mother for her commitment to breastfeeding, empathize with her loss, and be present to her not as a breastfeeding expert but as a caring professional.

Meanwhile, the physical discomforts of overdistention are difficult. The woman may be tempted to use the pump to relieve her feeling of fullness, so it is important to explain that continued use of the pump will not help her to stop lactating. Instruct the woman to gradually wean herself from the pump by decreasing first the duration of pumping episodes and then the frequency. To relieve her feelings of fullness, suggest that she stand in the shower to allow the milk to escape, then use ice to reduce the congestion.

EXPRESSING HUMAN MILK

The word *expression* is often used to connote obtaining milk from the breasts using the hands.

Technically, however, the term *expression* means using one's hands or a pump to obtain the milk. Expressing is indicated for both maternal and infant reasons. Likely indications include (1) when the mother needs to stimulate her breasts to initiate or increase her supply, (2) when the infant is unable to adequately suckle at the breast and the mother needs more stimulation, and (3) when the infant is separated from the mother.

Women who are separated from their infants have many options. They can (1) express and discard their milk (sometimes called "pump and dump"); (2) express, collect, and store their milk; or (3) express their milk, discarding sometimes and saving other times. The option a woman chooses depends on the infant's needs and health status, her own time constraints, and the situation that is causing the separation. For example, a working mother may have a very short break and prefer to pump and dump her milk. The disadvantage of this, of course, is that her infant will probably need to receive artificial milk in her absence. Other women prefer to express their milk and feed it to their infants later. The obvious advantage is that the infant will reap the benefits of human milk, whether he is sick or well. Milk that has dripped from one breast while the infant feeds at the other, called *drip milk*, is lower in calories, may become contaminated, and should not be collected for later use.

There are two basic methods of expression: *hand expression* and *mechanical expression* (pumping). Both have advantages and disadvantages; ideally, lactating women are taught to use both methods.

Hand Expression

In this text the term *hand expression* is synonymous with *manual expression,* although some people use manual expression to mean using a manual pump as opposed to an electric or battery-operated one. Hand expression should be in every lactating woman's repertoire of skills. A woman may have inadvertently left her manual pump at her sister's house across town, or a power failure may render her electric pump useless, but hands are always readily available! Contrary to popular belief, hand expression is not necessarily time consuming; it is a skill that simply needs to be acquired. Once she has mastered it, the woman who hand expresses may be every bit as speedy obtaining milk as her pump-toting contemporaries.

Hand expression costs nothing and is a skill that can be mastered with only a little practice. A procedure for hand expression is found in Table 14-4. Mothers who are reluctant to try hand expression because previous attempts have been unsuccessful usually have had inadequate instruction. Two good strategies help overcome this. First, teach hand expression when success is most likely—when the woman is engorged or when the infant is feeding on the contralateral breast. She will quickly see the results of her efforts! Otherwise, suggest that the woman stand in a warm shower, leaning forward. Both the warmth and the force of gravity will aid in her efforts. Teach the woman to massage her breasts and hand express just before using a pump; doing so aids in milk ejection.[45] This is particularly important for mothers of preterm infants who are not suckling at the breast; massaging improves milk volume, presumably because it provides tactile stimulation[46] (see Research Highlight box).

If hand expression is not entirely successful, troubleshoot for the reason. The correct technique for hand expression is shown in Fig. 14-1. Typically, women fail to push inward toward the chest and place their fingers somewhere other than over the lactiferous sinuses. Check for these two problems.

Table 14-4 PROCEDURE FOR HAND EXPRESSION

Purpose/Rationale
Hand expression can be used whenever the mother needs to express milk from her breast. Milk expressed by hand has relatively few bacteria, and the procedure is easy to learn. Hand expression can be used in place of or in conjunction with a pump.

Equipment
- Warm compresses (towel or diaper wet with warm water and wrung out works well)
- Collection container (sterile or clean container, depending on age and health status of infant)
- Nursing funnel if available or preferred

Procedure	Rationale/Key Points
Instruct the mother to thoroughly wash her hands	Handwashing is the single most effective means of preventing infection
Apply warm compresses to the breast	Increases vascularity; this stimulation may result in milk-ejection reflex
Massage breast; in each quadrant, start with gentle tactile stimulation until fully massaging tissue; repeat in other quadrants	Tactile stimulation facilitates milk-ejection reflex
Place thumb and forefingers in direct opposition to each other (e.g., 12 o'clock and 6 o'clock), about 1 to 1½ inch behind the nipple	Note that 1 to 1½ inch behind the nipple may or may not be at the outer edge of the areola
Push straight against the chest wall (for large breasts, first lift and then push into chest wall)	Mimic peristaltic motion of the infant's tongue
Lean over and direct sprays of milk into container (or funnel, if preferred and available)	To save milk that sprays
Occasionally massage distal areas	To drain distal lobules
Repeat above sequences at different position (e.g., 9 o'clock and 3 o'clock)	All quadrants of breast should be drained
Store collected milk per hospital policy	To give to infant

Also, provide patient education media; several are listed in Appendix B. The pamphlet by Marmet and the videotape by Frantz are superb.

Hand expression works well in several situations. Suggest hand expression to soften an engorged nipple/areola complex before the infant latches on; it is much less complicated than teaching a woman to use a pump for only a few milliliters of milk. Reassure the mother of a preterm infant that hand expression is *safe* for her infant because it harbors relatively few bacteria[47,48,110] and because hand expression better retains appropriate sodium levels, which are important factors for preterm infants.[49] However, hand expression is less time *efficient,* partly because women can express from only one breast at a time. (They can use a pump on both breasts at the same time.) Hand expression can be used as an adjunct to pumping when the pump is unavailable or not working. As one expert notes, "Although hand expression is not used frequently in the United States, mothers should be taught the principles and be encouraged to practice the technique as a back-up strategy in the event that they are separated from their breast pump, the pump malfunctions, or there is an electrical or battery power failure."[50]

Pumping
Breast Pumps

Pumping can be used in place of or in addition to hand expression. Consumer education should be aimed at helping the mother both choose and use a pump. The following sections are intended to compare the different types of pumps available and to give tips for using the pump.

There are some fundamental differences between pumps and infants. The main difference lies in which type of pressure is primarily used—negative pressure or mechanical pressure (negative pressure is like a vacuum cleaner; mechanical pressure is like sweeping with a broom). At the breast, the infant obtains milk primarily through mechanical pressure (i.e., the oral musculature does the "work" of stripping milk from the lactiferous sinuses); negative pressure is used primarily to hold the nipple/areola in place. In contrast, a pump relies primarily on negative pressure, while having little, if any, mechanical pressure.

Similarities between the pump and the infant are desirable. No pump is ideal, but features that are important to consider include efficiency, comfort, convenience, sterility, and miscellaneous other factors. Features of the "ideal" pump are described in Box 14-5. Actually, the ideal pump is one that most closely mimics the action of the infant. Specific information describing the capabilities and limitations of nearly every pump currently on the market is available.[51,52]

Mothers often ask which pump is best. There is no easy answer to this question. Some pumps are better under a certain set of circumstances, or for a certain woman.[53] The nurse needs to assist the mother to choose a pump that offers the most advantages for her circumstances; what might work well for a mother who suckles a healthy infant may not work for a mother who has no stimulation from infant suckling. The two best questions to use in helping the mother determine what is best for her circumstances are as follows: (1) How frequently and for how long will she use the pump? and (2) How much time does she have to complete the pumping session? (This is probably a greater issue for the working mother.) Suggestions for pump use are shown in Table 14-5. Pumps can be described in terms of two general categories: manual and motor driven.

Manual Pumps. Manual pumps are those that are not automated in any way. There are three categories of manual pumps: bulb pumps, cylinder pumps, and trigger pumps. Bulb pumps are not efficient and have only a 5-ml collecting chamber that needs to be emptied frequently. More important, they harbor bacteria even when boiled. These pumps are inappropriate for mothers in any circumstance.[54] Trigger pumps create a vacuum by using the trigger handle, as seen in Fig. 14-2. Cylinder pumps consist of two cylinders, as shown in Fig. 14-3. The inner one fits inside of the outer one, and they create a vacuum when the mother pulls the outer cylinder down. The outer cylinder collects milk; later a nipple can be screwed on, and the outer cylinder doubles as a feeding device. Except for the gasket, which must

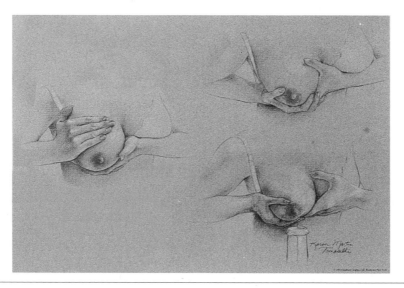

FIGURE **14-1** Hand massage *(left)* and expression *(right)*. *(Courtesy Karen Martin. Childbirth Graphics, Waco, TX.)*

RESEARCH HIGHLIGHT

Simultaneous Pumping with Massage Works Best

Citation: Jones E, Dimmock PW, Spencer SA. A randomised controlled trial to compare methods of milk expression after preterm delivery. *Arch Dis Child Fetal Neonatal Ed* 2001;85:F91-F95.

FOCUS

Jones and colleagues conducted a controlled trial "to compare sequential and simultaneous breast pumping on volume of milk expressed and its fat content." A secondary objective was to measure the effectiveness of breast massage on milk volume and fat content. Mothers who expressed at least five times per day before the beginning of the study were eligible to participate. The number of those who were eligible is not reported, but 52 mothers consented to participate in the study conducted in the United Kingdom.

Subjects were randomly assigned to sequential ("single") or simultaneous ("double") pumping groups. The groups were again divided according to gestation and parity. These six groups were studied for 4 consecutive days. Mothers were randomly assigned to massage on days 1 and 2, or on days 3 and 4. However, data from the first "massage day" was not analyzed in an attempt to give the mother an oppor-

tunity to master the massage technique. The breast massage was done with gentle, tactile rolling of the knuckles downward over the breasts. The pump was the electric Egnell Ameda Elite (United Kingdom). Flange inserts were used when appropriate to insure a snug fit of the flange in all cases. Mothers were instructed to pump at least 8 times during a 24-hour period.

Of the original 52, only 36 mothers completed the study; others withdrew for a variety of reasons, including death of the infant. Subjects had given birth to infants whose mean gestation was 29.97 weeks and whose mean weight was 1.5 kg. Contrary to instructions, mothers pumped for a mean of 5.2 times in a 24-hour period.

RESULTS

Simultaneous pumping was more effective than sequential pumping ($p < .01$), and massaging before pumping was more effective than nonmassage ($p < .01$) in terms of total milk volume obtained and total fat in grams ($p < .01$). As might be expected, fat concentration per expression was about the same, because with more fat and more volume, concentra-

be removed for cleaning, no part of the cylinder pump harbors bacteria, and all parts can be easily disassembled and cleaned. Popular brands include the Kaneson, Evenflo, Gerber, and Medela Manualectric.

Manual pumps typically have less suction power than automated pumps. The mother controls the number of "suck cycles" by the number of times she pulls the outer cylinder (of a cylinder pump) and the distance she pulls it. The amount of suction exerted increases, however, as the cylinder fills. Manual pumps do offer several advantages. They are less expensive than other types of pumps—usually less than $30. They are also lightweight and easily portable. They work well for a fully lactating mother with an abundant supply who occasionally needs a pump for a term, healthy infant who also suckles regularly. For example, mothers who are going out for the evening are good candidates for a hand pump. One study showed that among women who delivered earlier than 35 weeks, there was no difference in the volume of milk obtained, or the amount of milk fat obtained, between a manual pump with a soft flange and an electric pump with a hard flange. Whether these results can be

RESEARCH HIGHLIGHT—CONT'D

Simultaneous Pumping with Massage Works Best

tion is about the same. Total fat yield was significantly higher. Results of the questionnaire showed that scores rating the pump were about average; median was 4, with a range of 0 to 8, indicating that mothers were satisfied with comfort and efficiency of the pump. Similarly, the median score for massage was 4, with a range of 0 to 8. Interestingly, mothers who were assigned to massage on days 1 and 2 of the study were reluctant to give it up on days 3 and 4. Mothers who did simultaneous pumping reported greater satisfaction than mothers who did sequential pumping. Researchers also looked at the groups in terms of how long they continued breastfeeding. Two mothers had breast involution before the infants reached 37/40 weeks corrected age; both were in the sequential pumping group. However, 15 of the 36 mothers were fully breastfeeding or expressing when their infants reached 37/40 weeks corrected age, which reflected 5 to 13 weeks since giving birth.

STRENGTHS, LIMITATIONS OF THE STUDY

A notable strength of this study was the random assignment and the design that enabled investigators to look at massaging in addition to expressing. Another strength was that maternal self reports were considered in addition to objective measurements of volume and fat content. There were some limitations. First, it is unclear how many mothers were eligible for the study but did not agree to participate; similarly, only 36 of the original 52 completed the study. This may have created sampling bias. Second, no data on how many minutes the mothers pumped at each session or how many total minutes of pumping they achieved over the 24-hour period are available. Third, it was unclear on which day postpartum the woman actually entered the study.

CLINICAL APPLICATION

This study has significant clinical implications. First, the results of this study, which clearly showed that milk yield is greater when mothers of nonsuckling preterm infants pump simultaneously, are consistent with previous studies.[59,61] Breast massage, a practice that is frequently ignored or not encouraged, may provide the tactile stimulation that compensates for the lack of a suckling infant. This practice should be strongly encouraged when mothers are not suckling their infants.

Modified from Biancuzzo M. *Breastfeeding Outlook* 2001;2:6.

Box 14-5   The Ideal Breast Pump

EFFICIENCY

- Removes milk as rapidly as 75 ml/10 min with fat part of milk retained
- Container accommodates at least 4 oz (120 ml)
- Pump adapts and/or converts to infant nurser

COMFORT

Pressure Control

Amount and length of vacuum is selected by mother and automated to provide suction equivalent to healthy term infant. Infants apply suction for less than 1 second at a time with a mean *negative pressure* of –50 to –155 mm Hg at a rate of 42 to 60 times per minute. Initial suction would be at least –200 mm Hg to stimulate milk flow.

Pressure Exertion

Pressure exertion is –50 to –155 mm Hg, with a maximum of –240 mm Hg to stimulate milk flow.

Size and Shape of Flange ("Breast Cup")

A flange that fits properly surrounds the areola so that the nipple can move back and forth easily during pumping. The nipple should have room to be drawn out, and the flange should be adequate to transmit pressure or milking action to the collecting ampulae under the areola. The smaller the flange, the greater the pressure exerted directly on the mother's nipple tip. Conversely, the larger and deeper the flange, the greater the stimulation of the alveolar region of the breast, which may contribute to activation of the let-down reflex during pumping. Ideal range is:

    68-72 mm of the outer diameter
    35-40 mm depth of the flange

Flange Is Flexible

Flexibility is thought to provide more stimulation to lactiferous sinuses through areolar compression.

Cycling

A pump that cyles, rather than maintains constant negative pressure, is less likely to cause trauma to the nipple or areola.

CONVENIENCE

- Readily available; mother can purchase or rent at local drugstore or company can ship pump and/or accessories within 24 hours; spare parts easily available
- Easy to assemble, having as few parts as possible
- Portable
- Easy to handle
- Provides visual feedback to mother: can she see the amount of milk in the collecting chamber?
- Attaches to bottle with universal thread so that milk can be expressed directly into the container and capped with a tight-fitting lid

STERILITY/CLEANLINESS

- Sterility should be easily maintained with less than 1400 colonies/ml. This can be accomplished when all the parts of the pump that are in contact with the milk can be safely boiled or put into an electric dishwasher, or by using disposable parts.
- Avoid pumps that have several small nooks and crannies that are difficult to reach when cleaning.
- Closed systems do not allow ambient air into the milk, which could potentially introduce bacteria into the system, thereby reducing cross-contamination from one user to the other.

OTHER

- Pump should be appropriate to circumstances.
- Good instructions provided. The instructions should show importance of handwashing, how to assemble, how to sterilize, and how to use. Instructions should use simple language and give graphic or pictorial illustrations.
- Can mother afford this pump, or will insurance or Medicaid or WIC give assistance with the pump?

Table **14-5** PRIMARY USES OF AUTOMATED AND NONAUTOMATED PUMPS

	Pump Dependent	Part-Time Pumping	Occasional Use	Comments
Examples of Nonautomated Pumps				
Natural Mother Breast Pump Kit (Evenflo)			✓	Cylinder style
Happy Family (International Design)			✓	Cylinder style
Kaneson Comfort Plus (Omron)			✓	Cylinder style
Manual Breast Pump (Medela)			✓	Cylinder style
Manual Breast Pump (White River)			✓	Cylinder style
Ameda One-Hand Breast pump (Hollister)			✓	Handle style
Isis breast pump (Avent America)			✓	Handle style
Lupuco LTD			✓	Trigger style
Manual Breast Pump (Gerber)			✓	Trigger style
Examples of Automated Pumps				
MagMag Battery Pump (Omron)			✓	Single user; 5 cycles/min
Battery or Electric Breast Pump Kit (Gerber)			✓	Single user; 6 cycles/min
Nuture III (Bailey Medical)		✓	✓	Single user; 24 cycles/min
Miniclectric (Medela)		✓	✓	Single user; 30-38 cycles/min
Battery-electric breast pump (White River) #4850		✓		Single user
Pump-In-Style (Medela)		✓		Single user; 48 cycles/min
Ameda Purely Yours (Hollister)		✓		Single user; 30-60 cycles/min
Electric pump 8900 (White River)	✓	✓		Single user or multiuser; 20-30 cycles/min
Ameda Elite (Hollister)	✓	✓		Single user or multiuser; variable to 60 cycles/min
Ameda Lact-E (Hollister)	✓	✓		Single user or multiuser; 48 cycles/min
Lactina (Medela)	✓	✓		Single user or multiuser; 42-60 cycles/min
Lactina Plus (Medela)	✓	✓		Single user or multiuser; 42-60 cycles/min
Electric Pump 9600 (White River)	✓	✓		Single user or multiuser; 54-60 cycles/min
Ameda SMB (Hollister)	✓			Multiuser; 48 cycles/min
Classic 015 (Medela)	✓			Multiuser; 48 cycles/min
Electric Pump 9050 (White River)	✓			Multiuser; 60 cycles/min
Electric Pump 2000 (White River) wall unit	✓			Multiuser; 60 cycles/min

From Biancuzzo M. *J Obstet Gynecol Neonatal Nurs* 1999;28:417-426.
Note: This table is intended to provide examples of available products but is not intended to be comprehensive. The author and the publisher do not endorse products listed nor disparage those that are not listed.
Categories were assigned largely by input from the manufacturer's literature or representatives.

generalized to other brands or types of flanges is uncertain. Also, mothers who express milk only occasionally may have difficulty with their milk-ejection reflex, but this is not the fault of the pump.

Motor-Driven Pumps. Motor-driven pumps can be categorized as small motor, moderate-size motor, or large motor. They are either battery operated or electric. The size of the motor generally determines the suction power, cycles per minute, and suck/release. Small-motor pumps have limited suction power, and the suck/release interval is fairly long—about 10 to 20 per minute.

Battery-Operated Pumps. Generally, smaller or moderately sized motor-driven pumps are battery operated, as shown in Fig. 14-4. Battery-operated pumps are designed for use with a battery, but they may be equipped with a power

adapter. Battery-operated pumps vary tremendously from one brand to another—from those that exert little negative pressure and are very inefficient to those that are nearly as efficient as electric pumps—so it is difficult to categorize the advantages and disadvantages in terms of their efficiency. However, there are a few commonalties. Many battery-operated pumps convert or attach to a nurser, they are lightweight and clean, and cost less than $100. A possible disadvantage, however, is that the pump may be noisy, and a woman may hesitate to use it in a room where she does not want to be noticed. The batteries are fairly expensive and wear down quickly, so this may be a disadvantage for some mothers. A battery-operated pump is very appropriate for a fully lactating mother who needs the pump on a semi-regular basis and has a term, healthy infant who also suckles.

Electric Pumps. Hospital-grade, full-size electric pumps are the gold standard for pumps. Generally, the maternity floor has at least one that is wheeled from room to room, such as the one shown in Fig. 14-5, or wall-mounted units for individual patient rooms, as shown in Fig. 14-6. Hospital-grade pumps are most efficient because the motor—not the mother—applies the mechanical effort. Electric pumps usually yield a greater volume of fat than handheld pumps,[56] which is

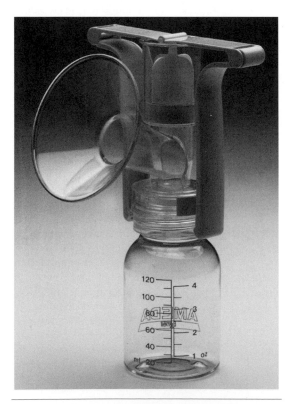

FIGURE **14-2** Hand-operated pump, trigger style. *(Courtesy Hollister Incorporated, distributor of Ameda Breastfeeding Products, Libertyville, Ill.)*

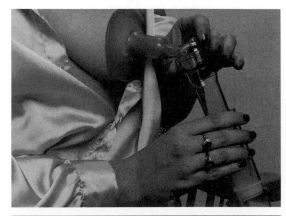

FIGURE **14-3** Hand-operated pump, cylinder style. *(Courtesy White River Concepts, Temecula, Calif.)*

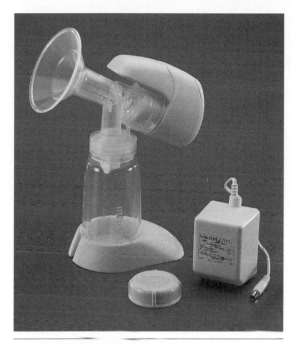

FIGURE **14-4** Battery-operated pump. *(Courtesy Medela, Inc., McHenry, Ill.)*

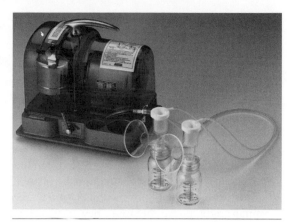

FIGURE **14-5** Electric pump, hospital grade. This pump can be placed on a bedside stand or a portable stand and wheeled from room to room. *(Courtesy Hollister Incorporated, distributor of Ameda Breastfeeding Products, Libertyville, Ill.)*

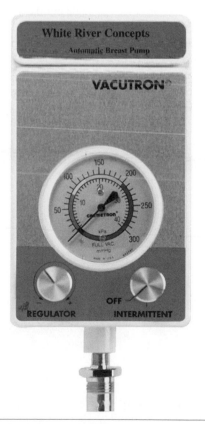

FIGURE **14-6** Electric pump, hospital grade, with wall mount. *(Courtesy White River Concepts, Temecula, Calif.)*

especially beneficial for critically ill infants. Currently, some smaller versions of hospital-grade pumps are nearly as efficient, such as that shown in Fig. 14-7. Some anecdotal reports have suggested that some smaller versions are less efficient, but research has not confirmed this.

Electric pumps and some battery-operated pumps can be fitted with a bilateral accessory kit; that is, there are two flanges, and the machine pumps both breasts at the same time (also called *double pumping*), as shown in Fig. 14-8. The electric pump with a double accessory kit appears to result in higher prolactin levels and thus higher volumes of milk than other methods of pumping,[57-59] and it takes less time than the single accessory kit.[60] Bilateral pumping has been shown to improve volume.[46,61]

A new electric device for expressing milk is made by Whittlestone (Fig. 14-9). It relies primarily on mechanical, pulsatile action, rather than the negative pressure that most pumps use. Because the product was not distributed until August of

2001, no studies that address its efficacy are published in peer-reviewed journals. However, computer and mathematical models have shown that theoretically, compression that mimics the peristaltic-like motion of the infant should yield greater milk flow.[62,63]

Although electric pumps have many advantages, a disadvantage is the cost for the accessory kit and related paraphernalia. The accessory kit for the mother costs from about $25 to $50, depending on whether she uses the unilateral or the bilateral kit. Most women would be unwilling to purchase a hospital-grade pump because they cost several hundred dollars. Most mothers can afford to rent a hospital-grade pump, however, and sometimes insurance will pay for the rental. Typically, renting for short term (3 months or less) costs about $2.50 per day; intermediate-term rentals (about 3 to 6 months) is about $1.50 to $2.00 per day; long-term rentals (more than 6 months) is about $1 per day. The local Women, Infants, and Children (WIC) office sometimes has pumps available for WIC participants, and most pump depots have a program available for mothers who would otherwise be unable to pay for using the pump. Socially disadvantaged women may have more difficulty renting these pumps, either because they cannot afford it or because a credit card is required by the rental facility.

If the infant is seriously compromised and not expected to suckle directly at the breast for some time, a hospital-grade pump is recommended. Mothers of infants who suckle frequently and vigorously, however, often want to avoid the expense of the electric pump when a manual pump or hand expression is adequate for the task.

How to Express Using a Pump

Show the mother how to operate the pump. To reinforce teaching, provide her with written instructions or videotapes specific to the particular pump she is using. Ideally, the mother should do a return demonstration.

There has been much controversy over whether it is necessary or advisable to discard the first 5 ml of milk expressed. The original rationale for this practice was to decrease the bacteria that accumulate just inside the nipple. Although Meier and Wilks[64] recommended this technique, no further evidence indicates that it is beneficial. HMBANA has determined that discarding the first 5 ml of milk is unnecessary if the milk is being given to the mother's own infant; donor milk is another matter.[54] Their recommendation came after a thorough analysis of the existing research. Furthermore, there is a practical side to this question: The mother of a preterm infant may have expressed only a few milliliters immediately after birth. Whatever benefit there may be to decreasing bacteria is outweighed by the value of the colostrum itself.[65]

There is no set rule for how long to express milk on each side. Mothers of well infants should express whenever the infant would usually be at the breast (and their breasts feel full). Expressing until a few minutes after the sprays diminish on one side and then switching to the other side (if using a single set-up) is effective.

If the infant cannot go to the breast for a prolonged period (i.e., the infant is unable to suckle), the goal is to achieve a minimum of 100 minutes of expressing per day during at least five

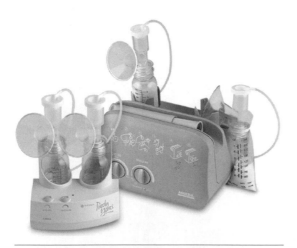

FIGURE 14-7 Electric pump, hospital grade, but lightweight for portability. Can be used with battery or built-in rechargeable battery. *(Courtesy Hollister Incorporated, distributor of Ameda Breastfeeding Products, Libertyville, Ill.)*

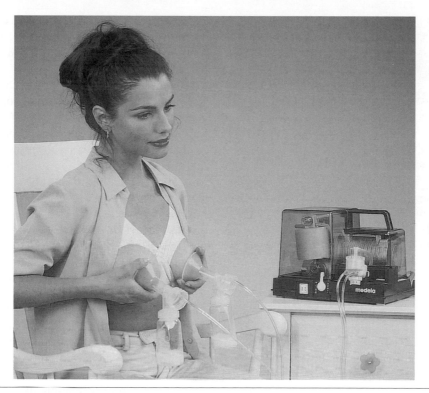

FIGURE **14-8** Woman expressing milk with a hospital-grade electric pump fitted with a double accessory kit. *(Courtesy Medela, Inc., McHenry, Ill.)*

sessions.[66] (In other words, the interval is less important than the minimum number of sessions and the total time achieved.) These guidelines represent the *minimum;* more stimulation is always better. Older studies have documented that mothers who delivered between 28 and 37 weeks of gestation can expect to pump about 342 ml ±229 ml per 24 hours.[67] The lower end of this range is considerably less than the amount produced by the fully lactating mother (i.e., the mother who has an infant suckling at the breast), who produces an average of nearly 700 ml per day during the first month,[68,69] but it is likely that nowadays, with better pumps and better support, women would be able to express more than these amounts.

Problems Expressing Milk

Even with the best pumps, mothers can and do encounter problems. The most common problems include the following.

Difficulty Letting Down to the Pump. Regardless of the type of pump used, some mothers may encounter problems. Help the mother to remember "great *results with* stimulation," or *gravity, relaxation, warmth,* and *stimulation.* The following are some ideas that may help to elicit the milk-ejection reflex:

- *Gravity:* Lean forward to maximize the use of gravity.
- *Warmth:* Apply warm compresses. Or start by leaning forward while using a hand pump in a warm shower.
- *Relaxation:* Dim the lights and play soft music. When mothers of low-birth-weight or very-low-birth-weight infants listened to a 20-minute audio tape designed to promote relaxation, they could pump up to 121% more than those who did not.[70] Also, keep a picture of the infant nearby. Have skin-to-skin contact as often as possible.

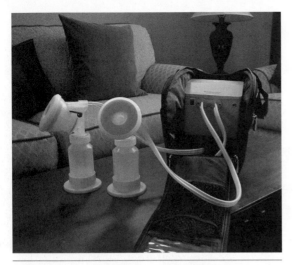

FIGURE **14-9** Breast expresser with double collection kit. (*Courtesy Whittlestone, Inc., Antioch, Calif.*)

- *Stimulation:* Gently hand massage; this aids in ejection of milk already stored in acini.[45] The hand massage is especially useful when the mother is pump dependent.[46]

Discouragement. Women who express their milk often have feelings of frustration, futility, and discouragement. Even with excellent education, the first few times expressing often do not go as well as mothers had hoped, and they often stop, citing "insufficient milk" and "too time consuming" as reasons for quitting.[32] It is important to realize that expressing is a skill to be mastered, and it may take four or five times before the woman is able to do it with relative ease and confidence. Furthermore, women may perceive a pump as messy and mechanical, with resulting feelings of embarrassment and awkwardness.[71]

These feelings can be frustrating and are best managed through sensitivity and anticipatory guidance. Help the woman overcome some of these feelings by doing the following: (1) Warn her ahead of time that she may obtain only drops the first few days after delivering, and anything more should be considered a bonus; (2) accentuate feelings of relaxation and confidence by presenting expression as easy and manageable; and (3) store milk in small containers, which will make it look like a greater volume.

Sore Breasts/Sore Nipples. Assuming that there is no direct breastfeeding, sore nipples or sore breasts are caused by improper use of the pump. A simple but commonly overlooked cause is that the mother has removed the pump from her breast with the suction still applied. If this is the case, instruct her to shut the suction off first, or to break the suction with her hand. A cracked nipple or an excoriated areola can also be caused by unrelieved or excessive negative pressure or improper positioning of the flange. Start problem solving by making sure that the mother is using the pump as directed. Turning the pressure volume up too high (or too soon) can be the root of the problem. Failing to center the flange over the nipple is another possibility. After the problem is corrected, it may take a few days for the soreness to disappear. In the meantime, recommend warmth, hand massage, and some hand expression before using the pump so that less negative pressure is needed to begin expressing. Sometimes a plugged duct occurs when a woman is pumping; this happens because one of the milk ducts is not being properly drained. A good remedy is massage and hand expression.

Insufficient Milk Supply. Insufficient milk supply can be a real problem among mothers who are expressing their milk, particularly if their infants are unable to accomplish vigorous, regular suckling. Several factors appear to be related to milk volume. First, stress can impede milk production and ejection, and this is especially true among mothers of preterm infants.[72,73] Sometimes, mothers must express milk for long periods when the infant is unable to suckle; this is a special challenge and requires some special management strategies.[74] Achieving an adequate milk volume requires some basic management strategies, such as those described in Chapter 7, and some specialized techniques for the pump-dependent mother. In general, mothers who are pump dependent generally need more stimulation to maintain supply.

COLLECTING AND COLLECTION DEVICES

Collecting and storing milk for well infants has few rules or regulations. Well newborns can better tolerate a loss of nutrients or the presence of pathogens. Collecting and storing milk for ill infants, however, requires more thought. Milk should be thought of as "white gold," and each drop should be saved and put in a container that preserves it best. Typically, mothers obtain very little milk the first day. A few tips are useful in preserving both the milk and the mother's positive perception:

- Hold a medicine cup to just beneath the nipple when removing the flange. This will help preserve those drops of colostrum or milk that would otherwise be lost when the flange is removed from the breast.
- Use a large-bore needle (18 gauge or larger) to get drops of milk out of the bottom of the collection container.
- Save colostrum into a 3- or 5-ml syringe. Seeing a syringe full or nearly full is much more encouraging to a mother than seeing a 4-oz bottle with only a tiny film on the bottom.

Choosing the Right Container

No one container is perfect for all circumstances; instead, a variety of containers have specific advantages and disadvantages for a particular set of circumstances. Ideally, the container would accommodate the amount of milk that the infant would consume at one feeding; would not harbor bacteria; and would preserve the protein, carbohydrate, fat, micronutrients, macronutrients, and other components of the milk.

Size

The container should hold about as much milk as the infant will consume at one feeding. Therefore this varies with the age and health of the infant. During the first few days after birth, the mother of a critically ill infant will want to start expressing milk but may burst into tears when she sees how little colostrum or milk she has obtained. She will be more encouraged by seeing her milk nearly filling a 3-ml syringe than seeing it lost in a 4-oz bottle.

Materials

Containers for human milk are made of either glass or plastic. Plastic containers can generally be categorized as polycarbonate, polystyrene, polypropylene, or polyethylene; a comparison is found in Table 14-6. Clear, hard plastic bottles—so clear they resemble glass—are made of *polycarbonate;* an example is the Evenflo bottle. Dull or cloudy hard plastic bottles are either *polystyrene* or *polypropylene.* An example of *polystyrene* is the Volu-feed bottle. Using these as containers for storage eliminates the need for pouring milk from another container to feed infants whose intake is less than 60 ml and must be precisely measured. An example of the *polypropylene* container is the storage bottle by Medela. The plastic bags specially designed for holding human milk are made out of *polyethylene.*

Some NICUs purchase 50-ml plastic centrifuge tubes for milk storage. The tubes are available from a number of manufacturers. Corning Co-Star manufactures several types; the most convenient ones for human milk storage are the polypropylene, presterilized centrifuge tubes with pointed bottoms that stand upright in a rack. These rigid, opaque tubes have tight-fitting lids, and their small size is convenient for storing small amounts of milk.

Any discussion of collection and collecting devices somewhat overlaps with a discussion about storage because collection and storage both affect the preservation of milk components and the pathogens that may enter the milk. Three factors influence preservation of milk components: container material, temperature, and time. (Temperature and time are addressed in the section on storage.)

Table **14-6**   COMPARISON OF MATERIALS USED FOR HUMAN MILK STORAGE CONTAINERS

Plastic	Looks Like	Examples	Comments
Polystyrene	Cloudy plastic	Volu-feed (Ross)	When frozen milk becomes heated, polymers are unstable. Very little research available to determine effects on milk.
Polypropylene	Milky white plastic	Accufeed (Wyeth)	Freezing in this container decreases lysozyme and lactoferrin.[75] Some loss (29%) of vitamin C, but this is not statistically significant.[76]
Polyethylene		Bags from Medela Bags from Ameda Bags from Platex	Bags can puncture easily; they are not designed for freezing. Not all are alike; some brands have nylon between the polyethylene layers, which prevents puncture and adherence. Loss of fat is significant. Does not interact with water- and fat-soluble nutrients such as vitamin A, zinc, iron, copper, sodium, and protein nitrogen. Up to 60% lower secretory IgA antibodies (specific for *E. coli* polysaccharides) are lost; these adhere to the polyethylene.[75]
Polycarbonate	Sturdy; clear plastic; looks just like glass	Cherubs bottle (Platex) Clear storage bottles by Evenflo Ameda Hygenikit	Very little research available to determine effects on milk. Can be autoclaved.
Glass	Clear	Pyrex	Leukocytes are destroyed when frozen milk is reheated because of the freezing/thawing, not the glass. Does not interact with water- and fat-soluble nutrients.[75,77] Storage results in adherence of cells with plastics and with glass, but more cells are "released" and become functional when milk is stored in glass.[75,78] Colostral cells do not adhere to glass.[77]

Modified from Biancuzzo M. *Comparison of materials used for human milk storage containers.* Conference Promoting Successful Breastfeeding for the Premature Neonate, Rochester, NY; 1992.

The effects of the container, temperature, and length of storage on milk components and potential pathogens are summarized in Table 14-7. Consider the advantages and disadvantages of glass and plastic, as well as the health of the infant who will be receiving the milk (i.e., a well infant will be less affected by less-than-optimal conditions than a sick infant will).

Even though there are distinct advantages and disadvantages, in general, milk may be safely stored in either glass[79] or hard plastic. Leukocytes stick to the glass, but their phagocytic ability is unaffected.[80] Investigators in India examined cells in terms of total cell count, the viability of cells, and whether they adhere to the container. Their findings showed that milk and colostrum stored in glass containers yielded a desirable percentage of free-living cells in suspension.[78]

Polyethylene. Commercial breast milk bags, shown in Fig. 14-10, are made primarily of polyethylene. The practical disadvantage of these containers is that they can leak or are punctured easily. A relatively simple solution is to double-bag or put the filled bags into a rigid container during storage. However, a more important disadvantage is that secretory IgA specific to *Escherichia coli* polysaccharides adheres to the polyethylene bags and is reduced by as much as 60%, so these bags are less than optimal for preterm infants.[75]

Polycarbonate. Studies have not investigated the effects of polycarbonate bottles, but there are no documented adverse effects from using them in clinical practice.

Polystyrene. Polystyrene was not designed to store human milk, and its effect on breast milk storage has not been studied.

How to Collect Milk

First, choose the type of container that best fits the needs of the situation, based on information in the previous section. The question may arise about whether the container needs to be sterile. "Clean" containers—those that have been through the dishwasher cycle or are deemed clean enough for food storage—are adequate for storing milk for term, healthy infants. The optimal practice is to store milk for hospitalized ill or preterm infants in sterilized containers.[54] Sometimes, however, the mother expresses her milk at home and suddenly discovers that she does not have a sterile container and instead uses a clean container. Unless there is some reason to suspect that this milk is contaminated, the milk should be given to the infant. (Furthermore, the flange, tubing, and other apparatus are only cleaned, but not steril-

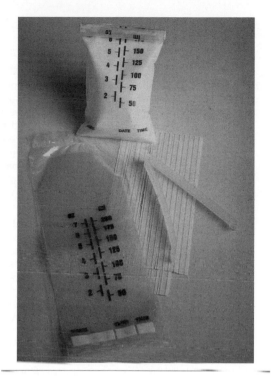

FIGURE **14-10** Plastic bags for storing milk.

ized, between pumping sessions.) After the infant is discharged from the hospital, clean containers are certainly adequate for storage of the mother's milk.

Whether milk can be "layered" depends on the circumstance. If the infant is hospitalized, avoid adding a layer of milk to a previously frozen sample.[54] The layering itself is not the problem; rather, opening and closing the container each time creates the possibility of contamination. If the infant is at home, however, this practice is probably acceptable, but teach the mother to chill the latest addition before she adds the fresh milk to the frozen sample. This reduces the possibility of bacterial growth.

The collected milk should be capped tightly; it should not be stored with only the nipple atop the container because this provides an entry for pathogens[100] and leads to oxidation of milk components, a deleterious effect. The container should be labeled with the infant's name and the date it

Table 14-7 EFFECTS OF CONTAINER TYPE, TEMPERATURE, AND TIME ON MILK COMPONENTS AND POTENTIAL PATHOGENS

		Comments/Findings	Source
Components of milk	Cellular components	Lymphocytes were decreased	48
	Fats	Losses occur with gavage feedings	81,82
		Altered when frozen or refrigerated, rather than fresh	83-85
		Decreases when stored in polyethylene bags	86
		Hospital-grade pump with automatic cycling best maintains the fat content of the milk	47,48,56,85,87
	Proteins		
	• Lactalbumin	No changes reported	
	• Lactoferrin	Decreases if milk is in polypropylene and glass	75
		Decreases across time	75
	• Lysozyme	Decreases if milk is in polyethylene bags	75
		Decreases across time	88
		Activity reduced 97% after boiling	89
		Decreases if milk is thawed in microwave	90
	• sIgA	Decreases with heat treatment	89
	• sIgA specific to E. coli	Decreases when milk is stored in polyethylene bags	75
		Decreases significantly when milk is thawed in microwave	90
	Carbohydrates	No changes reported	75
	Vitamins		
	• Fat soluble	Decreases if amount of fat decreases	
	• Water soluble	About 65% of vitamin C lost when milk is stored at excessive temperatures ($>37°$ C or $98.6°$ F)	85
		Vitamin C reduced; folacin, and vitamin B_6 significantly reduced when milk is pasteurized	76
	Minerals		
	• Major	No significant changes reported	
	• Micro	No significant changes reported	
Pathogens to milk	Bacterial	Storing beyond 4 hr at room temperature (approximately $22°$ C or $72°$ F) increases likelihood of bacterial contamination; study designs vary, and this is a conservative interpretation	86,91-95,112
		Milk stored in refrigerator beyond 48 hr can increase risk of bacterial growth	96,97
		Delaying milk expression after delivery of the infant has been associated with higher bacterial counts in early milk	30,66
		Most organisms in milk are normal flora	103, 111
	Viral	Cytomegalovirus and human immunodeficiency virus can be destroyed with pasteurization	98

was collected. (Stamping labels ahead of time with the patient's identifying data is a good way to label the containers.) Then milk should be used in the order it was collected. There is no need to routinely culture mother's own milk. (Donor milk is another matter; it is discussed in Chapter 15.)

Nurses often question whether human milk should be treated as a "body fluid" and therefore whether the usual precautionary measures should be observed when pouring or handling the milk. Human milk is not a bodily excretion—it is a secretion—and it is not listed by the Occupational Safety and Health Administration (OSHA) as a reason for gloving ("Occupational Exposure to Bloodborne Pathogens"; OSHA regulation 29 CFR 1910.1030). OSHA states: "Breast milk is not included in the standard's definition of other potentially infectious materials. Therefore contact with breast milk does not constitute occupational exposure, as defined by the standard. This determination was based on the Centers for Disease Control and Prevention's findings that human breast milk has not been implicated in the transmission of the human immunodeficiency virus (HIV) or the hepatitis B virus (HBV) to workers, although it has been implicated in perinatal transmission of HIV and the hepatitis surface antigen has been found in the milk of mothers infected with HBV. For this reason, gloves should be worn by health-care workers in situations where exposures to breast milk might be frequent, for example, in milk banking."[101] Some practical guidelines for the handling of human milk are listed in Box 14-6.

SAVING AND STORING

A simple checklist, intended for consumers, that describes the how-to of expressing, storing, using, and reheating mothers' milk is shown in Box 14-7. A more detailed list, outlined in Box 14-8, highlights key instruction points for implementing a teaching plan for mothers. These key points apply to all mothers regardless of their circumstances. Recommendations for expressing and storing human milk are different for term, healthy neonates than for those who are sick. A comparison is found in Table 14-8.

Box 14-6   Practical Recommendations for Handling Human Milk

- Refer to your agency's infection control manual to gain more information on "body fluids."
- Human milk is not on the OSHA list of "body fluids" that transmit HIV.
- Gloves are not *required* when in contact with women's nipples, but gloves are *recommended* to prevent the transmission of microorganisms from patient to patient.
- Gloves are not required when handling human milk (e.g., pouring human milk from one container to another).
- Washing hands, before and after patient contact, is the most important infection control action.

Mother's own milk that is saved or stored is often incorrectly referred to as *banked milk*. This term should be used only when referring to banked *donor* milk. In this chapter the focus is on storing the mother's own milk (i.e., the woman who saves and stores the milk for her own infant). In saving and storing mother's own milk, three things must be considered: (1) *temperature* (refrigerating, freezing), (2) *processing* (heat-treating or freezing the milk), and (3) *material* of the container. Table 14-7 highlights the effects of temperature, processing, and container material on milk components and possible pathogens. Storage of mother's own milk differs from that of other situations.[102]

Whereas the container material primarily affects the *components of milk*, as discussed previously, storage temperature and processing are more likely to affect *pathogens*. The titer of secretory IgA for *E. coli* polysaccharides occurs because it adheres to the side of some polyethylene bags; this is clinically important. Expert authors and clinicians have differing opinions about using these bags to store milk for compromised infants, but HMBANA strongly recommends not using them for this purpose.[54]

Bacterial contamination can happen at any time during expressing, collecting, or storing milk. And "there is no consensus about the bacteriological

Box 14-7 Guidelines for Consumer Education: Expressing, Collecting, Storing, Using, and Reheating Mothers' Milk

ASSEMBLING THE EQUIPMENT
- ❏ Washcloth, towels, or diapers.
- ❏ Clean or sterile plastic or glass container.
- ❏ Pump and related equipment (e.g., flange, tubing).

PREPARING THE BREASTS
- ❏ Wash hands.
- ❏ Put a washcloth, towel, or diaper under very warm running water until it is thoroughly soaked. Squeeze out water. Put on breast.
- ❏ Massage breasts: Begin with gentle finger stimulation and gradually increase to stroking and then massage.
- ❏ Begin at outer edges of each breast quadrant and move toward the nipple.
- ❏ Hand express a few drops, just to get the milk flowing.

PUMPING THE BREASTS
- ❏ Follow manufacturer's directions for operating pump.
- ❏ Follow manufacturer's directions for cleaning. For most, this involves simply cleaning the flange and tubing with soapy water and rinsing thoroughly after each use (or wash and rinse in electric dishwasher).

STORING IN REFRIGERATOR
- ❏ Put in refrigerator immediately.
- ❏ Refrigerator temperature should be ≤39° F (5.5° C).
- ❏ Use within 48-72 hours; otherwise transfer to freezer.
- ❏ Previously frozen breast milk may be refrigerated for up to 24 hours.

STORING IN FREEZER
- ❏ Use within 2-4 weeks if in freezer compartment in a refrigerator (old-fashioned type).
- ❏ Use within 3 months if in freezer section of refrigerator at less than −20° C (−4° F) (judge by hardness of ice cream).
- ❏ Use within 6 months if in deep freezer.

USING/THAWING/REWARMING
- ❏ Use oldest milk first.
- ❏ Thaw in refrigerator or in bowl of lukewarm water.
- ❏ Slower thaw is better.
- ❏ Warm in basin of water.

criteria for untreated human milk fed to babies in neonatal units."[91] However, most of the organisms that have been found in human milk are normal flora.[92,103]

Room Temperature

Whether or not milk may be stored at room temperature is largely dependent on the infant who is going to receive it. Early research suggested that mature milk can stand at room temperature for up to 6 hours[93,94] before being given to a well infant. This directive has been further refined; milk may stand at room temperature for up to 4 hours if the room temperature is no warmer than 25° C (77° F) or up to 24 hours if the room is no warmer than 15° C (59° F).[86] Colostrum may stand without likelihood of contamination for up to 24 hours,[94] presumably because of its large amount of antiinfective properties. Apart from concerns about pathogens, milk may also stand at room tempera-

ture of 15° to 25° C (59° to 77° F) without a decrease in the important digestive enzymes lipase and amylase.[104]

Refrigeration

There is no significant bacterial colonization of milk that has been stored in the refrigerator for up to 48 hours.[95] Milk should be stored at temperatures colder than 4° C (39° F)[105] for up to 24[86] to 48 hours,[106] because there is no significant bacterial colonization of milk before then.[95] Storage in glass containers at 4° C (39° F) for 48 hours causes a decrease in the viability of the cells and in macrophage and neutrophil concentration. Lymphocyte concentration is not affected.[107]

Freezing

Storing and feeding from the same bottle decreases contamination that can occur if the milk is poured

Box 14-8 PROVIDING HUMAN MILK FOR ALL INFANTS: KEY INSTRUCTION POINTS

GENERAL

- Once a day, rinse your breasts with water while bathing or showering. It is not necessary to wash breasts or nipples before each pumping session.
- Wash your hands well with soap and water each time before you express your milk. Use a nail brush to clean under fingernails once a day or if hands are especially soiled or nails especially long.

EXPRESSING MILK

- Use a method of expression that is appropriate to your circumstances.
- Express milk into a container.
- Thoroughly wash pump parts that are removable and those parts that have touched the milk. Use hot, soapy water and rinse well, place parts on a clean towel, cover them with another clean towel, and allow them to air dry. You may also dry them with a clean towel or put all of the removable parts through the dishwasher cycle.

COLLECTING

- Select a container that is appropriate, depending on how you express and your infant's circumstances.
- Package milk in amounts that the infant takes at one feeding.

- Pour the milk only once to decrease risk of contamination.
- Label the milk.

STORING

- Store the milk in the back of the refrigerator or the freezer, not in the door.
- Storage recommendations differ according to whether the infant is well or sick. See accompanying recommendations.
- Make sure the lid is solid, not a nipple with a hole.

TRANSPORTING

- Milk can be transported in an insulated bag or chest.

THAWING/REHEATING

- Place in the refrigerator for a day.
- For a quick thaw, hold the frozen milk container under cool or lukewarm running tap water or place it in a bowl of lukewarm water.
- Gently rotate the milk container. The cream part will be separated from the rest of the milk, and rotating the container mixes it together. Do not shake vigorously.
- Never microwave. Hot spots can develop because heating is uneven. Additionally, this reduces the levels of IgA, decreases the activity of lysozyme, and encourages growth of *E. coli.*

Developed from Human Milk Banking Association of North America. *Recommendations for collection, storage and handling of a mother's milk for her own infant in the hospital setting.* 3rd ed. Denver: HMBANA; 1999.

from the storage container to the feeding bottle, so this approach is commonly used. It is best to collect milk into hard-sided containers—either glass or plastic—instead of bags because they are not susceptible to puncturing. (Other disadvantages of plastic bags have been discussed earlier in the chapter.)

Freezing destroys living cells such as antimicrobial factors.[91] Therefore milk should be given fresh when possible. If it is not practical to provide fresh milk, milk may be safely stored in the freezer for different amounts of time, depending on the type of freezer. Milk can be safely stored in old-fashioned freezers—the type with the freezing compartment inside the refrigerator—for up to 1 month. Most households, however, have a separate freezing compartment above, below, or beside the refrigerator section. Milk can be safely stored in these freezers for up to 3 months. The freezer should be kept at approximately –20° C (–4° F) or cooler. Milk may be safely stored in deep freezers for up to 6 months. These times are optimal, but until a year has elapsed, it is better to use "outdated" human milk than artificial milk.

Temperature affects human milk, whether it is heat or cold. The important thing, however, is that the nutrients of the milk remain essentially unchanged; the bioactive factors are more altered by temperature and storage.[79]

Table 14-8 Providing Mother's Milk for Well or Sick Infants: A Comparison

		Term, Healthy Infant	Infant in Intensive Care Unit
Expressing	Initiation	• Put term, healthy newborn, not pump, to breast	• Pump early (within first 6 hr) to increase milk production and reduce bacteria
	Frequency	• Pump as often as the infant would breastfeed	• Pump at least 5 times per day
	Duration	• Pump until the sprays diminish and the breast feels soft (usually 10-15 min)	• Pump at least 100 min per 24 hr with an *electric* pump
	Method	• Short-term, does not matter	• Electric hospital-grade pump
Collecting	Routine screening for bacteria	• Not necessary	• Not necessary
	Discarding first few milliliters	• Not necessary	• Not necessary
	Containers	• Any clean container is acceptable	• Small, sterile containers; centrifuge containers (50 ml) work best for tiny infants; use glass or hard-sided plastic
	Labeling	• If infant is at home, label with date	• Label with date, time, infant's name, and nursery location, ID number, other pertinent identifying data
	Quantity	• Put into one container only what infant is likely to consume in one feeding; for infants less than 1 mo old this will be about 2-3 oz	• Put into one container only what infant is likely to consume in one feeding; the amount will vary dramatically from one infant to the other, depending on health status; consult with staff
	Layering	• Probably okay	• Not advised; bacterial contamination is more likely
Storing	Room temperature	• Store up to 4 hr	• Not advised
	Refrigerator <4° C (39° F)	• Store up to 72 hr	• Store up to 48 hr
	Freezer compartment <−20° C (−4° F)	• Store up to 3 mo	• Store up to 3 mo
	Deep freezer <−20° C (−4° F)	• Store up to 6 mo	• Store up to 3 mo; preferable to use outdated human milk rather than artificial milk
Transporting	Refrigerated milk	• In its own container	• In insulated box or chest
	Frozen milk	• In insulated box or chest, no ice	• In insulated box or chest, no ice
Delivery	Thawing	• Thaw in refrigerator for 24 hr; for quick thaw, run under lukewarm tap water	• Thaw in refrigerator for 24 hr; for quick thaw, run under tap water
	Pasteurizing	• Not recommended for mother's own milk	• Not recommended for mother's own milk
	Continuous gavage	• Does not apply	• Change tubing every 4 hr • Shorten feeding tube (see text)

Developed from Human Milk Banking Association of North America. *Recommendations for collection, storage and handling of a mother's milk for her own infant in the hospital setting.* 3rd ed. Denver: HMBANA; 1999.

TRANSPORTING

Milk may be transported in the collection container, and the container put into an insulated chest or carrying case; adding ice to frozen milk is unnecessary. On a long trip it may be wise to add commercially made ice packs to the container to transport refrigerated milk. The more expensive chests that hold six-packs work well, but disposable Styrofoam carriers are adequate.

THAWING AND REHEATING

It is always best to give the milk fresh.[91] If that is not possible, however, it should be frozen and thawed in amounts that the infant is likely to consume at one feeding. For tiny preterm newborns, this may be only a few milliliters. Healthy, term infants will consume less than 3 oz per feeding during the first month of life.

Milk can be thawed in one of two ways. The preferred method is to thaw it in the refrigerator overnight because secretory IgA is best preserved through this method.[108] If this is not possible, put the container of milk under lukewarm water (<44° to 49° C; 111° to 120° F) until it has thawed.[108]

Milk or other foods for infants should never be microwaved. Microwaving at high temperatures decreases the amount of antiinfective factors present, and the safety of microwaving at lower temperatures has not been established.[90] Case reports show that infants have been severely burned by food that has been "warmed" in the microwave.[109]

SUMMARY

Separation often can and does occur and may be either planned or unplanned. The key to an optimal experience for both the mother and her infant is to develop a plan to maintain lactation. For the well infant who is away from his mother intermittently, the mother can devise a plan well ahead of time to ensure that lactation continues as planned. For the compromised infant, the nurse often needs to initiate a plan to help the mother get started lactating and then, along with the mother, develop a more precise plan about how to express, save, store, transport, and collect her milk. Above all, the nurse must help the woman see that expressing and storing her milk is a realistic and rewarding alternative.

REFERENCES

1. Elander G, Lindberg T. Short mother-infant separation during first week of life influences the duration of breast-feeding. *Acta Paediatr Scand* 1984;73:237-240.
2. Bureau of Labor Statistics. Employment status of the civilian population by sex and age. May 3, 2002. Retrieved May 14, 2002, from http://www.bls.gov/news.release/empsit.t01.htm.
3. Gielen AC, Faden RR, O'Campo P et al. Maternal employment during the early postpartum period: effects on initiation and continuation of breast-feeding. *Pediatrics* 1991;87:298-305.
4. Littman H, Medendorp SV, Goldfarb J. The decision to breastfeed. The importance of father's approval. *Clin Pediatr Phila* 1994;33:214-219.
5. Noble S. Maternal employment and the initiation of breast-feeding. *Acta Paediatr* 2001;90:423-428.
6. Visness CM, Kennedy KI. Maternal employment and breast-feeding: findings from the 1988 National Maternal and Infant Health Survey. *Am J Public Health* 1997;87:945-950.
7. Ryan AS, Martinez GA. Breast-feeding and the working mother: a profile. *Pediatrics* 1989;83:524-531.
8. Hammer LD, Bryson S, Agras WS. Development of feeding practices during the first 5 years of life. *Arch Pediatr Adolesc Med* 1999;153:189-194.
9. Kearney MH, Cronenwett L. Breastfeeding and employment. *J Obstet Gynecol Neonatal Nurs* 1991;20:471-480.
10. Morse JM, Bottorff JL. Intending to breastfeed and work. *J Obstet Gynecol Neonatal Nurs* 1989;18:493-500.
11. Lindberg L. Trends in the relationship between breastfeeding and postpartum employment in the United States. *Soc Biol* 1996;43:191-202.
12. Novotny R, Hla MM, Kieffer EC et al. Breastfeeding duration in a multiethnic population in Hawaii. *Birth* 2000;27:91-96.
13. Fein SB, Roe B. The effect of work status on initiation and duration of breast-feeding. *Am J Public Health* 1998;88:1042-1046.
14. Bar-Yam NB. Workplace lactation support. Part II: working with the workplace. *J Hum Lact* 1998;14:321-325.
15. Corbett-Dick P, Bezek SK. Breastfeeding promotion for the employed mother. *J Pediatr Health Care* 1997;11:12-19.
16. McIntyre E, Hiller JE, Turnbull D. Determinants of infant feeding practices in a low socio-economic area: identifying environmental barriers to breastfeeding. *Aust NZ J Public Health* 1999;23:207-209.
17. Cohen R, Mrtek MB, Mrtek RG. Comparison of maternal absenteeism and infant illness rates among breast-feeding

and formula-feeding women in two corporations. *Am J Health Promot* 1995;10:148-153.

18. Valdes V, Pugin E, Schooley J et al. Clinical support can make the difference in exclusive breastfeeding success among working women. *J Trop Pediatr* 2000;46:149-154.

19. Knowles M. *The modern practice of adult education.* New York: Associated Press; 1980.

20. Meek JY. Breastfeeding in the workplace. *Pediatr Clin North Am* 2001;48:461-474.

21. Vogel A, Hutchison BL, Mitchell EA. Factors associated with the duration of breastfeeding. *Acta Paediatr* 1999;88:1320-1326.

22. Frederick IB, Auerbach KG. Maternal-infant separation and breast-feeding. The return to work or school. *J Reprod Med* 1985;30:523-526.

23. Auerbach KG. Employed breastfeeding mothers: problems they encounter. *Birth* 1984;11:17-20.

24. Hills-Bonczyk SG, Avery MD, Savik K et al. Women's experiences with combining breast-feeding and employment. *J Nurse Midwifery* 1993;38:257-266.

25. Janke JR. The incidence, benefits and variables associated with breastfeeding: implications for practice. *Nurse Pract* 1993;18:22-23, 28, 31-32.

26. Gates DM, O'Neill NJ. Promoting maternal-child wellness in the workplace. *AAOHN J* 1990;38:258-263.

27. Bell EH, Geyer J, Jones L. A structured intervention improves breastfeeding success for ill or preterm infants. *MCN Am J Matern Child Nurs* 1995;20:309-314.

28. Hunkeler B, Aebi C, Minder CE et al. Incidence and duration of breast-feeding of ill newborns. *J Pediatr Gastroenterol Nutr* 1994;18:37-40.

29. Hill PD, Brown LP, Harker TL. Initiation and frequency of breast expression in breastfeeding mothers of LBW and VLBW infants. *Nurs Res* 1995;44:352-355.

30. Asquith MT, Pedrotti PW, Harrod JR et al. The bacterial content of breast milk after the early initiation of expression using a standard technique. *J Pediatr Gastroenterol Nutr* 1984;3:104-107.

31. Baker BJ, Rasmussen TW. Organizing and documenting lactation support of NICU families. *J Obstet Gynecol Neonatal Nurs* 1997;26:515-521.

32. Forte A, Mayberry LJ, Ferketich S. Breast milk collection and storage practices among mothers of hospitalized neonates. *J Perinatol* 1987;7:35-39.

33. Kirsten GF, Bergman NJ, Hann FM. Kangaroo mother care in the nursery. *Pediatr Clin North Am* 2001;48:443-452.

34. Cattaneo A, Davanzo R, Bergman N et al. Kangaroo mother care in low-income countries. International Network in Kangaroo Mother Care. *J Trop Pediatr* 1998 44:279-282.

35. Cattaneo A, Davanzo R, Uxa F et al. Recommendations for the implementation of kangaroo mother care for low birth-weight infants. International Network on Kangaroo Mother Care. *Acta Paediatr* 1998;87:440-445.

36. Whitelaw A, Heisterkamp G, Sleath K et al. Skin to skin contact for very low birthweight infants and their mothers. *Arch Dis Child* 1988;63:1377-1381.

37. Bier JA, Ferguson AE, Morales Y et al. Comparison of skin-to-skin contact with standard contact in low-birth-weight infants who are breast-fed. *Arch Pediatr Adolesc Med* 1996;150:1265-1269.

38. Hurst NM, Valentine CJ, Renfro L et al. Skin-to-skin holding in the neonatal intensive care unit influences maternal milk volume. *J Perinatol* 1997;17:213-217.

39. Syfrett EB, Anderson GC, Behnken M. Early and virtually continuous kangaroo care for lower risk preterm infants: effect on temperature, breastfeeding, supplementation, and weight. In *Proceedings of the Biennial Conference on the Council of Nurse Researchers, American Nurses Association.* Washington DC: American Nurses Association; 1993.

40. Anderson GC. Current knowledge about skin-to-skin (kangaroo) care for preterm infants. *J Perinatol* 1991;11:216-226.

41. Durand RHS, LaRock S. The effect of skin-to-skin breast-feeding in the immediate recovery period on newborn thermoregulation and blood glucose values. *Neonatal Intensive Care* 1997;23:23-29.

42. Koepke JE, Bigelow AE. Observations of newborn suckling behavior. *Infant Behavior and Development* 1997;20:93-98.

43. Widstrom AM, Marchini G, Matthiesen AS et al. Nonnutritive sucking in tube-fed preterm infants: effects on gastric motility and gastric contents of somatostatin. *J Pediatr Gastroenterol Nutr* 1988;7:517-523.

44. Hann M, Malan A, Kronson M et al. Kangaroo mother care. *S Afr Med J* 1999;89:37-39.

45. Yokoyama Y, Ueda T, Irahara M et al. Releases of oxytocin and prolactin during breast massage and suckling in puerperal women. *Eur J Obstet Gynecol Reprod Biol* 1994;53:17-20.

46. Jones E, Dimmock PW, Spencer SA. A randomised controlled trial to compare methods of milk expression after preterm delivery. *Arch Dis Child Fetal Neonatal Ed* 2001;85:F91-F95.

47. Tyson JE, Edwards WH, Rosenfeld AM et al. Collection methods and contamination of bank milk. *Arch Dis Child* 1982;57:396-398.

48. Liebhaber M, Lewiston NJ, Asquith MT et al. Comparison of bacterial contamination with two methods of human milk collection. *J Pediatr* 1978;92:236-237.

49. Lang S, Lawrence CJ, Orme RL. Sodium in hand and pump expressed human breast milk. *Early Hum Dev* 1994;38:131-138.

50. Bocar DL. Combining breastfeeding and employment: increasing success. *J Perinat Neonatal Nurs* 1997;11:23-43.

51. Frantz K. *Breastfeeding product guide 1994.* Los Angeles: Geddes Productions; 1994.

52. Frantz K. *Breastfeeding products guide supplement.* Los Angeles: Geddes Productions; 1999.

53. Biancuzzo M. Selecting pumps for breastfeeding mothers. *J Obstet Gynecol Neonatal Nurs* 1999;28:417-426.

54. Arnold LDW, editor. *Recommendations for collection, storage, and handling of a mother's milk for her own infant in the hospital setting.* 3rd ed. Denver: Human Milk Banking Association of North America; 1999.

55. Fewtrell MS, Lucas P, Collier S et al. Randomized trial comparing the efficacy of a novel manual breast pump with a standard electric breast pump in mothers who delivered preterm infants. *Pediatrics* 2001;107:1291-1297.

56. Green D, Moye L, Schreiner RL et al. The relative efficacy of four methods of human milk expression. *Early Hum Dev* 1982;6:153-159.

57. Zinaman MJ, Hughes V, Queenan JT et al. Acute prolactin and oxytocin responses and milk yield to infant suckling and artificial methods of expression in lactating women. *Pediatrics* 1992;89:437-440.

58. Auerbach KG. Sequential and simultaneous breast pumping: a comparison. *Int J Nurs Stud* 1990;27:257-265.

59. Hill PD, Aldag JC, Chatterton RT. The effect of sequential and simultaneous breast pumping on milk volume and prolactin levels: a pilot study. *J Hum Lact* 1996;12:193-199.

60. Groh-Wargo S, Toth A, Mahoney K et al. The utility of a bilateral breast pumping system for mothers of premature infants. *Neonatal Netw* 1995;14:31-36.

61. Hill PD, Aldag JC, Chatterton RT. Effects of pumping style on milk production in mothers of non-nursing preterm infants. *J Hum Lact* 1999;15:209-216.

62. Zoppou C, Barry SI, Mercer GN. Comparing breastfeeding and breast pumps using a computer model. *J Hum Lact* 1997;13:195-202.

63. Zoppou C, Barry SI, Mercer GN. Dynamics of human milk extraction: a comparative study of breast feeding and breast pumping. *Bull Math Biol* 1997;59:953-973.

64. Meier P, Wilks S. The bacteria in expressed mothers' milk. *MCN Am J Matern Child Nurs* 1987;12:420-423.

65. Carroll L, Osman M, Davies DP. Does discarding the first few millilitres of breast milk improve the bacteriological quality of bank breast milk? *Arch Dis Child* 1980;55:898-899.

66. Hopkinson JM, Schanler RJ, Garza C. Milk production by mothers of premature infants. *Pediatrics* 1988;81:815-820.

67. DeCarvalho M, Anderson DM, Giangreco A et al. Frequency of milk expression and milk production by mothers of nonnursing premature neonates. *Am J Dis Child* 1985;139:483-485.

68. Lonnerdal B, Forsum E, Hambraeus L. A longitudinal study of the protein, nitrogen, and lactose contents of human milk from Swedish well-nourished mothers. *Am J Clin Nutr* 1976;29:1127-1133.

69. DeCarvalho M, Robertson S, Merkatz R et al. Milk intake and frequency of feeding in breast fed infants. *Early Hum Dev* 1982;7:155-163.

70. Feher SD, Berger LR, Johnson JD et al. Increasing breast milk production for premature infants with a relaxation/imagery audiotape. *Pediatrics* 1989;83:57-60.

71. Morse JM, Bottorff JL. The emotional experience of breast expression. *J Nurse Midwifery* 1988;33:165-170.

72. Chatterton RT Jr, Hill PD, Aldag JC et al. Relation of plasma oxytocin and prolactin concentrations to milk production in mothers of preterm infants: influence of stress. *J Clin Endocrinol Metab* 2000;85:3661-3668.

73. Lau C. Effects of stress on lactation. *Pediatr Clin North Am* 2001;48:221-234.

74. Stockdale HJ. Long-term expressing of breastmilk. *Breastfeed Rev* 2000;8:19-22.

75. Goldblum RM, Garza C, Johnson C et al. Effects of container upon immunologic factors in mature milk. *Nutr Res* 1981;1:449-459.

76. VanZoeren-Grobben D, Schrijver J, Van den Berg H et al. Human milk vitamin content after pasteurisation, storage, or tube feeding. *Arch Dis Child* 1987;62:161-165.

77. Garza C, Butte NF. Energy concentration of human milk estimated from 24-h pools and various abbreviated sampling schemes. *J Pediatr Gastroenterol Nutr* 1986;5:943-948.

78. Williamson MT, Murti PK. Effects of storage, time, temperature, and composition of containers on biologic components of human milk. *J Hum Lact* 1996;12:31-35.

79. Lawrence RA. Storage of human milk and the influence of procedures on immunological components of human milk. *Acta Paediatr Suppl* 1999;88:14-18.

80. Paxson CL Jr, Cress CC. Survival of human milk leukocytes. *J Pediatr* 1979;94:61-64.

81. Mehta NR, Hamosh M, Bitman J et al. Adherence of medium-chain fatty acids to feeding tubes during gavage feeding of human milk fortified with medium-chain triglycerides. *J Pediatr* 1988;112:474-476.

82. Stocks RJ, Davies DP, Allen F et al. Loss of breast milk nutrients during tube feeding. *Arch Dis Child* 1985;60:164-166.

83. Bitman J, Wood DL, Mehta NR et al. Lipolysis of triglycerides of human milk during storage at low temperatures: a note of caution. *J Pediatr Gastroenterol Nutr* 1983;2:521-524.

84. Friend BA, Shahani KM, Long CA et al. The effect of processing and storage on key enzymes, B vitamins, and lipids of mature human milk. I. Evaluation of fresh samples and effects of freezing and frozen storage. *Pediatr Res* 1983;17:61-64.

85. Garza C, Johnson CA, Harrist R et al. Effects of methods of collection and storage on nutrients in human milk. *Early Hum Dev* 1982;6:295-303.

86. Hamosh M, Ellis LA, Pollock DR et al. Breastfeeding and the working mother: effect of time and temperature of short-term storage on proteolysis, lipolysis, and bacterial growth in milk. *Pediatrics* 1996;97:492-498.

87. Minder W, Roten H, Zurbrugg RP et al. Quality of breast milk: its control and preservation. *Helv Paediatr Acta* 1982;37:115-137.

88. Garza C, Nichols BL. Studies of human milk relevant to milk banking. *J Am Coll Nutr* 1984;3:123-129.

89. Welsh JK, May JT. Anti-infective properties of breast milk. *J Pediatr* 1979;94:1-9.

90. Quan R, Yang C, Rubinstein S et al. Effects of microwave radiation on anti-infective factors in human milk. *Pediatrics* 1992;89:667-669.

91. Pardou A, Serruys E, Mascart Lemone F et al. Human milk banking: influence of storage processes and of bacterial contamination on some milk constituents. *Biol Neonate* 1994;65:302-309.

92. Sosa R, Barness L. Bacterial growth in refrigerated human milk. *Am J Dis Child* 1987;141:111-112.

93. Nwankwo MU, Offor E, Okolo AA et al. Bacterial growth in expressed breast-milk. *Ann Trop Paediatr* 1988;8:92-95.

94. Pittard WR, Anderson DM, Cerutti ER et al. Bacteriostatic qualities of human milk. *J Pediatrics* 1985;107:240-243.

95. Larson E, Zuill R, Zier V et al. Storage of human breast milk. *Infect Control* 1984;5:127-130.

96. Berkow SE, Freed LM, Hamosh M et al. Lipases and lipids in human milk: effect of freeze-thawing and storage. *Pediatr Res* 1984;18:1257-1262.

97. Jensen RG, Jensen GL. Specialty lipids for infant nutrition. I. Milks and formulas. *J Pediatr Gastroenterol Nutr* 1992;15:232-245.

98. Dworsky M, Stagno S, Pass RF et al. Persistence of cytomegalovirus in human milk after storage. *J Pediatr* 1982;101:440-443.

99. Pittard WB 3rd, Geddes KM, Brown S et al. Bacterial contamination of human milk: container type and method of expression. *Am J Perinatol* 1991;8:25-27.

100. Wilks S, Meier P. Helping mothers express milk suitable for preterm and high-risk infant feeding. *MCN Am J Matern Child Nurs* 1988;13:121-123.

101. Clark RA. Breast milk does not constitute occupational exposure as defined by standard. 1992. Retrieved May 14, 2002, from ttp://www.osha.gov/pls/oshaweb/owadisp. show_document?p_table=INTERPRETATIONS &p_id=20952

102. Williams-Arnold LD. *Storage for healthy infants and children.* Sandwich MA: Health Education Associates; 2000.

103. Law BJ, Urias BA, Lertzman J et al. Is ingestion of milk-associated bacteria by premature infants fed raw human milk controlled by routine bacteriologic screening? *J Clin Microbiol* 1989;27:1560-1566.

104. Hamosh M, Henderson TR, Ellis LA et al. Digestive enzymes in human milk: stability at suboptimal storage temperatures. *J Pediatr Gastroenterol Nutr* 1997;24:38-43.

105. Lavine M, Clark RM. The effect of short-term refrigeration of milk and addition of breast milk fortifier on the delivery of lipids during tube feeding. *J Pediatr Gastroenterol Nutr* 1989;8:496-499.

106. Lemons PM, Miller K, Eitzen H et al. Bacterial growth in human milk during continuous feeding. *Am J Perinatol* 1983;1:76-80.

107. Pittard WB 3rd, Bill K. Human milk banking. Effect of refrigeration on cellular components. *Clin Pediatr Phila* 1981;20:31-33.

108. Sigman M, Burke KI, Swarner OW et al. Effects of microwaving human milk: changes in IgA content and bacterial count. *J Am Diet Assoc* 1989;89:690-692.

109. Hibbard RA, Blevins R. Palatal burn due to bottle warming in a microwave oven. *Pediatrics* 1989;82:382-384.

110. Boo NY, Nordiah AJ, Alfizah H et al. Contamination of breast milk obtained by manual expression and breast pumps in mothers of very low birthweight infants. *J Hosp Infect* 2001;49:274-281.

111. Jones CA. Maternal transmission of infectious pathogens in breast milk. *J Paediatr Child Health* 2001;37:576-582.

112. Igumbor EO, Mukura RD, Makandiramba B et al. Storage of breast milk: effect of temperature and storage duration on microbial growth. *Cent Afr J Med* 2000;46:247-251.

CHAPTER 15

Nutritional Sources for Newborns

Throughout this text, there has been a clear emphasis on the idea that direct, exclusive breastfeeding is the ideal source of nutrition for newborns, whether they are well or compromised. When the newborn is not feeding directly at the breast or when supplementation is medically indicated, other alternatives must be explored.

The aim of this chapter is to describe the indications, advantages, and limitations of four basic sources of nutrition for the infant who is not breastfeeding directly: (1) fresh mother's milk—either modified or unmodified; (2) previously stored mother's milk—modified or unmodified; (3) donor milk; and (4) artificial milk. A basic understanding of these nutritional sources enables the nurse to provide better consumer education and to advocate for human milk as the ideal source for maintaining homeostasis in the infant.

HUMAN MILK

Human milk is unquestionably the gold standard for infant nutrition.[1,2] Ideally, the healthy, term infant experiences direct, exclusive breastfeeding; the milk itself and the act of feeding provide many advantages, as described in previous chapters.

When direct breastfeeding is not possible—for whatever reason—fresh milk or previously stored mother's milk is the next best choice. Expressed milk varies in the amount of benefits it provides for the infant. Freshly expressed mother's own milk offers the most benefit, followed by previously stored mother's own milk, and then donor milk. Artificial milk ("formula") is always inferior to human milk.

Mother's Own Milk: Fresh

Fresh milk comes from the infant's own mother and is given immediately or almost immediately—without processing or storing—to the infant. By definition, fresh milk is from the mother, never from donors. Milk from the infant's own mother, or mother's own milk (MOM, or expressed mother's milk [EMM]) is best when given fresh to the infant (as opposed to refrigerated or frozen). Of course, the infant gets fresh milk when feeding directly at the breast (direct breastfeeding), but he may also receive fresh milk if the mother expresses the milk and gives it to him to consume via some other method, as described in Chapter 16. More than milk that has been processed or stored, fresh milk has the greatest nutritional value for the infant.

During the early days of breastfeeding, healthy, term newborns should be given mother's milk only. Artificial milk supplements should be given only when medically indicated. Acceptable medical reasons for supplementing healthy, term newborns are found in Box 8-3.

Mother's Own Milk: Previously Stored

When mother's own milk is not given to the infant immediately (or almost immediately), it is stored, usually in either the refrigerator or the freezer. Previously stored milk may be more practical to use in some situations. For example, the employed mother may wish to leave milk in the refrigerator for her infant, or the mother of a critically ill infant may live many miles from a tertiary care center and may need to leave her milk for the infant to consume later. Previously stored milk can be used for either well or compromised newborns. However, the requirements for saving and storing are more rigorous for compromised infants than for well infants, as described in Chapter 14.

However, temperature, the type of container, and the length of storage influence the milk. Milk that is not promptly fed to infants may be altered. First, storage can diminish some of the components of the milk. Even if milk is not exposed to extremes in temperature, exposing it to light results, within 3 hours, in a 50% reduction in riboflavin content and 70% loss of vitamin A.[3] Second, pathogens may enter stored milk. The operative word here is *may* because stored milk, although it *may* be vulnerable to these limitations, is an excellent alternative to fresh milk.

Modified Mother's Own Milk

The American Academy of Pediatrics (AAP) states, "Human milk is the preferred feeding for *all* infants, including premature and sick newborns, with rare exception."[1] However, very-low-birth-weight (VLBW) infants will need to have mother's milk "modified" in some way; for example, the infant may need expressed milk with an added fortifier. The fortifier may be added to either fresh or previously stored milk.

Adding fortifier to human milk is sometimes confusing to parents. They have heard, over and over, that human milk has everything that the infant needs. The nurse often has the duty of explaining this apparent contradiction. Preterm mother's milk does have everything that the preterm infant needs, and theoretically, her milk alone would support both basal metabolism and growth. If the infant could consume an adequate volume of human milk, indeed he could receive enough proteins, fats, carbohydrates, and calories without modification or artificial supplementation. (Calcium and phosphorus would still be insufficient.) However, the VLBW infant has a very small stomach capacity, a limited ability to suckle, or a high metabolic rate (or a combination of thereof) along with several other factors to be considered. Therefore human milk alone may not meet his nutritional needs in some circumstances.

Fortified Human Milk

VLBW infants cannot thrive on their mother's milk only. Since 1983, consuming human milk only (i.e., without fortifier) has been associated with poor growth rates and unmet nutritional needs during hospitalization and thereafter.[4] To overcome this, commercially prepared products can be added to the mother's own milk. These are called *human milk fortifiers* (HMFs) because the products fortify human milk with extra nutrients, especially calcium, phosphorus, and protein, as well as carbohydrates, sodium, potassium, and magnesium. Some contain zinc, copper, and vitamins. Some contain fat.

There are two types of HMFs: powdered and liquid. Powdered fortifier is likely to be prescribed when a sufficient volume of mother's milk is available but the infant needs more calories and other nutrients than what he consumes from the human milk. Similarly, if volume needs to be restricted, the powder is preferable because more human milk can be given. In addition, parents seem to prefer the powder over the liquid.[5] Table 15-1 shows the volume of human milk, with and without fortification, that the newborn would need to consume to meet the suggested daily requirements.

Indications. Generally, fortifiers are indicated when the infant's birth weight is less than 1500 g (or 1800 g, depending on the hospital's protocol). When VLBW infants can tolerate human milk at greater than 100 ml/kg/day, supplementation using a human milk fortifier is started.[6] The volume is maintained for 2 to 4 days while the concentration is gradually increased. Usually, the fortifier is added gradually until the ideal "dose" is achieved, often referred to as *full fortification*. Full fortification is a 1:1 concentration for the liquid product, and four packets of the powdered product per deciliter (100 ml). The goal is to achieve a weight gain of approximately 15 g/kg/day. Fortification continues until the infant is taking all feedings from the breast directly or weighs 1800 to 2000 g, depending on the nursery protocol.

Efficacy of Human Milk Fortifier. HMF, whether in powdered or liquid form, improves growth, bone accretion, and neurodevelopmental outcomes. Schanler and colleagues assert, "The

Table 15-1 VOLUME (ml) NEEDED TO MEET ESTIMATED DAILY NUTRIENT REQUIREMENTS PER KILOGRAM OF INFANT BODY MASS

Nutrient	Estimated Daily Requirements per Kilogram	Human Milk Only	Human Milk Plus 4 Packets of Enfamil HMF/100 ml	Human Milk Plus 4 Packets Similac HMF/100 ml	Human Milk Fortified with Similac Natural Care (1:1 dilution)
Kilocalories	120 kcal	176 ml	146	146	160
Protein	≥3 g	286	140	146	184
Calcium	200 mg	714	169	138	201
Phosphorus	100 mg	714	169	123	202
Sodium	2 mEq	256	159	139	174
Potassium	2 mEq	149	108	68	99

This table shows the volume needed to meet estimated daily nutrient requirements per kilogram of infant body mass. For example, the infant would need to consume 176 ml of human milk per kg per day to obtain a requirement of 120 kcal/kg/day, based on a 120 kcal/kilogram/day estimate. In some situations, this is not possible. Through fortification of the milk, however, the infant could consume less volume (e.g., 146 or 160 ml) and meet the requirement. (Values listed are subject to change; refer to product label or packaging for most current information. Composition of human milk varies with maternal diet, stage of lactation, diurnally, and among mothers.)

use of fortified human milk generally provides the premature infant adequate growth, nutrient retention, and biochemical indices of nutritional status when fed at approximately 180 mL/kg/day compared with unfortified human milk"[7] (p. 379). The Cochrane Database Systematic Review has analyzed multiple randomized controlled trials describing the effects of HMF and has determined that HMF is associated with better short-term outcomes when compared with human milk only.[8] It is unlikely that further trials will be forthcoming because the advantages of fortified milk versus unfortified milk is now well established.

The more salient question now is whether fortified human milk is superior to artificial milk designed for preterm infants. Until recently, no studies making this comparison have existed. Schanler and colleagues' study showed that VLBW infants who were fed fortified human milk were discharged earlier and had fewer incidences of necrotizing enterocolitis and late-onset sepsis when compared with infants who were fed preterm formula.[9] Infants appear to tolerate fortified human milk well.[10]

Atkinson states that "the ideal amount and balance of supplemental nutrients to add to mother's milk for small premature infants remain unknown"[11] (p. 235). Although tissue growth occurs in early life in response to fortifying mother's milk, this early growth may not be as important as the long-term growth that occurs in these infants. Morley and Lucas point out that "the preterm period is not a critical window for nutritional programming on growth"[12] (p. 822). It will be helpful to have more clinical trials that address these issues.

Limitations and Considerations. Currently, two brands of powdered HMF are available. The one that has been in use for many years is the Enfamil Human Milk Fortifier (Mead Johnson, Evansville, IN), and more recently, the Similac Human Milk Fortifier (Ross Laboratories, Columbus, OH) has been used. Recently, a summary[13] of concerns with the Enfamil Human Milk Fortifier were noted. Problems noted in terms of the components included the protein content,[14] highly soluble calcium and phosphorus salts,[6] and high osmolality.[15] Schanler and Abrams observed that recipients of fortifier that contained highly soluble calcium and phosphorus demonstrated poorer fat absorption compared with recipients of HMF containing insoluble calcium and phosphorus.[6] More practical

RESEARCH HIGHLIGHT

Fortified Human Milk Is More Beneficial Than Preterm Formula

Citation: Schanler RJ, Shulman RJ, Lau C. Feeding strategies for premature infants: beneficial outcomes of feeding fortified human milk versus preterm formula. *Pediatrics* 1999;103:1150-1157.

FOCUS

Schanler and colleagues studied 108 infants whose gestational age was 26 to 30 weeks, with a mean birth weight around 1070 g. These infants were fed either predominantly fortified human milk ($N = 62$) or only preterm formula ($N = 46$). The aim of this prospective study was to describe "the role of diet by comparing the growth, feeding tolerance, health outcomes, biochemical indices of nutritional status, and nutrient absorption and retention" when the infants were fed either the fortified human milk (FHM) or the preterm formula (PF).

RESULTS

Infants fed FHM were discharged earlier (73 days ± 19 vs. 88 days ± 47). They had a significantly lower incidence of necrotizing enterocolitis and late-onset sepsis compared with the PF group. Infants in the FHM group took significantly fewer days to complete tube feedings and to reach 2000 g of body weight. Feeding tolerance was about the same between the groups. Infants fed FHM took greater volumes of milk during the study period but had significantly slower rates of weight gain and linear growth measurements. Intakes of nitrogen and copper were higher and magnesium and zinc were lower in the FHM milk group. Interestingly, parents of the FHM infants visited more frequently than parents of infants fed PF.

STRENGTHS, WEAKNESSES OF THE STUDY

Although the infants did not necessarily receive human milk exclusively (because of the mother's milk supply), the investigators tracked the volume of milk fed throughout the study so that they could confidently report that the infant had been fed predominantly fortified human milk.

CLINICAL APPLICATION

Although the rates of weight gain were slower in infants fed FHM, the investigators question what they really mean because the overall health of the infant was better when fed FHM. The lower incidence of necrotizing enterocolitis found in this study is consistent with the findings in several previous studies. It is of interest to see that 13% of the mothers in the study said that they did not plan to breastfeed if their infants had been born at term, but when informed of the potential benefits of human milk for their infants, they changed their minds. Nurses and other health care providers should help parents make informed feeding decisions.

---

problems involve difficulty with mixability and separation of human milk fat with continuous tube feedings.[16] Concerns about growth have also emerged. Concerns about fortifier, however, should not prevent it from being used.[17]

A recent study compared the two powdered fortifiers commercially available in the United States.[13] (Another study compared the Ross product with the Wyeth product, which is commercially available abroad.[18]) The Similac Human Milk Fortifier contained more protein, fat, calcium, phosphorus, magnesium, sodium, potassium, chloride, manganese, zinc, copper, and vitamins than the Enfamil Human Milk Fortifier. Greater growth was noted in the infants who were fed Similac Human Milk Fortifier. Milk intakes were similar.

Administering Feedings with Fortifier. To administer a feeding using the *powdered* fortifier, dissolve the powder in the mother's milk. Check the order to be sure the amount is within acceptable limits. A typical order might start with adding one or two packets per 100 ml of mother's milk, then progressing to two packets, three packets, and then four packets. The four packets per 100 ml of milk (or one packet per 25 ml of milk) provide approximately 82 kcal/100 ml (24 kcal/oz) to the infant; this is usually the maximum amount ordered. To dissolve the powder, first run the milk under water until it reaches about 37° C (98° F). Add the fortifier and shake (avoid overshaking). Warming the milk helps, but the fortifier can be difficult to dissolve.

Liquid fortifier (Similac Natural Care) is most likely to be used when the mother does not have a sufficient volume of milk. It provides volume as well as nutrients. Human milk at full fortification with Natural Care has a lower osmolarity than human milk with powdered HMF. It also provides less energy; 75 versus 82 kcal/ml and less calcium and phosphorus than the HMF supplemented human milk as shown in Table 15-2. The liquid fortifier provides a lesser amount of calories, calcium, and phosphorus than the powdered fortifier, as shown in Table 15-2.

Before administering a feeding using the liquid fortifier, check the order to make sure it is within acceptable limits. A typical order might start with adding 1 part liquid fortifier to 2 parts human milk; if the infant can tolerate this for at least 24 hours, he can advance to "full fortification" (i.e., 1 part liquid fortifier to 1 part human milk). When human milk is in a 1:1 ratio with the Natural Care, however, it provides about 22 kcal/oz. Some nursery protocols may allow a little powdered fortifier to be added after the mother's milk is diluted 1:1 with the liquid fortifier to increase the calories and nutrients without further diluting the human milk.

Until recently, newborns were not discharged to home while using fortifier. Discharge nutrition is a controversial issue at this point, with some centers discharging infants to home while still using the fortifier. One possible rationale for using liquid fortifier at home is if the mother has especially low milk volume. If the neonatal team determines that there are substantial benefits to this practice, the newborn may be discharged with an order to continue fortification of his mother's milk. If this is the case, discharge planning needs to include specific instructions about how to combine the fortifier with human milk. The cost of the fortifier should be considered, however, as well as its availability. Often, these products are both cost prohibitive and difficult to obtain. Furthermore, the extra expense is borne by the parents, not by their health insurance company.

Hindmilk Only

It is often difficult for compromised newborns to get the hindmilk while at the breast, particularly if they tire easily. Expressing milk and giving hindmilk only is one strategy for providing extra fat and calories. This is a relatively new concept, and little research has been done on the efficacy of this practice. However, recently, low-birth-weight (LBW) infants made significantly greater weight gains when given hindmilk only.[19]

Donor Milk: Human Milk Banking

Donor milk is milk that has been expressed by a lactating mother for an infant other than her own. She donates this milk to a donor milk bank, and it is distributed to infants whose mothers cannot provide human milk. Donor milk is processed, whereas the mother's own milk is not. This is important because processing human milk usually through heat-treating—affects the components and potential pathogens of human milk. Donor milk is often "pooled," meaning that it may have come from several different women. Donor milk has been recognized by the AAP as a desirable source of nutrition.[2,20]

Indications

If the mother's own milk is unavailable—the mother is unable or unwilling to lactate—donor milk, although less desirable than mother's own milk, is preferable to artificial milk. However, banked donor milk must be prescribed. A frequent reason for prescribing it is prematurity. Preterm infants who are fed pasteurized donor milk have better outcomes than those who are fed artificial milk.[21] (However, multiple other reasons have been reported for using donor milk, as described in Box 15-1.) Donor milk is a cost-effective strategy for preterm infants because of improved outcomes.[22,23]

Limitations and Considerations

Donor milk is processed. Technically, refrigerating, freezing, and thawing are ways of processing human milk, but here the discussion is limited to the more detrimental effects of processing that

Table **15-2**　Nutrients Provided by Human Milk Fortified with Similac Natural Care (NF), Enfamil Human Milk Fortifier (HMF), and Similac HMF per 100 ML

Ratio	Natural Care Only	Human Milk with Similac Natural Care				Human Milk	Human Milk with Enfamil Fortifier				Human Milk with Similac Human Milk Fortifier			
	Alone	1:3	1:2	1:1	2:1	Alone	1 pkt/dl	2 pkt/dl	3 pkt/dl	4 pkt/dl	1 pkt/dl	2 pkt/dl	3 pkt/dl	4 pkt/dl
Kcal	81.00	77.75	76.67	75.00	72.33	68.00	72.00	75.00	79.00	82.00	71.50	75	78.50	82.00
CHO (g)	8.61	8.26	8.14	7.91	7.67	7.20	7.48	7.75	8.03	9.30	7.65	8.1	8.55	9.00
Protein(g)	2.20	1.91	1.82	1.63	1.43	1.05	1.33	1.60	1.88	2.15	1.30	1.55	1.80	2.05
Fat (g)	4.41	4.28	4.24	4.16	4.07	3.90	4.06	4.23	4.39	4.55	3.99	4.08	4.17	4.26
Ca (mg)	171.00	135.25	123.33	99.50	75.67	28.00	50.50	73.00	95.50	118.00	57.25	86.50	115.75	145.00
P (mg)	85.00	67.25	61.33	49.50	37.67	14.00	25.3	36.50	47.8	59.00	30.75	47.50	64.25	81.00
Na (mg)	34.66	30.48	29.08	26.30	23.51	17.93	20.68	23.43	26.18	28.93	21.68	25.43	29.18	32.93
K (mg)	103.97	91.08	86.78	78.18	69.59	52.40	57.40	62.40	67.40	72.40	68.15	83.90	99.65	115.40
Vitamin D	122.00	91.50	81.99	62.00	42.00	2.00	39.5	77.00	114.50	152.00	32.00	62.00	92.00	122.00
		← Increasing Concentrations →					← Increasing Concentrations →				← Increasing Concentrations →			

This table shows the amount of nutrient provided by human milk alone and when it is combined with fortifier. For example, when 1 packet of human milk fortifier is added to 1 dl (100 ml) of human milk, it provides 0.72 kcal per ml (approximately 22 kcal/oz). NB: The recommended dilution is 1:1 for Natural Care; more concentrated feedings are not recommended except in unusual circumstances. The recommended dilution for HMF is 4 packets per deciliter (100 ml). Values are based on manufacturer's product information.
Data are derived from product information. Values listed are subject to change; refer to product label or packaging for most current information.

Box 15-1 CLINICAL USES OF DONOR MILK

NUTRITIONAL USES

Prematurity
Failure to thrive
Malabsorption syndromes
Short-gut syndrome
Renal failure
Feeding intolerance
Inborn errors of metabolism
Postsurgical nutrition
Cardiac problems
Bronchopulmonary dysplasia
Pediatric burn cases

MEDICINAL/THERAPEUTIC USES

Treatment for infectious diseases (intractable diarrhea, gastroenteritis, infantile botulism, sepsis, pneumonia, hemorrhagic conjunctivitis)

Postsurgical healing (omphalocele, gastroschisis, intestinal obstruction/bowel fistula, colostomy repair)
Immunodeficiency diseases (severe allergies, IgA deficiencies, HIV)
Inborn errors of metabolism
Solid organ transplants (including adults)
Noninfectious intestinal disorders (ulcerative colitis, irritable bowel syndrome)
Topical burn treatment

PREVENTIVE USES

Necrotizing enterocolitis
Crohn's disease
Colitis
Allergies to bovine and soy milks/feeding intolerance
During immune suppression therapy

Data from the Human Milk Banking Association of North America, 1998.

typically occur with donor milk, namely, pasteurization and lyophilization. (These processes are never recommended for mother's own milk.) Subjecting milk to pasteurization or lyophilization alters three basic factors: (1) immune factors—immunoglobulins,[24] antibodies to *Escherichia coli*, lactoferrin,[25] and viable lymphocytes[26]; (2) antiviral factors (cytomegalovirus [CMV], human immunodeficiency virus [HIV]); and (3) bacteria.

The processing fee for human milk varies from bank to bank but is usually about $2.75 (plus shipping) per ounce. Whether the woman is covered by the Woman, Infants, and Children (WIC) program; Medicaid; or private insurance determines whether she may receive reimbursement for this processing fee. Currently, WIC does not cover this fee. Medicaid determines whether this cost is covered on a case-by-case basis, and private insurances may cover the cost depending on whether the milk is on their formulary and whether there is a justified medical necessity for donor milk.

In the last decade or so, there have been concerns about the possibility of transmission of disease from donor milk. However, there are no published reports of disease transmission of pasteurized donor milk since the inception of donor milk banking in the United States in 1911.

Transmission of disease is certainly possible—perhaps even likely—if individual mothers simply "share" their milk with one another.

Pasteurization. Pasteurization is a heating process whereby organisms in milk are destroyed. The Human Milk Banking Association of North America (HMBANA) standard is to pasteurize human milk at a temperature of $62.5°$ C for 30 minutes. Pasteurizing milk destroys its cellular content, including lymphocytes,[27] and decreases immunoglobulin and antiinfective properties.

Lyophilization. Lyophilization is the "rapid freezing and dehydration of the frozen product under high-vacuum-freeze drying."[28] This process is undertaken to destroy pathogens, but it results in some destruction of cells as well. Lyophilization is not currently used in the United States, but it is sometimes used in other countries.

Donor Milk Banks

The term *human milk bank* refers to those hospitals that operate and staff a formal donor milk bank and accept milk not only from mothers of hospitalized infants but from donors as well. (The term *banked milk,* which appears frequently in research studies, can be misleading; it may correctly refer to donor milk or incorrectly to the mother's own milk that has

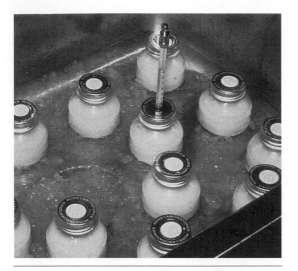

FIGURE 15-1 Processing donor milk at human milk bank. Note water bath with bottle containing monitoring thermometer.

simply been stored. This terminology is important because donor milk is processed, as shown in Fig. 15-1, whereas mother's own milk usually is not.)

HMBANA has defined the characteristics of a donor human milk bank; the definition and the contact information are listed in Appendix A. Donor milk banks in North America belong to the HMBANA. Among other goals, HMBANA develops standards for milk banking practices and reviews those guidelines annually to see that they conform with current research.

For recipients, the benefits of donor human milk are many, and the risks are negligible. Only expressed breast milk is suitable for donation. Dripped milk—milk that drips from the contralateral breast while the infant is feeding at the other breast—is unacceptable because the energy value is low and contamination is likely.[29] Furthermore, milk is accepted only from healthy lactating women who meet the criteria to become donors. (Sometimes, potential donors are excluded only temporarily, for example, if they are receiving short-term medication therapy.) Working closely with the Centers for Disease Control and Prevention and the U.S. Food and Drug Administration, HMBANA has established four screening processes to prevent contaminated milk from being dispensed: (1) A thorough health history

is obtained from the potential donor, (2) volunteer donors undergo serologic testing, (3) donated milk is pasteurized, and (4) donated milk is tested for bacteria both before and after pasteurization, and milk is not dispensed unless its bacterial count is at zero.

Milk banks provide benefits for donors, also. Some mothers make one-time donations when they have an unused supply in storage. This may happen when an older infant is consuming more solids than milk. The mother finds many containers of her milk occupying the freezer space but cannot bring herself to discard the milk; donating the milk overcomes both obstacles. Sometimes, the mother of a critically ill infant has expressed and saved many ounces of milk for her own infant who later dies. She may gain some sense of consolation by donating her milk with the hope that it will help another survive. More typically, a woman volunteers to regularly express milk for the milk bank. In this case the woman is producing more milk than her infant wants or needs to suckle; she therefore donates the oversupply to the bank. As advocates, we can help donors and recipients reap the benefits of donor milk banks as described in Box 15-2.

ARTIFICIAL MILK AND OTHER SUPPLEMENTS

Artificial milk differs significantly from human milk, as described in earlier chapters. The *standard* formula differs particularly with respect to concentrations of phosphorus and calcium and renal solute load.

Standard Formula

Standard formulas are designed for healthy, term newborns. Although some purport to be like the mother's milk, none are; all artificial milk is inferior to human milk. These artificial substitutes may be either (1) milk protein based (casein predominant or whey predominant), (2) soy protein based, (3) protein hydrolysate based, or (4) amino acid based.

Milk-Based Artificial Milk

The standard product provides 20 calories per ounce. The source of protein differs, depending on whether the formula is casein predominant or whey predominant. Carbohydrate is provided in

Box 15-2   How Can We Help Potential Donors and Recipients?

- Approach the physician in charge of the patient's care and urge him or her to consider ordering donor human milk. If the physician agrees, he or she should then contact the HMBANA office (see Appendix A). Office personnel will direct the physician or other prescriber to the milk bank that is either geographically closest or the bank that has the best supply of donor milk on hand. The physician must then write a prescription for the milk. Prescriptions may be faxed and followed with a hard copy to the milk bank.

- Help the prescriber gather pertinent details before sending the prescription to the milk bank. For example, the prescription must note the condition for which the donor milk is being prescribed and the number of ounces required per day. Generally, the milk is shipped in batches for a 1- to 2-week supply.

- Oppose anyone who says that donor milk is not an option because the milk bank is too far away from the recipient. The milk can be shipped anywhere in the country. Multiple methods of transport have been used; if there is a substantial distance involved, the milk is usually shipped frozen with dry ice by overnight delivery service.

- Encourage women to become donors if their infants cannot use all of their milk. Refer women who wish to become donors to the HMBANA to see if they meet the eligibility criteria for becoming donors.

- Reassure potential donors that getting their milk to a milk bank is a realistic option. If the mother lives near a milk bank, she or a family member can drive the milk to the bank, or the bank sometimes has a volunteer pick up milk from local residents. If the mother does not live near a milk bank, however, she should consider donating to a milk bank that accepts out-of-state donations. Whether or not banks accept milk from out-of-state donors depends on their supply, which can vary dramatically from month to month. These banks nearly always pay for shipping the milk and for the cost of donor serologic screening. If the donor has had blood drawn at her local hospital, she should ship a sample with the milk in order to spare the bank the cost.

- Persuade policy makers to make donor milk the social norm. For example, encourage physicians to order a "stock" supply of donor milk. The physician can order a certain number of ounces of donor milk for the inpatient facility rather than for an individual patient. In this way, the donor milk is immediately available, and it deters staff from giving artificial milk.

- Become involved in legislation modeled after the New York State law that entitles all infants access to human milk. The public health law says, ". . . any and all infants requiring human breast milk be assured access to sufficient quantities of wholesome human breast milk, donated by concerned lactating mothers on a continual and systematic basis." (See Appendix D-5 for full text and citation.)

- Incorporate the topic of donor milk into childbirth classes. When parents become aware of this alternative, they will begin to ask their health care providers to prescribe it. Similarly, mothers who have unused milk are likely to consider donating it if they recognize how their gift could be a lifesaver for another. Both the supply and demand could increase if only there was more awareness of donor human milk banks.

Modified from Biancuzzo M. *Childbirth Instructor,* September/October, 1998.

---

the form of lactose from fat-free cow's milk. Fat is usually provided from vegetable sources. The formulas also contain minerals, vitamins, taurine, inositol, choline, and one or more stabilizers or emulsifiers. All formulas contain some iron, but those with at least 1 mg/100 kcal are referred to as *iron fortified.*

The most widely available casein-predominant formula in the United States is Similac. The ratio of whey to casein still falls short of the low casein ratio found in human milk. Until recently, three whey-predominant formulas were available in the United States: Enfamil (Mead Johnson/Bristol-Myers Squibb), SMA (Wyeth), and Similac PM

60/40 (Ross Laboratories). However, SMA is no longer available in the United States.

The benefits of polyunsaturated long-chain fatty acids in human milk, especially arachidonic acids (AA) and docosahexaenoic acid (DHA), have long been associated with improved growth and development, particularly neurodevelopment and visual acuity. To mimic their effects in human milk, DHA and AA have been added to artificial milks marketed outside of the United States. Beginning in February 2002, DHA and AA are now being added to artificial milks marketed in the United States. Whether improved outcomes can be *solely* attributed to DHA or AA in breastfed infants is uncertain.[30] Hence, the efficacy of adding these fatty acids to artificial milk is questionable. In a randomized, double-blind study, the addition of DHA and AA to artificial milk was not associated with better outcomes in *term* infants,[31] but it has been associated with better outcomes in *preterm* infants.[32] Further studies are needed before any clear conclusions can be drawn.

Soy-Based Artificial Milk

Isolated soy protein–based artificial milks are free of cow's milk protein and lactose. They provide 20 kcal/oz. The protein is supplemented with L-methionine (improves nitrogen balance, weight gain, urea nitrogen excretion, and albumin synthesis), L-carnitine (optimizes mitochondrial oxidation of long-chain fatty acids), and taurine (functions as an antioxidant and, along with glycine, is a major conjugate of bile acids in early infancy).[33] The carbohydrate component is lactose free, and instead is corn starch or other saccharides. The fat is vegetable based, rather than cholesterol based. (For a discussion of the benefits of cholesterol for newborns, see Chapter 4.)

In most cases, milk-based artificial milks are preferred when human milk is unavailable. Soy-based artificial milks are indicated for infants with galactosemia and hereditary lactase deficiency. Unless there is a strong medical indication for soy-based formulas, however, they should not be given. Parents or providers who casually give soy-based formulas may not understand the concerns surrounding plant estrogens called *isoflavones* that are present in soy-based formulas.

Dietary consumption of isoflavones—well known for altering menstrual cycles and lowering cholesterol to improve health in adults—calls into question how these effects might be detrimental to the infant's sexual development or brain growth. The daily intake of isoflavones in infants who are exclusively fed soy-based infant formulas has been shown to be 5 to 10 times higher than a comparable dose (per kilogram of body weight) used to achieve hormonal regulation in adults.[34] Furthermore, plasma levels of isoflavones in these infants are 13,000 to 22,000 times higher than plasma estriol that naturally occurs in early human life.[35] It is uncertain what effects, if any, the isoflavones exert on infant growth, sexual development, bone density, and serum lipids. However, Setchell and colleagues observe that "it is difficult to believe that isoflavones, circulating at these high concentrations, are biologically inert in infants, particularly given their weaker binding to serum proteins."[36]

A recent study has suggested that there are few, if any, adverse outcomes in infants who are fed soy-based formulas,[37] but the methodology and reporting of outcomes in this study has been criticized.[38] Experts point out that adverse outcomes of isoflavones have not been demonstrated in clinical practice or research studies, presumably because of the isoflavone's low affinity for the infant's estrogen receptors.[39] However, Badger and colleagues emphasize the importance of confirming the few existing studies related to soy-based infant formulas and urge that new studies are needed "to investigate the more subtle effects that could occur during development or that could surface later in life."[40]

Artificial milks that are soy based are not designed or recommended for preterm infants who weigh less than 1800 g.[33] The aluminum content is at least 20 times greater than that in human milk, and because aluminum competes with calcium for absorption, the preterm infant becomes even more at risk for decreased skeletal bone mineralization.

The mother who is breastfeeding may have heard myths that soy-based artificial milks are better for breastfed infants than milk-based formulas. This is simply untrue. A few points, noted from the official position of the AAP,[33] provide a sound basis for answering questions raised by breastfeeding mothers:

- Isolated soy protein–based formula has no advantage over cow's milk protein–based formula as a supplement for the breastfed infant.
- The routine use of isolated soy protein–based formula has no proven value in the prevention or management of infantile colic.
- The routine use of isolated soy protein–based formula has no proven value in the prevention of atopic disease in healthy or high-risk infants.

Protein Hydrolysate–Based Formulas

Protein hydrolysate–based formulas, such as Alimentum, Nutramigen, and Pregestimil, contain nitrogen in the form of enzymatically hydrolyzed protein. Parents sometimes erroneously assume these are better substitutes for human milk than milk protein–based formulas. To the contrary, these formulas were not designed for routine use. They were intended for infants with specific problems, including food protein–induced enterocolitis and atopic reactions to milk or isolated soy proteins.

Amino Acid–Based Formulas

Currently, there is formula for newborns that consists of 100% amino acids (Neocate). An amino acid–based formula is indicated for infants who have symptoms of severe food allergy. Although clinical trials of Neocate have been conducted,[41-49] these are not meant to be used without testing and the clear clinical judgment of the problem and treatment options. (See Chapter 11 for a discussion of these formulas as related to colic.)

"Special Formula"

Preterm formula (e.g., Similac Special Care 20 and Similac Special Care 24, Enfamil Premature Formula 20 and Enfamil Premature Formula 24, and Preemie SMA) is designed for preterm or LBW newborns. Those labeled "20" provide 20 kcal/oz, and those labeled "24" have 24 kcal/oz. (Nutrient content of most formulas are listed on the website of the manufacturer.)

Formulas designed for preterm infants support bone accretion rates when the infant is fed at least 120 kcal/kg/day. Preterm formula is designed for feeding preterm infants who weigh less than 2000 g and who are rapidly growing. Other special formulas (e.g., NeoSure and Enfacare) have been designed for infants who were born at low birth weight and have been started on the preterm formula but who are no longer experiencing the rapid growth that occurs directly after birth and are approaching hospital discharge. These so-called postdischarge formulas appear to be beneficial for infants who are born before term.[50-52]

It is permissible and even desirable to "inoculate" artificial milk with a "dose" of colostrum. It may be impractical to give such a small amount of colostrum to the infant, especially if it needs to go through a feeding tube. By "inoculating" the feeding, one provides the antiinfective and immune benefits of the colostrum to the infant. This practice, once more prevalent, has recently fallen out of favor because some clinicians have misinterpreted a research study about mixing artificial milk with human milk. The study showed significantly decreased lysozyme activity when equal parts of formula and human milk were mixed.[53] This finding cannot be generalized to "inoculating" a feeding with milk or colostrum.

Other Supplemental Feeding Substances

Sterile water and glucose water are sometimes given, but there is no real indication for these substances, as discussed in Chapter 8. Teas, herbs, and so forth are routinely given in some cultures for ritual purposes.

Vitamin and Mineral Supplements

Whether breastfed infants need vitamin and mineral supplements has been a topic of debate. With so much emphasis on human milk as the "perfect" food, skeptics have argued that the greater amounts of some vitamins and minerals in artificial milk are "better" compared with the smaller amounts in human milk; this reflects a more-is-better assumption. However, vitamins or minerals in human milk are more easily absorbed, and hence smaller amounts are ideal for breastfed infants but inadequate for formula-fed infants.

Since 1961, vitamin K has been routinely given as an intramuscular supplement at delivery to prevent hemorrhage in the newborn. (Because it is a fat-soluble vitamin, infants who have more fat content in their diet will naturally get more vitamin K.) The AAP Committee on Nutrition states, "Of course, all infants, including breastfed infants, must receive a vitamin K supplement at birth."[2]

Vitamin D deficiency results in rickets, which is uncommon but possible in breastfed infants. A recent report from North Carolina described a total of 30 breastfed African-American infants who developed nutritional rickets because of a vitamin D deficiency.[54] (The report does not specify whether these children were exclusively or partially breast-fed.) The authors concluded that dark-skinned infants should be given vitamin D supplements and taken out into the sunlight more frequently. These recommendations are based on an under-standing that because of the high melanin (which acts as a neutral filter and absorbs solar radiation) in their skin, dark-skinned children are risk for vitamin D deficiency. In an accompanying editor-ial, Welch[55] questions why there is any objection to giving vitamin D to *all* children, and he notes that it is currently available only in the form of drops that contain vitamins A and C as well. The case report he is reacting to, however, reports rickets only in African-American infants, and whether vitamin D supplements are appropriate for other populations has not been determined. It is likely that the AAP will gather data on this topic and issue a recommendation to address this question.

Vitamin A deficiency rarely occurs in breastfed infants, but it can be a topic for discussion because it is commonly paired with vitamin D in commer-cial supplements. Vitamin B deficiencies are rela-tively rare in the United States. Several case reports describe vitamin B_{12} deficiency in infants whose mothers are strict vegetarians. However, vitamin B_1 (thiamin) deficiency can also occur in breastfed infants of thiamin-deficient mothers, but this usu-ally occurs only in developing countries.

Iron deficiency rarely develops before 4 to 6 months of age in breastfed infants because new-borns have a store of iron to meet their needs dur-ing this period. Although human milk has lesser iron than iron-fortified formula, breastfed new-borns rarely have *nutritional* anemia. The AAP[56]

states that "iron found in human milk is far more bioavailable, resulting in much lower rates of iron-deficiency anemia compared with low-iron cow milk formula. Nevertheless, 6% to 20% of exclu-sively breastfed infants remain at risk for reduced iron stores."[57,58] In one study, however, none of the infants who were *exclusively* breastfed for 7 months or more were anemic.[57] (Artificial milk is fortified with iron.)

Fluoride supplements are not needed for healthy breastfed infants.[2] Evidence has shown that there is adequate fluoride in human milk.

The AAP Committee on Nutrition states that "Under usual circumstances, the healthy, breastfed, full-term infant requires little or no vitamin and mineral supplementation."[2] In general, vitamin and mineral supplementation for the healthy for-mula-fed infant can conveniently be given in the formula, and later, in cereals. Preterm infants who consume less than 300 kcal per day or weigh less than 2.5 kg have individualized needs for vitamins and minerals, and these are often given as a multi-vitamin supplement or as a specific nutrient sup-plement.

SUMMARY

When direct breastfeeding is not possible, the par-ents, as well as the health care team, need a thor-ough understanding of the options. The mother's own fresh milk is always the first choice. The mother's own milk, previously stored, is an excel-lent choice. Whether given fresh or frozen, the mother's own milk may be more beneficial if it is given with fortifiers or given as hindmilk only to some compromised infants. Donor milk, available from donor milk banks, may have lost some of its goodness because of the high heat required for the pasteurization process, but it is still a good alternative for infants whose mothers are unable to provide their own milk. Artificial milk, in all circum-stances, is inferior to human milk.

REFERENCES

1. American Academy of Pediatrics. Work Group on Breastfeeding. Breastfeeding and the use of human milk. *Pediatrics* 1997;100:1035-1039.

2. Committee on Nutrition American Academy of Pediatrics. *Pediatric nutrition handbook*. 4th ed. Elk Grove Village, IL: American Academy of Pediatrics; 1998.

3. Bates CJ, Liu DS, Fuller NJ et al. Susceptibility of riboflavin and vitamin A in breast milk to photodegradation and its implications for the use of banked breast milk in infant feeding. *Acta Paediatr Scand* 1985;74:40-44.

4. Atkinson SA, Radde IC, Anderson GH. Macromineral balances in premature infants fed their own mothers' milk or formula. *J Pediatr* 1983;102:99-106.

5. Fenton TR, Tough SC, Belik J. Breast milk supplementation for preterm infants: parental preferences and postdischarge lactation duration. *Am J Perinatol* 2000;17:329-333.

6. Schanler RJ, Abrams SA. Postnatal attainment of intrauterine macromineral accretion rates in low birth weight infants fed fortified human milk. *J Pediatr* 1995;126: 441-447.

7. Schanler RJ, Hurst NM, Lau C. The use of human milk and breastfeeding in premature infants. *Clin Perinatol* 1999; 26:379-398, vii.

8. Kuschel CA, Harding JE. Multicomponent fortified human milk for promoting growth in preterm infants. *Cochrane Database Syst Rev* 2000:CD000343.

9. Schanler RJ, Shulman RJ, Lau C. Feeding strategies for premature infants: beneficial outcomes of feeding fortified human milk versus preterm formula. *Pediatrics* 1999;103: 1150-1157.

10. Moody GJ, Schanler RJ, Lau C et al. Feeding tolerance in premature infants fed fortified human milk. *J Pediatr Gastroenterol Nutr* 2000;30:408-412.

11. Atkinson SA. Human milk feeding of the micropremie. *Clin Perinatol* 2000;27:235-247.

12. Morley R, Lucas A. Randomized diet in the neonatal period and growth performance until 7.5-8 y of age in preterm children. *Am J Clin Nutr* 2000;71:822-828.

13. Reis BB, Hall RT, Schanler RJ et al. Enhanced growth of preterm infants fed a new powdered human milk fortifier: a randomized, controlled trial. *Pediatrics* 2000;106:581-588.

14. Carlson SE. Long-chain polyunsaturated fatty acids and development of human infants. *Acta Paediatr Suppl* 1999;88:72-77.

15. De Curtis M, Candusso M, Pieltain C et al. Effect of fortification on the osmolality of human milk. *Arch Dis Child Fetal Neonatal Ed* 1999;81:F141-F143.

16. Sankaran K, Papageorgiou A, Ninan A et al. A randomized, controlled evaluation of two commercially available human breast milk fortifiers in healthy preterm neonates. *J Am Diet Assoc* 1996;96:1145-1149.

17. Schanler RJ. The use of human milk for premature infants. *Pediatr Clin North Am* 2001;48:207-219.

18. Porcelli P, Schanler R, Greer F et al. Growth in human milk-fed very low birth weight infants receiving a new human milk fortifier. *Ann Nutr Metab* 2000;44:2-10.

19. Valentine CJ, Hurst NM, Schanler RJ. Hindmilk improves weight gain in low-birth-weight infants fed human milk. *J Pediatr Gastroenterol Nutr* 1994;18:474-477.

20. American Academy of Pediatrics and the American College of Obstetrics and Gynecology. *Guidelines for perinatal care*. 4th ed. Elk Grove Village, IL: American Academy of Pediatrics; 1997.

21. Lucas A, Morley R, Cole TJ et al. A randomised multicentre study of human milk versus formula and later development in preterm infants. *Arch Dis Child*. 1994;70:F141-F146.

22. Wight NE. Donor human milk for preterm infants. *J Perinatol* 2001;21:249-254.

23. Arnold LDW. The cost-effectiveness of using banked donor milk in the neonatal intensive care unit: prevention of necrotizing enterocolitis. *J Hum Lact* 2002;18:172-177.

24. Sigman M, Burke KI, Swarner OW et al. Effects of microwaving human milk: changes in IgA content and bacterial count. *J Am Diet Assoc* 1989;89:690-692.

25. Ford JE, Marshall VME, Reiter B. Influence of the heat treatment of human milk on some of its protective constituents. *J Pediatr* 1977;90:29-35.

26. Davies DP. Human milk banking. *Arch Dis Child* 1982;57: 3-5.

27. Liebhaber M, Lewiston NJ, Asquith MT et al. Alterations of lymphocytes and of antibody content of human milk after processing. *J Pediatr* 1977;91:897-900.

28. Lawrence RA, Lawrence RM. *Breastfeeding: a guide for the medical profession*. 5th ed. St. Louis: Mosby; 1999.

29. Stocks RJ, Davies DP, Carroll LP et al. A simple method to improve the energy value of bank human milk. *Early Hum Dev* 1983;8:175-178.

30. Innis SM, Gilley J, Werker J. Are human milk long-chain polyunsaturated fatty acids related to visual and neural development in breast-fed term infants? *J Pediatr* 2001; 139:532-538.

31. Auestad N, Halter R, Hall RT et al. Growth and development in term infants fed long-chain polyunsaturated fatty acids: a double-masked, randomized, parallel, prospective, multivariate study. *Pediatrics* 2001;108: 372-381.

32. O'Connor DL, Hall R, Adamkin D et al. Growth and development in preterm infants fed long-chain polyunsaturated fatty acids: a prospective, randomized controlled trial. *Pediatrics* 2001;108:359-371.

33. American Academy of Pediatrics Committee on Nutrition. Soy protein-based formulas: recommendations for use in infant feeding. *Pediatrics* 1998;10:148-153.

34. Cassidy A, Bingham S, Setchell KD. Biological effects of a diet of soy protein rich in isoflavones on the menstrual cycle of premenopausal women. *Am J Clin Nutr* 1994;60:333-340.

35. Setchell KD, Zimmer-Nechemias L, Cai J et al. Exposure of infants to phyto-oestrogens from soy-based infant formula. *Lancet* 1997;350:23-27.

36. Setchell KD, Zimmer-Nechemias L, Cai J et al. Isoflavone content of infant formulas and the metabolic fate of these phytoestrogens in early life. *Am J Clin Nutr* 1998;68:1453S-1461S.

37. Strom BL, Schinnar R, Ziegler EE et al. Exposure to soy-based formula in infancy and endocrinological and reproductive outcomes in young adulthood. *JAMA* 2001;286:807-814.

38. Goldman LR, Newbold R, Swan SH. Exposure to soy-based formula in infancy. *JAMA* 2001;286:2402-2403.

39. Zung A, Reifen R, Kerem Z et al. Phytoestrogens: the pediatric perspective. *J Pediatr Gastroenterol Nutr* 2001;33:112-118.

40. Badger TM, Ronis MJ, Hakkak R et al. The health consequences of early soy consumption. *J Nutr* 2002;132:559S-565S.

41. Hill DJ, Cameron DJ, Francis DE et al. Challenge confirmation of late-onset reactions to extensively hydrolyzed formulas in infants with multiple food protein intolerance. *J Allergy Clin Immunol* 1995;96:386-394.

42. Hill DJ, Heine RG, Cameron DJ et al. The natural history of intolerance to soy and extensively hydrolyzed formula in infants with multiple food protein intolerance. *J Pediatr* 1999;135:118-121.

43. de Boissieu D, Matarazzo P, Dupont C. Allergy to extensively hydrolyzed cow milk proteins in infants: identification and treatment with an amino-acid-based formula. *J Pediatr* 1997;131:744-747.

44. de Boissieu D, Dupont C. Time course of allergy to extensively hydrolyzed cow's milk proteins in infants. *J Pediatr* 2000;136:119-120.

45. Niggemann B, Binder C, Dupont C et al. Prospective, controlled, multi-center study on the effect of an amino-acid-based formula in infants with cow's milk allergy/intolerance and atopic dermatitis. *Pediatr Allergy Immunol* 2001;12:78-82.

46. Isolauri E, Tahvanainen A, Peltola T et al. Breast-feeding of allergic infants. *J Pediatr* 1999;134:27-32.

47. Hill DJ, Heine RG, Cameron DJ et al. Role of food protein intolerance in infants with persistent distress attributed to reflux esophagitis. *J Pediatr* 2000;136:641-647.

48. Estep DC, Kulczycki A Jr. Colic in breast-milk-fed infants: treatment by temporary substitution of Neocate infant formula. *Acta Paediatr* 2000;89:795-802.

49. Estep DC, Kulczycki A Jr. Treatment of infant colic with amino acid-based infant formula: a preliminary study. *Acta Paediatr* 2000;89:22-27.

50. Carver JD, Wu PY, Hall RT et al. Growth of preterm infants fed nutrient-enriched or term formula after hospital discharge. *Pediatrics* 2001;107:683-689.

51. Lucas A, Fewtrell MS, Morley R et al. Randomized trial of nutrient-enriched formula versus standard formula for post-discharge preterm infants. *Pediatrics* 2001;108:703-711.

52. Worrell LA, Thorp JW, Tucker R et al. The effects of the introduction of a high-nutrient transitional formula on growth and development of very-low-birth-weight infants. *J Perinatol* 2002;22:112-119.

53. Quan R, Yang C, Rubinstein S et al. The effect of nutritional additives on anti-infective factors in human milk. *Clin Pediatr Phila* 1994;33:325-328.

54. Kreiter SR, Schwartz RP, Kirkman HN et al. Nutritional rickets in African American breast-fed infants. *J Pediatr* 2000;137:153-157.

55. Welch TR, Bergstrom WH, Tsang RC. Vitamin D-deficient rickets: the reemergence of a once-conquered disease. *J Pediatr* 2000;137:143-145.

56. American Academy of Pediatrics Committee on Nutrition. Iron fortification of infant formulas. *Pediatrics* 1999;104:119-123.

57. Pisacane A, De Vizia B, Valiante A et al. Iron status in breast-fed infants. *J Pediatr* 1995;127:429-431.

58. Duncan B, Schifman RB, Corrigan JJ Jr et al. Iron and the exclusively breast-fed infant from birth to six months. *J Pediatr Gastroenterol Nutr* 1985;4:421-425.

CHAPTER

16 *Techniques for Delivering Human and Artificial Milk*

Under most circumstances, the healthy infant who has ready access to his mother can meet all of his nutritional and fluid needs by suckling her breasts. (Medical indications for supplementation[1] are described in Chapter 8.) When the infant does not have ready access to his mother's breasts, as described in Chapter 14, or if the infant is not completely well, nourishment may need to be given some other way. When the newborn is not feeding directly at the breast or when supplementation is medically indicated, the question then becomes: How exactly should this nourishment be delivered to the infant?

The aim of this chapter is to describe ways to deliver enteral or oral feedings of human milk or artificial milk. Infants who cannot obtain all of their nourishment at the breast can be viewed as being on a continuum from those who cannot tolerate oral feedings at all to those who vigorously suckle the breast but occasionally obtain their nourishment by some other means. Furthermore, preterm infants can sometimes suckle the breast and then receive the remainder of their feeding by gavage if they become fatigued.

It is often assumed that the infant who is not suckling must have artificial milk. This is entirely untrue; *what* is given is an issue entirely separate from *how* it is given. Fig. 16-1 shows a flowchart that separates issues of what from how. Human milk, as well as artificial milk, may be given by a variety of methods. All methods have distinct advantages and disadvantages for the infant, the mother, or both.[2] Table 16-1 summarizes the advantages and disadvantages of several feeding options. It is the nurse's responsibility to facilitate indirect breastfeeding in a way that preserves the breastfeeding relationship to the greatest extent possible. Priorities for care during nonexclusive breastfeeding are presented in Box 16-1.

GAVAGE FEEDINGS

If the infant's gastrointestinal tract is completely unable to tolerate food, nourishment is given parenterally (i.e., intravenously, including total parenteral nutrition[3]). If the infant's gastrointestinal tract can tolerate food, however, he may nonetheless be unable to ingest the food orally, for one of many reasons. Infants are unable to take oral feedings if they have anomalies of the digestive tract (see Chapter 11), an inability to coordinate suck/swallow, severe debilitation, respiratory distress, or unconsciousness. Rather than being fed orally, these infants are fed enterally (i.e., through the stomach or small intestine). A gastrostomy feeding—feeding through a tube passed directly into the stomach from the abdominal wall—is initiated if the infant has an anomaly of the mouth, pharynx, esophagus, or cardiac sphincter of the stomach. Enteral feedings have special implications for extremely low-birth-weight infants.[4] More frequently, however, newborns are fed by *gavage* feedings.

Gavage feeding is accomplished by passing a small tube via the nares (nasogastric gavage [NG]) or via the mouth (orogastric gavage [OG]) directly into the stomach. The tube may contain either human or artificial milk, but preterm infants tolerate enteral feeding of human milk sooner than artificial milk.[5] Usually, if only a few gavage feedings are anticipated, the tube is inserted for each feeding. For very ill infants, however, the tube is usually indwelling (i.e., not removed for each

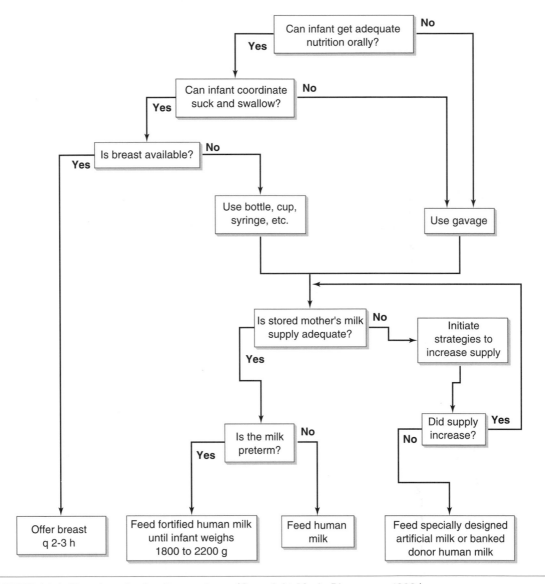

FIGURE **16-1** Flowchart for feeding options. *(Copyright Marie Biancuzzo, 1998.)*

feeding). The feeding may be given by bolus (intermittent gavage) or administered continuously (continuous gavage; i.e., the feeding is infused via a pump). The rate of the infusion depends on the infant's general health status. (A complete discussion of how to provide enteral feedings is found in most pediatric textbooks.)

Infants who are very sick or preterm typically have continuous OG or NG feedings, and the human milk or artificial milk is given via an electronic infusion pump, similar to those used to deliver intravenous fluids. Typically, infants who weigh more than 1000 g are more likely to be gavaged by an intermittent bolus about every 3 hours, whereas those who weigh less are usually fed by continuous pump. Energy expenditure appears to be greater when intermittent feedings are used.[6] However, outcomes appear comparable; among very-low-birth-weight (VLBW) infants, growth rates and macronutrient retention rates and lengths of hospital stay are similar whether they are fed by continuous or intermittent gavage.[7]

Although gavage feedings are always invasive, oxygen desaturation is three times more likely with bottle-feedings than with bolus gavage feedings.[8] In VLBW infants, intermittent gavage can lead to respiratory difficulties,[9] but growth rate and length of hospitalization do not differ significantly whether the gavage feedings are continuous or intermittent.[7]

Continuous slow-infusion feedings of human milk can result in losses of the milk's components.[10-12] Weight loss may occur because lipids (high in caloric value) may stick to the sides of the tubes.[10-12] Therefore it is critical to monitor for weight loss if infants are receiving continuous gavage feedings of human milk. Calcium and phosphorus are also lost.[13]

Administration Responsibilities for Delivering Human Milk via Gavage

Continuous infusion can potentially decrease lipid delivery and increase pathogens. Therefore several evidence-based clinical implications emerge for the nurse.

- Place the syringe *below* the isolette with the tip pointed upward so that the fat will rise and be pushed through the tube first. The fat that has accumulated during a continuous feeding will rise toward the end of the feeding; a 25- to 40-degree angle is best.[14] This improves fat delivery to the infant.
- Watch for weight loss. Fat and protein losses occur with continuous gavage,[12] and a slow rate of infusion magnifies the problem.[11] Milk that is fortified with medium-chain triglycerides adheres to the feeding tube.[15] Homogenized milk seems to lower the fat loss during tube feedings.[16]
- Reduce the threat of infection and nutrient loss by infusing the milk over 10 to 20 minutes for an intermittent feeding (depending on what is safe for the newborn) and deliver milk through minibore tubing rather than standard-bore tubing, to better preserve the creamatocrit[17]; use short feeding tubes. (*Creamatocrit* is the percentage of cream in human milk.[18])

- Ensure adequate fat intake. Advocate for measuring human milk creamatocrit at least once a day[19] to estimate the caloric value. Collect the sample from the distal end of the infusion set. As described in Chapter 10, parents can perform this task as well as providers.[20]
- Change the syringe and tubing at least every 4 hours.[21,22] Less frequent tubing changes may result in excessive bacteria.
- Develop an appropriate protocol that is implemented by well-trained staff; this has been shown to reduce contamination.[23]

Nonnutritive Sucking during Gavage Feeding

In the late 1980s, studies led to the practice of encouraging VLBW infants to suck on a pacifier when being gavage fed. VLBW infants more quickly made the transition from gavage to oral feeding when they used a pacifier, presumably because of an accelerated maturation of the sucking reflex.[74] Whether pacifier use during tube feedings improves weight gain is uncertain; some researchers suggest that it does.[24-26] When infants suck on a pacifier during intermittent gavage feedings, they exhibit less behavioral distress while maintaining physiologic parameters.[27]

In planning care for the gavage-fed newborn, however, there may be a better alternative than pacifiers. The mother's breast, after being "emptied," gives the infant the benefits of warmth, comfort, and the soothing sound of the mother's heartbeat. Furthermore, sucking on the mother's breast gives the needed stimulation to improve her milk supply and offers the mother an opportunity to actively participate in her infant's care. When newborns are allowed to suck on the mother's breast in this manner, feeding at the breast is the next logical step in the infant's growth and development. Besides the obvious physiologic benefits for both mother and infant, those who use this practice are more likely to continue breastfeeding for a longer period than those who do not.[28]

Infants who no longer need gavage feedings can make a gradual transition to oral feedings. LBW and VLBW infants are typically unable to consume the volume needed to support their needs for maintenance and growth. The goal is for the infant

Table **16-1**   Effect of Feeding Options on Mother and Child

Feeding Options	Will Promote Goal of Long-Term Breastfeeding	Is Infant Actually Breastfeeding?	What Is Infant's Energy/Time Expenditure?	Does Infant Receive Human Milk?
Continue frequent breastfeeding	Possibly	Yes	High	Yes
Supplement after breast (bottle, cup, dropper)	No	Yes	High	If uses pumped human milk
Temporarily bottle-feed pumped human milk, then resume breastfeeding	Possibly	No	Low	Yes
Bottle-feed pumped human milk	No	No	Low	Yes
Feeding tube device with pumped human milk	Yes	Yes	Low	Yes
Feeding tube device with formula	Yes	Yes	Low	Half
Finger feeding by tube/syringe on finger	No	No	High, if slow feeder	If uses pumped human milk
Quit breastfeeding for bottle-feeding	No	No	Low	No

Copyright Kittie Frantz, 1992.

Box **16-1**   Priorities for Care: Nonexclusive Breastfeeding

- Determine why indirect breastfeeding and/or artificial milk supplementation has been initiated and proceed with clinical management and counseling as appropriate.
- Build the mother's confidence in herself and her ability to nourish her infant. Avoid any implication that the supplement is just as good or superior to her own milk.
- Facilitate consumption of human milk, if appropriate.
- If it is not possible for the infant to receive human milk, suggest ways to make the supplements more similar to human milk. "Inoculating" artificial milk with human milk helps the newborn associate feeding with the smell of human milk. Warm artificial milk so that it is about the same temperature as milk directly from the breast. Suggest other ways to simulate the breastfeeding experience, including positioning, skin-to-skin contact, and eye contact.
- Identify and correct breastfeeding problems that can be solved by better clinical management. Usually, this means assisting infants who are not latched on correctly.
- Give specific information to parents of infants who are ill or unable to suckle. Emphasize that supplementation is usually a temporary strategy, and estimate how long supplementation is expected to continue. Meanwhile, devise a plan to facilitate full breastfeeding.
- Reassure mothers who wish to (e.g., the employed mother) or need to supplement that supplementation will not "ruin" breastfeeding. Do not try to starve the reluctant nurser into submission. Help the family choose a supplementation method that works for them.
- When possible, choose a method for delivering milk that is least disruptive to the breastfeeding relationship.
- Show families the technique for the chosen method; require a return demonstration and provide positive and negative feedback to help them master the technique.
- Reinforce the importance of expressing to maintain milk supply.
- Evaluate the infant's weight gain, the family's comfort level, and the mother's lactation status. Do not assume that all is well!

Is Infant Gaining Weight?	Is It Safe for Infant?	What Is Effect on Milk Supply?	What Is Maternal Time Expenditure?
May be poor	Yes, if weight monitored	Decreases	High
Yes	Yes (cup = aspiration danger)	Decreases	High
Yes, if enough milk pumped	Yes	Decreases	Medium
Yes, if enough milk pumped	Yes	Decreases if long term	Medium
Yes, if enough milk pumped	Yes	Good	Medium to high
Yes	Yes	Good	Medium
Not always	Aspiration danger	Decreases	High
Yes	Yes	Gone	Low

to consume at least 150 ml/kg/day (equivalent to at least 100 kcal/kg/day of human milk). Gradually increasing the amount of volume given through indirect feedings, as shown in Table 16-2, helps achieve this goal. Human milk, however, may also be given directly to infants who weigh less than 1500 g, as described in Chapter 10. A combination of direct and indirect feedings often works well. If infants have not been completely weaned from the nasogastric tube, it should be removed during feedings; oxygen desaturation is greater (in VLBW infants) when the tube is left in place.[29]

ORAL FEEDINGS

Oral feedings are clearly best because the biologic, psychologic, and cultural values associated with feedings are preserved. Oral feedings are not invasive and provide a time for interaction between the infant and caregiver. However, the compromised infant is often unable to get all of the nourishment he needs at the breast, and hence the professional or parent must ask, *How* can we best deliver human milk (or artificial milk, if human milk is unavailable) orally? Several alternatives.

Bottles

Bottles are widely used in the United States to provide nourishment to newborns. Many professionals presume they have no negative effects, but this is untrue. Lau and colleagues[30] point out that standard bottles have two factors that may hamper feeding performance: "(1) net hydrostatic pressure generated by the presence of the milk, which tends to increase flow rate and (2) a gradual build-up in negative pressure or vacuum inside the bottle, which tends to retain milk within" (p. 454). The newer angled bottles appear to offer physiologic advantages,[31] presumably because they allow the infant to self-pace the feeding.[30,32] Decreasing the flow rate appears to be helpful.[33]

Bottle-feeding disrupts the infant's vital signs. The effects of respiratory compromise are perhaps the most significant disadvantage to artificial nippling, especially for preterm infants. The decrease in oxygen saturation for preterm infants while bottle-feeding is well documented.[34-36] Cardiac status is adversely affected by bottle-feeding as compared with breastfeeding.[37] Systolic blood pressure changed significantly when healthy, term breastfed infants between 24 and 92 hours of age were offered a bottle. Bottle-fed infants also had an increase in their basal blood pressure when they began sucking the bottle, but the change was not as dramatic.[38] The position that the infant is in, however, may affect physiologic stability.[39] When VLBW infants have sucking bursts of 30 or more sucks per burst, oxygen desaturation is likely; infants should not be allowed to hold their breath for more than 10 seconds when they do this, which requires careful observation and intervention by the caregiver.[29]

Table **16-2**   GUIDELINES FOR INITIATING ORAL FEEDINGS OF HUMAN MILK FOR LBW AND VLBW INFANTS

The suggested guidelines below may be considered for inclusion in hospital protocols but should not be used without approval from the neonatologist. The goal is for the infant to consume a minimum of 150 ml/kg/day (equivalent to a minimum of 100 mg/kg/day of human milk).

Infant's Birth Weight	Begin Feedings*	Continue Feedings
750-1000 g	2 ml human milk × 4 feedings 3 ml human milk × 4 feedings 4 ml human milk × 4 feedings 4 ml human milk × 4 feedings	Continue to advance 2 ml every 4 feedings until the newborn is consuming at least 150 ml/kg/day
1001-1250 g	3 ml human milk × 4 feedings 4 ml human milk × 4 feedings 6 ml human milk × 4 feedings 8 ml human milk × 4 feedings	Continue to advance 2 ml every 4 feedings until the newborn is consuming at least 150 ml/kg/day
1251-1500 g	6 ml human milk × 4 feedings 8 ml human milk × 4 feedings 10 ml human milk × 4 feedings 12 ml human milk × 4 feedings 14 ml human milk × 4 feedings 16 ml human milk × 4 feedings	Continue to advance 2-3 ml every 4 feedings until the newborn is consuming at least 150 ml/kg/day
1501-1800 g	6 ml human milk × 4 feedings 9 ml human milk × 4 feedings 12 ml human milk × 4 feedings 15 ml human milk × 4 feedings 18 ml human milk × 4 feedings 21 ml human milk × 4 feedings	Continue to advance 3-4 ml every 4 feedings until the newborn is consuming at least 150 ml/kg/day
1801-2100 g	10 ml human milk × 4 feedings 15 ml human milk × 4 feedings 20 ml human milk × 4 feedings 25 ml human milk × 4 feedings	Continue to advance 5 ml every 4 feedings until the newborn is consuming at least 150 ml/kg/day
2101-2500 g	15 ml human milk × 4 feedings 20 ml human milk × 4 feedings 25 ml human milk × 4 feedings 30 ml human milk × 4 feedings	Continue to advance 5-10 ml every 4 feedings until the newborn is consuming at least 150 ml/kg/day
Over 2500 g	Begin with 25-45 ml human milk (indirect or direct feedings); if tolerated, feed ad lib	If tolerated feed ad lib

Source: University of Rochester Medical Center, Rochester, NY.
*These quantities apply to human milk only, not to fortified milk. Human milk is always given full strength, never diluted.

Bottle-feeding also takes more energy. Newborns show a higher sucking frequency when they suck the bottle as compared with the breast,[40] which requires a greater expenditure of energy. Furthermore, when those same newborns were fed human milk from a bottle and artificial milk from a bottle, there was no difference in either sucking frequency or sucking pressure.[40] Therefore it appears that the act of sucking at the bottle—not the fluid that is consumed—determines the suck and breathing patterns of newborns. Bottle-feeding has also been associated with ear infections.[41]

Term and preterm infants differ distinctly in how they tolerate oral feedings given by bottle.[42] Although gestation alone does not appear to predict the infant's ability to exclusively breastfeed, it

- Clenched fists
- Hyperextension of the head, back, and legs
- Elevated shoulders
- Facial grimace
- Milk spilled from the mouth
- Gulping sounds as the infant swallows
- Uneven respirations
- Breath holding, with eventual pauses between swallows to breathe

Source: Weber F, Woolridge MW, Baum JD. *Devel Med Child Neurol* 1986;28:19-24.

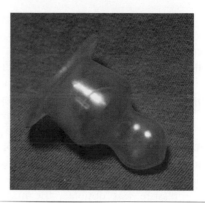

FIGURE **16-2** Nuk-style nipple.

does appear to directly influence his ability to master bottle-feeding techniques.[43] Preterm infants who are nippling have a clear "transitional" pattern of sucking[44,45] and seem to benefit from having the caregiver provide jaw support.[46] They may also benefit from nonnutritive sessions before bottle-feeding.[47] Perhaps most important, the person feeding the preterm infant also must use a developmentally appropriate approach for feeding.[48] Whether in preterm or term infants, a too-fast flow can be stressful for the infant, and it must be detected and corrected by the parent or caregiver. Box 16-2 lists signs that milk flow from the bottle is too fast for the infant to handle adequately.

The effect of bottle and nipple use on breast-feeding continuation has not been well studied. One study conducted in the United States showed that continuation of breastfeeding was more likely if infants were given fewer than two bottles per week during the second to the sixth week postpartum.[49] A study in Switzerland, however, showed that at 6 months, there was no difference in breastfeeding incidence.[50] Both of these studies have notable limitations. Any future trials need to find ways to study the effect of the supplement (filling the newborn's stomach) apart from the effect of sucking the teat, and this will be difficult. Multiple studies have shown short-term and long-term adverse outcomes that can be directly attributed to

artificial teats, however, including dental malocclusion, dental caries, and otitis media.

Nipples

Although there are several variations, three basic styles of artificial nipples are available: standard, preterm, and Nuk. (There are also specialized styles.) The styles differ from one another in shape, size, consistency (malleability), distensibility (ability to elongate when sucked), and the size and configuration of the nipple hole. (The nipple hole may be plain or crosscut, and some holes are larger than others.) Most artificial nipples are less compressible than the human nipple.[51]

Any claim that an artificial nipple is "just like mother" is false. Although one artificial nipple can deliver milk posteriorly to the foramen cecum region of the tongue and can elongate 120% from its resting state, the human nipple elongates 200% from its resting state.[52] Often, consumers and health care providers promote the Nuk type of nipple (Fig. 16-2) for breastfed infants, but in one expert's words, "The Nuk type . . . is promoted as being similar in shape to the human nipple, but the functional superiority of these nipples is yet to be proved."[53] Mothers often need to experiment a bit to find a nipple that works well for their individual infant. Mothers may perceive that some artificial nipples are better than others, but *different* would be a more appropriate descriptor than *better*.

One study examined different nipple units to evaluate the milk flow characteristics of artificial nipples on the market. An apparatus was set up to mimic infant sucking, and two different amounts of negative pressure were tested. Preterm nipple units required fewer "sucks" than the standard nipple units to yield the same amount of milk. Nuk nipple units required more "sucks" than the standard nipple units. Larger nipple holes and greater distensibility resulted in greater milk flow rate. However, the nipple unit itself was only one part of the equation in the evaluation of the nipple unit; the amount of negative pressure exerted was the other part of the equation. When the amount of negative pressure was doubled, the number of needed sucks decreased significantly.[54] Infants who suck a Nuk-style nipple have a very different sucking style than those sucking standard nipples.[55]

Before the advent of the Baby-Friendly Hospital Initiative, healthy, term breastfed newborns were routinely given artificial nipples atop formula bottles when they were supplemented. Nipple confusion, although not a term fully accepted by the medical community, may hinder successful breastfeeding for term or preterm newborns.[56] However, there is evidence that jaw development is hindered by bottle-feeding; masseter muscle activity is significantly reduced in bottle-fed infants who are 2 to 6 months old.[57]

Infants who have difficulty switching between the breast and bottle may benefit from a few simple strategies. Positioning the infant upright[59] using a reusable bottle (rather than a disposable bag), and a nipple that is round[51] and soft[58] can be helpful.[59] A high-flow nipple, which may be beneficial for either term or preterm bottle-feeding infants,[30,33,60] may be "confusing" for the breastfed infant who must adapt to a flow that is quite unlike the flow he experiences from the breast.[59]

Several special feeding devices with special nipples have been invented. A widely used one is the Haberman Feeder, as shown in Fig. 16-3. Multiple reports have described the usefulness of this device in infants with clefts, including in one recent experimental study.[61] I have used it more frequently in infants with neurologic defects.

In most cases, bottles and artificial nipples are not the ideal methods for delivering oral nutrition to infants, particularly preterm infants. Artificial bottles and nipples adversely affect vital signs, energy expen-

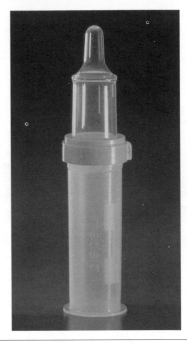

FIGURE **16-3** The Haberman feeder can be used for infants with cleft or other infants who have difficulty using a standard nipple. *(Courtesy Medela, Inc., McHenry, Ill.)*

diture, and potentially, other aspects of the infant's well-being. If direct breastfeeding is not possible, the first step is to develop a plan for moving toward direct breastfeeding. In the meantime, alternative strategies for delivering the feeding should be explored.

Alternatives to Bottles

Oral feedings of human milk or artificial milk can be given by a bottle or, preferably, by one of several alternative methods. Such methods have distinct advantages and disadvantages. One factor to especially consider is that of personal preference; some methods are considered awkward or undesirable simply because the nurse, mother, or other caregiver simply does not like to use them. The priority is to generate alternatives and to choose one that is most practical and least objectionable. When the pediatrician prescribes supplementation, he or she usually does not specify how it should be given, but it is important to muster his or her support for the method chosen. More often, it is the mother who has strong feelings about which method she uses. Ideally, after being pre-

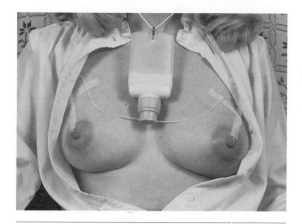

FIGURE **16-4** Supplemental Nursing System. *(Courtesy Medela, Inc., McHenry, Ill.)*

sented with multiple options, the mother should choose one method of supplementation, and the entire health care team should support that decision. It is counterproductive for several individuals to recommend or teach several methods; the mother is unlikely to choose or use any of them when seemingly conflicting recommendations are given.

Nursing Supplementers

Nursing supplementers are devices with tubes that are placed on the mother's nipple; the infant suckles both the human nipple and the tube. Hence, the infant who has a weak suck or who requires extra calories gets more reward for his efforts by using this device, which can be filled with either human milk or artificial milk.

The nursing supplementer may be useful for infants who have poor oral motor functions, such as those with neurologic impairments, because the flow of milk helps organize their suck/swallow reflex. It can also be used successfully for mothers who have a low milk supply because the infant is suckling the breast, which stimulates better production. This device can also be used for adoptive mothers. The most popular of these devices are the Supplemental Nursing System (Fig. 16-4) and the Starter Supplemental Nursing System by Medela and the Lact-Aid Nursing Trainer System by Lact-Aid International (Fig. 16-5). Although these devices are similar, they are not identical.

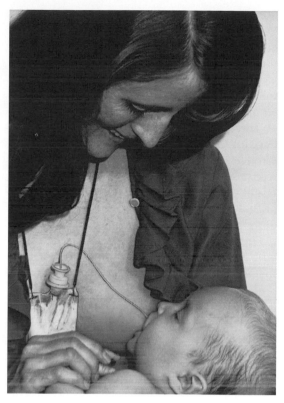

FIGURE **16-5** Lact-Aid Nursing Trainer System. *(Courtesy Jimmie Lynn Avery, Lact-Aid International, Athens, Tenn.)*

Most notably, the Lact-Aid Training System has a collapsible bag, which is usually positioned so that its bottom is below the infant's chin. (The device may also be hung so that gravity assists in milk delivery for special circumstances.) Thus the infant obtains milk without having to overcome the vacuum created in a rigid container. By using the collapsible bag, pressure is the same as atmospheric pressure. There is one tube coming from the container, and it is available in one size. It does not have to be positioned in the exact center of the infant's lower lip. Instructions are included for adjusting flow to accommodate more viscous artificial milk.

The Supplemental Nursing System uses a rigid container and is hung from the mother's neck. There are two tubes coming from the container: one to the right breast and one to the left. The one not in use is clamped off while the one going to the infant remains open. Thus milk flows by the negative pressure exerted by the infant, with assistance from gravity. The device comes with tubes of three different sizes; the larger tubes better accommodate the thicker viscosity of artificial milk. The tube to the infant should be positioned in the center of his lower lip.

These devices offer many advantages, as outlined in Table 16-1. Most important, the infant can receive human milk and the mother's breast can receive stimulation. Furthermore, the flow of milk from the device actually stimulates the suck/swallow response. Swallowing is really a continuation of the sucking reflex. Hence, in situations in which the infant is unable to organize this suck/swallow response with the breast only, or only when the mother has a milk-ejection response, the nursing supplementer may help to better organize the infant's response.

The major disadvantage is that mothers may consider the device somewhat of a nuisance to get on and off. The Lact-Aid is somewhat less obtrusive, whereas it may be difficult or impossible to camouflage the Supplemental Nurser System under the woman's clothing. Some practical problems can arise in using the supplementer. Potential problems, as well as possible solutions, are listed in Table 16-3. Furthermore, the nursing supplementer should not serve as a substitute for good breastfeeding management.

Cup-Feeding

Cup-feeding has become popular in the last few years, but its use dates back several decades.[62,63] More recent reports have shown that it has been

Table 16-3   POTENTIAL PROBLEMS AND SOLUTIONS WITH SUPPLEMENTAL DEVICES

Possible Problem	Possible Strategies
Infant rejects tube because he has previously been fed with a nasogastric tube and responds to the noxious presence of the tube	Try kangaroo care before trying the nursing supplementer; this will give the infant a sense of familiarity with being near the breast, smelling the milk, etc. Pull the tube up slightly so that infant is able to feel the breast first
Difficulty getting milk to drip well	Ask mother to first practice (without the infant) using water in the system Other suggestions include the following: • Check for any blockage in system • Determine whether this is the right size tubing • Adjust the height according to the flow desired
Breast skin breakdown; tape on skin	Lact-Aid generally does not require tape; for Supplemental Nursing System use paper tape (hair-setting tape found in most drugstores also works well and is inexpensive) Applying a warm cloth to the skin after removing the tape may be soothing
Formula too thick to go through tubing	For Supplemental Nursing System use largest size tubing For Lact-Aid refer to instructions included with the device Devise a makeshift supplementary system: use a no. 5 feeding tube; tape to mother's nipple and attach other end to syringe; slowly push formula through the tube with the syringe Determine whether infant can have human milk for one feeding instead of artificial milk
Infant unable to suck tube successfully (e.g., has cleft palate)	For Lact-Aid see product instructions for gravity-assisted flow

successful in preterm infants, including preterm twins[64] and those with cleft defects.[65] Less mature infants "lap" the milk, whereas the more mature infants "sip" the milk.[65] Cup-feeding can begin quite early; one report described an infant of 29 weeks of gestation, whose birth weight was 900 g, as using the cup successfully.[66] A very recent descriptive study looked at the lapping and sipping mechanisms used by preterm infants during cup-feeding, as well as their ability to coordinate milk intake with breathing.[67] The authors state, "Our findings that breathing and oxygen saturation remain stable during bursts of laps and sips suggests that cup-feeding as performed in this study is safe for preterm infants" (p. 17). They caution, however, that spillage can be a potential problem. Although they question if cup-feeding is "an optimal technique for facilitating breastfeeding in preterm infants" they did not compare it against or suggest alternatives.

Not surprisingly, one study showed that breast-feeding is less physiologically stressful than cup-feeding.[68] Curiously, the investigators concluded that cup feeding "should not be considered a safe or simple feeding method in respect to preterm infants," but this conclusion cannot be reasonably drawn from the data collected for the study. (They did not compare cup-feeding with other non-breastfeeding options, for example, bottle-feeding.)

When compared with bottle-feeding, cup-feeding is less physiologically stressful and offers other advantages as well. A carefully conducted study by Howard and colleagues was most impressive[69] (see Research Highlight box). They showed that cup-feeding provided more physiologic stability (heart rate, respiratory rate, and oxygen saturation) compared with bottle-feeding. A later study confirmed this.[70] Length of stay is reduced for infants who cup-feed.[71] Preterm newborns are more likely to be exclusively breastfeeding at discharge when they have been cup-fed rather than bottle-fed.[65]

Oddly, well-respected, knowledgeable breast-feeding experts have dismissed cup-feeding as being based on "ideology" while not mentioning the existing evidence.[72] At least one prominent nursing organization has taken a stand against cup-feeding by misinterpreting the available study results. Skeptics should read and interpret the existing studies carefully, thinking of both the subjects and the methodology used. For example, study results for healthy, term infants[69,71] cannot necessarily be used as a basis for care of the preterm infants, and vice versa. Similarly, one study explicitly said that the milk was "poured" into the infant's mouth. This practice, presumed to be physiologically stressful, is not recommended by clinical experts.[73]

There are some problems with cup-feeding, however. Spillage has been reported as a problem[74,75] but may be correctable with adequate staff education. A protocol, based on related research, has been developed for using cup-feeding in the neonatal intensive care setting[76]; Table 16-4 suggests appropriate assessments, contraindications, implementation, and evaluation for cup-feeding. Cup-feeding the newborn is a simple procedure, as shown in Fig. 16-6; Appendix B lists resources for the how-to. The key is for the infant, not the caregiver, to control the rate at which the feeding is given.

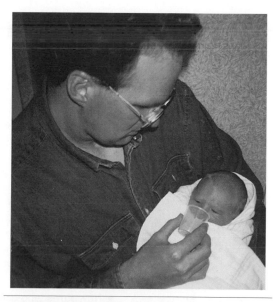

FIGURE **16-6** Cup-feeding. *(Courtesy Martha Schult, Boise, Idaho.)*

Syringe

A variety of syringes can be used to give oral feedings. Any syringe can be filled with artificial or human milk and then squirted slowly and gently into the newborn's mouth, allowing time for infant swallowing. An appropriate-sized syringe should be used to accommodate the amount of milk that the newborn is anticipated or required to consume. For example, a very preterm infant may consume only a few milliliters of colostrum, so a 3-ml syringe would work well. A preterm infant who is required to consume at least 18 ml per feeding could be fed with a 20-ml syringe. Similar to the regular syringe found at the nurse's station, an Asepto-type syringe can also be used. It is consid-erably larger and therefore more useful for a term infant who is unable to breastfeed but is capable of consuming 50 ml in a feeding. A piece of pediatric catheter tubing attached to the end of any syringe is sometimes helpful. The caregiver is in control of this method of feeding, however, and must be extremely cautious not to overwhelm the infant with too much volume.

Periodontal syringes, with a curved end (Fig. 16-7) improve the "aim" of the caregiver but offer no other distinct advantage and are not designed for nutritional purposes. Occasionally, some hospitals require a written physician's order for using the periodontal syringe, although this is often not the case.

Table 16-4   SAMPLE PROTOCOL: CUP-FEEDING A NEWBORN

Title: Cup-Feeding a Newborn
Purpose: To provide human milk or artificial milk (formula) to a newborn who has a weak or inadequate suck or who is separated from his mother
Level: Independent; does not require a physician's order for implementation
Supportive Data: Clinical cases and research studies show that cup-feeding improves the likelihood that newborns will be exclusively breastfeeding at time of hospital discharge. This alternative to bottle-feeding is noninvasive, and although research is ongoing, thus far cup-feeding has not been shown to have any adverse effects for either term or preterm infants.
Contents

Key Words	Nursing/Clinical Care
Initial Assessment	**General** • Any infant who can tolerate oral feedings is a potential candidate for cup-feeding. This includes both breastfed and bottle-fed newborns. • A newborn does not necessarily need to "prove himself" by sucking a rubber nipple or suckling a breast before the initiation of cup-feeding. Feeding cues are a signal for cup-feedings. • The infant must have a gag reflex present and tongue movement. **The Term Infant** • Any infant whose mother is unavailable for breastfeeding. • When infant requires feeding or supplement for medical reasons, as determined by the physician. **The Preterm Infant** • Demonstrates coordination of lips/tongue and swallowing, but does not need to coordinate bottle sucking with swallow before cup-feeding is initiated. Initiate at nurse's discretion. **Other Situations** • Newborns who cannot form an adequate seal, exert adequate suction, or suck effectively (at the breast or with the bottle) may use cup-feeding. This may include newborns with clefts or other defects.

Table 16-4 SAMPLE PROTOCOL: CUP-FEEDING A NEWBORN—CONT'D

Contraindications	• Any newborn who is likely to aspirate is not a candidate for cup-feeding. Newborns with a poor gag reflex, those who are lethargic in general, or others who have marked neurologic deficits should be excluded. • Newborns who are less than 35 weeks of gestation should be evaluated on a case-by-case basis for respiratory and other conditions that may affect safety.
Ongoing Assessment and Implementation	• Cup can contain human milk, human milk with fortifiers, or artificial milk. • Use in conjunction with nasogastric or orogastric feeding, as appropriate. • Wrap infant securely to prevent his hands from interfering with the cup. • Support infant in an upright position. • Tip cup so cup just touches lips. • *Do not pour:* Allow the rim of the cup to touch or rest on lower lip, tip the cup, and wait for the infant to sip. Do not apply pressure to lower lip. • Allow infant to set the pace. Do not offer more until infant swallows.
Evaluation	• Determine whether infant consumes required number of milliliters each feeding (if ordered). • If the infant refuses cup-feeding (or is "not interested"), consider gavage. • Check for spillage on the bib or clothing.
Documentation	• Record volume consumed "via cup" on infant Kardex.
References	List four or fewer references that you and your colleagues believe best substantiate the protocol you create.

1. _____
2. _____
3. _____
4. _____

Approval/review/revision
Person, title, and/or committee _____ Approval date _____ By _____
Revision date (date last reviewed) _____ Anticipated review date _____

Distribution
Persons receiving copies _____
Location _____

Modified from Biancuzzo M. *Mother Baby Journal* 1997;2:27-33.

Finger-Feeding

Finger-feeding is a method in which the mother or other caregiver allows the infant to suck on a finger while food is being delivered, as shown in Fig. 16-8. It can be accomplished using a periodontal syringe or a feeding tube.

How or if finger-feeding is implemented is a matter of personal preference and dexterity. Some clinicians prefer this method because it does offer advantages, including clear sensory signals to the trigeminal nerve via the hard palate.[77] I have never become comfortable with finger-feeding because I am unable to simultaneously hold the infant, keep a stiff finger in the infant's mouth, and regulate the syringe.

Perhaps an easy way to accomplish finger-feeding is to attach a feeding tube to a finger of the caregiver's dominant hand and instruct her to insert it, pad side up, toward the infant's palate. In this way, the infant can use his tongue in an undulating motion to suck (on a finger) and swallow about every third suck as the caregiver delivers about 0.5 ml of milk. The infant should not exert suction on the tube; the idea is to have a troughed

RESEARCH HIGHLIGHT

Cups Are a Good Alternative to Bottles; Direct Breastfeeding Best

Citation: Howard CR, de Blieck EA, ten Hoopen CB et al. Physiologic stability of newborns during cup- and bottle-feeding. *Pediatrics* 1999;104:1204-1207.

FOCUS

This comparative study reminds clinicians that cup-feeding may or may not be a way to prevent so-called nipple confusion. The phenomenon of nipple confusion has not been clearly established, and if such a phenomenon does exist, it is only one of many factors that should be considered when deciding how to best administer a feeding. This is the first randomized trial to measure the physiologic stability of infants fed by cup in comparison with those fed by bottle, aged 1 to 3 days. Nurses administered artificial milk from a cup ($N = 51$) or a bottle ($N = 47$) to newborns 1 to 3 days old while mothers breastfed their own 1- to 3-day-old infants ($N = 25$). Heart rate, respiratory rate, and oxygen saturation rates were monitored in all of the infants. Investigators also measured the amounts ingested and the length of time it took to complete the feedings.

RESULTS

There was no significant difference in heart rates, respiratory rates, or oxygen saturation rates between the cup-fed and the bottle-fed groups. The breastfed infants, however, had significantly better heart rates, respiratory rates, and oxygen saturation rates. Quite apart from the physiologic data, this study also showed that newborns who cup-fed ingested as much and in about the same amount of time as those who were bottle-fed. Breastfed newborns spent more time during their feeding.

STRENGTHS, LIMITATIONS OF THE STUDY

The authors point out that a possible limitation of the study is that the mothers held and fed infants at the breast, whereas nurses fed the artificially fed infants. More important, however, one might wonder if the artificial milk influenced results because a previous study has shown that artificial milk itself contributes to less physiologic stability.[37]

CLINICAL APPLICATION

It was not surprising to find that these healthy, term infants were generally more physiologically stable when breastfeeding than when feeding by a bottle because previous studies have shown this to be true with preterm infants.[34,35] Unfortunately, many clinicians have had difficulty creating hospital protocols to support the use of a cup because of the fears that cup-feeding is unsafe.[76] Interestingly, bottle-feeding has never come under such scrutiny, and this study has shown bottle-feeding is no more physiologically advantageous than cup-feeding.

Modified from Biancuzzo M. *Breastfeeding Outlook* 2000;1:6.

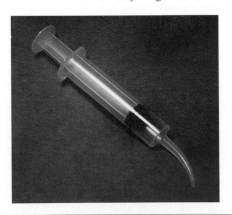

FIGURE **16-7** Periodontal syringe.

tongue much like breastfeeding. (If the infant does not first lower and then trough his tongue, apply slight downward pressure on the posterior part of the tongue, then release.) As the infant sucks, the caregiver can gently push about 0.5 ml of milk from the attached syringe into the infant's mouth about every third suck. The feeding should be unhurried and should continue for about 20 to 30 minutes.

Other Devices

Various other devices have been used for supplementing infants. Medicine droppers work fairly well for newborns. They offer the advantage of easy handling and a way to measure the volume given, and

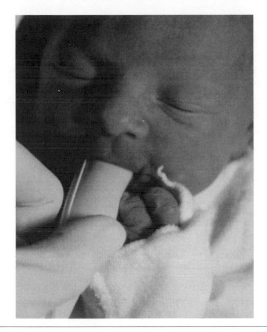

FIGURE **16-8** Finger-feeding. *(Copyright Debi Bocar, Lactation Consultant Services, Oklahoma City, Okla.)*

they can be easily sterilized in the autoclave if hospital policy requires them to be sterile. A disadvantage is that they do not provide the infant with much, if any, tactile stimulation to the oral cavity, and they may limit the infant's ability to control the feeding.

Variations of the spoon have also been used, including the Rosti bottle, used in the United Kingdom, and the SoftFeeder (Fig. 16-9), manufactured by Medela. Both have a spoonlike device at the end of a handle and are convenient for administering feedings. Alternative feeding devices help to uphold the World Health Organization's directive to "give no artificial bottles or teats,"[78] as discussed in Chapter 8.

THE TRANSITION TO DIRECT AND EXCLUSIVE BREASTFEEDING

The aim of this book has been to provide strategies that facilitate direct breastfeeding for the newborn. It seems fitting, therefore, to realize that although sick infants may initially have no oral feedings, or have indirect feedings, the whole idea is to help them make the transition from gavage feedings to breastfeedings, or from nonsuckling oral methods to direct suckling at the breast. Interestingly, infants who have been supplemented by gavage, rather than by bottle, tend to have an increased likelihood of breastfeeding at discharge, 3 days, 3 months, and 6 months.[79]

Parents may want to know how long it will take infants before they can suckle at the breast. This tends to vary; it will take longer for newborns who

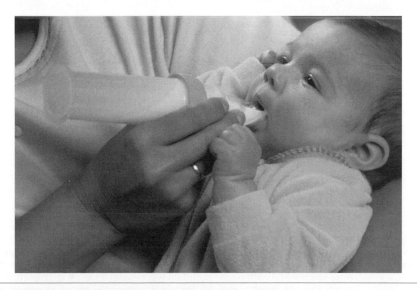

FIGURE **16-9** SoftFeeder. *(Courtesy Medela, Inc., McHenry, Ill.)*

have been especially ill.[80] Full nippling takes longer when it is limited by neurodevelopmental capacities, including respiratory control.[81]

In some cases infants may not have had oral feedings until 2 months after birth,[82] and this poses quite a challenge. When they eventually do have the opportunity to nipple feed, their ability to do so is not enhanced by having had prior exposure to the nonnutritive sucking of a pacifier. Sucking behavior does, however, improve with practice.[82] Usually, these sorts of situations occur with preterm infants,

and a detailed explanation of breastfeeding as a first oral experience is covered in Chapter 10.

All of the techniques for delivering nourishment described in this chapter are inferior to direct breastfeeding. Ideally, then, the situation of indirect breastfeeding or supplementing the infant with artificial milk should be considered temporary. A teaching plan for parents of preterm infants is presented in Chapter 10. A plan for the transition from indirect or supplemental feedings to exclusive direct feeding is found in Table 16-5.

Table **16-5** TRANSITION TO EXCLUSIVE DIRECT BREASTFEEDING

Nursing Responsibility	Clinical Strategy	Rationale
Determine readiness to breastfeed	Introduce breastfeedings before bottle-feedings	There is no need for an infant to "prove himself" by sucking a bottle before going to breast. Traditional criteria—arbitrary minimum weights, tolerance of bottle feedings, gestational age, stability of body temperature, or impending discharge—are not supported by scientific research. Ability to coordinate suckling and swallowing with minimal changes in cardiorespiratory response (bradycardia, apnea, hypoxemia) is the current criteria for initiating breastfeeding (until further research-based criteria are identified). Criteria for "breastfeeding" and "bottle-feeding" should be restated as ability to tolerate oral feedings.
Prepare infant for first direct breastfeedings	Teach infant to associate mother with feedings (e.g., place mother's breast pad in isolette)	Infant will begin to associate maternal odors with feedings (discourage use of perfume by parents).
	Remove nasogastric tube when doing oral feedings	This improves suckling efforts
	Gavage with nipple in infant's mouth	Sucking improves oxygenation of infant. Infant associates suckling with satiety.
	Practice kangaroo care	Practice may be associated with increased weight gains.[24-26] Increases mother's confidence in holding infant. Increases infant's familiarity with mother's breast and nipple. Nuzzling previously pumped breast before planned feedings optimizes experience. Diminishes the "event" atmosphere of first feeding. Reduces mother's anxiety.
	Maximize mother's milk production before first feedings	Easier for infant to transfer milk with an abundant milk supply compared with milk trickling from breast. If milk flows too forcefully, pump 2-3 minutes before feeding to reduce flow rate.
	Gently stimulate lips and mouth	Stimulating mouth and lips (e.g., having parent perform mouth care) helps infant become aware of his oral cavity. Avoiding bottle nipples reduces possibility of infant developing confusion between breast and bottle nipples.
Initiate first feedings	Establish reasonable expectations—tolerating the positioning and opening wide may be only expectation for very first feed	Parents almost always have expectations that infant will breastfeed like a champion the very first time. Helping the parent to anticipate small gains encourages rather than disappoints them.

Table **16-5** TRANSITION TO EXCLUSIVE DIRECT BREASTFEEDING—CONT'D

Nursing Responsibility	Clinical Strategy	Rationale
	Provide reassurance and optimal environment	Staying with mother and giving help optimizes feeding interactions.
		Providing warm, comfortable, private location free from visual and auditory distractions and drafts helps with maternal relaxation (and hence milk ejection) and helps stabilize infants' vital signs and temperature.
	Position the mother; use footstool and pillows as appropriate	Comfortable position that facilitates good alignment, areolar grasp, areolar compression, and audible swallowing, as described in Chapter 7, facilitates milk transfer.
	Stimulate infant-use alerting techniques (see Chapter 7)	Helps infant to be in an optimal state for feeding.
	Maintain thermoneutral environment; monitor infant temperature according to unit protocol	Mother's breasts are warmer than the rest of her body.
		If necessary, supplemental heat (overhead warmer, heat lamp) can be used to increase ambient temperature during the feeding experience.
	Use most optimal position for infant	"Nesting" infant with physical boundaries (e.g., pillows, towel rolls) helps hypotonic infant maintain postural control and conserve energy.
		Transitional hold allows for good control of infant and good visibility of preterm or hypotonic infant.
	Cue the infant to suckle	Gently touching the lips with the nipple helps the infant open wide.
	Entice infant to suck • Express milk onto lips • Elicit milk-ejection reflex • Offer breast with easier flow first • Instill a *few* drops of milk in the infant's mouth via feeding tube to elicit suckle-swallow reflex	Gentle perioral stimulation before infant is ready for first feed, as described above, helps infant become aware of his oral cavity. The suckle-swallow reflex is a chained response. By having the milk readily available and in abundant supply, the infant is more likely to get into the rhythm of the chained suckle-swallow response.
	Monitor infant physiologic responses to breastfeeding	Alterations in heart rate, respiratory rate, oxygen saturation, body temperature, color (especially perioral cyanosis) are signs of distress.
	Determine whether milk transfer is occurring	Infants can suck without actually obtaining milk. A reassuring sign is when infants have audible swallowing. Perform prefeeding and postfeeding weight assessments.
	Continue feeding, unless otherwise indicated	Unless the infant shows signs of fatigue or stress cues, the feeding may be continued until he is satiated. Allowing infants to rest can be restorative. Interrupting a feeding on the "first" side may result in cessation of breastfeeding for that session.
Facilitate transition to cue-based feeding	Develop nursery protocols that support cue-based feedings before discharge	Term infants consume more milk and grow faster when fed frequently and in response to hunger cues. Preterm infant may be on "modified" cue-based feeding plan (see Chapter 10). Cue-based feedings in the hospital help prepare mothers and infants for cue-based feedings at home

Source: Bocar D. *Breastfeeding educator resource notebook.* Oklahoma City, OK: Lactation Consultant Services; 1998.

SUMMARY

Ideally, all infants will breastfeed directly and exclusively. In circumstances when they do not, however, alternative methods for delivering nourishment must be explored. Ideally, the nourishment delivered should be human milk, but artificial milk may be given if desired or medically indicated. Multiple devices, each having its own advantages and disadvantages, can be used to give nourishment to the infant who is not exclusively breastfeeding.

REFERENCES

1. World Health Organization. Acceptable medical reasons for supplementation. Baby-Friendly Hospital Initiative: Part II: hospital-level implementation. Promoting breast-feeding in health facilities. A short course for administrators and policy-makers. Geneva: WHO; 1996.
2. Frantz KB. The slow-gaining breastfeeding infant. *NAACOGS Clin Iss Perinat Womens Health Nurs* 1992;3:647-655.
3. Pinchasik D. From TPN to breast feeding—feeding the premature infant—2000: Part I. Parenteral nutrition. *Am J Perinatol* 2001;18:59-72.
4. Newell SJ. Enteral feeding of the micropremie. *Clin Perinatol* 2000;27:221-234.
5. Simmer K, Metcalf R, Daniels L. The use of breastmilk in a neonatal unit and its relationship to protein and energy intake and growth. *J Paediatr Child Health* 1997;33:55-60.
6. Grant J, Denne SC. Effect of intermittent versus continuous enteral feeding on energy expenditure in premature infants. *J Pediatr* 1991;118:928-932.
7. Silvestre MA, Morbach CA, Brans YW et al. A prospective randomized trial comparing continuous versus intermittent feeding methods in very low birth weight neonates. *J Pediatr* 1996;128:748-752.
8. Poets CF, Langner MU, Bohnhorst B. Effects of bottle feeding and two different methods of gavage feeding on oxygenation and breathing patterns in preterm infants. *Acta Paediatr* 1997;86:419-423.
9. Blondheim O, Abbasi S, Fox WW et al. Effect of enteral gavage feeding rate on pulmonary functions of very low birth weight infants. *J Pediatr* 1993;122:751-755.
10. Brooke OG, Barley J. Loss of energy during continuous infusions of breast milk. *Arch Dis Child* 1978;53:344-345.
11. Greer FR, McCormick A, Loker J. Changes in fat concentration of human milk during delivery by intermittent bolus and continuous mechanical pump infusion. *J Pediatr* 1984;105:745-749.
12. Stocks RJ, Davies DP, Allen F et al. Loss of breast milk nutrients during tube feeding. *Arch Dis Child* 1985;60:164-166.
13. Bhatia J, Rassin DK. Human milk supplementation. Delivery of energy, calcium, phosphorus, magnesium, copper, and zinc. *Am J Dis Child* 1988;142:445-447.
14. Narayanan I, Singh B, Harvey D. Fat loss during feeding of human milk. *Arch Dis Child* 1984;59:475-477.
15. Mehta NR, Hamosh M, Bitman J et al. Adherence of medium-chain fatty acids to feeding tubes during gavage feeding of human milk fortified with medium-chain triglycerides. *J Pediatr* 1988;112:474-476.
16. Rayol MR, Martinez FE, Jorge SM et al. Feeding premature infants banked human milk homogenized by ultrasonic treatment. *J Pediatr* 1993;123:985-988.
17. Brennan-Behm M, Carlson GE, Meier P et al. Caloric loss from expressed mother's milk during continuous gavage infusion. *Neonatal Netw* 1994;13:27-32.
18. Lucas A, Gibbs JA, Lyster RL et al. Creamatocrit: simple clinical technique for estimating fat concentration and energy value of human milk. *Br Med J* 1978;1:1018-1020.
19. Lemons JA, Schreiner RL, Gresham EL. Simple method for determining the caloric and fat content of human milk. *Pediatrics* 1980;66:626-628.
20. Griffin TL, Meier PP, Bradford LP et al. Mothers' performing creamatocrit measures in the NICU: accuracy, reactions, and cost. *J Obstet Gynecol Neonatal Nurs* 2000;29:249-257.
21. Lemons PM, Miller K, Eitzen H et al. Bacterial growth in human milk during continuous feeding. *Am J Perintol* 1983;1:76-80.
22. Botsford KB, Weinstein RA, Boyer KM et al. Gram-negative bacilli in human milk feedings: quantitation and clinical consequences for premature infants. *J Pediatr* 1986;109:707-710.
23. Patchell CJ, Anderton A, Holden C et al. Reducing bacterial contamination of enteral feeds. *Arch Dis Child* 1998;78:166-168.
24. Bernbaum JC, Pereira GR, Watkins JB et al. Nonnutritive sucking during gavage feeding enhances growth and maturation in premature infants. *Pediatrics* 1983;71:41-45.
25. Field T, Ignatoff E, String ES et al. Nonnutritive sucking during tube feedings: effects on preterm neonates in an intensive care unit. *Pediatrics* 1982;70:381-384.
26. Ernst JA, Rickard KA, Neal PR et al. Lack of improved growth outcome related to nonnutritive sucking in very low birth weight premature infants fed a controlled nutrient intake: a randomized prospective study. *Pediatrics* 1989;83:706-716.
27. DiPietro JA, Cusson RM, Caughy MO et al. Behavioral and physiologic effects of nonnutritive sucking during gavage feeding in preterm infants. *Pediatr Res* 1994;36:207-214.
28. Narayanan I, Mehta R, Choudhury DK et al. Sucking on the 'emptied' breast: non-nutritive sucking with a difference. *Arch Dis Child* 1991;66:241-244.
29. Shiao SY. Comparison of continuous versus intermittent sucking in very-low-birth-weight infants. *J Obstet Gynecol Neonatal Nurs* 1997;26:313-319.

30. Lau C, Schanler RJ. Oral feeding in premature infants: advantage of a self-paced milk flow. *Acta Paediatr* 2000;89:453-459.

31. Farber SD, VanFossen RL, Koontz SW. Quantitative and qualitative video analysis of infant feeding: angled and straight-bottle feeding systems. *J Pediatr* 1995;126:S188-S124.

32. Lau C, Sheena HR, Shulman RJ et al. Oral feeding in low birth weight infants. *J Pediatr* 1997;130:561-569.

33. Schrank W, Al-Sayed LE, Beahm PH et al. Feeding responses to free-flow formula in term and preterm infants. *J Pediatr* 1998;132:426-430.

34. Meier P. Bottle- and breast-feeding: effects on transcutaneous oxygen pressure and temperature in preterm infants. *Nurs Res* 1988;37:36-41.

35. Blaymore Bier JA, Ferguson AE, Morales Y et al. Breastfeeding infants who were extremely low birth weight. *Pediatrics* 1997;100:E3.

36. Chen CH, Wang TM, Chang HM et al. The effect of breast- and bottle-feeding on oxygen saturation and body temperature in preterm infants. *J Hum Lact* 2000;16:21-27.

37. Butte NF, Smith EO, Garza C. Heart rates of breast-fed and formula-fed infants. *J Pediatr Gastroenterol Nutr* 1991;13:391-396.

38. Cohen M, Witherspoon M, Brown DR et al. Blood pressure increases in response to feeding in the term neonate. *Dev Psychobiol* 1992;25:291-298.

39. Mizuno K, Inoue M, Takeuchi T. The effects of body positioning on sucking behaviour in sick neonates. *Eur J Pediatr* 2000;159:827-831.

40. Mathew OP, Bhatia J. Sucking and breathing patterns during breast- and bottle-feeding in term neonates. Effects of nutrient delivery and composition. *Am J Dis Child* 1989;143:588-592.

41. Brown CE, Magnuson B. On the physics of the infant feeding bottle and middle ear sequela: ear disease in infants can be associated with bottle feeding. *Int J Pediatr Otorhinolaryngol* 2000;54:13-20.

42. Lau C, Hurst N. Oral feeding in infants. *Curr Probl Pediatr* 1999;29:105-124.

43. Lau C, Alagugurusamy R, Schanler RJ et al. Characterization of the developmental stages of sucking in preterm infants during bottle feeding. *Acta Paediatr* 2000;89:846-852.

44. Palmer MM. Identification and management of the transitional suck pattern in premature infants. *J Perinat Neonat Nurs* 1993;7:66-75.

45. Palmer MM, VandenBerg KA. A closer look at neonatal sucking. *Neonatal Netw* 1998;17:77-79.

46. Hill AS, Kurkowski TB, Garcia J. Oral support measures used in feeding the preterm infant. *Nurs Res* 2000;49:2-10.

47. Pickler RH, Frankel HB, Walsh KM et al. Effects of nonnutritive sucking on behavioral organization and feeding performance in preterm infants. *Nurs Res* 1996;45:132-135.

48. Shaker CS. Nipple feeding preterm infants: an individualized, developmentally supportive approach. *Neonatal Netw* 1999;18:15-22.

49. Cronenwett L, Stukel T, Kearney M et al. Single daily bottle use in the early weeks postpartum and breast-feeding outcomes. *Pediatrics* 1992;90:760-766.

50. Schubiger G, Schwarz U, Tonz O. UNICEF/WHO baby-friendly hospital initiative: does the use of bottles and pacifiers in the neonatal nursery prevent successful breastfeeding? Neonatal Study Group. *Eur J Pediatr* 1997;156:874-877.

51. Nowak AJ, Smith WL, Erenberg A. Imaging evaluation of artificial nipples during bottle feeding. *Arch Pediatr Adolesc Med* 1994;148:40-42.

52. Nowak AJ, Smith WL, Erenberg A. Imaging evaluation of breast-feeding and bottle-feeding systems. *J Pediatr* 1995;126:S130-S134.

53. Mathew OP. Science of bottle feeding. *J Pediatr* 1991;114:511-519.

54. Mathew OP. Nipple units for newborn infants: a functional comparison. *Pediatrics* 1988;81:688-691.

55. Sakashita R, Kamegai T, Inoue N. Masseter muscle activity in bottle feeding with the chewing type bottle teat: evidence from electromyographs. *Early Hum Dev* 1996;45:83-92.

56. Neifert M, Lawrence R, Seacat J. Nipple confusion: toward a formal definition. *J Pediatr* 1995;126:S125-S129.

57. Inoue N, Sakashita R, Kamegai T. Reduction of masseter muscle activity in bottle-fed babies. *Early Human Dev* 1995;42:185-193.

58. Palmer B. The influence of breastfeeding on the development of the oral cavity: a commentary. *J Hum Lact* 1998;14:93-98.

59. Kassing D. Bottle-feeding as a tool to reinforce breastfeeding. *J Hum Lact* 2002;18:56-60.

60. Walden E, Prendergast J. Comparison of flow rates of holes versus cross-cut teats for bottle-fed babies. *Prof Care Mother Child* 2000;10:7-8.

61. Turner L, Jacobsen C, Humenczuk M et al. The effects of lactation education and a prosthetic obturator appliance on feeding efficiency in infants with cleft lip and palate. *Cleft Palate Craniofac J* 2001;38:519-524.

62. Davis HV, Sears RR, Miller HC et al. Effects of cup, bottle and breast feeding on oral activities of newborn infants. *Pediatrics* 1948;2:549-558.

63. Fredeen RC. Cup feeding of newborn infants. *Pediatrics* 1948;2:544-548.

64. Biancuzzo M. Breastfeeding preterm twins: a case report. *Birth* 1994;21:96-100.

65. Lang S, Lawrence CJ, Orme RL. Cup feeding: an alternative method of infant feeding. *Arch Dis Child* 1994;71:365-369.

66. Gupta A, Khanna K, Chattree S. Cup feeding: an alternative to bottle feeding in a neonatal intensive care unit. *J Trop Pediatr* 1999;45:108-110.

67. Dowling DA, Meier PP, DiFiore JM et al. Cup-feeding for preterm infants: mechanics and safety. *J Hum Lact* 2002;18:13-20.

68. Freer Y. A comparison of breast and cup feeding in preterm infants: effect on physiological parameters. *J Neonat Nursing* 1999;5:16-21.

69. Howard CR, de Blieck EA, ten Hoopen CB et al. Physiologic stability of newborns during cup- and bottle-feeding. *Pediatrics* 1999;104:1204-1207.

70. Marinelli KA, Burke GS, Dodd VL. A comparison of the safety of cupfeedings and bottlefeedings in premature infants whose mothers intend to breastfeed. *J Perinatol* 2001;21:350-355.

71. Brown SJ, Alexander J, Thomas P. Feeding outcome in breast-fed term babies supplemented by cup or bottle. *Midwifery* 1999;15:92-96.

72. Meier PP. Breastfeeding in the special care nursery. Prematures and infants with medical problems. *Pediatr Clin North Am* 2001;48:425-442.

73. Kuehl J. Cup feeding the newborn: what you should know. *J Perinat Neonatal Nurs* 1997;11:56-60.

74. Dowling DA. Physiological responses of preterm infants to breast-feeding and bottle-feeding with the orthodontic nipple. *Nurs Res* 1999;48:78-85.

75. Malhotra N, Vishwambaran L, Sundaram KR et al. A controlled trial of alternative methods of oral feeding in neonates. *Early Hum Dev* 1999;54:29-38.

76. Biancuzzo M. Creating and implementing a protocol for cup feeding. *Mother Baby Journal* 1997;2:27-33.

77. Hazelbaker AK. In defense of finger feeding. *Rental Roundup* 1997;14:10-11.

78. WHO and UNICEF. *Protecting, promoting, and supporting breast-feeding: the special role of maternity services.* Geneva: World Health Organization; 1989.

79. Kliethermes PA, Cross ML, Lanese MG et al. Transitioning preterm infants with nasogastric tube supplementation: increased likelihood of breastfeeding. *J Obstet Gynecol Neonatal Nurs* 1999;28:264-273.

80. Mandich M, Ritchie SK. Transition times to oral feeding in premature infants with and without apnea. *J Obstet Gynecol Neonatal Nurs* 1995;25:771-776.

81. Pridham K, Brown R, Sondel S et al. Transition time to full nipple feeding for premature infants with a history of lung disease. *J Obstet Gynecol Neonatal Nurs* 1998;27:533-545.

82. Mizuno K, Ueda A. Development of sucking behavior in infants who have not been fed for 2 months after birth. *Pediatr Int* 2001;43:251-255.

Appendixes

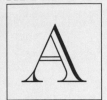

APPENDIX

A

Community Breastfeeding Support

This appendix provides a way to contact organizations that provide products or services that help mothers initiate or continue breastfeeding. Mothers have direct access to these organizations. Mention of these organizations does not constitute endorsement of their services or products by the author or the publisher. This list is not intended to be all-inclusive. Other local or national organizations may also be helpful to the breastfeeding mother.

A-1 *Support Groups for Parents*

La Leche League International

La Leche League International (LLLI), started by a group of breastfeeding women in 1957, continues today as an international organization that focuses on consumer support and advocacy for breastfeeding. LLLI also provides materials, continuing education, and products for professionals. There are more than 3500 local chapters in about 50 countries throughout the world. To contact local chapters, contact La Leche League International and ask for the chapter in your area.

La Leche League International
PO Box 4079
Schaumburg, IL 60168-4079
Phone: (847) 519-7730
Toll-free: (800) LALECHE
Fax: (847) 519-0035
Web site: http://www.lalecheleague.org

Cleft Palate Foundation

The Cleft Palate Foundation (CPF) was founded in 1973 by its parent, the American Cleft Palate–Craniofacial Association (ACPA), to be the public service arm of the professional association. CPF is a nonprofit organization that aims to enhance the quality of life for individuals with congenital facial deformities and their families through education, research support, and facilitation of family-centered care. CPF's major activities include the operation of CleftLine and the dissemination of CPF publications. To contact local chapters, call the following hotline, and ask for the chapter in your area.

The Cleft Palate Foundation
104 South Estes Dr., Suite 204
Chapel Hill, NC 27514
Phone: (919) 933-9044
Toll-free: (800) 24-CLEFT
Fax: (919) 933-9604
Web site: http://www.cleftline.org
E-mail: cleftline@aol.com

National Down Syndrome Society

The National Down Syndrome Society (NDSS) was established in 1979 to increase public awareness about Down syndrome, to assist families in addressing the needs of children born with this genetic condition, and to sponsor and encourage scientific research. NDSS supports research, sponsors symposia, advocates on behalf of families, provides information and referral services through their toll-free number, and develops and distributes educational materials.

National Down Syndrome Society
666 Broadway, 8th Floor
New York, NY 10012-2317
Phone: (212) 460-9330
Toll-free: (800) 221-4602
Fax: (212) 979-2873
Web site: http://www.ndss.org
E-mail: info@ndss.org

National Organization of Mothers of Twins Clubs

The National Organization of Mothers of Twins Clubs, Inc. (NOMOTC), was founded in 1960 to promote the special aspects of child development related specifically to multiple-birth children. NOMOTC is a network of about 475 local clubs, representing more than 21,000 individual parents of multiples. NOMOTC is funded by dues, donations, and grants.

National Organization of Mothers of Twins
  Clubs
PO Box 438
Thompsons Station, TN 37179-0438
Phone: (615) 595-0936
Toll-free: 877-540-2200
Web site: http://www.nomotc.org
E-mail: INFO@nomotc.org

Multiple Births Canada

Multiple Births Canada, formerly The Parents of Multiple Births Association of Canada, exists to improve the quality of life for multiple-birth individuals and families in Canada. With an extensive network of local chapters, health care professionals, and organizations, Multiple Births Canada is the source for information on multiple births in Canada. It is a nonprofit organization of parents of multiples across Canada.

Multiple Births Canada Business Office
PO Box 432
Wasaga Beach, Ontario L0L 2P0
Canada
Phone: (705) 429-0901
Toll-free (in Canada): (866) 228-8824
Fax: (705) 429-9809
Web site: http://www.multiplebirthscanada.org
E-mail: office@multiplebirthscanada.org

A-2 Equipment Companies

Many companies in the United States and abroad manufacture breast pumps and related equipment. Companies who provided photos for or whose product is mentioned in this book are listed here:

Bailey Medical Engineering
2216 Sunset Dr.
Los Osos, CA 93402
Phone: (805) 528-5781
Toll-free: (800) 413-3216
Fax: (805) 528-1461
Web site: http://www.baileymed.com
E-mail: folks@baileymed.com

Hollister
Customer Care Department
2000 Hollister Dr.
Libertyville, IL 60048
Phone: (847) 918-5882
Toll-free: (800) 323-4060
Web site: http://www.hollister.com

Kendall
15 Hampshire St.
Mansfield, MA 02048
Phone: (508) 261-8000
Toll-free: (877) GEL-DISCS
Fax: (508) 261-8271
Web site: http://www.kendallhq.com
E-mail: maternimates@owd.com

Lact-Aid International
PO Box 1066
Athens, TN 37371-1066
Phone: (423) 744-9090
Fax: (423) 744-9116
Web site: http://www.lact-aid.com
E-mail: orders@lact-aid.com

Maternal Concepts
130 S. Public St.
Elmwood, WI 54740
Phone: (715) 639-4050
Toll-free: (800) 310-5817
Fax: (715) 639-2435
Web site: http://www.maternalconcepts.com
E-mail: sales@maternalconcepts.com

Medela
PO Box 660
McHenry, IL 60051-0660
Phone: (815) 363-1166
Toll-free: (800) 435-8316
Toll-free fax: (800) 995-7867
Web site: http://www.medela.com
E-mail: customer.service@medela.com

Prolac Inc.
10 W. Genesee St.
PO Box 117
Skaneateles, NY 13152
Phone: (315) 685-1955
Toll-free: (888) 410-2547
Fax: (315) 685-6304
Web site: http://www.prolac.com
E-mail: sales@blis.com

Puronyx (Formerly, Maturna)
990 Park Center Dr., Suite E
Vista, CA 92083
Phone: (760) 597-1464
Toll-free: (800) 944-4006
Fax: (760) 597-1466
Web site: http://www.puronyx.com
E-mail: info@puronyx.com

White River Concepts
41715 Enterprise Circle North, Suite 204
Temecula, CA 92590
Phone: (909) 296-0081
Fax: (909) 296-0083
Web site: http://www.whiteriver.com
E-mail: custsvc@whiteriver.com

Whittlestone
PO Box 2237
Antioch, CA 94531
Phone: (707) 748-4010
Toll-free: (877) 608-6455
Fax: (707) 748-4193
Web site: http://www.whittlestone.com
E-mail: bmckendry@whittlestone.com

A-3 *Donor Human Milk Banks in North America*

A donor human milk bank is defined by the Human Milk Banking Association of North America (HMBANA) as a service established for the purpose of collecting, screening, processing, storing, and distributing donated human milk to meet the specific needs of individuals for whom human milk is prescribed by physicians. (Further information is given in Chapter 15.) Relatively few donor milk banks exist in North America; more are established in Europe. To find out how to become a donor or a recipient of human milk from a HMBANA bank, contact:

Human Milk Banking Association of
   North America*
Web site: http://www/hmbana.com

*Their web site provides contact information for the individual members of HMBANA.

APPENDIX

B

Parent Education Media

This appendix is designed to identify selected materials for parent education. Materials listed here can be obtained by contacting the respective publishers, producers, and distributors of these materials as listed in Appendix E, or—in the case of paperback books and some other material—by visiting a bookstore. Many items are available from vendors other than those listed; only vendors in the United States are listed here. The author welcomes suggestions about other places where these materials may be easily obtained. Readers or vendors may send comments to:

bookcomments@wmc-worldwide.com

All materials are in English; additional languages are listed. All videotapes are in NTSC for-mat; additional formats may be available. Materials listed in this appendix do not necessarily constitute endorsement by the author or the publisher, and this list is not intended to be all-inclusive. The author and the publisher have made every attempt to verify the information listed herein. However, availability is subject to change, and prices are approximate and in most cases do not include shipping and handling charges. The author has determined that the resources listed in this appendix are aimed primarily at a consumer audience but acknowledges that some of these materials may be helpful for professionals also.

B-1 *Motivating Women to Breastfeed*

The following audio, visual, and audiovisual materials are designed to motivate women to breastfeed by discussing benefits or debunking myths about breastfeeding. In general, these are most helpful when used during the prenatal period, but it is never too late to provide them.

Key words are listed to help the reader quickly focus on pertinent aspects of the education materials. All media listed are in English; every attempt is made to list other language versions when available. Prices are approximate and are subject to change; in addition, in most cases prices do not include shipping and handling.

Key Word/Target Population	Media	Length	Additional Languages	Author	Date
Advantages	Videotape	22 min		Best Start	1996
Advantages	Videotape	14 min	Spanish	Lawrence, RA	2001
Advantages	Pamphlet	Multifold	Spanish, Cambodian, Russian, French, Vietnamese	Health Education Associates	
Advantages	Pamphlet	Multifold		Health Education Associates	
Advantages	Pamphlet	Multifold		Health Education Associates	
Advantages	Pamphlet	Multifold		Health Education Associates	
Advantages	Pamphlet	Multifold	Spanish, Vietnamese	Health Education Associates	
Advantages	Pamphlet	Multifold		Health Education Associates	
Advantages	Videotape	22 min		Not listed	1999
Advantages	Book	62 pages	Creole, French, Spanish	Wiggins, PK	1995
Advantages	Videotape	19 min	Spanish	Not listed	1998
African-American	Videotape	14 min		Office of the Maryland WIC Program; features Anita Baker	1993
African-American	Videotape	14 min		Office of the Maryland WIC Program	1997
Allergies	Pamphlet	Multifold		Health Education Associates	
Anticipation	Book	128 pages		Cook, CB	2002
Cow's milk	Pamphlet	Multifold	Spanish	Health Education Associates	

Title	Publisher/Producer	Available from	Price
Loving Our Children, Loving Ourselves	Best Start	Best Start	$25
The Benefits of Breastfeeding	Eagle Video Productions Inc.	Eagle Video Productions Inc., LLLI	$59 plus $5 S&H
Breastfeeding: Best for Baby and You	Health Education Associates	Health Education Associates	$1 ≤24; quantity discounts available
Breastfeeding: It's More Than Just Food	Health Education Associates	Health Education Associates	$1 ≤24; quantity discounts available
Have You Thought about Breastfeeding?	Health Education Associates	Health Education Associates	$1 ≤24; quantity discounts available
Is It Worth It to Breastfeed?	Health Education Associates	Health Education Associates	$1 ≤24; quantity discounts available
Nursing Is Easy When You Know How	Health Education Associates	Health Education Associates	$1 ≤24; quantity discounts available
Why Do Mothers Breastfeed?	Health Education Associates	Health Education Associates	$1 ≤24; quantity discounts available
The Breastfeeding Game: Benefits (Volume 1)	InJoy	InJoy Videos	$224.80 for all 4 volumes
Why Should I Nurse My Baby?	L. A. Publishing	Bookstores, Publisher	$6; bulk rate available
Breastfeeding: Part I, Why-to	Vida Health Communications	Vida Health Communications	$195
Giving You the Best That I've Got, Baby	Maryland Dept. of Health and Mental Hygiene and Johns Hopkins University School of Public Health	Johns Hopkins Center for Communication	$20
Learning How to Breastfeed Your Baby	Maryland Dept. of Public Health and Mental Hygiene and Johns Hopkins University School of Public Health	Johns Hopkins Center for Communication	$15
Breastfeeding Advice for Families with Allergies	Health Education Associates	Health Education Associates	$1 ≤24; quantity discounts available
What to Expect When Breastfeeding	Random House, London	Bookstores	$13.95
No Cow's Milk in the First Year	Health Education Associates	Health Education Associates	$1 ≤24; quantity discounts available

Continued

Key Word/Target Population	Media	Length	Additional Languages	Author	Date
Embarrassment	Pamphlet	Bifold	Spanish, Native American	Best Start	1997
Family	Pamphlet	Multifold		Health Education Associates	
Family	Pamphlet	Multifold	Spanish	Health Education Associates	
Family, sexuality	Pamphlet	Multifold	Spanish	Health Education Associates	
Fathers	Videotape	8 min		Not listed	1999
Lifestyle	Pamphlet	Bifold	Native American, Spanish	Best Start	1997
Public health	Videotape	3 min		Spangler, A	1996
Support	Pamphlet	Bifold	Spanish, Native American	Best Start	1997
Teens	Videotape	22 min	Spanish	Best Start	1993
Teens	Pamphlet	Multifold		Health Education Associates	
Teens	Pamphlet	Multifold		Health Education Associates	
Teens	Videotape/ manual	20 min	Spanish	Not listed	1998

Title	Publisher/Producer	Available from	Price
Embarrassment? Don't Shy Away from Breastfeeding	Best Start	Best Start	$0.17 ≤1000; quantity discounts available
If Your Grandchild Is Breastfed	Health Education Associates	Health Education Associates	$1 ≤24; quantity discounts available
Men Ask about Breastfeeding	Health Education Associates	Health Education Associates	$1 ≤24; quantity discounts available
Fathers Ask Questions about Breastfeeding	Health Education Associates	Health Education Associates	$1 ≤24; quantity discounts available
Breastfeeding and Basketball	InJoy	InJoy Videos	$79.95
Busy Moms: Breastfeeding Works Around my Schedule	Best Start	Best Start	$0.17 ≤1000; quantity discounts available
Through Their Eyes: Breastfeeding the Gift for Life	Amy Spangler	Childbirth Graphics	$16.50
Encouragement: Give a Breastfeeding Mom Your Loving Support	Best Start	Best Start	$0.17 ≤1000; quantity discounts available
Nobody Loves Them Like You	Best Start	Best Start	$25
Breastfeeding: Too Good to Miss out on! (comic book format)	Health Education Associates	Health Education Associates	$1 ≤24; quantity discounts available
Teens Can Breastfeed	Health Education Associates	Health Education Associates	$ 1 ≤24; quantity discounts available
Teen Breastfeeding, the Natural Choice. Volume 1: Why Breastfeed?	InJoy Productions	InJoy Videos	$79.95 (2-volume sets, $139.95)

B-2 *Managing Breastfeeding in Wellness Situations*

The following audio, visual, and audiovisual materials are designed to help the clinician manage breastfeeding for well infants and their mothers. One key word has been assigned to help the reader quickly identify pertinent points, but multiple points are usually covered in the media. Prices are approximate and are subject to change; in addition, most do not include shipping and handling.

Key Word/Target Population	Media	Length	Additional Languages	Author	Date
Advantages	Pamphlet	Multifold	Spanish, Vietnamese	Health Education Associates	
Attachment	Pamphlet	Multifold		Health Education Associates	
Attachment	Videotape	20 min		Glove, R	2002
Attachment, milk supply	Pamphlet	Multifold	French, Cambodian, Vietnamese, Russian, Spanish	Health Education Associates	
Attachment, positioning	Book	240 pages		Renfrew, M; Fisher, C	2000
Attachment, positioning	Videotape	14 min	Spanish	Frantz, K	1986
Attachment, positioning	Videotape	15 min		Frantz, K	1986
Attachment, positioning	Pamphlet	Multifold		Health Education Associates	
Attachment, positioning	Videotape	20 min		Royal College of Midwives/Fisher, C	1990
Attachment, positioning	Videotape	20 min	Spanish	Smith, L	1991
Burping	Videotape	18 min	Spanish	Frantz, K	1986
Drugs	Pamphlet	Multifold		Health Education Associates	
Early discharge	Videotape	25 min		Frantz, K	1996
Early discharge	Videotape	30 min		Royal College of Midwives/Fisher, C	1996
Early discharge	Videotape	30 min	Spanish	Not listed	1994
Early discharge	Videotape	31 min	Spanish	Not listed	2002
Early initiation	Videotape	9 min		Widstrom, A	1996
Early initiation	Videotape	6 min		Righard, L	1995
Embarrassment	Pamphlet	Multifold	Spanish, Vietnamese	Health Education Associates	

Title	Publisher/Producer	Available from	Price
Nursing Is Easy When You Know How	Health Education Associates	Health Education Associates discounts available	$1 ≤24; quantity discounts available
Learning about Breastfeeding	Health Education Associates	Health Education Associates	$1 ≤24; quantity discounts available
Follow Me Mum	Tapestry Film Productions	Rebecca Glover (reblact@iinet.net.au)	$60
How to Nurse Your Baby	Health Education Associates	Health Education Associates	$1 ≤24; quantity discounts available
Bestfeeding: Getting Breastfeeding Right for You	Celestial Arts	Bookstores	$15
Breastfeeding Techniques That Work! Volume 1: First Attachment	Geddes Productions	Geddes Productions	$39.95
Breastfeeding Techniques That Work! Volume 2: First Attachment in Bed	Geddes Productions	Geddes Productions	$39.95
An Easy Way to Get Started at Breastfeeding	Health Education Associates	Health Education Associates	$1 ≤24; quantity discounts available
Helping a Mother Breastfeed: No Finer Investment	Healthcare Productions LTD	Producer	$46.95
A Healthier Baby by Breastfeeding	Television Innovation Company	LLLI, Bright Futures	$29.95
Breastfeeding Techniques That Work! Volume 4: Burping the Baby	Geddes Productions	Geddes Productions	$39.95
Drugs and Medicine in Breast Milk	Health Education Associates	Health Education Associates	$1 ≤24; quantity discounts available
Breastfeeding Techniques That Work! Volume 8: The First Week	Geddes Productions	Geddes Productions	$39.95
Breastfeeding: Coping with the First Week	Royal College of Midwives	Growing with Baby	$79.95
Home before You Know It	Vida Health Communications	Vida Health Communications	$245
Hospital to Home	InJoy	InJoy	$250
Breastfeeding: The Baby's Choice	BGK Enterprises	ACE Graphics	$76.12
Delivery Self Attachment	Geddes Productions	Geddes Productions	$14.95
How to Nurse Modestly	Health Education Associates	Health Education Associates	$1 ≤24; quantity discounts available

Continued

Key Word/Target Population	Media	Length	Languages Additional	Author	Date
Expression, hand	Pamphlet	Multifold		Health Education Associates	
Feeding cues	Videotape	10 min		Cooperation with Texas WIC	1997
Feeding cues and behavior	Pamphlet	Multifold		Health Education Associates	
How-to	Book	400 pages		Colson, LJ (editor)	2002
How-to	Book	304 pages		Fredregill, S	2002
How-to	Book	304 pages		Tamaro, J	1998
How-to	Book	180 pages		King, FS	1992
How-to	Book	352 pages		Mark, AP	2000
How-to	Book	240 pages		Meeks, JY (editor)	2002
How-to	Book	105 pages	Spanish	Spangler, A	2000
How-to	Book	432 pages		Eiger, MS; Olds, SW	1999
How-to	Booklet	30 pages		Danner, SC	1997
How-to	Pamphlet	12 pages	Spanish	Danner, SC	1998
How-to	Book	480 pages	Spanish	La Leche League International	1997
How-to	Book	288 pages		Lothrop, H	1998
How-to	Book	256 pages		Huggins, K (editor)	1999
How-to	Videotape	16 min	Spanish	Not listed	2000
How-to	Book	176 pages		Kitzinger, S	1998
How-to	Book	176 pages		Wiggins, PK; Dettwyler, KA	1996
How-to	Book	288 pages		Sears, W; Sears, M	2000
How-to	Book	234 pages		Moody, J; Britten, J; Hogg, K	1997

Title	Publisher/Producer	Available from	Price
Breast Massage and Hand Expression of Breast Milk	Health Education Associates	Health Education Associates	$1 ≤24; quantity discounts available
Infant Cues: A Feeding Guide	Mark-It Television	Childbirth Graphics	$69.95
Breastfeeding: Those First Weeks at Home	Health Education Associates	Health Education Associates	$1 ≤24; quantity discounts available
Breastfeeding Sourcebook	Omnigraphics	Bookstores	$78
The Everything Breastfeeding Book	Adams Media Corporation	Bookstores	$12.95
So That's What They're for! Breastfeeding Basics (2nd ed.)	Adams Media Corporation	Bookstores	$10.95
Helping Mothers to Breastfeed (rev. ed.)	African Medical and Research Foundation	Publisher	$12
The Complete Idiot's Guide to Breastfeeding	Alpha Books	Bookstores	$16.95
The American Academy of Pediatrics New Mother's Guide to Breastfeeding	Bantam Books	Bookstores	$13.95
Amy Spangler's Breastfeeding: A Parent's Guide	Amy Spangler	Bookstores	$8.95
The Complete Book of Breastfeeding	Bantam Books	Bookstores	$6.50
Nursing Your Baby Beyond the First Days	Childbirth Graphics	Childbirth Graphics	$1.77 each (minimum of 50) or $1.53 (minimum of 250)
Nursing Your Baby for the First Time	Childbirth Graphics	Childbirth Graphics	$14.95 for pack of 50
The Womanly Art of Breastfeeding (6th ed.)	Dutton Plume	Bookstores, LLLI,	$15.95
Breastfeeding Naturally: A New Approach for Today's Mother	Fisher Books	Bookstores	$12.95
The Nursing Mothers Companion (4th ed.)	Harvard Common Press	Bookstores	$24.95 (hard cover); $12.95 (soft cover)
14 Steps to Better Breastfeeding	InJoy	InJoy Videos	$99.95
Breastfeeding Your Baby	Knopf	Bookstores	$20
Breastfeeding: A Mother's Gift	L. A. Publishing	Bookstores, Publisher	$10; quantity rate available
The Breastfeeding Book: Everything You Need to Know about Nursing Your Baby from Birth Through Weaning	Little, Brown & Company	Bookstores	$28.95 (hard cover); $14.95 (soft cover)
Breastfeeding Your Baby	Lothrop, Hannah	Bookstores	$13

Continued

Key Word/Target Population	Media	Length	Additional Languages	Author	Date
How-to	Book	336 pages		Rosenthal, MS; Arsenault, G	2000
How-to	Videotape	60 min	Spanish	Not listed	2000
How-to	Videotape	35 min	Spanish, French	Nylander, G	1994
How-to	Book	470 pages		Neifert, M	1998
How-to	Book	416 pages		Pryor, K; Pryor, G	1991
How-to	Book	464 pages		Newman, J; Pitman, T	2000
How-to	Book	336 pages		Martin, C (with Nancy Funnemark Krebs, MD, MS, RD, editor)	2000
How-to	Book	272 pages		Moran, E	2000
How-to	Videotape	75 min	Spanish, Cantonese, Mandarin	Livingstone, V	1994
How-to	Videotape	25 min	Spanish	Not listed	1998
Latch-on, milk transfer	Videotape	23 min		Not listed	1999
Nutrition	Pamphlet	Multifold		Health Education Associates	
Nutrition	Pamphlet	Multifold	Spanish, Vietnamese	Health Education Associates	
Positioning	Videotape	12 min		Woolridge, M; Johnson, D	1997
Prolonged breastfeeding	Videotape	21 min	Spanish	Not listed	1999
States of newborn behavior	Videotape	10 min		Danner, S	1994
Supporting breastfeeding	Videotape	45, 57 min		Not listed	1999
Telephone	Booklet	116 pages		Jolley, S	1996
Toddlers, extended breastfeeding	Book	308 pages		Bumgarner, NJ	2000
Weaning	Book	108 pages		Huggins, K; Ziedrich, L	1994
Weaning	Pamphlet	Multifold		Health Education Associates	

Title	Publisher/Producer	Available from	Price
The Breastfeeding Sourcebook: Everything You Need to Know (3rd ed.)	Lowell House	Bookstores	$17.95
First Days Home	Milner-Fenwick	Milner-Fenwick	Bulk pricing only
Breast Is Best	Norwegian Film Institute	INFACT Canada, Healthy Children	$60
Dr. Mom's Guide to Breastfeeding	Plume (Penguin Group)	Bookstores	$16
Nursing Your Baby	Pocket Books	Bookstores	$6.99
The Ultimate Breastfeeding Book of Answers: The Most Comprehensive Problem-Solution Guide to Breastfeeding	Prima Publishing	Bookstores	$16.95
The Nursing Mother's Problem Solver	Simon & Schuster	Bookstores	$13
Bon Appetit, Baby! The Breastfeeding Kit	Treasure Chest Publications	Bookstores	$24.95
The Art of Successful Breastfeeding (4 chapters)	University of British Columbia	Vancouver Breastfeeding Centre, Milner-Fenwick	$20 for home use, $99 for institutional price
Breastfeeding: Part II, How-to	Vida Health Communications	Vida Health Communications	$195 for single
Valerie's Diary: Beginning Breastfeeding (Volume 2)	InJoy	InJoy Videos	$224.80 for all 4 volumes
An Easy Diet for Breastfeeding Mothers	Health Education Associates	Health Education Associates	$1 ≤24; quantity discounts available
Nutrition for Breastfeeding Mothers	Health Education Associates	Health Education Associates	$1 ≤24; quantity discounts available
Breastfeeding: A Guide to Successful Positioning	Mark-It Television	Childbirth Graphics	$79.95
Straight Talk from Breastfeeding Moms: Beyond the Newborn (Volume 3)	InJoy	InJoy Videos	$224.80 (for all 4 volumes)
Baby Talk	State University of New York at Stonybrook	State University of New York at Stonybrook	$20
The Clinical Management of Breastfeeding for Health Professionals (2 parts)	Vida Health Communications	Vida Health Communications	$395 (both volumes)
Breastfeeding Triage Tool (3rd ed.)	Seattle-King County Department of Public Health	Childbirth Graphics	$10
Mothering Your Nursing Toddler	La Leche League International	Bookstores	$14.95
The Nursing Mother's Guide to Weaning	Harvard Common Press	Bookstores, LLLI	$11.95
Weaning Your Breastfed Baby	Health Education Associates	Health Education Associates	$1 ≤24; quantity discounts available

B-3 *Managing Breastfeeding in Wellness Situations with Special Focus*

The following audio, visual, and audiovisual materials are designed to help manage or prevent problems for mostly well infants or to provide advice about feeding the infant when special situations arise, for example, multiple gestation. (Because employed mothers deal mostly with issues of separation, employment is listed in the next section.) One key word has been assigned to help the reader quickly identify pertinent points, but multiple points are usually covered in the media. Prices are approximate and are subject to change; in addition, most do not include shipping and handling.

Key Word/Target Population	Media	Length	Additional Languages	Author	Date
Adoption	Book	141 pages		Peterson, DS	1999
Allergies	Pamphlet	Multifold		Health Education Associates	
Attachment	Videotape	6 min		Harris, H	1994
Cesarean	Videotape	26 min		Frantz, K	1986
Cesarean	Pamphlet	Multifold		Health Education Associates	
Diabetes	Pamphlet	Multifold		Health Education Associates	
Employment	Videotape	56 min		Frantz, K	1988
Engorgement	Pamphlet	Multifold		Bocar, D	1997
Hospital routines	CAI module	2 hr		Page-Goertz, S; McCamman, S	2001
How-to	Videotape	35 min	Spanish, French	Nylander, G	1994
How-to	Videotape	75 min	Spanish, Cantonese, Mandarin	Livingstone, V	1994
Hyperbilirubinemia	CAI module	90 min		Page-Goertz, S; McCamman, S	2001
Jaundice	Pamphlet	Multifold		Health Education Associates	
Legal rights	Packet	Multiple pages		La Leche League International	1991
Legal rights	Pamphlet	8 pages		La Leche League International	1991

Title	Publisher/Producer	Available from	Price
Breastfeeding the Adopted Baby	Corona Publishing Co.	Bookstores, LLLI	$12.95
Breastfeeding Advice for Families with Allergies	Health Education Associates	Health Education Associates	$1 ≤24; quantity discounts available
Mandy & Matt: A Solution for Breastfeeding Attachment through Co-Bathing	Midwifery Birthing Services	ACE Graphics	$18.41
Breastfeeding Techniques That Work! Volume 3: First Attachment after Cesarean	Geddes Productions	Geddes Productions	$39.95
Breastfeeding after a Cesarean	Health Education Associates	Health Education Associates	$1 ≤24; quantity discounts available
Breastfeeding and the Diabetic Mother	Health Education Associates	Health Education Associates	$1 ≤24; quantity discounts available
Breastfeeding Techniques That Work! Volume 5: Successful Working Mothers	Geddes Productions	Geddes Productions	$39.95
Engorgement	Lactation Consultant Services	Lactation Consultant Services	Special pricing
Breastfeeding Management Series: Creating Breastfeeding Friendly Environments	Jones and Bartlett	Publisher	$150
Breast Is Best	Norwegian Film Institute	INFACT Canada, Healthy Children	$60
The Art of Successful Breastfeeding (4 chapters)	University of British Columbia	Vancouver Breastfeeding Centre, Milner-Fenwick	$20 for home use; $99 for institutional price
Breastfeeding Management Series: Hyperbilirubinemia in the Breastfeeding Infant	Jones and Bartlett	Publisher	$150
Jaundice in Newborn Babies	Health Education Associates	Health Education Associates	$1 ≤24; quantity discounts available
Breastfeeding Rights Packet	La Leche League International	La Leche League International	$10
Legal Rights of Breastfeeding Mothers: USA Scene	La Leche League International	La Leche League International	$0.75

Continued

Key Word/Target Population	Media	Length	Additional Languages	Author	Date
Multiple gestation	Videotape	30 min		Gromada, K	1998
Multiple gestation	Pamphlet	Multifold		Health Education Associates	1993
Multiple gestation	Book	448 pages		Noble, E	1991
Multiple gestation	Book	380 pages		Gromada, K	1999
Problems	Pamphlet	Multifold		Health Education Associates	
Sore breasts, nipples	Videotape	24 min		Fisher, C; Inch, S	1997
Tandem	Pamphlet	20 pages		Berke, G	1989
Teens	Videotape/ manual	28/37 min	Spanish	Not listed	1998

Title	Publisher/Producer	Available from	Price
Double Duty: The Joys and Challenges of Caring for Newborn Twins	DLF Enterprises	Breastfeeding Support Network	Special pricing
Breastfeeding Your Twins	Health Education Associates	Health Education Associates	$1 ≤24; quantity discounts available
Having Twins: A Parent's Guide to Pregnancy, Birth & Early Childhood (2nd ed.)	Houghton Mifflin	Bookstores, LLLI	$18
Mothering Multiples: Breastfeeding and Caring for Twins or More (4th ed.)	La Leche League International	Bookstores	$14.95
Keeping Breastfeeding Easy	Health Education Associates	Health Education Associates	$1 ≤24; quantity discounts available
Breastfeeding: Dealing with the Problems	Royal College of Midwives	Childbirth Graphics	$79.95
Nursing for Two, Is It for You?	La Leche League International	La Leche League International	$2.50
Teen Breastfeeding, the Natural Choice. Volume 2: Starting Out Right	InJoy Productions	InJoy Videos	$79.95 (2-volume sets, $139.95)

B-4 *Preventing or Managing Breastfeeding Problems*

The following audio, visual, and audiovisual materials are designed to help manage breastfeeding for newborns or mothers who have special problems. Prices are approximate and are subject to change; in addition, most do not include shipping and handling.

Key Word/Target Population	Media	Length	Additional Languages	Author	Date
Ankyloglossia	Videotape	20 min		Jain, E	1996
Cleft	Pamphlet	16 pages		Danner, SC; Cerutti, ER	1996
Cleft	Videotape	16 min		Children's Mercy Hospital	1996
Cleft	Pamphlet	Foldover	Spanish	Cleft Palate Foundation	1999
Cleft	Booklet	31 pages	French	Herzog-Isler, C; Honigmann, K	1996
Cleft	Videotape	23 min	French	Herzog-Isler, C; Honigmann, K	1996
Down syndrome	Pamphlet	12 pages		Danner, SC; Cerutti, ER	1996
Kangaroo	Videotape	26 min		Bergman, N	2000
Kangaroo care	Videotape	8 min		Not listed	1999
Neurologically impaired	Pamphlet	8 pages		Danner, SC; Cerutti, ER	1996
Preterm	Videotape	12 min		Herzorg-Isler, C	1996
Preterm	Book	222 pages		Ludington-Hoe, SM; Golant, SK	1993
Preterm	Pamphlet	12 pages		Danner, SC; Cerutti, ER	1996
Preterm	Videotape	14 min		Not listed	1996
Preterm	Pamphlet	Multifold		Health Education Associates	1992
Preterm	Pamphlet	Multifold		Health Education Associates	
Preterm	Book	28 pages	Spanish	Gotsch, G	1999
Peterm	Videotape, DVD	35 plus 21 min		Morton, J	2002

Title	Publisher/Producer	Available from	Price
Tongue-Tie: Impact on Breastfeeding	(Unknown)	www.drjain.com	$60
Nursing Your Baby with Cleft Palate or Cleft Lip	Childbirth Graphics	Childbirth Graphics	$14.95 for pack of 50
The Special Touch Babies Need: Caring for the Infant with Cleft Lip/Palate	Children's Mercy Hospital	Children's Mercy Hospital	$45
Feeding an Infant with a Cleft	Cleft Palate Foundation	Cleft Palate Foundation	Single copy free to families
Give Us a Little Time	Medela	Medela, LLLI	$3
Samuel: Breastfed Infants with Cleft Lip and Cleft Palate	Medela	Medela, LLLI	$46
Breastfeeding Your Baby with Down Syndrome	Childbirth Graphics	Childbirth Graphics	$14.95 for pack of 50
Kangaroo Mother Care	Geddes Productions	Geddes Productions	$40
Breastfeeding and Kangaroo Care for Your NICU Baby	InJoy	InJoy Videos	$89.95
Nursing Your Neurologically Impaired Baby	Childbirth Graphics	Childbirth Graphics	$14.95 for pack of 50
Chiara, Mother's Milk for the Preterm Baby	Medela, Inc.	Medela, Inc.	Special pricing
Kangaroo Care: The Best You Can Do to Help Your Preterm Infant	Bantam Publishing Group	Bookstores	$15
Breastfeeding Your Premature Baby	Childbirth Graphics	Childbirth Graphics	$14.95 for pack of 50
Breastfeeding the Preterm Infant: A Positive Approach	Ameda (Hollister)	Ameda (Hollister)	$26.50
Breastfeeding Your Premie	Health Education Associates	Health Education Associates	$1 ≤24; quantity discounts available
Your Premie Needs You	Health Education Associates	Health Education Associates	$1 ≤24; quantity discounts available
Breastfeeding Your Premature Baby	La Leche League	Bookstores, LLLI	$6.50
A Premie Needs His Mother	Breastmilk Solutions	Breastmilk Solutions (http://www.breastmilk solutions.com/order.html)	$125

B-5 *Introducing Supplements and Facilitating Indirect Breastfeeding during Separation Periods*

The following audio, visual, and audiovisual materials are designed to help mothers success- fully breastfeed even when they are separated from their newborns or supplementation is required. The word *expression* is listed as a key word, but it includes pumps and pumping. Prices are approximate and subject to change; in addition, most do not include shipping and handling.

Key Word/Target Population	Media	Length	Additional Languages	Author	Date
Employment, pump, problems	Videotape	33 min		Not listed	1999
Employment	Book	224 pages		Wilkoff, WG	2002
Employment	Videotape/ manual	30 min		Not listed	1996
Employment	Book	160 pages		Grams, M	1985
Employment	Videotape	56 min		Frantz, K	1988
Employment	Book	208 pages		Pryor, G	1997
Employment	Pamphlet	4 pages		HMHB Breastfeeding Promotion Committee	1998
Employment	Pamphlet	13 pages	Spanish	HMHB Breastfeeding Promotion Committee	1997
Employment	Pamphlet	7 pages		La Leche League International	1991
Employment	Pamphlet	8 pages		Bocar, D	1997
Employment	Book	256 pages		Mason, DJ; Ingersoll, D	1997
Engorgement	Pamphlet	Multifold		Bocar, D	1997
Expression	Pamphlet	16 pages		Danner, S	1997
Expression	Pamphlet	Multifold		Health Education Associates	1991
Expression	Pamphlet	12 pages		Bernshaw, N	1991

Title	Publisher/Producer	Available from	Price
Simple Solutions: Making It Work (Volume 4)	InJoy Videos	InJoy Videos	$224.80 (for all 4 volumes)
Maternity Leave Breast Feeding Plan: How to Enjoy Nursing for 3 Months and Go Back to Work Guilt-Free	Fireside	Bookstores	$12
Working and Breastfeeding? Yes, You Can Do It!	Not listed	Childbirth Graphics	$65
Breastfeeding Success for Working Mothers	Achievement Press	Bookstores	$15
Breastfeeding Techniques That Work! Volume 5: Successful Working Mothers	Geddes Productions	Geddes Productions	$39.95
Nursing Mother, Working Mother: The Essential Guide for Breastfeeding and Staying Close to Your Baby after You Return to Work	Harvard Common Press	Bookstores	$10.95
What Gives These Companies a Competitive Edge: Worksite Support for Breastfeeding Employees	Healthy Mothers Healthy Babies	Healthy Mothers Healthy Babies	Single copies free
Working and Breastfeeding	Healthy Mothers Healthy Babies	Best Start	Single pamphlet free; $0.51 in bulk
Practical Hints for Working and Breastfeeding	La Leche League International	La Leche League International	$0.75
Combining Breastfeeding and Employment: A Planning Checklist	Lactation Consultant Services	Lactation Consultant Services	Special pricing
Breastfeeding and the Working Mother: The Complete Guide for Today's Nursing Mother	St. Martin's Press	Bookstores	$12
Engorgement	Lactation Consultant Services	Lactation Consultant Services	Special pricing
Expressing Breast Milk	Childbirth Graphics	Childbirth Graphics	$0.82; quantity discounts available
When Your Baby Needs Your Milk	Health Education Associates	Health Education Associates	$1 ≤24; quantity discounts available
A Mother's Guide to Milk Expression and Breast Pumps	La Leche League International	La Leche League International	$0.95

Continued

Key Word/Target Population	Media	Length	Additional Languages	Author	Date
Expression	Pamphlet	4 pages	Spanish	Marmet, C	1988
Expression, hand	Videotape	18 min	Spanish	Frantz, K	1988
Supplementation	Pamphlet	Multifold		Health Education Associates	
Supplementation	Videotape	23 min	Spanish	Frantz, K	1989

Title	Publisher/Producer	Available from	Price
Manual Expression of Breast Milk: Marmet Technique	Lactation Institute	Lactation Institute	Free at www.lactationinstitute.org
Breastfeeding Techniques That Work! Volume 6: Hand Expression	Geddes Productions	Geddes Productions	$39.95
Combining Breast and Bottle Feeding	Health Education Associates	Health Education Associates	$1 ≤24; quantity discounts available
Breastfeeding Techniques That Work! Volume 7: Using a Supplemental Nursing System	Geddes Productions	Geddes Productions	$39.95

B-6 *Other Problems and Related Resources*

Media for other problems are listed here.

Key Word/Target Population	Media	Length	Additional Languages	Author	Date
Advantages	Videotape	15 min		Georgetown University Institute for Reproductive Health	1993
Baby-friendly	Videotape	33 min		U. S. Committee for UNICEF	1994
Bonding	Book	272 pages		Klaus, PH; Klaus, MH; Kennel, JH	2000
Breast self-exam	Videotape	8.5 min		Doughty, L	2000
Child spacing	Book	208 pages		Kippley, S	1999
Consoling	Book	237 pages		Sears, W; Sears, M	1996
Counseling	Videotape/ manual	8 min		Best Start	1997
Counseling	Videotape	20 min		Fisher, C	1994
Crying	Book	416 pages		Orenstein, J	1997
Crying	Videotape	38 min	Spanish	Karp, H	2002
Cup-feeding	Videotape	10 min		Lang, S	1995
Feminism	Book	272 pages		Ward, JD	2000
Feminism	Book	AU: pages		Ward, JD	2000

Title	Publisher/Producer	Available from	Price
Breastfeeding: Protecting a Natural Resource	Georgetown University Institute for Reproductive Health	Academy for Educational Development	$20
Learning to Be Baby Friendly: One Hospital's Experience	U.S. Committee for UNICEF	Baby-Friendly U.S.A.	$13
Bonding: Building the Foundations of Secure Attachment and Independence	Perseus	Bookstores	$16
Breast Self-Exam during Pregnancy and Lactation	Health Midwest	Menorah Medical Center Auxiliary	$49.95 plus S&H
Breastfeeding and Natural Child Spacing: How Ecological Breastfeeding Spaces Babies	Couple to Couple League	Bookstores	$9.95
The Fussy Baby Book: Parenting Your High-Need Child from Birth to Five Years	Little, Brown & Company	Bookstores	$12.95
Best Start 3-Step Counseling Strategy Module (includes What Difference Does It Make and a new training manual)	Best Start	Best Start	$72 (includes manual and guide)
She Needs You—Chloe Fisher at the Swedish Breastfeeding Institute	Swedish Breastfeeding Institute	Health Education Associates	$39.95
365 Ways to Calm Your Crying Baby	Adams Media Corporation	Bookstores	$7.95
The Happiest Baby on the Block: The New Way to Calm Crying and Help Your Baby Sleep Longer	The Happiest Baby, Inc.	The Happiest Baby, Inc. (http://www.thehappiestbaby.com)	$18.95; also in DVD, $25.95
The Baby Feeding Cup	Ameda	Ameda	Special pricing
At the Crossroads of Medicine, Feminism, and Religion	La Leche League	Bookstores, La Leche League	$14.35
La Leche League: At the Crossroads of Medicine, Feminism, and Religion	University of North Carolina Press	Bookstores, La Leche League	$39.95 (hard cover); $15.95 (soft cover)

Continued

Key Word/Target Population	Media	Length	Additional Languages	Author	Date
Feminist issues	Book	296 pages		Blum, LM	2000
General	Book	162 pages		Jones, S; Tompson, M; Ziedrich, L	1992
Lactational amenorrhea	Videotape	26 min		Georgetown Institute for Reproductive Health	1996
Mammaplasty	Book	328 pages		West, D	2001
Maternal nutrition	Book	220 pages		Dalley, J; Dalley, J; Dalley, NS	1997
Maternal weight loss	Book	235 pages		Behan, E	1992
Newborn behavior	Videotape	30 min		Klaus, M; Keefe, M	1998
Nipple trauma	CAI module	2 hr		Page-Goertz, S; McCamman, S	2001
Recipes	Book	125 pages		Frissell-Deppe, T	2002
Sleep	Book	312 pages		Jackson, D	1999
Sleep	Pamphlet	Multifold		Health Education Associates	
Sleep	Pamphlet	Multifold		Health Education Associates	
Sleep	Audio tape	33 min		Not listed	

Title	Publisher/Producer	Available from	Price
At the Breast: Ideologies of Breastfeeding and Motherhood in the Contemporary United States	Beacon Press	Bookstores	$30 (hard cover); $18 (soft cover)
Crying Baby, Sleepless Nights	Penguin Books	Bookstores	$12.95
Taking the First Steps: The Lactational Amenorrhea Method for Family Planning	Georgetown University	Academy for Educational Development	$20
Defining Your Own Success: Breastfeeding after Breast Reduction Surgery	Bookstores, La Leche League	Bookstores	$39.95 (hard cover); $24.95 (soft cover)
The Meat & Potatoes of Breastfeeding: Easy Nutritional Guidelines for Breastfeeding Moms	Footprint Press	Bookstores	$15
Eat Well, Lose Weight While Breastfeeding: Complete Nutrition Book for Nursing Mothers, Including a Healthy Guide to Weight Loss Your Doctor Promise	Villard Books	Bookstores	$14.95
Amazing Talents of the Newborn	Johnson & Johnson	Johnson & Johnson Pediatric Institute	$10
Breastfeeding Management Series: Nipple Trauma	Jones and Bartlett	Publisher	$150
A Breastfeeding Mother's Secret Recipes: Breastmilk Recipes, Fun Food for Kids and Quick Dishes!	J.E.D. Publishing	Bookstores	$14.95
Three in a Bed	Bloomsbury Publishers	Bookstores	$14.95
Helping Your Baby Sleep through the Night	Health Education Associates	Health Education Associates	$1 ≤24; quantity discounts available
Sleep Patterns of Breastfed Babies	Health Education Associates	Health Education Associates	$1 ≤24; quantity discounts available
Baby-go-to-Sleep Audiotape or CD	Winning Edge	Winning Edge, discount department stores	$15.90

B-7 *Media Critique*

It is difficult, if not impossible, to find a videotape, pamphlet, or book that is ideal for all parents. Furthermore, several people, rather than one individual, usually choose the patient education media to be stocked in the hospital or clinic. The following template is a useful tool for each member of the interdisciplinary team to note the media's pertinent criteria. If each member of the group looks for each point listed here, a lively discussion afterward can help the group to determine which media should be stocked.

Title

BACKGROUND

Produced by:

Compliments of:

Intended audience:

Length of media:

Content expert:

PURPOSE OF MEDIA:

CONTENT:

CRITIQUE OF MEDIA:

Rating Scale:

0 = Totally unacceptable
1 = Acceptable, but needing modification
2 = Generally acceptable
3 = Superb

_____ Purpose fits needs of intended audience

_____ Conservative and realistic

_____ Appropriate for our population: terminology, cultural aspect, etc.

_____ Tone/approach

_____ Pictures

_____ Organization

_____ Content relevant

_____ Content complete

_____ Content accurate

_____ Explanations clear

_____ Overall rating of this media

Is purpose of media evident to clinician? _____

What is the greatest strength of this media? _____

What is the greatest weakness of this media? _____

Price: _____

Other comments:

APPENDIX

C

Professional Development and Support

This appendix seeks to provide a starting point for professionals who wish to find material and human resources to support breastfeeding.

C-1 *Organizations and Associations*

Following are organizations whose main mission is to assist health care professionals. All attempts have been made to provide the latest contact information.

Academy of Breastfeeding Medicine
191 Clarksville Rd.
Princeton Junction, NJ 08550
Phone: (609) 799-4900
Toll-free: (877) 836-9947
Fax: (609) 799-7032
Web site: http://www.bfmed.org

African Medical and Research Foundation
PO Box 30125
Nairobi, Kenya
Phone: (254) 250-1301
Fax: (254) 260-9518
Web site: http://www.amref.org/
E-mail: amrefhq@users.africaonline.co.ke

American Academy of Family Physicians
11400 Tomahawk Creek Parkway
Leawood, KS 66211-2672
Phone: (913) 906-6000
Web site: http://www.aafp.org
E-mail: fp@aafp.org

American Academy of Pediatrics
141 Northwest Point Blvd.
Elk Grove Village, IL 60007-1098
Phone: (847) 434-4000
Toll-free: (800) 433-9016
Fax: (847) 434-8000
Web site: http://www.aap.org
E-mail: kidsdoc@aap.org

American College of Nurse-Midwives
818 Connecticut Ave., N.W., Suite 900
Washington, DC 20006
Phone: (202) 728-9860
Fax: (202) 728-9897
Web site: http://www.midwife.org
E-mail: info@acnm.org

American College of Obstetricians &
  Gynecologists
409 12th St., S.W.
Washington, DC 20024-6920
Toll-free: (800) 762-2264
Fax: (202) 554-3490
Web site: http://www.acog.org
E-mail: several; refer to web site

American Dietetic Association
216 W. Jackson Blvd.
Chicago, IL 60606-6995
Phone: (312) 899-0040
Toll-free: (800) 877-1600
Fax: (312) 899-1979
Web site: http://www.eatright.org
E-mail: sales@eatright.org

American Hospital Association
1 N. Franklin
Chicago, IL 60606-3421
Phone: (312) 422-3000
Fax: (312) 422-4796
Web site: http://www.aha.org

American Public Health Association
800 I St., N.W.
Washington, DC 20001-3710
Phone: (202) 777-APHA
Fax: (202) 777-2534
Web site: http://www.apha.org
E-mail: comments@apha.org

Association of Women's Health, Obstetric and
Neonatal Nurses
2000 L St., N.W., Suite 740
Washington, DC 20036
Phone: (202) 261-2400
Toll-free: (800) 673-8499
Fax: (202) 728-0575
Web site: http://www.awhonn.org

Baby-Friendly USA
8 Jan Sebastian Way Unit #22
Sandwich, MA 02563
Phone: (508) 888-8092
Fax: (508) 888-8050
Web site: http://www.babyfriendlyusa.org
E-mail: info@babyfriendlyusa.org

British Columbia Breastfeeding Society
9131 Evancio Crescent
Richmond, British Columbia V7E 5J2
Canada

British Dietetic Association
5th Floor, Charles House
148/9 Great Charles Street Queensway
Birmingham, B3 3HT
United Kingdom
Phone: 0121-200-8080
Fax: 0121-200-8081
Web site: http://www.bda.uk.com
E-mail: info@bda.uk.com

British Paediatric Association
5 St. Andrews Place
Regents Park
London, NW1 4LB
United Kingdom
Phone: 0171-486-6151
Fax: 0171-486 6009

Cleft Palate Foundation
104 South Estes Dr., Suite 204
Chapel Hill, NC 27514
Phone: (919) 933-9044
Toll-free: (800) 24-CLEFT
Fax: (919) 933-9604
Web site: http://www.cleftline.org
E-mail: cleftline@aol.com

Coalition for Improving Maternity Services
PO Box 2346
Ponte Vedra Beach, FL 32004
Phone: (904) 285-1613
Toll-free: (888) 282-CIMS
Fax: (904) 285-2120
Web site: http://www.motherfriendly.org
E-mail: info@motherfriendly.org

Dietitians of Canada
480 University Ave., Suite 604
Toronto, Ontario M5G 1V2
Canada
Phone: (416) 596-0857
Fax: (416) 596-0603
Web site: http://www.dietitians.ca

Doulas of North America
PO Box 626
Jasper, IN 47547
Toll-free: (888) 788-DONA
Fax: (812) 634-1491
Web site: http://www.dona.com
E-mail: doula@dona.org

Human Milk Banking Association of North
   America*
Web site: http://www.hmbana.com

INFACT Canada
6 Trinity Square
Toronto, Ontario M5G 1B1
Canada
Phone: (416) 595-9819
Fax: (416) 591-9355
Web site: http://www.infactcanada.ca
E-mail: info@infactcanada.ca

Institute for Reproductive Health
Georgetown University Medical Center
3 PHC, Room 3004
3800 Reservoir Rd., N.W.
Washington, DC 20007
Phone: (202) 687-1392
Fax: (202) 687-6846
Web site: http://www.irh.org
E-mail: irhinfo@georgetown.edu

International Childbirth Education Association
PO Box 20048
Minneapolis, MN 55420
Phone: (952) 854-8660
Toll-free: (800) 624-4934
Fax: (952) 854-8772
Web site: http://www.icea.org
E-mail: info@icea.org

International Confederation of Midwives
   Eisenhowerlaan 138
2517 KN The Hague
The Netherlands
Phone: 31-70-3060520
Fax: 31-70-3555651
Web site: http://www.internationalmidwives.org
E-mail: info@internationalmidwives.org

International Federation of Gynecology &
   Obstetrics
FIGO Secretariat
70 Wimpole St.
London W1G8AX
United Kingdom
Phone: +44 20-7224-3270
Fax: +44 20-7935-0736
Web site: http://www.figo.org
E-mail: figo@figo.org

International Lactation Consultant Association
1500 Sunday Dr., Suite 102
Raleigh, NC 27607
Phone: (919) 787-5181
Fax: (919) 787-4916
Web site: http://www.ilca.org
E-mail: info@ilca.org

International Pediatric Association
Hopital Necker-Enfants Malades
149, rue de Sèvres, 75743
Paris, France
Phone: 33-1-42-19-26-45
Fax: 33-1-42-19-26-44
Web site: http://www.ipa-france.net
E-mail: IntPedAss@aol.com

International Society for Research on Human
   Milk & Lactation
Perinatal Center
202 S. Park St.
Madison, WI 53715
Phone: (608) 262-6561
Fax: (608) 267-6377
Web site: http://www.isrhml.org
E-mail: frgreer@facstaff.wisc.edu

*Their web site provides contact information for the individual
members of HMBANA.

Lactation Study Center
URMC Box 777
601 Elmwood Ave.
Rochester, NY 14642
Phone: (585) 275-0088
Fax: (585) 461-3614
E-mail: Linda_Friedman@urmc.rochester.edu

Lactation Support Service
British Columbia Children's Hospital
4480 Oak St.
Vancouver, British Columbia V6H 3V4
Canada
Phone: (604) 875-2345, ext. 7607

Lamaze International
2025 M Street, N.W., Suite 800
Washington, DC 20036-3309
Phone: (202) 367-1128
Toll-free: (800) 368-4404
Fax: (202) 367-2128
Web site: http://www.lamaze.org
E-mail: lamaze@dc.sba.com

Maternity Center Association
281 Park Ave., South
5th Floor
New York, NY 10010
Phone: (212) 777-5000
Fax: (212) 777-9320
Web site: http://www.maternity.org
E-mail: info@maternitywise.org

National Alliance for Breastfeeding Advocacy
National Breastfeeding Promotion Office
9684 Oak Hill Dr.
Ellicott City, MD 21042-6321
Phone: (410) 995-3726
Fax: (410) 992-1977
Web site: http://naba-breastfeeding.org
E-mail: barbara@naba-breastfeeding.org

National Alliance for Breastfeeding Advocacy,
    Office of Educational Services
254 Conant Rd.
Weston, MA 02193-1756
Phone: (617) 893-3553
Fax: (617) 893-8608
E-mail: marsha@naba-breastfeeding.org

National Association of Childbearing Centers
3123 Gottschall Rd.
Perkiomenville, PA 18074
Phone: (215) 234-8068
Fax: (215) 234-8829
Web site: http://www.birthcenters.org
E-mail: ReachNACC@BirthCenters.org

National Association of Neonatal Nurses
4700 W. Lake Ave.
Glenview, IL 60025-1485
Toll-free: (800) 451-3795
Fax: (888) 477-6266
Web site: http://www.nann.org
E-mail: info@nann.org

National Down Syndrome Society
666 Broadway
New York, NY 10012-2317
Phone: (212) 460-9330
Toll-free: (800) 221-4602
Fax: (212) 979-2873
Web site: http://www.ndss.org
E-mail: info@ndss.org

National Healthy Mothers, Healthy Babies
    Coalition
121 N. Washington St., Suite 300
Alexandria, VA 22314
Phone: (703) 836-6110
Fax: (703) 836-3470
Web site: http://www.hmhb.org
E-mail: info@hmhb.org

National Perinatal Association
3500 E. Fletcher Ave., Suite 205
Tampa, FL 33613-4712
Phone: (813) 971-1008
Toll-free: (888) 971-3295
Fax: (813) 971-9306
Web site: http://www.nationalperinatal.org
E-mail: npa@nationalperinatal.org

National WIC Association (formerly, National
    Association of WIC Directors)
2001 S St., N.W., Suite 580
Washington, DC 20009-3355
Phone: (202) 232-5492
Fax: (202) 387-5281
Web site: http://www.nwica.org

Royal College of Midwives
15 Mansfield St.
London, W1G 9NH
United Kingdom
Phone: +44 (0)20 7312 3535
Fax: +44 (0)20 7312 3536
Web site: http://www.rcm.org.uk
E-mail: info@rcm.org.uk

Royal College of Obstetricians and Gynaecologists
27 Sussex Place
Regent's Park
London, NW1 4RG
United Kingdom
Phone: +44 (0)20-7772-6200
Fax: +44 (0)20-7723-0575
Web site: http://www.rcog.org.uk

UNICEF
3 United Nations Plaza
New York, NY 10017
Phone: (212) 326-7000
Fax: (212) 887-7465
Web site: http://www.unicef.org
E-mail: netmaster@unicef.org

United States Breastfeeding Committee
Web site: http://www.usbreastfeeding.org
E-mail: info@usbreastfeeding.org

U.S. Fund for UNICEF
333 E. 38th St.
New York, NY 10016
Phone: (212) 686-5522
Toll-free: (800) FOR-KIDS
Web site: http://www.unicefusa.org
E-mail: webmaster@unicefusa.org

Wellstart International
PO Box 80877
San Diego, CA 92138-0877
Phone: (619) 295-5192
Fax: (619) 574-8159
Web site: http://www.wellstart.org
E-mail: info@wellstart.org

World Alliance for Breastfeeding Advocacy
PO Box 1200
10850 Penang
Malaysia
Phone: +60-4-6584816
Fax: +60-4-6572655
Web site: http://www.waba.org.br
E-mail: secr@waba.po.my

World Health Organization (WHO)
Avenue Appia 20
1211 Geneva 27
Switzerland
Phone: +41-22-791-2111
Fax: +41-22-791-3111
Web site: http://www.who.int
E-mail: info@who.int

C-2 *Suggested Library for Professionals*

References that may be helpful for those involved in breastfeeding management are listed in this section. This list is not meant to be all-inclusive and is not meant to endorse any product. Rather, it has been compiled to identify media that the author or her colleagues have found helpful in clinical practice. All videotapes are in NTSC format; additional formats may be available. Prices are approximate, and most do not include shipping and handling

Key Word/Target Population	Media	Length	Additional Languages	Author	Date
Advantages	Videotape	15 min		Georgetown University Institute for Reproductive Health	1993
Ankyloglossia	Videotape	20 min		Jain, E	1996
Attachment, positioning	Videotape	20 min		Royal College of Midwives/Fisher, C	1990
Baby-Friendly	Videotape	33 min		U.S. Committee for UNICEF	1994
Clinical management	Videotape	57 min		AWHONN	1999
Clinical management	Videotape	45 min		AWHONN	1999
Counseling	Videotape	20 min		Fisher, C	1994
Counseling	Videotape/manual	8 min		Best Start	1997
Early initiation	Videotape	17 min		Not listed	1993
Early initiation	Videotape	6 min		Righard, L	1995
Employment	Pamphlet	4 pages		HMHB Breastfeeding Promotion Committee	1993
Hospital routines	CAI module	2 hr		Page-Goertz, S; McCamman, S	2001
How-to	Videotape	75 min	Spanish, Cantonese, Mandarin	Livingstone, V	1994
Hyperbilirubinemia	CAI module	90 min		Page-Goertz, S; McCamman, S	2001

charges. Many items are available from vendors other than those listed; only vendors in the United States are listed here. The author welcomes suggestions about other places where these materials may be easily obtained. Readers or vendors may send comments to bookcommentswmc-world-wide.com. Contact information for vendors is listed in Appendix E.

Videotapes/Pamphlets/Booklets

Title	Publisher/Producer	Available from	Price
Breastfeeding: Protecting a Natural Resource	Georgetown University Institute for Reproductive Health	Academy for Educational Development	$20
Tongue-Tie: Impact on Breastfeeding	(Unknown)	www. drjain.com	$60
Helping a Mother Breastfeed: No Finer Investment	Healthcare Productions LTD	Producer	$46.95
Learning to Be Baby Friendly: One Hospital's Experience	U.S. Committee for UNICEF	Baby-Friendly U.S.A.	$13
Clinical Management of Breastfeeding for Health Professionals: Part II	Vida Communications	Producer	$150
Clinical Management of Breastfeeding for Health Professionals: Part I	Vida Communications	Producer	$150
She Needs You—Chloe Fisher at the Swedish Breastfeeding Institute	Swedish Breastfeeding Institute	Health Education Associates	$39.95
Best Start Training Program (includes What Difference Does it Make and a new training manual)	Best Start	Best Start	$72 (includes manual and guide)
Baby's choice	BGK Enterprises	ACE Graphics	$50
Delivery Self Attachment	Geddes Productions	Geddes Productions	$14.95
What Gives These Companies a Competitive Edge: Worksite Support for Breastfeeding Employees	Healthy Mothers Healthy Babies	Healthy Mothers Healthy Babies	Free
Breastfeeding Management Series: Creating Breastfeeding Friendly Environments	Jones and Bartlett	Publisher	$150
The Art of Successful Breastfeeding (4 chapters)	University of British Columbia	Vancouver Breastfeeding Centre, Milner-Fenwick	$20 for home use, $99 for institutional price
Breastfeeding Management Series: Hyperbilirubinemia in the Breastfeeding Infant	Jones and Bartlett	Publisher	$150

Continued

Key Word/Target Population	Media	Length	Additional Languages	Author	Date
Lactational amenorrhea	Videotape	26 min		Georgetown Institute for Reproductive Health	1996
Nipple trauma	CAI module	2 hr		Page-Goertz, S; McCamman, S	2001
Preterm	Videotape	29 min	French, Spanish	UNICEF	
Preterm	Videotape	14 min	Spanish	UNICEF	
Sore breasts, nipples	Videotape	24 min		Fisher, C; Inch, S	1997
States of consciousness	Videotape	25 min		Blackburn, S	1991
States of newborn behavior	Videotape	10 min		Danner, S	1994
Supporting breastfeeding	Videotape	45, 57 min		Not listed	1999

Title	Publisher/Producer	Available from	Price
Taking the First Steps: The Lactational Amenorrhea Method for Family Planning	Georgetown University	Academy for Educational Development	$20
Breastfeeding Management Series: Nipple Trauma	Jones and Bartlett	Publisher	$150
Feeding Low Birth Weight Babies	UNICEF	UNICEF	Special pricing
Mother Kangaroo, A Light of Hope	UNICEF	UNICEF	Special pricing
Breastfeeding: Dealing with the Problems	Royal College of Midwives	Childbirth Graphics	$79.95
Early Parent-Infant Relationships	March of Dimes	March of Dimes	Special pricing
Baby Talk	State University of New York at Stonybrook	State University of New York at Stonybrook	$20
The Clinical Management of Breastfeeding for Health Professionals (2 parts)	Vida Health Communications	Vida Health Communications	$395 (both volumes)

Books and Other Hard Copy

American Academy of Pediatrics and the American College of Obstetrics and Gynecology. *Guidelines for perinatal care.* 4th ed. Elk Grove Village, IL: American Academy of Pediatrics; 1997.

Biancuzzo, M, ed. *Breastfeeding Outlook,* a quarterly newsletter that provides up-to-the-minute information on legislation, resources for parents and professionals, media reviews, breaking research, and other events in the lactation community.

Biancuzzo M. *Helping Mothers choose and initiate breastfeeding.* WMC Worldwide; 2001.

Biancuzzo M. *Sore nipples: prevention and problem solving.* Herndon VA: WMC Worldwide; 2000.

Briggs GG, Freeman RK, Yaffe SJ. *Drugs in pregnancy and lactation.* 6th ed. Baltimore: Williams & Wilkins; 2001.

Cadwell K, ed. *Reclaiming breastfeeding for the United States: protection, promotion and support.* Sudbury, MA: Jones and Bartlett; 2002.

Cadwell K et al. *Maternal and infant assessment for breastfeeding and human lactation: a guide for the practitioner.* Sudbury, MA: Jones and Bartlett; 2002.

Committee on Nutrition. American Academy of Pediatrics. *Pediatric nutrition handbook.* 4th ed. Elk Grove Village, IL: American Academy of Pediatrics; 1998.

Enkin M et al. *Guide to effective care in pregnancy and childbirth.* 3rd ed. Cary, NC: Oxford University Press; 2000.

Fomon SJ. *Nutrition of normal infants.* St. Louis: Mosby; 1993.

Frantz K. *Breastfeeding product guide 1994.* Los Angeles: Geddes Productions; 1994.

Frantz K. *Breastfeeding products guide supplement.* Los Angeles: Geddes Productions; 1999.

Goldman AS, Atkinson SA, Hanson LA. *Human lactation 3. The effects of human milk on the recipient infants.* New York: Plenum Press; 1987.

Hale T. *Medications & mothers' milk: a manual of lactational pharmacology.* 10th ed. Amarillo, TX: Pharmasoft Publishing; 2002.

Hamosh M, Goldman AS. *Human lactation 2. Maternal and environmental factors.* New York: Plenum Press; 1986.

Henschel D. *Breastfeeding: a guide for midwives.* Cheshire, England: Books for Midwives Press; 1996.

Institute of Medicine. *Nutrition during lactation.* Washington, DC: National Academy Press; 1991.

Jensen RG, Neville MC. *Human lactation. Milk components and methodologies.* New York: Plenum Press; 1985.

Jensen RG, ed. *Handbook of milk composition.* San Diego: Academic Press; 1995.

Koletzko B, Michaelsen KF, Hernell OL, eds. *Short and long term effects of breast feeding on child health.* New York: Kluwer Academic/Plenum Publishers; 2000.

La Leche League International. *The womanly art of breastfeeding.* 6th ed. Schaumburg, IL: La Leche League International; 1997.

Labbok M, Cooney C, Coly S. *Guidelines: breastfeeding, family planning and the lactational amenorrhea method—LAM.* Washington, DC: Georgetown University Institute for Reproductive Health; 1994.

Lauwers J, Shinskie D. *Counseling the nursing mother.* 3rd ed. Sudbury, MA: Jones and Bartlett; 2000.

Lawrence RA. *A review of the medical benefits and contraindications to breastfeeding in the United States.* Arlington, VA: National Center for Education in Maternal and Child Health; 1997. Available at http://www.ncemch.org/pubs/PDFs/BreastfeedingTIB.pdf. 1-888-Ask HRSA (275-4772).

Lawrence RA, Lawrence RM. *Breastfeeding: a guide for the medical profession.* 5th ed. St. Louis: Mosby; 1999.

Minchin M. *Breastfeeding matters.* 4th ed. Victoria, Australia: Australia Alma Publications; 1998.

Mohrbacher N, Stock J. *The breastfeeding answer book.* 2nd ed. Schaumburg, IL: La Leche League International; 1996.

Newton N. *Newton on breastfeeding.* Seattle: Birth & Life Bookstore; 1987.

Palmer G. *The politics of breastfeeding.* London: Pandora Press; 1994.

Riordan J, Auerbach KG. *Breastfeeding and human lactation.* 2nd ed. Sudbury, MA: Jones and Bartlett; 1998.

Sokol EJ. *The code handbook: a guide to implementing the International Code of Marketing of Breastmilk Substitutes.* Penang, Malaysia: IBFAN; 1997.

Spisak S, Gross SS. *Second followup report: the Surgeon General's Workshop on Breastfeeding and Human Lactation.* Washington, DC: National Center for Education in Maternal and Child Health; 1991.

Stuart-Macadam P, Dettwyler KA, eds. *Breastfeeding: biocultural perspectives.* Hawthorne, NY: Aldine de Gruyter; 1995.

U.S. Department of Health and Human Services. *Report of the Surgeon General's Workshop on Breastfeeding and Human Lactation.* Rockville, MD: Health Resources and Services Administration; 1984.

U.S. Department of Health and Human Services. HHS blueprint for action on breastfeeding. Washington, DC: Office on Women's Health, U.S. Department of Health and Human Services; 2000.

World Health Organization. *Hypoglycaemia of the newborn.* Geneva: World Health Organization; 1997.

World Health Organization and UNICEF. *Innocenti Declaration: 30 July to 1 Aug, 1990, Florence Italy.* Geneva: Author; 1990.

World Health Organization. *A common review and evaluation framework.* Geneva: World Health Organization; 1996.

World Health Organization. *International Code of Marketing of Breast-Milk Substitutes.* Geneva: World Health Organization; 1981.

Worthington-Roberts B, Williams SR. *Nutrition in pregnancy and lactation.* 6th ed. Madison, WI: Brown Benchmark; 1997.

C-3 *Sources of Continuing Education for Professionals*

Continuing education can be offered through multiple formats, including in-person contact with the instructor and self-learning programs. In-person contact through conferences and seminars is the time-honored way of providing and obtaining continuing education for nurses, as well as other health care providers.

Self-learning packages require a word of caution. Many self-learning packages are created using an existing book or tape that was not intended for self-learning; objectives and test questions are later retrofitted, and the participant is not guided through the learning process. Self-learning packages that rely solely on one piece of previously existing media are usually inferior to self-learning packages that include several types of learning activities that are designed for independent learning. Furthermore, a self-learning package that relies on one piece of existing media does not guarantee that the book's original author or authors were involved in the preparation of the self-learning package. For example, without the knowledge or participation of the author or publisher, a self-learning package using the first edition of this book was developed and sold. If this book's author is involved in creating a self-learning package that uses this book, links for the product will be listed at http://www.mariebiancuzzo.com.

Multiple sources exist for continuing education in the United States. Sources listed here are those with which the author has had direct contact, which offer continuing education on a regular basis, and have been offering continuing education to professionals for more than 10 years.

American Dietetic Association
216 W. Jackson Blvd.
Chicago, IL 60606-6995
Phone: (312) 899-0040
Toll-free: (800) 877-1600
Fax: (312) 899-1979
Web site: http://www.eatright.org
E-mail: sales@eatright.org

Breastfeeding Support Consultants
228 Park Lane
Chalfont, PA 18914
Phone: (215) 822-1281
Fax: (215) 997-7879
Web site: http://www.bsccenter.org
E-mail: info@bsccenter.org

Geddes Productions
PO Box 41761
Los Angeles, CA 90041-0761
Phone: (323) 344-8045
Fax: (323) 257-7209
Web site: http://www.geddesproduction.com
E-mail: orders@geddesproduction.com

Healthy Children Project's Center for
    Breastfeeding
8 Jan Sebastian Way #13
Sandwich, MA 02563-2359
Phone: (508) 888-8044
Toll-free: (888) 888-8077
Fax: (508) 888-8050
Web site: http://www.healthed.cc
E-mail: hea@capecod.net

Lactation Associates
254 Conant Rd.
Weston, MA 02192
Phone: (871) 893-3553
Fax: (871) 893-8608
E-mail: marshalact@aol.com

Lactation Consultant Services
11320 Shady Glen Rd.
Oklahoma City, OK 73162
Phone: (405) 722-2163
Fax: (405) 722-2197
Web site: http://lactation-consultant-services.com
E-mail: dbocar@aol.com

Lactation Education Resources
3621 Lido Place
Fairfax, VA 22031
Phone: (703) 691-2069
Fax: (703) 691-3983
Web site: http://www.LERon-line.com
E-mail: LERonline@yahoo.com

Lactation Institute
16430 Ventura Blvd., Suite 303
Encino, CA 91436
Phone: (818) 995-1913
Fax: (818) 995-0634
Web site: http://www.lactationinstitute.org
E-mail: info@lactationinstitute.org

Wellstart International
PO Box 80877
San Diego, CA 92138-0877
Phone: (619) 295-5192
Fax: (619) 574-8159
Web site: http://www.wellstart.org
E-mail: info@wellstart.org

WMC Worldwide, L. L. C.
PO Box 387
Herndon, VA 20172
Phone: (703) 758-0092
Fax: (703) 758-0891
Web site: http://www.wmc-worldwide.com
E-mail: mbiancuzzo@wmc-worldwide.com

APPENDIX D

Breastfeeding Protection and Promotion

This appendix gives a broad overview of political, legislative, and regulatory actions that have protected, promoted, and supported breastfeeding.

D-1 *International Code of Marketing of Breast-Milk Substitutes: Summary of Provisions*

The International Code of Marketing was developed in 1981 by the World Health Organization. The United States endorsed the principles of this International Code in 1994 but has not fully embraced the Code; for example, manufacturers of artificial milk continue to advertise to U.S. consumers in clear violation of Article 5. The Code is an essential part of the Baby-Friendly Hospital Initiative, and a summary of its provisions follows. The Code in its entirety can be purchased from the World Health Organization (see Appendix C-1 for address).

International Code of Marketing of Breast-Milk Substitutes (1981)

Summary of Provisions

Article 1: Aim of the Code. The aim of this code is to contribute to the provision of safe and adequate nutrition for infants by the protection and promotion of breastfeeding and by ensuring the proper use of breast-milk substitutes, when these are necessary, on the basis of adequate information and through appropriate marketing and distribution.

Article 2: Scope of the Code. The Code applies to the marketing, and practices related thereto, of the following products: breast-milk substitutes, including infant formula; other milk products; food; and beverages, including bottle-fed complementary foods, when marketed or otherwise represented to be suitable, with or without modification, for use as a partial or total replacement of breast milk, feeding bottles, and teats. It also applies to their quality and availability and to information concerning their use.

Article 3: Definitions. The Code defines the terms *breast-milk substitute, complementary food, container, distributor, health care system, health worker, infant formula, label, manufacturer, marketing, marketing personnel, samples,* and *supplies.* The distinction between samples and supplies of infant formula is especially relevant to hospital policies because the Code recommends that the former not be distributed, whereas the latter may be donated or sold at low cost to an institution or organization for social purposes (e.g., families in need) if they are not used as a sales inducement. These supplies should be given only to infants who have to be fed a breast-milk substitute and should be continued for as long as they are medically indicated.

Article 4: Information and Education for the Purposes of the Code. Governments should have the responsibility to ensure that objective and consistent information is provided on infant and young child feeding for use by families and those involved in the field of infant and young child nutrition. This responsibility should cover either the planning, provision, design and dissemination of information, or their control.

Article 5: The General Public and Mothers. There should be no advertising or other form of promotion to the general public of products within the scope of this Code. Manufacturers and distributors should not provide, directly or indirectly, to pregnant women, mothers, or members of their families samples of products within the scope of this Code.

Article 6: Health Care Systems. No facility of a health care system should be used for the purpose of promoting infant formula or other products within the scope of this Code.

Article 7: Health Workers. Health workers should encourage and protect breastfeeding. Information provided by manufacturers and distributors to health professionals regarding products should be restricted to scientific and factual matters. No financial or material inducements to promote products should be offered by manufacturers or distributors to health workers or members of their families, nor should these be accepted by health care workers. Samples of infant formula and other products—or of equipment or utensils for their preparation—or use should not be provided to health care workers except when necessary for the purpose of professional evaluation or research at the institutional level.

Article 8: Persons Employed by Manufacturers and Distributors. The volume of sales of products within the scope of this Code should not be included in the calculation of bonuses, nor should quotas be set specifically for sales of these products. Personnel employed in marketing products should not perform educational functions in relation to pregnant women or mothers.

Article 9: Labeling. Labels should be designed to provide the necessary information about the appropriate use of the product, so as not to discourage breastfeeding.

Article 10: Quality. Quality of products is an essential element for the protection of the health of infants and therefore should be of a high recognized standard. Food products should meet applicable standards recommended by the Codex Alimentarius Commission.

Article 11: Implementation and Monitoring. Governments should take action to give effect to the principles and aim of this Code, as appropriate to their social and legislative framework, including the adoption of national legislation, regulations or other suitable measures. Responsibility for monitoring the application of this Code lies with governments. Manufacturers and distributors and appropriate nongovernmental organizations, professional groups, and consumer organizations should collaborate with governments to this end. Independently of any other measures, manufacturers and distributors should regard themselves as responsible for monitoring their marketing practices according to the principles and aim of this Code and for taking steps to ensure that their conduct at every level conforms to them. Nongovernmental organizations, professional groups, institutions, and individuals concerned should have the responsibility of drawing the attention of manufacturers or distributors to activities that are incompatible with the principles and aim of this Code. The appropriate governmental authority should also be informed. Manufacturers and distributors should apprise their marketing personnel of the Code and their responsibilities under it. Member States shall communicate annually to the Director-General information on action taken to give effect to the principles and aim of this Code. The Director-General shall report in even years to the World Health Assembly on the status of implementation of the Code and shall provide technical support to Member States in implementation and furtherance of the principles and aim of this Code.

D-2 *Baby-Friendly™ Hospital Initiative*

The Baby Friendly™ Hospital Initiative is discussed in Chapters 1 and 8. Following are documents that are central to the Baby-Friendly initiative.

Hospital Self-Appraisal

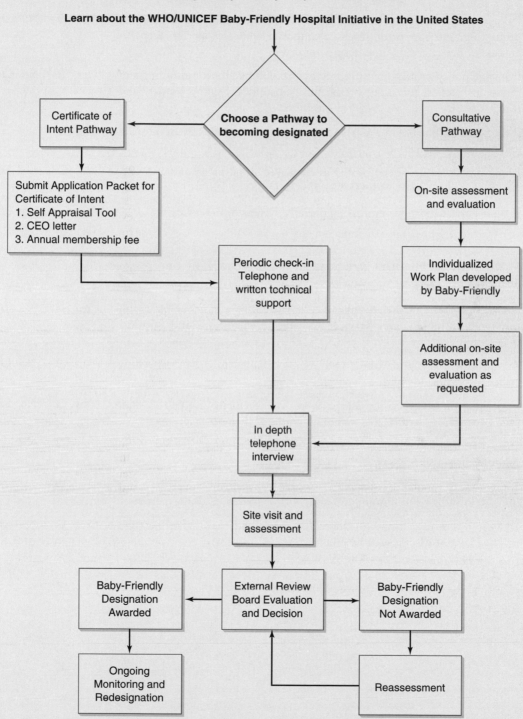

Becoming a Baby-Friendly Hospital or Birth Center

Learn about the WHO/UNICEF Baby-Friendly Hospital Initiative in the United States

Choose a Pathway to becoming designated

Certificate of Intent Pathway

Consultative Pathway

Submit Application Packet for Certificate of Intent
1. Self Appraisal Tool
2. CEO letter
3. Annual membership fee

On-site assessment and evaluation

Periodic check-in Telephone and written technical support

Individualized Work Plan developed by Baby-Friendly

Additional on-site assessment and evaluation as requested

In depth telephone interview

Site visit and assessment

Baby-Friendly Designation Awarded

External Review Board Evaluation and Decision

Baby-Friendly Designation Not Awarded

Ongoing Monitoring and Redesignation

Reassessment

STEP 1. Have a Written Breastfeeding Policy That Is Routinely Communicated to All Health Care Staff

1.1 Does the health facility have an explicit written policy for protecting, promoting, and supporting breastfeeding that addresses all Ten Steps to Successful Breastfeeding in maternity services?   Yes ❑   No ❑

1.2 Does the policy protect breastfeeding by prohibiting all promotion of and group instruction for using breast-milk substitutes, feeding bottles, and teats?   Yes ❑   No ❑

1.3 Is the breastfeeding policy available so that all staff who take care of mothers and babies can refer to it?   Yes ❑   No ❑

1.4 Is the breastfeeding policy posted or displayed in all areas of the health facility that serve mothers, infants, and/or children?   Yes ❑   No ❑

1.5 Is there a mechanism for evaluating the effectiveness of the policy?   Yes ❑   No ❑

STEP 2. Train All Health Care Staff in Skills Necessary to Implement This Policy

2.1 Are all staff aware of the advantages of breastfeeding and acquainted with the facility's policy and services to protect, promote, and support breastfeeding?   Yes ❑   No ❑

2.2 Are all staff caring for women and infants oriented to the breastfeeding policy of the hospital on their arrival?   Yes ❑   No ❑

2.3 Is training on breastfeeding and lactation management given to all staff caring for women and infants within 6 months of their arrival?   Yes ❑   No ❑

2.4 Does the training cover at least eight of the Ten Steps to Successful Breastfeeding?   Yes ❑   No ❑

2.5 Is the training on breastfeeding and lactation management at least 18 hours in total, including a minimum of 3 hours of supervised clinical experience?   Yes ❑   No ❑

2.6 Has the health care facility arranged for specialized training in lactation management of specific staff members?   Yes ❑   No ❑

STEP 3. Inform All Pregnant Women about the Benefits and Management of Breastfeeding

3.1   Does the hospital include an antenatal care clinic or an antenatal inpatient ward?   Yes ❑   No ❑

3.2   If yes, are most pregnant women attending these antenatal services informed about the benefits and management of breastfeeding?   Yes ❑   No ❑

3.3   Do antenatal records indicate whether breastfeeding has been discussed with the pregnant woman?   Yes ❑   No ❑

3.4   Is a mother's antenatal record available at the time of delivery?   Yes ❑   No ❑

3.5   Are pregnant women protected from oral or written promotion of group instruction for artificial feeding?   Yes ❑   No ❑

3.6   Does the health care facility take into account a woman's intention to breastfeed when deciding on the use of a sedative, an analgesic, or an anesthetic (if any) during labor and delivery?   Yes ❑   No ❑

3.7   Are staff familiar with the effects of such medicaments on breastfeeding? Yes ❑   No ❑

3.8   Does a woman who has never breastfed or who has previously encountered problems with breastfeeding receive special attention and support from the staff of the health care facility?   Yes ❑   No ❑

STEP 4. Help Mothers Initiate Breastfeeding within a Half Hour of Giving Birth

4.1   Are mothers whose deliveries are normal given their babies to hold, with skin contact, within a half hour of completion of the second stage of labor and allowed to remain with them for at least the first hour?   Yes ❑   No ❑

4.2   Are the mothers offered help by a staff member to initiate breastfeeding during this first hour?   Yes ❑   No ❑

4.3   Are mothers who have had cesarean deliveries given their babies to hold, with skin contact, within a half hour after they are able to respond to their babies?   Yes ❑   No ❑

4.4   Do the babies born by cesarean stay with their mothers, with skin contact, at this time for at least 30 minutes?   Yes ❑   No ❑

STEP 5. Show Mothers How to Breastfeed and How to Maintain Lactation, Even if They Should Be Separated from Their Infants

5.1　Does nursing staff offer all mothers further assistance with breastfeeding within 6 hours of delivery?　　Yes ❑　No ❑

5.2　Are most breastfeeding mothers able to demonstrate how to correctly position and attach their babies for breastfeeding?　　Yes ❑　No ❑

5.3　Are breastfeeding mothers shown how to express their milk or given information on expression and/or advised of where they can get help should they need it?　　Yes ❑　No ❑

5.4　Are staff members or counselors who have specialized training in breastfeeding and lactation management available full-time to advise mothers during their stay in health care facilities and in preparation for discharge?　　Yes ❑　No ❑

5.5　Does a woman who has never breastfed or who has previously encountered problems with breastfeeding receive special attention and support from the staff of the health care facility?　　Yes ❑　No ❑

5.6　Are mothers of babies in special care helped to establish and maintain lactation by frequent expression of milk?　　Yes ❑　No ❑

STEP 6. Give Newborn Infants No Food or Drink Other Than Breast Milk, Unless Medically Indicated

6.1　Do staff have a clear understanding of what the few acceptable reasons are for prescribing food or drink other than breast milk for breastfeeding babies?　　Yes ❑　No ❑

6.2　Do breastfeeding babies receive no other food or (than breast milk) unless medically indicated?　　Breast milk only　Yes ❑

6.3　Are any breast-milk substitutes, including special formulas, that are used in the facility, purchased in the same way as any other foods or medicines?　　Some other food/drink　No ❑

6.4　Do health facility and health care workers refuse free or low-cost* supplies of breast-milk substitutes, paying close to retail market price for any?　　Yes ❑　No ❑

6.5　Is all promotion of infant foods or drinks other than breast milk absent from the facility?　　Yes ❑　No ❑

*Low-cost: below 80% open-market retail cost. Breast-milk substitutes intended for experimental use or "professional evaluation" should also be purchased at 80% or more of retail prices.

STEP 7. Practice Rooming-in—Allow Mothers and Infants to Remain Together—24 Hours a Day

7.1   Do mothers and infants remain together (rooming-in or bedding-in) 24 hours a day, except for periods of up to an hour for hospital procedures or if separation is medically indicated?   Yes ❑   No ❑

7.2   Does rooming-in start within an hour of a normal birth?   Yes ❑   No ❑

7.3   Does rooming-in start within an hour of when a cesarean mother can respond to her baby?   Yes ❑   No ❑

STEP 8. Encourage Breastfeeding on Demand

8.1   By placing no restrictions on the frequency or length of breastfeedings, do staff show they are aware of the importance of breastfeeding on demand?   Yes ❑   No ❑

8.2   Are mothers advised to breastfeed their babies whenever their babies are hungry and as often as their babies want to breastfeed?   Yes ❑   No ❑

STEP 9. Give No Artificial Teats or Pacifiers (Also Called *Dummies* or *Soothers*) to Breastfeeding Infants

9.1   Are babies who have started to breastfeed cared for without any bottle feedings?   Yes ❑   No ❑

9.2   Are babies who have started to breastfeed cared for without use of pacifiers?   Yes ❑   No ❑

9.3   Do breastfeeding mothers learn that they should not give any bottles or pacifiers to their babies?   Yes ❑   No ❑

9.4   By accepting no free or low-cost feeding bottles, teats, or pacifiers, do the facility and the health workers demonstrate that these should be avoided?   Yes ❑   No ❑

STEP 10. Foster the Establishment of Breastfeeding Support [Groups] and Refer Mothers to Them on Discharge from the Hospital or Clinic

10.1 Does the hospital give education to key family members so that they can support the breastfeeding mother at home?   Yes ❑   No ❑

10.2 Are breastfeeding mothers referred to breastfeeding support groups, if any are available?   Yes ❑   No ❑

10.3 Does the hospital have a system of follow-up support for breastfeeding mothers after they are discharged, such as early postnatal or lactation clinic checkups, home visits, or telephone calls?   Yes ❑   No ❑

10.4 Does the facility encourage and facilitate the formation of mother-to mother or health care worker-to-mother support groups?   Yes ❑   No ❑

10.5 Does the facility allow breastfeeding counseling by trained mother support group counselors in its maternity services?   Yes ❑   No ❑

Becoming a Baby-Friendly Hospital

HOSPITAL DATA   Date _____

If no nursery for normal well newborns exists, write "none" in space provided.

Hospital Name: _____

Address: _____

City, District, or Region _____ Country: _____

Name of Chief Hospital Administrator: _____ Telephone: _____

Names of Senior Nursing Officers (or other personnel in charge):

For the Facility: _____ Telephone: _____

For the Maternity Ward: _____ Telephone: _____

For the Antenatal Service: _____ Telephone: _____

Name of person to be contacted for additional information: _____

Type of Hospital: Government   Private—Not for profit   Private—For profit
                         Mission   Teaching   Other: _____

HOSPITAL CENSUS DATA

Total bed capacity: _____
_____ in labor and delivery area
_____ in the maternity ward
_____ in the normal nursery
_____ in the special care nursery
_____ in other areas for mothers and children

Total deliveries for 12 months ending _____
_____ were by cesarean   Cesarean rate _____%
_____ were low-birth-weight babies (<2500 g)   Low-birth-weight rate _____%
_____ were in special care   Special care rate _____%

Infant feeding data for deliveries from records or staff reports:
_____ mother/infant pairs discharged in the past month
_____ mother/infant pairs breastfeeding at discharge in the past month   _____%
_____ mother/infant pairs breastfeeding exclusively from birth to discharge in the past month   ____%
_____ infants discharged in the past month who have received at least one bottlefeed since birth ____%

How was the infant feeding data obtained?
_____ From records
_____ Percentages are an estimate, provided by: _____

Name of person(s) filling out this form:

Ten Steps to Successful Breastfeeding

The Baby-Friendly Hospital Initiative promotes, protects, and supports breastfeeding through The Ten Steps to Successful Breastfeeding for Hospitals as outlined by UNICEF and WHO. The steps for the United States are as follows:

1. Have a written breastfeeding policy that is routinely communicated to all health care staff.
2. Train all health care staff in skills necessary to implement this policy.
3. Inform all pregnant women about the benefits and management of breastfeeding.
4. Help mothers initiate breastfeeding within an hour of birth.*
5. Show mothers how to breastfeed and how to maintain lactation even if they should be separated from their infants.
6. Give newborn infants no food or drink other than breast milk, unless medically indicated.
7. Practice "rooming-in" by allowing mothers and infants to remain together 24 hours a day.
8. Encourage breastfeeding on demand.
9. Give no artificial teats, pacifiers, dummies, or soothers to breastfeeding infants.
10. Foster the establishment of breastfeeding support groups and refer mothers to them on discharge from the hospital or birthing center.

D-3 *Innocenti Declaration*

On the Protection, Promotion and Support of Breastfeeding:

Recognising that Breastfeeding is a unique process that:

- provides ideal nutrition for infants and contributes to their healthy growth and development;

- reduces incidence and severity of infectious diseases, thereby lowering infant morbidity and mortality;
- contributes to women's health by reducing the risk of breast and ovarian cancer, and by increasing the spacing between pregnancies;
- provides social and economic benefits to the family and the nation;
- provides most women with a sense of satisfaction when successfully carried out; and that Recent research has found that:
- these benefits increase with increased exclusiveness[1] of breastfeeding during the first 6 months of life, and thereafter with increased duration of breastfeeding with complementary foods; and
- programme interventions can result in positive changes in breastfeeding behaviour;

We therefore declare that

As a global goal for optimal maternal and child health and nutrition, all women should be enabled to practise exclusive breastfeeding and all infants should be fed exclusively on breast milk from birth to 4-6 months of age. Thereafter, children should continue to be breastfed, while receiving appropriate and adequate complementary foods, for up to 2 years of age or beyond. This child-feeding ideal is to be achieved by creating an appropriate environment of awareness and support so that women can breastfeed in this manner.

Attainment of the goal requires, in many countries, the reinforcement of a "breastfeeding culture" and its vigorous defence against incursions of a "bottle-feeding culture." This requires commitment and advocacy for social mobilization, utilizing to the full the prestige and authority of acknowledged leaders of society in all walks of life.

Efforts should be made to increase women's confidence in their ability to breastfeed. Such empowerment involves the removal of constraints and influences that manipulate perceptions and behaviour towards breastfeeding, often by subtle and indirect means. This requires sensitivity, continued vigilance, and a responsive and comprehensive

---

*When written in 1989, this step required breastfeeding initiation with the first *half* hour. Research in the 1990s showed that the natural sequence of behavior is for suckling to occur within the first hour. Therefore this step was modified for U.S. hospitals. (From Baby-Friendly USA.)

[1]Exclusive breastfeeding means that no other drink or food is given to the infant; the infant should feed frequently and for unrestricted periods.

communications strategy involving all media and addressed to all levels of society. Furthermore, obstacles to breastfeeding within the health system, the workplace and the community must be eliminated.

Measures should be taken to ensure that women are adequately nourished for their optimal health and that of their families. Furthermore, ensuring that all women also have access to family planning information and services allows them to sustain breastfeeding and avoid shortened birth intervals that may compromise their health and nutritional status, and that of their children.

All governments should develop national breastfeeding policies and set appropriate national targets for the 1990s. They should establish a national system for monitoring the attainment of their targets, and they should develop indicators such as the prevalence of exclusively breastfed infants at discharge from maternity services, and the prevalence of exclusively breastfed infants at 4 months of age.

National authorities are further urged to integrate their breastfeeding policies into their overall health and development policies. In so doing they should reinforce all actions that protect, promote and support breastfeeding within complementary programmes such as prenatal and perinatal care, nutrition, family planning services, and prevention and treatment of common maternal and childhood diseases. All healthcare staff should be trained in the skills necessary to implement these breastfeeding policies.

Operational Targets:

All governments by the year 1995 should have:

- appointed a national breastfeeding coordinator of appropriate authority, and established a multisectoral national breastfeeding committee composed of representatives from relevant government departments, non-governmental organizations, and health professional associations;
- ensured that every facility providing maternity services fully practises all ten of the *Ten Steps to Successful Breastfeeding* set out in the

[2]World Health Organization, Geneva, 1989.

joint WHO/UNICEF statement[2] "Protecting, promoting and supporting breast-feeding: the special role of maternity services";

- taken action to give effect to the principles and aim of all Articles of the International Code of Marketing of Breast-Milk Substitutes and subsequent relevant World Health Assembly resolutions in their entirety; and
- enacted imaginative legislation protecting the breastfeeding rights of working women and established means for its enforcement.

We also call upon international organizations to:

- draw up action strategies for protecting, promoting and supporting breastfeeding, including global monitoring on evaluation of their strategies;
- support national situation analyses and surveys and the development of national goals and targets for action; and
- encourage and support national authorities in planning, implementing, monitoring and evaluating their breastfeeding policies.

The Innocenti Declaration was produced and adopted by participants at the WHO/UNICEF policy makers' meeting on "Breastfeeding in the 1990s: A Global Initiative," cosponsored by the United States Agency for International Development (AID) and the Swedish International Development Authority (SIDA), held at the Spedale degli Innocenti, Florence, Italy, on 30 July to 1 August 1990. The Declaration reflects the content of the original background document for the meeting and the views expressed in group and plenary sessions.

D-4 *Acceptable Medical Reasons for Supplementation**

A few medical indications in a maternity facility may require that individual infants be given fluids or food in addition to, or in place of, breast milk.

*From World Health Organization. Acceptable medical reasons for supplementation. Baby-Friendly Hospital Initiative: Part II: hospital-level implementation. Promoting breast-feeding in health facilities. A short course for administrators and policymakers. Geneva; 1996.

It is assumed that severely ill babies, babies in need of surgery, and very-low-birth-weight infants will be in a special care unit. Their feeding will be individually decided, given their particular nutritional requirements and functional capabilities, although breast milk is recommended whenever possible. These infants in special care are likely to include the following:

- Infants with very low birth weight (less than 1500 g) who are born before 32 weeks of gestational age
- Infants with severe dysmaturity with potentially severe hypoglycemia or those who require therapy for hypoglycemia and who do not improve through increased breastfeeding or by being given breast milk

For infants who are well enough to be with their mothers on the maternity ward, there are very few indications for supplements. To assess whether a facility is inappropriately using fluids or breast-milk substitutes, any infants receiving additional supplements must have been diagnosed as follows:

- Infants whose mothers have severe maternal illness (e.g., psychosis, eclampsia, shock)
- Infants with inborn errors of metabolism (e.g., galactosemia, phenylketonuria, maple syrup urine disease)
- Infants with acute water loss, for example, during phototherapy for jaundice, whenever increased breastfeeding or use of expressed breast milk cannot provide adequate hydration
- Infants whose mothers require medication that is contraindicated when breastfeeding (e.g., cytotoxic drugs, radioactive drugs, and antithyroid drugs other than propylthiouracil)

When breastfeeding has to be temporarily delayed, interrupted, or supplemented, mothers should be helped to establish or maintain lactation, for example, through manual or hand-pump expression of milk, in preparation for the moment when full breastfeeding may be begun or resumed. If the interruption is due to problems with the infant, milk can be expressed, stored if necessary, and provided to the infant as soon as medically advisable. If it is due to a maternal medication or disease that negatively affects the quality of milk, the milk should be pumped and discarded.

D-5 Legislation Related to Breastfeeding

State Legislation Related to Breastfeeding

Following is a summary of legislation that has occurred at the state level. The intention is to identify legislation that has been passed or is pending in each of the 50 states. No attempt has been made to specify the language or extent of the legislation that has been passed. Readers are referred to http://www. supportbreastfeeding.com and http://www. lalecheleague.org/LawBills.html for the details (these are the sources for the information summarized in the following table). Updates on legislation at the state level can be viewed at http://thomas.gov.loc.

- *Year legislation first enacted* refers to the first year that the state government enacted legislation concerning a breastfeeding issue; additional legislation may have occurred thereafter. *Failed* means that a bill was introduced, but the bill did not pass, or did not carry over into the next year to be voted upon. Some of the laws address the importance and benefits of breastfeeding.
- *Explicit right to breastfeed in public* means that a law has been passed that explicitly states the woman's right to breastfeed in public. (Breastfeeding is not "illegal" in any state.) Readers are encouraged to read the *exact* language of the law because it varies substantially from one state to another. Some simply state the woman's right, for example, "anywhere a woman and her child have a right to be," whereas other language is restrictive, such as "in a discreet manner."
- *Employment situations* refers to legislation that has been designed to help women breastfeed in the workplace. This is a broad heading, and the nature of what was addressed varies substantially from state to state.
- *Jury duty exemption* refers to legislation that exempts the woman who is breastfeeding from jury duty; again, the stipulations vary from

	Year Legislation First Enacted	Explicit Right to Breastfeed in Public	Jury Duty Exemption	Employment Situations	Family Law	Other
Alabama						
Alaska	1998	✓				
Arizona						
Arkansas						
California	1995	✓	✓	✓		Hospitals must have a lactation consultant available
Colorado						
Connecticut	1997	✓		✓		
Delaware	1997	✓		✓		
Florida	1993	✓		✓		
Georgia	1999	✓		✓		
Hawaii	1999	✓		✓		
Idaho	1996	✓		✓		
Illinois	1995	✓		✓		
Indiana						
Iowa	1994	✓	✓			
Kansas						
Kentucky	Failed					
Louisiana	2001	✓				
Maine	1999	✓				
Maryland	2001					Exempts breastfeeding equipment from sales tax
Massachusetts	Pending					
Michigan	1994	✓				
Minnesota	1997	✓	✓	✓		
Mississippi						
Missouri	1999	✓				
Montana	1999	✓				
Nebraska						
Nevada	1995	✓				
New Hampshire	1999	✓				
New Jersey	1997	✓				
New Mexico	1999	✓				
New York	1994	✓				Allows breastfeeding in prison
North Carolina	1993	✓				
North Dakota						
Ohio						
Oklahoma						
Oregon	1999	✓	✓			
Pennsylvania						
Rhode Island	1998	✓				
South Carolina						
South Dakota						
Tennessee	1999	✓		✓		
Texas	1995	✓		✓		
Utah	1995	✓				
Vermont	Pending					
Virginia	1994	✓				
Washington	2001	✓				
West Virginia						
Wisconsin	1995	✓				
Wyoming	Failed					

state to state, and readers should check the exact language.

- *Family law* refers to state law that require accommodating breastfeeding in situations such as divorce and visitation, or similar matters.

Public Health Law: New York State

In addition to legislation that protects the woman and her infant, the Public Health Law in New York State provides for human milk for infants, as described here.

Availability of Human Milk.

State of New York. An Act to amend the public health law, in relation to the availability of human breast milk for infant consumption.

The people of the State of New York, represented in Senate and Assembly, do enact as follows:

§1. Legislative findings. The legislature hereby finds and declares that human breast milk, the preferred food for all infants, provides a superior, well-tolerated nutritional source because of its unique components. It contains substances, lacking in other forms of infant nutrition, which help control infection and aid in preventing infant disease. For premature infants or those with low birth weight or infants who are allergic to cow's milk and infant formulas, human breast milk is essential.

It shall be the declared policy of the state of New York that any and all infants requiring human breast milk be assured access to sufficient quantities of wholesome human breast milk, donated by concerned lactating mothers on a continual and systematic basis. The availability of such a supply of human breast milk should be made known to the public so that health providers and families of infants with particular need for human breast milk will be aware of its accessibility.

§2. The public health law is amended by adding a new section twenty-five hundred five to read as follows:

§2505. Human breast milk; collection, storage, and distribution; general powers of the commissioner. The commissioner is hereby empowered to:

(a) Adopt regulations and guidelines including, but not limited to donor standards, methods of collection, and standards for storage, and distribution of human breast milk;

(b) Conduct educational activities to inform the public and health care providers of the availability of human breast milk for infants determined to require such milk and to inform potential donors of the opportunities for proper donation;

(c) Establish rules and regulations to effectuate the provisions of this section.

§3 This act shall take effect immediately.

New York State Health Code in Support of Breastfeeding (Added 1984)*

Chapter V, Subchapter A, Article 2, Part 405
Hospitals—minimum standards
(Statutory authority: Public Health law §2803)
405.8 Maternal, child health and newborn services

(10) (i) The hospital, with the advice of the maternity staff, shall formulate a program of instruction and provide assistance for each maternity patient(s) in the fundamentals of (normal) infant care including infant feeding choice and techniques, post-pregnancy care and family planning.

(ii) The hospital shall provide instruction and assistance to each maternity patient who has chosen to breast-feed and shall provide information on the advantages and disadvantages of breastfeeding to women who are undecided as to the feeding method for their infants. As a minimum:

(a) the hospital shall designate at least one person who is thoroughly trained in breast-feeding physiology and management to be responsible for ensuring the implementation of an effective breast-feeding program; and

*From Office of Health Systems Management, Bureau of Standards Development, New York State Department of Health, Empire State Plaza, Albany, NY; 1984.

(b) policies and procedures shall be developed to assist the mother to breast-feed which shall include, but not be limited to:

(1) prohibition of the application of standing orders for antilactation drugs;

(2) placement of the infant for breast-feeding immediately following delivery, unless contraindicated;

(3) restriction of the infant's supplemental feedings to those indicated by the medical condition of the infant or of the mother;

(4) provision for the infant to be fed on demand; and

(c) assurance that an educational program has been given as soon after admission as possible which shall include but not be limited to:

(1) the nutritional and physiological aspects of human milk;

(2) the normal process for establishing lactation, including care of breasts, common problems associated with breast-feeding and frequency of feeding;

(3) dietary requirements for breast-feeding;

(4) diseases and medication or other substances which may have an effect on breast-feeding;

(5) sanitary procedures to follow in collecting and storing human milk; and

(6) sources for advice and information available to the mother following discharge.

California

In February 2002, a bill was introduced in California that would prohibit the indiscriminate distribution of formula gifts often given to mothers. Introduced by Goldberg, Bill #AB-2447 begins with a preamble declaring how these packs, which are seemingly innocuous, can potentially undermine breastfeeding. The bill states, "No man-ufacturer of infant formula shall distribute in this state free samples of infant formula to a mother, an expectant mother, or family members of a mother or expectant mother, unless these samples are requested in a written form that she has signed that clearly states information about both the risk associated with feeding infant formula to a baby and the benefits of breastfeeding." It also specifies that not only are manufacturers prohibited from doing this, but also *hospitals and health care professionals* are prohibited from this practice unless the mother gives informed consent as stated. Under this bill, hospitals would also not be allowed to share information with infant formula manufacturers about how to reach mothers or expectant mothers.

Although this bill may appear to be the answer to eliminating free "gifts" to mothers, it will need to be accompanied by strong patient education. Mothers often sign informed consent forms quickly and eagerly. However, California's bill could be used as a model to introduce similar legislation in other states.

Federal Legislation Related to Breastfeeding

The following highlights federal legislation related to breastfeeding. Updates to federal legislation can be found by visiting the Government Printing Office's web site at http://www.access.gpo.gov and searching for the keyword "breastfeeding."

Special Supplemental Nutrition Program for Women, Infants, and Children (WIC)

The Special Supplemental Nutrition Program for Women, Infants, and Children (WIC) was legislated by Congress in 1972 as a pilot program and authorized as a permanent program in 1975. For eligible women, infants, and children, WIC provides supplemental foods that are high in protein, iron, vitamins A and C, and calcium. In 1989 the U.S. Department of Agriculture set aside $8 million for breastfeeding promotion each year, which WIC state agencies were required to spend on breastfeeding promotion and support. Furthermore, each WIC state agency is required to designate a breastfeeding coordinator. A brief description of the history of WIC and its involvement in breastfeeding promotion is found in Chapter 1.

Healthy Meals for Healthy Americans Act (1994) Public Law 103-448

Healthy Meals for Healthy Americans Act, passed by Congress in 1994, revised the formula for determining the amount of funds to be spent for WIC breastfeeding promotion and support. The act replaced the $8 million target level with a national maximum for breastfeeding promotion and support expenditures of $21 for each pregnant and breastfeeding woman. The $21 is adjusted annually based on inflation.

Family and Medical Leave Act (FMLA) (1993), 29 CFR Part 825, Public Law 103-3, 107

The FMLA generally requires private-sector employers of 50 or more employees and public agencies to provide up to 12 work weeks of unpaid, job-protected leave to eligible employees for certain specified family and medical reasons; to maintain eligible employees' preexisting group health insurance coverage during period of FMLA leave; and to restore eligible employees to their same or an equivalent position at the conclusion of the FMLA leave. This is WH Publication #1419 and can be obtained by contacting Division of Policy Analysis, Wage and Hour Division, Employment Standards Administration, U.S. Department of Labor, Room S-3506, 200 Constitution Avenue, NW, Washington, DC 20210; phone: (202) 219-8412.

Federal Legislation Related Specifically to Breastfeeding

Several bills have been introduced into the federal legislation that specifically relate to breastfeeding. A summary of bills that have recently been enacted, or pending, follows.

Name of Bill	Purpose	Rationale	Status
Right to Breastfeed Act (H.R. 1848, 106th Congress)	Ensures a woman's right to breastfeed anywhere on federal property where she and her child are authorized to be.	In the past, women who have breastfed in museums, parks, and the U.S. Capitol have been asked to leave.	Enacted into law September 1999 as part of the Treasury-Postal Appropriations bill (H.R. 24900). See http://thomas.loc.gov.
Breastfeeding Promotion Act (H.R. 285, 107th Congress)	Purpose is (1) to clarify the Pregnancy Discrimination Act to protect women, under civil rights law, from being fired or discriminated against for expressing milk in the workplace; (2) to provide tax incentives for employers who provide an optimal environment, equipment, or personnel for breastfeeding at the work site; (3) to require the FDA to develop minimum quality standards for breast pumps ensure that products on the market are safe and effective; and (4) to allow breastfeeding equipment to a tax-deductible medical expense.	Companies who have already invested in lactation programs have found that it saves them money in health care costs and employee turnover. Because breast pumps have not been regulated, they may not provide the optimal mechanism for expressing milk on a regular basis, and hence, mothers who use them are likely to experience a low milk supply and other problems.	Introduced in the House by Carolyn Maloney (D-NY).

Modified from Biancuzzo M. *Breastfeeding Outlook*, 2000;2:5.

Helpful Government Web Sites

Agency for Health Care Policy and Research (AHCPR)   http://www.ahcpr.gov

Department of Health and Human Services   http://www.hhs.gov

Department of Labor   http://www.dol.gov

Federal Legislation   http://thomas.loc.gov

Food and Drug Administration (FDA)   http://www.fda.gov

Government Printing Office   http://www.gpo.gov

Health Care Financing Administration (HCFA)   http://www.hcfa.gov

Health Resources and Services Administration (HRSA)   http://www.hrsa.dhhs.gov

Healthy People 2010 Initiative   http://www.health.gov/healthypeople/

National Institutes of Health   http://www.nih.gov

National Institutes of Health (contains old Surgeon
  General's statements)   http://sgreports.nlm.nih.gov/NN/

U.S. Department of Agriculture—WIC   http://www.usda.gov/FCS/wic.htm

D-6 *Statements on Breastfeeding*

Following are position statements issued by various organizations and associations that pertain to the promotion of breastfeeding. Most of the position papers are found in the organization's official journal as listed here. Unless otherwise noted, the remainder can be obtained by visiting the organization's web site or by contacting the organization*; the organization's address is found in Appendix C-1.

American Academy of Pediatrics Work Group on Breastfeeding. Breastfeeding and the Use of Human Milk. *Pediatrics* 1997;100:1035–1039. Earlier statements were issued in 1980 and 1982.

American Academy of Family Physicians. Leawood, KS: American Academy of Family Physicians. Available from the American Academy of Family Physicians (AAFP) and online at http://www.aafp.org/policy/x1641.xml.

*A web site address is provided for statements that are more difficult to obtain. Before ordering a print copy, check the organization's home page to determine whether electronic versions of official statements can be downloaded by members or nonmembers.

American Academy of Pediatrics and the American College of Obstetrics and Gynecology. *Guidelines for perinatal care*. 4th ed. Elk Grove Village, IL: American Academy of Pediatrics; 1997.

American College of Nurse Midwives. Statement on breast-feeding. *J Nurse Midwifery* 1993;38:4.

American College of Obstetricians and Gynecologists. *Breastfeeding: maternal and infant aspects*. ACOG Educational Bulletin #258. Washington DC: American College of Obstetricians and Gynecologists; 2000.

American Dietetic Association. Position of the American Dietetic Association: promotion of breast-feeding. *J Am Diet Assoc* 1997;97:662–666.

American Hospital Association. *Something to think about . . . promotion of breastfeeding*. Chicago: American Hospital Association; 1992.

American Medical Association. *AMA policy compendium*. Chicago: American Medical Association; 1990.

American Public Health Association. Position paper 8022: Infant feeding in the United States. *Am J Public Health* 1981;71:207–211.

Association of Women's Health, Obstetric and Neonatal Nurses (AWHONN). *Position statement: breastfeeding; 1998. Washington, DC: AWHONN.

British Pediatric Association. Statement of the Standing Committee on Nutrition. *Arch Dis Child* 1994;71:376–380.

Holy Father. (1995.) *Papal statement on breastfeeding.* Vatican City. Available at http://www. ewtn.com/library/PAPALDOC/JP2FEED.HTM.

International Childbirth Education Association. *ICEA position paper on infant feeding.* 1992. Minneapolis: ICEA.

International Federation of Gynecology and Obstetrics. Recommendations of the International Federation of Gynecology and Obstetrics for action to encourage breastfeeding. *Int J Gynaecol Obstet* 1982;20:171–172.

International Lactation Consultant Association. *Position paper on infant feeding.* Raleigh, NC: International Lactation Consultant Association; 1994.

Lamaze International. *Position paper on infant feeding.* Washington, DC: Lamaze International; 1995.

National Association of WIC Directors. *Guidelines for breastfeeding promotion and support in the WIC program.* Washington, DC: National Association of WIC Directors; 1994.

National Association of Pediatric Nurse Associates and Practitioners. NAPNAP policy statement on breastfeeding. *J Pediatr Health Care* 1988;2:314.

National Perinatal Association (NPA). Position statement on breastfeeding. Tampa: NPA (in progress).

Spisak S, Gross SS. *Second followup report: the Surgeon General's Workshop on Breastfeeding and Human Lactation.* Washington, DC: National Center for Education in Maternal and Child Health; 1991. Available at http://sgreports.nlm. nih.gov/NN/B/C/S/W/.

US Breastfeeding Committee. *Protecting, promoting, supporting breastfeeding in the United States: a national agenda.* Available at http://www. usbreastfeeding.org.

US Department of Health and Human Services. *Report of the Surgeon General's Workshop on Breastfeeding and Human Lactation.* Rockville, MD: Health Resources and Services Administration; 1984. Available http://sgreports.nlm.nih. gov/NN/B/C/G/F/.

US Department of Health and Human Services. *Followup report: the Surgeon General's Workshop on Breastfeeding and Human Lactation.* Rockville, MD: Health Resources and Services Administration; 1985. Available at http://sgreports.nlm.nih.gov/NN/B/C/T/H/.

US Department of Health and Human Services. *HHS blueprint for action on breastfeeding.* Washington, DC: Office on Women's Health, US Department of Health and Human Services; 2000.

US Department of Health and Human Services. *Healthy People 2010: national health promotion and disease prevention objectives.* Washington, DC: Government Printing Office; 2002. Available at http://www.health.gov/healthypeople.

WHO and UNICEF. *Innocenti Declaration: 30 July to 1 Aug. 1990, Florence, Italy.* Geneva: Author; 1990. Available from http://www.waba.org.br/inno.htm.

WHO and UNICEF. *Protecting, promoting, and supporting breast-feeding: the special role of maternity services.* Geneva: World Health Organization; 1989. Available from WHO Publications Center. (See Appendix E.)

World Health Organization. *International code of marketing of breast-milk substitutes.* Geneva: World Health Organization; 1981.

Publishers/Producers/Distributors

Contact list for publishers, producers, and distributors who carry breastfeeding media are listed in other appendices in this book. Every effort has been made to ensure accuracy of the contact information listed here; however, this information changes rapidly. Suggestions from readers or vendors are welcomed; please send comments to bookcommentswmc-worldwide.com.

Academic Press
525 B St., Suite 1900
San Diego, CA 92101-4495
Phone: (619) 231-0926
Customer Ecare: (888) 677-7357

Academy for Educational Development
1825 Connecticut Ave., NW
Washington, DC 20009-5721
Phone: (202) 884-8822
Fax: (202) 884-8400
Web site: http://www.aed.org
E-mail: admindc@aed.org

ACE Graphics
PO Box 173
Sevenoaks Kent TN14 5ZT
United Kingdom
Phone: (01959) 524 622
Fax: (01959) 525 800
Web site: http://www.acegraphics.com.au
E-mail: ukinfo@acegraphics.com.au

African Medical and Research Foundation
PO Box 30125
Nairobi
Kenya
Phone: 254-2-605331
Fax: 254-2-609518
Web site: http://www.amref.org
E-mail: amref.inf@amref.org

American Academy of Pediatrics
141 Northwest Point Blvd.
Elk Grove Village, IL 60007-1098
Phone: (847) 434-4000
Toll-free: (800) 433-9016
Fax: (847) 434-8000
Web site: http://www.aap.org
E-mail: kidsdoc@aap.org

American Dietetic Association
216 W. Jackson Blvd.
Chicago, IL 60606-6995
Phone: (312) 899-0040
Toll-free: (800) 877-1600
Fax: (312) 899-1979
Web site: http://www.eatright.org
E-mail: sales@eatright.org

Avery Publishing Group
120 Old Broadway
Garden City Park, NY 11040-5000
Phone: (516) 741-2155
Toll-free: (800) 548-5757
Fax: (516) 742-1892
E-mail: averypubg@aol.com

Baby-Friendly USA
8 Jan Sebastian Way Unit #22
Sandwich, MA 02563
Phone: (508) 888-8092
Fax: (508) 888-8050
Web site: http://www.babyfriendlyusa.org
E-mail: info@babyfriendlyusa.org

Best Start Social Marketing
4809 E. Busch Blvd., Suite 104
Tampa, FL 33617
Phone: (813) 971-2119
Toll-free: (800) 277 4975
Fax: (813) 971-2280
E-mail: beststart@beststartinc.org

Breastfeeding Support Network
2050 W. 9th Ave.
Oshkosh, WI 54904
Phone: (920) 231-1611
Toll-free: (888) 666-7224
Web site: http://www.momsbags.com
E-mail: toman@momsbags.com

Birth & Life Bookstore
Division of Cascade HealthCare Products
141 Commercial Street, N.E.
Salem, OR 97301
Phone: (503) 378-7545
Toll-free: (800) 443-9942
Fax: (503) 371-5395
Web site: http://www.1cascade.com

Breastfeeding Support Consultants
228 Park Lane
Chalfont, PA 18914-3135
Phone: (215) 822-1281
Fax: (215) 997-7879
Web site: http://www.bsccenter.org
E-mail: info@bsccenter.org

Bright Future Lactation Resource Centre
6540 Cedarview Ct.
Dayton, OH 45459
Phone: (937) 438-9458
Toll-free: (888) 235-7201
Fax: (937) 438-3229
Web site: http://www.bflrc.com
E-mail: lindaj@bflrc.com

Celestial Arts
Division of Ten Speed Press
Box 7123
Berkeley, CA 94707
Phone: (510) 559-1600
Toll-free: (800) 841-BOOK
Fax: (510) 559-1629
Web site: http://www.tenspeed.com
E-mail: order@tenspeed.com

Childbirth Graphics
PO Box 21207
Waco, TX 76702-1207
Phone: (254) 776-6461, ext. 287
Toll-free: (800) 299-3366, ext. 287
Fax: (254) 776-1428
Web site: http://www.childbirthgraphics.com
E-mail: sales@wrsgroup.com

Children's Mercy Hospital
2401 Gillham Rd.
Kansas City, MO 64108
Phone: (816) 234-3000
Web site: http://www.childrens-mercy.org
E-mail: webmaster@cmh.edu

Cleft Palate Foundation
104 South Estes Dr., Suite 204
Chapel Hill, NC 27514
Phone: (919) 933-9044
Toll-free: (800) 24-CLEFT
Fax: (919) 933-9604
Web site: http://www.cleftline.org
E-mail: cleftline@aol.com

Eagle Video Productions Inc.
2201 Woodnell Dr.
Raleigh, NC 27603-5240
Phone: (919) 779-7891
Toll-free: (800) 838-5848
Fax: (919) 779-7284
Web site: http://www.eaglevideo.com
E-mail: bruce@eaglevideo.com

Geddes Productions
PO Box 41761
Los Angeles, CA 90041-0761
Phone: (323) 344-8045
Fax: (323) 257-7209
Web site: http://www.geddesproduction.com
E-mail: orders@geddesproduction.com

Growing with Baby
1230 Marsh St.
San Luis Obispo, CA 93401
Phone: (805) 543-6988
Toll-free: (800) 524-9554
Fax: (805) 543-6692
Web site: http://www.growingwithbaby.com
E-mail: aherron178@aol.com or elsabird@
    pacbell.net

Hanley & Belfus, Inc.
210 South 13th St.
Philadelphia, PA 19107
Phone: (215) 546-7293
Toll-free: (800) 962-1892
Fax: (215) 790-9330
Web site: http://www.hanleyandbelfus.com
E-mail: custserv@hanleyandbelfus.com

Harvard Common Press
535 Albany St.
Boston, MA 02118
Phone: (617) 423-5803
Toll-free: (888) 657-3755
Fax: (617) 695-9794
Web site: http://www.harvardcommonpress.com
E-mail: orders@harvardcommonpress.com

Health Education Associates
8 Jan Sebastian Way #13
Sandwich, MA 02563-2359
Phone: (508) 888-8044
Toll-free: (888) 888-8077
Fax: (508) 888-8050
Web site: http://www.healthed.cc
E-mail: hea@capecod.net

Health Sciences Center for Educational Resources
University of Washington
Box 357161
Seattle, WA 98195-7161
Phone: (206) 685-1158
Fax: (206) 543-8051
Web site: http://www.cer.hs.washington.edu
E-mail: center@u.washington.edu

Healthy Mothers Healthy Babies
121 North Washington St., Suite 300
Alexandria, VA 22314
Phone: (703) 836-6110
Fax: (703) 836-3470
Web site: http://www.hmhb.org
E-mail: info@hmhb.org

Hollister
Customer Care Department
2000 Hollister Drive
Libertyville, IL 60048
Phone: (847) 918-5882
Fax: (800) 323-4060
Web site: http://www.hollister.com

INFACT Canada
6 Trinity Square
Toronto, Ontario M5G 1B1
Canada
Phone: (416) 595-9819
Fax: (426) 591-9355
Web site: http://www.infactcanada.ca
E-mail: orders@infactcanada.ca

InJoy Productions
1435 Yarmouth, Suite 102
Boulder, CO 80304
Phone: (303) 447-2082
Toll-free: (800) 326-2082
Fax: (303) 449-8788
Web site: http://www.injoyvideos.com
E-mail: custserv@injoyvideos.com

International Childbirth Education Association
PO Box 20048
Minneapolis, MN 55420
Phone: (952) 854-8660
Toll-free: (800) 624-4934
Fax: (952) 854-8772
Web site: http://www.icea.org
E-mail: info@icea.org

International Lactation Consultant Association
1500 Sunday Dr., Suite 102
Raleigh, NC 27607
Phone: (919) 787-5181
Fax: (919) 787-4916
Web site: http://www.ilca.org
E-mail: ilca@erols.com

Johns Hopkins Center for Communications
111 Market Place, Suite 310
Baltimore, MD 21202-4024
Phone: (410) 659-6300
Fax: (410) 659-6266
Web site: http://www.jhuccp.org
E-mail: webadmin@jhuccp.org

Jones and Bartlett Publishers
40 Tall Pine Dr.
Sudbury, MA 01776
Phone: (978) 443-5000
Toll-free: (800) 832-0034
Fax: (978) 443-8000
Web site: http://www.jbpub.com
E-mail: custserv@jbpub.com

L. A. Publishing
PO Box 773
Franklin, VA 23851
Phone: (757) 562-5017
Toll-free: (800) 397-5833
Fax: (757) 569-1447
Web site: http://lapub.com
E-mail: lapco@fastrus.com

Lactation Associates
254 Conant Rd.
Weston, MA 02192
Phone: (871) 893-3553
Fax: (871) 893-8608
E-mail: marshalact@aol.com

Lactation Consultant Services
11320 Shady Glen Rd.
Oklahoma City, OK 73162
Phone: (405) 722-2163
Fax: (405) 722-2197
Web site: http://lactation-consultant-services.com
E-mail: dbocar@aol.com

Lactation Institute
16430 Ventura Blvd., Suite 303
Encino, CA 91436
Phone: (818) 995-1913
Fax: (818) 995-0634
Web site: http://www.lactationinstitute.org
E-mail: info@lactationinstitute.org

Lakeview Breastfeeding Clinic
6628 Crowchild Trail, S.W.
Calgary, Alberta T3E 5R8
Canada
Phone: (403) 246-7076
Fax: (403) 249-0156
Web site: http://www.drjain.com
E-mail: drjain@drjain.com

Lifecircle
4452 Rustic Rd.
Yorba Linda, CA 92886
Phone: (714) 524-0080

Lippincott Williams & Wilkins
PO Box 1600
Hagerstown, MD 21741
Phone: (410) 528-4000
Toll-free: (800) 638-3030
Fax: (301) 223-2400
Web site: http://www.lww.com
E-mail: custserv@lww.com

Maryland WIC Administration
201 West Preston St.
Baltimore, MD 21201
Phone: (410) 767-6902
Fax: (410) 333-5243
Web site: http://mdwic.org

Medela
PO Box 660
McHenry, IL 60051-0660
Phone: (815) 363-1166
Toll-free: (800) 435-8316
Fax: (800) 995-7867
Web site: http://www.medela.com
E-mail: customer.service@medela.com

Milner-Fenwick
2125 Greenspring Dr.
Timonium, MD 21093
Phone: (410) 252-1700
Toll-free: (800) 432-8433
Fax: (410) 252-6316
Web site: http://www.milner-fenwick.com

Mosby
11830 Westline Industrial Dr.
St. Louis, MO 63146
Toll-free (domestic): (800) 545-2522
Phone (nondomestic): (314) 453-7010;
    (800) 460-3110 (Italy, Spain, Germany, and
    United Kingdom)
Fax: (314) 453-7095
Fax toll-free (domestic): (800) 568-5136
Web site:
http://www.us.elsevierhealth.com/Mosby/

National Academy Press
2101 Constitution Ave., N.W.
Lockbox 285
Washington, DC 20055
Phone: (202) 334-3313
Toll-free: (888) 624-8373
Fax: (202) 334-2451
Web site: http://www.nap.edu
E-mail: zjones@nas.edu

National Center for Education in Maternal and
    Child Health
2000 15th Street, N., Suite 701
Arlington, VA 22201-2617
Phone: (703) 524-7802
Fax: (703) 524-9335
Web site: http://www.ncemch.org
E-mail: info@ncemch.org

Noodle Soup
4614 Prospect Ave., Suite 328
Cleveland, OH 44103-4314
Phone: (216) 881-7177
Toll-free: (800) 795-9295
Fax: (216) 881-0083
Web site: http://www.noodlesoup.com
E-mail: vicky@noodlesoup.com

Northwestern Memorial Hospital
333 East Superior St.
Chicago, IL 60611
Phone: (312) 908-7398

Oxford University Press
2001 Evans Rd.
Cary, NC 27513
Phone: (919) 677-0977
Toll-free: (800) 451-7556
Fax: (919) 677-1303
Web site: http://www.oup-usa.org

Pharmasoft Publishing
21 Tascocita Circle
Amarillo, TX 79124-7301
Phone: (806) 358-8138
Toll-free: (800) 378-1317
Fax: (806) 358-9480
Web site: http://www.ibreastfeeding.com
E-mail: books@ibreastfeeding.com

Plenum Publishing Corp.
233 Spring St.
New York, NY 10013
Phone: (212) 620-8000
Toll-free: (800) 221-9369
Web site: http://www.wkap.com

Royal College of Midwives
15 Mansfield St.
London W1G 9NH
United Kingdom
Phone: 44 (0)20-7312-3535
Fax: 44 (0)20-7312-3536
Web site: http://www.rcm.org.uk
E-mail: info@rcm.org.uk

Spangler, Amy
PO Box 501046
Atlanta, GA 31150-1046
Phone: (770) 913-9332
Fax: (770) 913-0822
Web site: http://www.daddymommyandme.com
E-mail: akspangler@aol.com

SUNY Stonybrook
School of Nursing, HSC
Stonybrook, NY 11794-8240

TENSOR
12008 W. 87th St. Parkway, Suite 303
Lenexa, KS 66215-2888
Phone: (913) 894-8885

UNICEF
3 United Nations Plaza
New York, NY 10017
Phone: (212) 326-7000
Fax: (212) 888-7465
Web site: http://www.unicef.org
E-mail: netmaster@unicef.org

Vancouver Breastfeeding Centre
611 West 11th Avenue
Vancouver, British Columbia V5Z 1M1
Canada
Phone: (604) 875-4678
Fax: (604) 876-5017
Web site: http://mypage.direct.ca/m/millerb/
E-mail: millerb@direct.ca

Vida Health Communications
6 Bigelow St.
Cambridge, MA 02139
Phone: (617) 864-1334
Toll-free: (800) 550-7047
Fax: (617) 864-7862
Web site: http://www.vida-health.com
E-mail: information@vida-health.com

Wellstart International
PO Box 80877
San Diego, CA 92138-0877
Phone: (619) 295-5192
Fax: (619) 574-8159
Web site: http://www.wellstart.org
E-mail: info@wellstart.org

World Health Organization (WHO)
CH-1211
Geneva 27
Switzerland
Phone: +41-22-791-2111
Fax: +41-22-791-3111
Web site: http://www.who.int
E-mail: info@who.int

World Health Organization Publications Center
49 Sheridan Ave.
Albany, NY 12210
Phone: (518) 436-9686
Fax: (518) 436-7433
Web site: http://www.who.int/dsa/cat98/zhow.htm
E-mail: qcorp@compuserv.com

Web Sites That Relate to Breastfeeding

It is not practical to list all of the web sites that related to breastfeeding. A few sites that have special relevance to this text, or those that provide multiple links to other sites, are listed. (Also see the helpful government web sites listed in Appendix D-5.)

Breastfeeding Protection

Following are a few sites that describe the legislated rights of women and children with respect to breastfeeding, as well as issues surrounding the marketing of human milk substitutes.

http://www.who.int/nut/documents/code_english	This site has a downloadable PDF file of the entire *Code of Marketing of Breast-milk Substitutes* written by the World Health Organization in 1981. (An abbreviated form of the Code is printed in Appendix D.)
http://thomas.loc.gov	This site tracks bills that are currently in the state legislature. Type in the word *breastfeeding* for latest updates.
http://www.lalecheleague.org/LawBills.html and http://www.supportbreastfeeding.com	These sites provide information regarding bills that have been passed or are pending.
http://www.usbreastfeeding.org/Publications.html	This site lists activities of the U.S. Breastfeeding Committee, as a downloadable PDF file of the *Strategic Plan for Breastfeeding* in the United States.
http://www.tdh.state.tx.us/lactate/media.htm	This is the site for the National Breastfeeding MediaWatch, sponsored by the Texas Department of Health, which is an ongoing project of the Bureau of Nutrition Services. This site shows how to write letters to publishers and producers when breastfeeding is shown in a negative way in the media.

Breastfeeding Promotion

Following are a few sites that describe the advantages of breastfeeding at the individual level (i.e., mother and infant). These sites as also discuss benefits to society and the global ecology.

http://www.cdc.gov/breastfeeding	This is the web site of the Centers for Disease Control and Prevention (CDC). The CDC has multiple links to other sites that protect, promote, and support breastfeeding.
http://www.breastfeeding.com	This site is designed for both parents and providers, and it has links to multiple other sites that protect, promote, and support breastfeeding.
http://www.fda.gov/medwatch	Information on formula and pump defects and recalls is posted on this site.
http://www.parentingweb.com/ lounge/whybf.htm#environmental	This site describes how bottle-feeding harms the environment, including the relationship of toxins to the entire food chain (not just human milk) and what we can do at the local and national levels to reduce environmental waste and contamination through breastfeeding.

Breastfeeding Support

Following are two sites that describe or provide links to evidence-based policies, practices, and programs that support breastfeeding initiation and duration.

http://www.aap.org/advocacy/bf/aapbrres.htm	This site provides links to multiple policy statements that have been written by the American Academy of Pediatrics and that are specific to, or relate to, breastfeeding.
http://www.breastfeedingoutlook.com	This site has a Click Here column that is online, rather than in the printed newsletter. The Click Here column lists web sites that are pertinent to current events in the lactation community or that relate to the articles in the printed newsletter.

Index

Page numbers followed by f indicate figures; t, tables; and b, boxes.